P9-CEM-262

ACP | MKSAP® 18
Medical Knowledge Self-Assessment Program®

General Internal Medicine

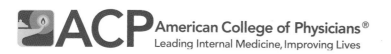

ACP American College of Physicians®
Leading Internal Medicine, Improving Lives

Welcome to the General Internal Medicine Section of MKSAP 18!

In these pages, you will find updated information on routine care of the healthy patient; patient safety and quality improvement; professionalism and ethics; palliative medicine; common symptoms, including chronic pain, medically unexplained symptoms, dyspnea, cough, fatigue, dizziness, syncope, insomnia, and lower extremity edema; musculoskeletal pain; dyslipidemia; obesity; men's and women's health; eye disorders; ear, nose, mouth, and throat disorders; mental and behavioral health; geriatric medicine; perioperative medicine; and other clinical challenges. All of these topics are uniquely focused on the needs of generalists and subspecialists in internal medicine.

The core content of MKSAP 18 has been developed as in previous editions—all essential information that is newly researched and written in 11 topic areas of internal medicine—created by dozens of leading generalists and subspecialists and guided by certification and recertification requirements, emerging knowledge in the field, and user feedback. MKSAP 18 also contains 1200 all-new peer-reviewed, psychometrically validated, multiple-choice questions (MCQs) for self-assessment and study, including 168 in General Internal Medicine. MKSAP 18 continues to include *High Value Care* (HVC) recommendations, based on the concept of balancing clinical benefit with costs and harms, with associated MCQs illustrating these principles and HVC Key Points called out in the text. Internists practicing in the hospital setting can easily find comprehensive *Hospitalist*-focused content and MCQs, specially designated in blue and with the 🄷 symbol.

If you purchased MKSAP 18 Complete, you also have access to MKSAP 18 Digital, with additional tools allowing you to customize your learning experience. MKSAP Digital includes regular text updates with new, practice-changing information, 200 new self-assessment questions, and enhanced custom-quiz options. MKSAP Complete also includes more than 1200 electronic, adaptive learning–enhanced flashcards for quick review of important concepts, as well as an updated and enhanced version of Virtual Dx, MKSAP's image-based self-assessment tool. As before, MKSAP 18 Digital is optimized for use on your mobile devices, with iOS- and Android-based apps allowing you to sync between your apps and online account and submit for CME credits and MOC points online.

Please visit us at the MKSAP Resource Site (mksap.acponline.org) to find out how we can help you study, earn CME credit and MOC points, and stay up to date.

On behalf of the many internists who have offered their time and expertise to create the content for MKSAP 18 and the editorial staff who work to bring this material to you in the best possible way, we are honored that you have chosen to use MKSAP 18 and appreciate any feedback about the program you may have. Please feel free to send any comments to mksap_editors@acponline.org.

Sincerely,

Patrick Alguire

Patrick C. Alguire, MD, FACP
Editor-in-Chief
Senior Vice President Emeritus
Medical Education Division
American College of Physicians

General Internal Medicine

Committee

Paul S. Mueller, MD, MPH, FACP, Section Editor[2]
Consultant, Division of General Internal Medicine
Professor of Medicine and Professor of Biomedical Ethics
Mayo Clinic College of Medicine and Science
Rochester, Minnesota

Karthik Ghosh, MD, MS, FACP[1]
Director, Breast Clinic
Consultant, Division of General Internal Medicine
Professor of Medicine
Mayo Clinic College of Medicine and Science
Rochester, Minnesota

Scott Herrle, MD, MS, FACP[1]
Assistant Professor of Medicine
University of Pittsburgh School of Medicine
Pittsburgh, Pennsylvania

Arya B. Mohabbat, MD, FACP[2]
Consultant, Division of General Internal Medicine
Assistant Professor of Medicine
Mayo Clinic College of Medicine and Science
Rochester, Minnesota

Kurt Pfeifer, MD, FACP[1]
Professor of Medicine
Division of General Internal Medicine
Medical College of Wisconsin
Milwaukee, Wisconsin

Mary Beth Poston, MD, FACP[1]
Associate Professor
Internal Medicine Residency Program Director
Palmetto Health
University of South Carolina
Columbia, South Carolina

Julie Rosenbaum, MD, FACP[2]
Associate Professor of Medicine
Yale University School of Medicine
New Haven, Connecticut

Jacob J. Strand, MD, FACP[1]
Consultant, Division of General Internal Medicine
Chair, Center for Palliative Medicine
Assistant Professor of Medicine
Mayo Clinic College of Medicine and Science
Rochester, Minnesota

Karna K. Sundsted, MD, FACP[1]
Consultant, Division of General Internal Medicine
Assistant Professor of Medicine
Mayo Clinic College of Medicine and Science
Rochester, Minnesota

Amy Tu Wang, MD, FACP[1]
Assistant Professor of Medicine
David Geffen School of Medicine at UCLA
Director, Employee Health Services
Associate Director, Internal Medicine Residency Program
Harbor-UCLA Medical Center
Torrance, California

Editor-in-Chief

Patrick C. Alguire, MD, FACP[2]
Senior Vice President Emeritus, Medical Education
American College of Physicians
Philadelphia, Pennsylvania

Deputy Editor

Robert L. Trowbridge, Jr., MD, FACP[2]
Associate Professor of Medicine
Tufts University School of Medicine
Maine Medical Center
Portland, Maine

General Internal Medicine Reviewers

Laura Greci Cooke, MD, FACP[1]
Preetivi Ellis, MD, FACP[1]
Major Frederick L. Flynt, MD, MC USAF, FACP[1]
Jason Higdon, MD, FACP[1]
Susan Hingle, MD, FACP[1]
Nadia Irshad, MD[2]
Michael LoCurcio, MD, FACP[1]
Ryan D. Mire, MD, FACP[1]
Anne Newland, MD, MPH, FACP[1]
Samuel C. Pan, MD[1]
Bonnie E. Gould Rothberg, MD, PhD, MPH[2]
Harlan L. South, MD, FACP[1]
Carola A. Tanna, MD[2]

Hospital Medicine General Internal Medicine Reviewers

Enyinnaya U. Abarikwu, MD[1]
Saaid T. Abdel-Ghani, MD, FACP[1]
Saaima Arshad, MD[1]
Captain Brian N. Bowes, MD, MC USN, FACP[1]

General Internal Medicine ACP Editorial Staff

Jackie Twomey[1], Senior Staff Editor
Megan Zborowski[1], Senior Staff Editor
Julia Nawrocki[1], Digital Content Associate/Editor
Joysa Winter[1], Staff Editor
Margaret Wells[1], Director, Self-Assessment and Educational Programs
Becky Krumm[1], Managing Editor, Self-Assessment and Educational Programs

ACP Principal Staff

Davoren Chick, MD, FACP[2]
Senior Vice President, Medical Education

Patrick C. Alguire, MD, FACP[2]
Senior Vice President Emeritus, Medical Education

Sean McKinney[1]
Vice President, Medical Education

Margaret Wells[1]
Director, Self-Assessment and Educational Programs

Becky Krumm[1]
Managing Editor

Valerie Dangovetsky[1]
Administrator

Ellen McDonald, PhD[1]
Senior Staff Editor

Megan Zborowski[1]
Senior Staff Editor

Jackie Twomey[1]
Senior Staff Editor

Randy Hendrickson[1]
Production Administrator/Editor

Julia Nawrocki[1]
Digital Content Associate/Editor

Linnea Donnarumma[1]
Staff Editor

Chuck Emig[1]
Staff Editor

Joysa Winter[1]
Staff Editor

Kimberly Kerns[1]
Administrative Coordinator

---

1. Has no relationships with any entity producing, marketing, reselling, or distributing health care goods or services consumed by, or used on, patients.

2. Has disclosed relationship(s) with any entity producing, marketing, reselling, or distributing health care goods or services consumed by, or used on, patients.

Disclosure of relationships with any entity producing, marketing, reselling, or distributing health care goods or services consumed by, or used on, patients.

Patrick C. Alguire, MD, FACP
Royalties
UpToDate

Davoren Chick, MD, FACP
Royalties
Wolters Kluwer Publishing
Consultantship
EBSCO Health's DynaMed Plus
Other: Owner and sole proprietor of Coding 101 LLC; research consultant (spouse) for Vedanta Biosciences Inc.

Nadia Irshad, MD
Other: Partnership of Hillside Urgent Care

Arya B. Mohabbat, MD, FACP
Research Grants/Contracts
Nestle Purina

Paul S. Mueller, MD, MPH, FACP
Board Member
Boston Scientific Patient Safety Advisory Board, Augsburg University, American Osler Society
Other: Associate Editor for Journal Watch, Massachusetts Medical Society
Honoraria
Medtronic Medical Education

Julie Rosenbaum, MD, FACP
Stock Options/Holdings
Pfizer, Merck, Monsanto

Bonnie E. Gould Rothberg, MD, PhD, MPH
Stock Options/Holdings
Butterfly Networks Inc., Hyperfine Technologies, LAM Therapeutics, Quantum-Si

Carola A. Tanna, MD
Stock Options/Holdings
Eli Lilly and Co.

Robert L. Trowbridge, Jr., MD, FACP
Consultantship
American Board of Internal Medicine

Acknowledgments

The American College of Physicians (ACP) gratefully acknowledges the special contributions to the development and production of the 18th edition of the Medical Knowledge Self-Assessment Program® (MKSAP® 18) made by the following people:

Graphic Design: Barry Moshinski (Director, Graphic Services), Michael Ripca (Graphics Technical Administrator), and Jennifer Gropper (Graphic Designer).

Production/Systems: Dan Hoffmann (Director, Information Technology), Scott Hurd (Manager, Content Systems), Neil Kohl (Senior Architect), and Chris Patterson (Senior Architect).

MKSAP 18 Digital: Under the direction of Steven Spadt (Senior Vice President, Technology), the digital version of MKSAP 18 was developed within the ACP's Digital Products and Services Department, led by Brian Sweigard (Director, Digital Products and Services). Other members of the team included Dan Barron (Senior Web Application Developer/Architect), Chris Forrest (Senior Software Developer/Design Lead), Kathleen Hoover (Senior Web Developer), Kara Regis (Manager, User Interface Design and Development), Brad Lord (Senior Web Application Developer), and John McKnight (Senior Web Developer).

The College also wishes to acknowledge that many other persons, too numerous to mention, have contributed to the production of this program. Without their dedicated efforts, this program would not have been possible.

MKSAP Resource Site (mksap.acponline.org)

The MKSAP Resource Site (mksap.acponline.org) is a continually updated site that provides links to MKSAP 18 online answer sheets for print subscribers; access to MKSAP 18 Digital; Board Basics® e-book access instructions; information on Continuing Medical Education (CME), Maintenance of Certification (MOC), and international Continuing Professional Development (CPD) and MOC; errata; and other new information.

International MOC/CPD

For information and instructions on submission of international MOC/CPD, please go to the MKSAP Resource Site (mksap.acponline.org).

Continuing Medical Education

The American College of Physicians is accredited by the Accreditation Council for Continuing Medical Education (ACCME) to provide continuing medical education for physicians.

The American College of Physicians designates this enduring material, MKSAP 18, for a maximum of 275 *AMA PRA Category 1 Credits*™. Physicians should claim only the credit commensurate with the extent of their participation in the activity.

Up to 36 *AMA PRA Category 1 Credits*™ are available from December 31, 2018, to December 31, 2021, for the MKSAP 18 General Internal Medicine section.

Learning Objectives

The learning objectives of MKSAP 18 are to:

- Close gaps between actual care in your practice and preferred standards of care, based on best evidence
- Diagnose disease states that are less common and sometimes overlooked and confusing
- Improve management of comorbid conditions that can complicate patient care
- Determine when to refer patients for surgery or care by subspecialists
- Pass the ABIM Certification Examination
- Pass the ABIM Maintenance of Certification Examination

Target Audience

- General internists and primary care physicians
- Subspecialists who need to remain up to date in internal medicine
- Residents preparing for the certifying examination in internal medicine
- Physicians preparing for maintenance of certification in internal medicine (recertification)

ABIM Maintenance of Certification

Check the MKSAP Resource Site (mksap.acponline.org) for the latest information on how MKSAP tests can be used to apply to the American Board of Internal Medicine (ABIM) for Maintenance of Certification (MOC) points following completion of the CME activity.

Successful completion of the CME activity, which includes participation in the evaluation component, enables the participant to earn up to 275 medical knowledge MOC points and patient safety MOC credits in the ABIM's MOC program. It is the CME activity provider's responsibility to submit participant completion information to ACCME for the purpose of granting MOC credit.

Earn Instantaneous CME Credits or MOC Points Online

Print subscribers can enter their answers online to earn instantaneous CME credits or MOC points. You can submit your answers using online answer sheets that are provided at mksap.acponline.org, where a record of your MKSAP 18 credits will be available. To earn CME credits or to apply for MOC points, you need to answer all of the questions in a test and earn a score of at least 50% correct (number of correct answers divided by the total number of questions). Please note that if you are applying for MOC points, you must also enter your birth date and ABIM candidate number.

Take either of the following approaches:

1. Use the printed answer sheet at the back of this book to record your answers. Go to mksap.acponline.org, access the appropriate online answer sheet, transcribe your answers, and submit your test for instantaneous CME credits or MOC points. There is no additional fee for this service.

2. Go to mksap.acponline.org, access the appropriate online answer sheet, directly enter your answers, and submit your test for instantaneous CME credits or MOC points. There is no additional fee for this service.

Earn CME Credits or MOC Points by Mail or Fax

Pay a $20 processing fee per answer sheet and submit the printed answer sheet at the back of this book by mail or fax, as instructed on the answer sheet. Make sure you calculate your score and enter your birth date and ABIM candidate number, and fax the answer sheet to 215-351-2799 or mail the answer sheet to Member and Customer Service, American College of Physicians, 190 N. Independence Mall West, Philadelphia, PA 19106-1572, using the courtesy envelope provided in your MKSAP 18 slipcase. You will need your 10-digit order number and 8-digit ACP ID number, which are printed on your packing slip. Please allow 4 to 6 weeks for your score report to be emailed back to you. Be sure to include your email address for a response.

If you do not have a 10-digit order number and 8-digit ACP ID number, or if you need help creating a username and password to access the MKSAP 18 online answer sheets, go to mksap.acponline.org or email custserv@acponline.org.

Disclosure Policy

It is the policy of the American College of Physicians (ACP) to ensure balance, independence, objectivity, and scientific rigor in all of its educational activities. To this end, and consistent with the policies of the ACP and the Accreditation Council for Continuing Medical Education (ACCME), contributors to all ACP continuing medical education activities are required to disclose all relevant financial relationships with any entity producing, marketing, reselling, or distributing health care goods or services consumed by, or used on, patients. Contributors are required to use generic names in the discussion of therapeutic options and are required to identify any unapproved, off-label, or investigative use of commercial products or devices. Where a trade name is used, all available trade names for the same product type are also included. If trade-name products manufactured by companies with whom contributors have relationships are discussed, contributors are asked to provide evidence-based citations in support of the discussion. The information is reviewed by the committee responsible for producing this text. If necessary, adjustments to topics or contributors' roles in content development are made to balance the discussion. Further, all readers of this text are asked to evaluate the content for evidence of commercial bias and send any relevant comments to mksap_editors@acponline.org so that future decisions about content and contributors can be made in light of this information.

Resolution of Conflicts

To resolve all conflicts of interest and influences of vested interests, ACP's content planners used best evidence and updated clinical care guidelines in developing content, when such evidence and guidelines were available. All content underwent review by peer reviewers not on the committee to ensure that the material was balanced and unbiased. Contributors' disclosure information can be found with the list of contributors' names and those of ACP principal staff listed in the beginning of this book.

Hospital-Based Medicine

For the convenience of subscribers who provide care in hospital settings, content that is specific to the hospital setting has been highlighted in blue. Hospital icons (🄷) highlight where the hospital-only content begins, continues over more than one page, and ends.

High Value Care Key Points

Key Points in the text that relate to High Value Care concepts (that is, concepts that discuss balancing clinical benefit with costs and harms) are designated by the HVC icon [HVC].

Educational Disclaimer

The editors and publisher of MKSAP 18 recognize that the development of new material offers many opportunities for error. Despite our best efforts, some errors may persist in print. Drug dosage schedules are, we believe, accurate and in accordance with current standards. Readers are advised, however, to ensure that the recommended dosages in MKSAP 18 concur with the information provided in the product information material. This is especially important in cases of new, infrequently used, or highly toxic drugs. Application of the information in MKSAP 18 remains the professional responsibility of the practitioner.

The primary purpose of MKSAP 18 is educational. Information presented, as well as publications, technologies, products, and/or services discussed, is intended to inform subscribers about the knowledge, techniques, and experiences of the contributors. A diversity of professional opinion exists, and the views of the contributors are their own and not those of the ACP. Inclusion of any material in the program does not constitute endorsement or recommendation by the ACP. The ACP does not warrant the safety, reliability, accuracy, completeness, or usefulness of and disclaims any and all liability for damages and claims that may result from the use of information, publications, technologies, products, and/or services discussed in this program.

Publisher's Information

Copyright © 2018 American College of Physicians. All rights reserved.

This publication is protected by copyright. No part of this publication may be reproduced, stored in a retrieval system, or transmitted in any form or by any means, electronic or mechanical, including photocopy, without the express consent of the ACP. MKSAP 18 is for individual use only. Only one account per subscription will be permitted for the purpose of earning CME credits and MOC points and for other authorized uses of MKSAP 18.

Disclaimer Regarding Direct Purchases from Online Retailers

CME and/or MOC for MKSAP 18 is available only if you purchase the program directly from ACP. CME credits and MOC points cannot be awarded to those purchasers who have purchased the program from non-authorized sellers such as Amazon, eBay, or any other such online retailer.

Unauthorized Use of This Book Is Against the Law

Unauthorized reproduction of this publication is unlawful. The ACP prohibits reproduction of this publication or any of its parts in any form either for individual use or for distribution.

The ACP will consider granting an individual permission to reproduce only limited portions of this publication for his or her own exclusive use. Send requests in writing to MKSAP® Permissions, American College of Physicians, 190 N. Independence Mall West, Philadelphia, PA 19106-1572, or email your request to mksap_editors@acponline.org.

MKSAP 18 ISBN: 978-1-938245-47-3
General Internal Medicine ISBN: 978-1-938245-55-8

Printed in the United States of America.

For order information in the U.S. or Canada call 800-ACP-1915. All other countries call 215-351-2600 (Monday to Friday, 9 AM – 5 PM ET). Fax inquiries to 215-351-2799 or email to custserv@acponline.org.

Errata

Errata for MKSAP 18 will be available through the MKSAP Resource Site at mksap.acponline.org as new information becomes known to the editors.

Table of Contents

General Internal Medicine High Value Care Recommendations

The American College of Physicians, in collaboration with multiple other organizations, is engaged in a worldwide initiative to promote the practice of High Value Care (HVC). The goals of the HVC initiative are to improve health care outcomes by providing care of proven benefit and reducing costs by avoiding unnecessary and even harmful interventions. The initiative comprises several programs that integrate the important concept of health care value (balancing clinical benefit with costs and harms) for a given intervention into a broad range of educational materials to address the needs of trainees, practicing physicians, and patients.

HVC content has been integrated into MKSAP 18 in several important ways. MKSAP 18 includes HVC-identified key points in the text, HVC-focused multiple choice questions, and, for subscribers to MKSAP Digital, an HVC custom quiz. From the text and questions, we have generated the following list of HVC recommendations that meet the definition below of high value care and bring us closer to our goal of improving patient outcomes while conserving finite resources.

High Value Care Recommendation: A recommendation to choose diagnostic and management strategies for patients in specific clinical situations that balance clinical benefit with cost and harms with the goal of improving patient outcomes.

Below are the High Value Care Recommendations for the General Internal Medicine section of MKSAP 18.

- High breast density alone does not necessitate adjunctive breast imaging other than routine screening mammography (see Item 154).
- Direct-to-consumer genomic testing contributes very little to overall disease risk.
- The U.S. Preventive Services Task Force does not recommend multivitamins or herbal supplements for the prevention of cardiovascular disease or cancer.
- Enteral or parenteral artificial nutritional support at the end of life does not improve survival, is invasive, and can cause side effects.
- No evidence supports the use of long-term opioid therapy in patients with chronic noncancer pain; long-term opioid use is associated with poorer overall functional status, worse quality of life, and worse pain.
- In patients with medically unexplained symptoms, clinicians should limit diagnostic tests to those deemed medically necessary.

- In patients with acute cough, chest radiography is not indicated in the absence of abnormal vital signs or abnormal lung examination findings.
- Treatment of acute cough is primarily symptomatic; antibiotics are not recommended without a clear bacterial cause.
- Routine imaging is not recommended for benign paroxysmal positional vertigo.
- In patients with central vertigo, MRI is more sensitive than CT in detecting ischemic stroke, whereas CT provides an expedited, cost-effective assessment for hemorrhagic stroke.
- The American College of Physicians recommends against routinely performing brain imaging in cases of syncope that do not involve objective focal neurologic findings.
- Diagnostic testing, such as polysomnography, is usually unnecessary in the evaluation of insomnia.
- Pharmacologic therapies for insomnia are associated with adverse effects and should only be initiated in patients with insomnia refractory to nonpharmacologic interventions.
- Most patients with nonspecific low back pain do not require imaging or other diagnostic testing.
- Most patients with neck pain do not require imaging studies.
- Most patients with rotator cuff disease do not require imaging studies.
- In patients with asymptomatic popliteal (Baker) cysts, no treatment is necessary.
- In patients in whom statin therapy is being considered, an alanine aminotransferase level should be obtained at baseline to evaluate for liver dysfunction; further hepatic monitoring is unnecessary if the baseline level is normal (see Item 148).
- There is little evidence that over-the-counter weight loss supplements are effective.
- Treatment is not indicated in patients with low testosterone levels only; it should be reserved for patients with a low testosterone level associated with symptoms.
- Routine laboratory testing for the diagnosis of menopause is not recommended.
- Medications have not been shown to be of benefit in the management of tinnitus.
- Acute rhinosinusitis is usually caused by viruses, allergies, or irritants, and avoidance of unnecessary antibiotics represents high value care.
- Patients with pharyngitis who present with fewer than three of the four Centor criteria do not need to be tested or treated for group A *Streptococcus* infection.

- In tobacco cessation, combining behavioral counseling with pharmacotherapy is more effective than either modality alone, and combining more than one type of nicotine replacement therapy (short- and long-acting) is more effective than monotherapy.
- Cognitive impairment is best measured with assessment examinations, such as the Mini-Cog and the Mini–Mental State Examination, rather than laboratory testing or imaging (see Item 48).
- No pharmacologic therapies are recommended for the treatment of stress urinary incontinence or functional incontinence.
- Hydrocolloid or foam dressings are superior to standard gauze dressings in the treatment of pressure injuries (see Item 118).
- Preoperative laboratory testing should be performed based on the patient's medical conditions, physical examination findings, and preoperative symptoms; routine laboratory panels expose patients to unnecessary testing and are not recommended.
- Patients with low cardiovascular risk (<1% risk for a perioperative major adverse cardiac event) may proceed to surgery without preoperative cardiac stress testing.
- Preoperative cardiac stress testing should generally be reserved for patients at elevated risk for a major adverse cardiac event with a functional capacity less than 4 metabolic equivalents, but only if the results of the test will change perioperative management (see Item 34).
- Routine electrocardiography is not indicated in asymptomatic patients undergoing low-risk surgical procedures.
- In patients with coronary artery disease, routine coronary angiography or revascularization should not be performed exclusively to reduce perioperative cardiovascular events.
- Preoperative chest radiography is indicated only in patients with signs or symptoms of pulmonary disease and in patients with underlying cardiac or pulmonary disease and new or unstable symptoms.
- Spirometry should not be routinely performed preoperatively except in patients undergoing lung resection.
- Asymptomatic carotid bruit is not predictive of perioperative stroke and requires no preoperative evaluation.
- Pregnant patients should undergo the same preoperative medical evaluation as nonpregnant patients; additional diagnostic testing is unnecessary.

General Internal Medicine

High Value Care in Internal Medicine

Although the United States spends more on health care than all other developed nations, it has higher rates of medical care–related mortality and shorter life expectancy. Compared with other high-income countries, patients in the United States pay more for prescription drugs, undergo more diagnostic tests, and pay the highest hospital and physician prices for procedures. In response to this unsustainable spending, health policy organizations and other expert groups advocate implementing a high value approach to patient care.

High value care is individualized care that delivers proven benefits while minimizing risks and unnecessary costs. It requires a careful evaluation to determine whether the benefits of a diagnostic test or intervention justify the harms and costs. Importantly, when determining value, clinicians should consider the benefits of a test or intervention before the cost. Focusing primarily on cost increases the tendency to avoid an expensive test or intervention regardless of outcome or to continue a low-cost intervention that provides no benefit. Notably, some costly or risky tests and interventions, such as screening colonoscopy, are high value because their benefits may be substantial. Similarly, some inexpensive and low-risk tests and interventions, such as routine daily laboratory testing in hospitalized patients, represent low value care. Examples of high value and low value care are provided in **Table 1**.

Shared decision making is essential to high value care, particularly because perceived patient demand is one driver of inappropriate testing and interventions. Including patients in the decision-making process provides opportunities to educate patients on balancing benefits with potential harms and costs and to incorporate their values and preferences into the care process.

Resources to help clinicians determine the value of common tests and interventions are available from the American College of Physicians (https://www.acponline.org/clinical-information/high-value-care), Alliance for Academic Internal Medicine, and Society of Hospital Medicine. In addition, the Choosing Wisely campaign, an initiative of the American Board of Internal Medicine Foundation with medical specialty societies, has published specialty-specific lists of commonly used tests or procedures whose necessity should be questioned and discussed by clinicians and patients (www.choosingwisely.org). *Consumer Reports* works with many of the Choosing Wisely partners to develop patient-friendly materials from the lists of recommendations and to disseminate them to consumers through a network of Choosing Wisely consumer partners.

TABLE 1.	Examples of High Value and Low Value Care Interventions		
Intervention		**Cost**	**Benefit**
High Value Care			
High-sensitivity D-dimer testing to exclude venous thromboembolism in patients with low likelihood of disease		Low	High negative predictive value
Influenza vaccination		Low	High benefit for reducing disease burden and complications
Low Value Care			
Antibiotic therapy in patients with upper respiratory tract infection		Low	No benefit for reducing duration or severity of illness
Carotid ultrasonography in patients with syncope		Intermediate	Low diagnostic value
Imaging studies in patients with low back pain in the absence of "red flag" findings (fever, involuntary weight loss, incontinence)		Intermediate	Low diagnostic value

KEY POINT

- High value care is individualized care that delivers proven benefits while minimizing risks and unnecessary costs.

HVC

Interpretation of the Medical Literature

Introduction

The science of medicine is constantly evolving, and peer-reviewed literature is the primary means of disseminating new medical knowledge. The application of this information to patient-centered medical decision making requires an understanding of different study designs and how to interpret statistical tests for significance. Although research in the basic sciences (including pharmacology and physiology) provides the basis for many clinical advances, this chapter will review interpretation of the literature that may be immediately applicable to the clinical setting.

Study Designs

Study designs can be divided into two broad categories: experimental studies and observational studies. The selection of a study design is guided by the suitability of the design to address the clinical question and the population being studied.

The validity, or trustworthiness, of a study's results may be limited by bias and/or confounders (see Validity of a Study).

Experimental Study Designs

Experimental studies systematically expose some or all of the individuals in the study to a potential causative or protective factor (the exposure, often a treatment) (**Table 2**). Exposed and unexposed participants are compared with respect to developing the outcome of interest. As an example, an experimental study might compare patients with diabetes mellitus treated with a statin to those treated with a placebo to determine whether patients receiving active treatment are more or less likely than untreated patients to experience cardiovascular events.

The process for allocating the exposure or treatment to the study participants affects the study strength and the validity of the findings. The strongest experimental design is the randomized controlled trial. By randomly allocating the treatment, confounders (both known and unknown) are randomly distributed in the treatment and control groups. The least rigorous experimental design is the quasi-experimental design, in which participants are not randomly assigned. One example of a quasi-experimental design is a pre–post trial, in which

TABLE 2. Experimental Study Designs				
Study Design	**Description**	**Best Uses**	**Common Limitations to Use/Validity**	**Common Measure of Association**
Quasi-experimental study	All participants receive treatment of interest Example: phase I drug trial	Establishing treatment effect, defining risks of adverse events	Difficult to clearly establish that treatment caused outcome Risk for confounding, especially for factors not known	Before-and-after comparison of outcome of interest
Non-randomized controlled trial	Treatment is allocated in a prespecified manner but not using randomization; comparison is made between different treatment groups or between treatment and control groups Example: study of surgical and nonsurgical treatment options in which enrolled participants are assigned to the treatment type they prefer to receive	When patients/participants may not be amenable to being randomly assigned to a treatment or when randomization is not ethically permitted	Risk for confounding, especially for factors not known Risk for selection bias if patients are allowed choice in treatment allocated	Difference between treatment groups in outcome of interest Measure reported varies depending on outcome of interest and statistical technique
Cluster randomized trial	Participants are randomly assigned as a unit instead of individually Example: study of effect of diabetic education on average hemoglobin A_{1c} value, in which participants are community primary care practices	Treatments for which randomization of individual patients is not feasible or ethical When effect at a level larger than an individual level (i.e., institution or health system) is being studied	Complicated statistical analysis May be difficult to ensure groups being compared are similar (risk for confounding)	Difference between treatment groups in outcome of interest Measure reported varies depending on outcome of interest and statistical technique
Randomized controlled trial	Participants are randomly assigned to one of the treatment options (including control/placebo group)	Considered to be highest level of evidence for treatment studies Confounding is minimized if study is large enough	Generalizability is limited to the population included in the trial Expensive and resource intensive to conduct	Difference between treatment groups in outcome of interest Measure reported varies depending on outcome of interest and statistical technique

all participants receive the studied treatment and results are obtained by comparing measurements taken before and after the outcome; thus, participants serve as their own internal controls. Because there is no external control group, the ability of the quasi-experimental design to determine cause and effect is limited.

Observational Study Designs

In observational studies, no treatment is imposed on the persons being studied. Instead, researchers observe naturally occurring events in individuals who have or have not been exposed to a risk factor or treatment. The relationships between risk factors and disease may be explored, but the ability to assess for causality is limited.

Common observational study designs include ecologic, cross-sectional, case-control, and cohort studies. Case reports or case series, which describe an individual case or a series of related cases, are not true studies but have the potential to identify new or unique relationships to be further studied.

Ecologic studies evaluate the prevalence or extent of an exposure across distinct populations. They are hypothesis generating and are used to identify compelling trends for an exposure of interest across different groups, which can be investigated subsequently in more focused studies. Ecologic studies cannot be used to determine causation. Incorrect assignment of causation based on ecologic study results is termed the ecologic fallacy.

Cross-sectional studies evaluate the relationship between exposures and health outcomes in a population of interest. These studies are characterized by the measurement of factors and outcomes at a single point in time. Because cross-sectional studies lack comparison groups and the temporal sequence is often unknown, these studies are best used to determine disease prevalence and generate hypotheses; they can also assess the relatedness between two exposures of interest. Surveys conducted by health services groups may serve as the basis for these studies. Examples include the National Health and Nutrition Examination Survey and the Behavioral Risk Factor Surveillance Survey, both conducted by the Centers for Disease Control and Prevention.

Case-control studies compare past exposures in patients with and without disease. The events being studied have already occurred; therefore, there is potential for recall bias, which arises when patients with the disease of interest are more likely to recall past exposures compared with controls. However, for the study of rare diseases, case-control studies may be the best way to collect enough data to determine meaningful relationships.

Cohort studies divide participants into groups based on the presence or absence of a critical exposure and evaluate for differences between the groups in the development of a disease or outcome. Cohort studies may enroll participants before the outcome develops and follow patients forward in time (prospective cohorts), or they may enroll participants after an event has occurred (retrospective cohorts). Cohort studies are ideal for studying diseases or outcomes that develop over time, evaluating the effect of rare potential causative factors, and performing time-to-event (survival) analyses; however, these studies are subject to losses to follow-up. Similar to case-control studies, retrospective cohorts may also be subject to recall bias.

Systematic Reviews and Meta-Analysis

Narrative review articles, a common source of information for clinicians, present an expert assessment of the known evidence on a certain topic. Although narrative reviews are valuable learning resources, the body of evidence they contain varies and is influenced by the experiences of the authors. In contrast, systematic reviews involve a systematic search of the literature using predefined criteria to collect all published and unpublished studies that address the topic. This systematic approach minimizes selection bias and increases the strength of the information presented. Systematic reviews that combine the results of the studies included in a statistical analysis are termed meta-analyses.

The value of meta-analysis often resides in the ability to pool data and increase sample size and statistical power, as the ability to detect a difference between two groups depends on the number of persons being studied. A larger sample size has a greater power to discriminate smaller differences between groups; however, larger studies carry a higher cost and are logistically more complicated to administer. Meta-analysis of high-quality randomized controlled trials is considered to be one of the highest levels of clinical evidence. Factors that limit the ability to combine study results meaningfully include differences in the study populations, research measures, and statistical techniques.

KEY POINTS

- Experimental studies systematically expose some or all of the individuals in the study to a potential causative or protective factor; the strongest experimental design is the randomized controlled trial. **HVC**

- Cross-sectional studies lack comparison groups, and the temporal sequence is often unknown; therefore, these studies are best used in determining disease prevalence and generating hypotheses. **HVC**

- Case-control studies compare past exposures in patients with and without disease; these studies are advantageous for the study of rare diseases. **HVC**

- Cohort studies are ideal for studying diseases or outcomes that develop over time, evaluating the effect of rare potential causative factors, and performing time-to-event (survival) analyses. **HVC**

Validity of a Study

Validity refers to the fidelity of the study results to what is correct or true. Validity can be further characterized as internal or external. Internal validity refers to how well study error is minimized and to what degree the results are true. External validity is the extent to which the study results can be applied to settings other than the study setting; it represents the generalizability of the study results. Threats to the validity of a study include systematic error and random error.

Systematic error is the influence of confounders and bias on the results of a study. Confounders, factors other than the variables being studied that are associated with the studied population and may affect the end point being assessed, are a common threat to validity. An observational study, for example, may show that patients receiving statin therapy have an increased risk for cardiovascular events compared with those not taking statin therapy. However, the presence of a powerful confounder, specifically that patients receiving statin therapy are at high risk for cardiovascular events, influences the outcome of the study. The impact of confounding can be reduced by design strategies, such as matching, and evaluation techniques, including stratification of the analysis and regression techniques (or regression adjustment).

Bias refers to the presence of factors that skew the study results in a specific direction. Bias can be introduced at any point in a study design, including patient recruitment and outcome measurement. Careful study design can decrease the likelihood of bias; however, once bias has been introduced into the study, it cannot be eliminated or minimized.

Random error is error that is introduced by random variability or purely by chance. The role of chance is expressed by the P value or confidence interval and is determined by statistical analysis. The likelihood of random error can be decreased by increasing study size and using precise measurement strategies.

Statistical Analysis

Statistical significance is reported using P values or confidence intervals, which express the probability that chance alone accounts for the result. A P value less than or equal to 0.05 ($\leq 5\%$ probability that chance alone accounts for the result) is often considered as indicating a statistically significant finding. However, this determination is arbitrary, and some researchers may opt for a different level (typically more stringent).

Confidence intervals express the range of values within which the true result falls; the 95% confidence interval means that there is 95% confidence that the true value is within the confidence interval range. Narrower ranges imply greater confidence, or certainty, that the reported value is closer to the true value.

Sensitivity, Specificity, and Predictive Values

Sensitivity and specificity reflect the accuracy of a diagnostic or screening test (**Table 3**). Sensitivity is the ability of the test to detect those who truly have a disease or condition, or the probability that the test result will be positive in a patient with the disease. Specificity is the ability of the test to correctly identify those without the disease, or the probability that the test result will be negative in a patient without the disease. Therefore, sensitive tests are those with minimal rates of false-negative results, and specific tests are those with minimal rates of false-positive results.

Positive and negative predictive values reflect the validity of a positive or negative test result for predicting the presence or absence of disease in a specific population. The positive predictive value is the proportion of those with a positive test result who truly have the disease. The negative predictive value is the proportion of those with a negative test result who are truly free of the disease. Predictive values are determined not only by sensitivity and specificity but also by the prevalence of the disease in the population.

Likelihood Ratios

Likelihood ratios (LRs) are used to translate the impact of sensitivity and specificity of a specific clinical finding on the probability of a disease or outcome in a given patient; they provide a measure of the strength of association between the clinical finding and the specific disease. Each clinical finding, inclusive of symptoms, physical findings, and laboratory and imaging results, has a positive and negative LR for a specific disease. The positive LR is used when the test result is positive, and the negative LR is used when the test result is negative.

LRs are used in conjunction with the pretest probability of disease (the probability of disease in the patient before the test result is considered). The interaction of the pretest probability and LR results in a posttest probability of disease. The posttest probability may then serve as the rationale for treating a patient for the disease in question (if the positive test resulted in a high posttest probability) or ruling out a diagnosis (if the negative test resulted in a very low posttest probability). Mathematically, the pretest probability (a percentage) is converted to pretest odds (a ratio), the odds are multiplied by the appropriate LR, and the posttest odds are converted to a posttest probability.

For ease of clinical use, several general LR rules apply. Positive LR values of 2, 5, and 10 correspond to an increase in disease probability by 15%, 30%, and 45%, respectively; negative LR values of 0.5, 0.2, and 0.1 correspond to a decrease in disease probability by 15%, 30%, and 45%, respectively. Larger positive LRs and smaller negative LRs are more apt to affect clinical decisions.

Clinical calculators that provide a quick means for calculating LRs and their effect on probability of disease, such as one from the Centre for Evidence-Based Medicine (https://www.cebm.net/2014/06/catmaker-ebm-calculators/), are widely available. Alternatively, nomograms may be used to extrapolate the posttest probability of disease from the pretest probability of disease based on the LR (**Figure 1**).

Absolute and Relative Risk Reduction

Absolute risk reduction and relative risk reduction are measures commonly used to report the efficacy of an intervention

TABLE 3. Common Terms Used in Interpretation of the Medical Literature for Diagnostic Tests

Term	Definition	Calculation	Notes
Prevalence (Prev)	Proportion of patients with the disease in the population	Prev = (TP + FN) / (TP + FP + FN + TN)	
Sensitivity (Sn)	Proportion of patients with the disease who have a positive test result	Sn = TP / (TP + FN)	
Specificity (Sp)	Proportion of patients without the disease who have a negative test result	Sp = TN / (FP + TN)	
Positive predictive value (PPV)	Proportion of patients with a positive test result who have the disease	PPV = TP / (TP + FP)	Increases with *increasing* prevalence
Negative predictive value (NPV)	Proportion of patients with a negative test result who do not have the disease	NPV = TN / (TN + FN)	Increases with *decreasing* prevalence
Positive likelihood ratio (LR+)	The ratio of the probability of a positive test result among patients with the disease to the probability of a positive result among patients without the disease	LR+ = Sn / (1 − Sp)	
Negative likelihood ratio (LR−)	The ratio of the probability of a negative test result among patients with the disease to the probability of a negative result in patients without the disease	LR− = (1 − Sn) / Sp	
Pretest odds	The odds that a patient has the disease before the test is performed	Pretest odds = pretest probability / (1 − pretest probability)	
Posttest odds	The odds that a patient has the disease after a test is performed	Posttest odds = pretest odds × LR	LR+ is used if result of test is positive; LR− is used if result of test is negative A nomogram is available to calculate posttest probability using pretest probability and LR without having to convert pretest probability to odds (see Figure 1)
Pretest probability	Proportion of patients with the disease before a test is performed	Pretest probability can be estimated from population prevalence, clinical risk calculators, or clinical experience if no evidence-based tools exist	
Posttest probability	Proportion of patients with the disease after a test is performed	Posttest probability = posttest odds / (1 + posttest odds)	

FN = false negative; FP = false positive; TN = true negative; TP = true positive.

(**Table 4**). Absolute risk reduction is the difference in the response to treatment between experimental and control groups. Absolute risk reduction is particularly relevant when the measure reported is the rate of development of a clinically meaningful end point, such as the incidence of cardiovascular events or death in studies of lipid-lowering therapy. Because these differences may seem small, investigators will often also report the relative risk or risk ratio (the ratio of the risk for the event in the experimental group to the risk for the event in the

control group) as well as relative risk reduction, or (1 − risk ratio) × 100%.

The difference in the magnitude of these measures can be illustrated with a study of lipid-lowering therapy in which the rate of acute coronary syndromes in 5 years is 3.6% in the treated group and 4.8% in the control group. The absolute risk reduction is 1.2%. The risk ratio, however, is 75%, and the relative risk reduction is 25%. Therefore, although the absolute difference in rates between the two groups is small (1.2%), the

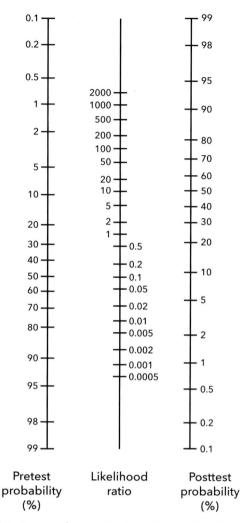

FIGURE 1. Nomogram for interpreting diagnostic test results. In this nomogram, a straight line drawn from a patient's pretest probability of disease (which is estimated from experience, local data, or published literature) through the likelihood ratio for the test result will indicate the posttest probability of disease.

Reproduced with permission from Fagan TJ. Letter: nomogram for Bayes theorem. N Engl J Med. 1975 Jul 31;293(5):257. [PMID: 1143310] Copyright 1975, Massachusetts Medical Society.

effect of a treatment may appear substantial when relative risk reduction (25%) is reported.

Numbers Needed to Treat and Harm

The clinical impact of an intervention can be further assessed by using the number needed to treat (NNT) and the number needed to harm (NNH). The NNT is the inverse of the absolute risk reduction. It represents the number of patients who must receive a treatment to cause one additional patient to benefit, and it provides a quantifiable measure of the treatment effect that is easily understood by physicians and patients. The acceptability of the NNT depends on the risks associated with the condition, the cost and side effects of the treatment, and other treatments available.

The NNH can be similarly calculated for studies measuring adverse outcomes, but it also needs to be considered in the context of the benefits of the treatment and the severity of the harm incurred.

> **KEY POINTS**
>
> - Sensitivity is the ability of the test to detect those who truly have a disease or condition, whereas specificity is the ability of the test to correctly identify those without the disease.
> - Likelihood ratios are used to translate the impact of sensitivity and specificity of a specific clinical finding on the probability of a disease or outcome in a given patient.
> - Absolute risk reduction is the difference in the response to treatment between experimental and control groups.
> - The number needed to treat is the inverse of the absolute risk reduction and represents the number of patients who must receive a treatment to cause one patient to benefit.

Levels of Evidence

Levels of evidence describe the strength and quality of study results and can aid in clinical decision making. Systematic reviews, with or without meta-analysis, provide the highest level of evidence, followed by large, multicenter randomized, blinded, placebo-controlled trials. Large, meticulously controlled studies generally provide a higher level of evidence than smaller studies. Experimental studies provide a higher level of evidence than observational studies, and reports of expert opinion provide the lowest acceptable level of evidence. The U.S. Preventive Services Task Force and other organizations have developed grading systems to rank the relative rigor of clinical studies (**Table 5**). The grading system used by the U.S. Preventive Services Task Force for levels of benefit is provided in Routine Care of the Healthy Patient.

Routine Care of the Healthy Patient

History and Physical Examination
Periodic Health Examination

The periodic health examination has played a central role in patient care for the past century, becoming an expectation for physicians and patients alike. Although evidence suggests periodic health examinations may improve surrogate outcomes, such as reduction in cardiovascular risk factors and increased receipt of preventive services, there is no evidence that they reduce mortality or other patient-important outcomes. A 2012 Cochrane systematic review confirmed that general health checks result in more diagnoses and medication prescriptions but do not reduce morbidity, hospitalizations, or mortality. The Danish Inter99 trial showed that screening for

TABLE 4. Common Terms Used in Interpretation of the Medical Literature for Therapeutics

Term	Definition	Calculation	Notes
Absolute risk (AR)	The probability of an event occurring in a group during a specified time period	AR = patients with event in group / total patients in group	Also known as event rate; can be for benefits or harms. Often, an experimental event rate (EER) is compared with a control event rate (CER)
Relative risk (RR)	The ratio of the probability of developing a disease with a risk factor present to the probability of developing the disease without the risk factor present	RR = EER / CER	Used in cohort studies and randomized controlled trials
Absolute risk reduction (ARR)	The difference in rates of events between experimental group (EER) and control group (CER)	ARR = | EER − CER |	
Relative risk reduction (RRR)	The ratio of absolute risk reduction to the event rate among controls	RRR = | EER − CER | / CER	
Number needed to treat (NNT)	Number of patients needed to receive a treatment for one additional patient to benefit	NNT = 1 / ARR	A good estimate of the effect size
Number needed to harm (NNH)	Number of patients needed to receive a treatment for one additional patient to be harmed	NNH = 1 / ARI	ARI is the absolute risk increase and equals | EER − CER | when the event is an unfavorable outcome (e.g., drug side effect)

TABLE 5. U.S. Preventive Services Task Force Hierarchy of Research Design

Level	Description
I	Properly powered and conducted RCT; well-conducted systematic review or meta-analysis of homogeneous RCTs
II-1	Well-designed controlled trial without randomization
II-2	Well-designed cohort or case-control analytic study
II-3	Multiple time series with or without the intervention; results from uncontrolled studies that yield results of large magnitude
III	Opinions of respected authorities, based on clinical experience; descriptive studies or case reports; reports of expert committees

RCT = randomized controlled trial.

Reproduced from U.S. Preventive Services Task Force. Procedure Manual. https://www.uspreventiveservicestaskforce.org/Page/Name/procedure-manual. November 2017. Accessed June 27, 2018.

ischemic heart disease and repeated counseling over 5 years for those at high risk had no effect on risks for ischemic heart disease, stroke, or mortality after 10-year follow-up. Periodic health examinations also have a substantial financial impact, costing $5.2 billion annually without including costs of additional testing, visits, or missed work, according to a 2007 estimate. Overdiagnosis and overtreatment are other potential drawbacks to periodic health checks. Therefore, the Society of General Internal Medicine, through the Choosing Wisely campaign, specifically recommends against performing general health checks that include a comprehensive examination and laboratory testing for asymptomatic adults.

Despite this evidence, the periodic health examination may offer value that is difficult to measure in clinical trials. It provides dedicated time for screening and counseling and strengthens physician-patient relationships, which may improve adherence to physician recommendations. Notably, Medicare covers an initial preventive physical examination once in a lifetime within the first 12 months of a patient's enrollment in Medicare and an annual wellness visit thereafter. These visits are described as a focused physical and health review rather than a comprehensive head-to-toe physical examination.

Routine History and Physical Examination

Obtaining a basic history is essential in establishing a clinician-patient relationship and understanding the patient's health history, concerns, and expectations (**Table 6**). Patients may be sensitive about sharing certain information, such as substance use and sexual practices, and open and nonjudgmental communication can encourage sharing. Clinicians should preface these inquiries by informing the patient that these questions are asked of everyone, the information is necessary to provide the best care, and responses are confidential.

A focused physical examination should always be performed to address the patient's concerns and relevant historical findings. Irrespective of gender presentation, physicians should provide care for the present anatomy in a

TABLE 6.	Components of the History

Past medical conditions and surgeries
   Hospitalizations
   Major childhood illnesses
   Allergies and corresponding reactions

Social history
   Alcohol use
   Tobacco use
   Illicit drug use
   Spirituality

Work and home situation
   Social support
   Safety
- Home safety: intimate partner violence and abuse, working smoke alarms, water heater set to ≤49 °C (120 °F), weapons safety
- Safety outside of the home: seatbelt use while driving, helmet use while motorcycling or bicycling, no electronic device use while driving

Diet

Physical activity

Family history

Medication history
   Prescription and over-the-counter medications
   Past and current hormone use for transgender patients
   Vitamins and supplements
   Herbal preparations and nontraditional therapies

Sexual history[a]
   Partners
- How many sex partners have you had in the past 2 months? 12 months?
- Have you had sex with men, women, or both?

   Practices
- What kind of sexual contact have you had? Vaginal (penis in vagina), anal (penis in rectum/anus), or oral sex (mouth on penis/vagina)?

   Protection/pregnancy
- Have you ever had a sexually transmitted infection?
- What do you do to protect yourself from sexually transmitted infections?
- Are you or your partner trying to get pregnant?
- What are you doing to prevent pregnancy?

Review of systems

[a]When taking a sexual history, do not assume heterosexuality, and use gender-neutral language when referring to partners ("partner" or "spouse" rather than "wife," "husband," "girlfriend," or "boyfriend").

sensitive, respectful, and affirming manner. In contrast to the focused physical examination, the value of the routine physical examination in asymptomatic patients has been debated.

Regularly obtaining height and weight (to calculate BMI) as well as blood pressure is universally recommended. Additionally, pulse palpation in individuals older than 65 years has been found effective for detection of atrial fibrillation. The U.S. Preventive Services Task Force (USPSTF) recommends against routine abdominal, testicular, and bimanual pelvic examinations for cancer screening. The USPSTF has also concluded that there is insufficient evidence to recommend routine cardiac and lung auscultation, thyroid palpation, skin examination, visual acuity assessment, and hearing assessment, although these evaluations may be appropriate as part of a comprehensive physical examination in persons at increased risk. Relatively no harms arise from these examinations save for the opportunity cost of providing another service that may be more valuable. Routine laboratory tests, such as screening complete blood count and urinalysis, are not recommended.

Preparticipation physical examination is required for adolescents before participation in organized sports. In conjunction with the American Academy of Family Physicians and several professional sports medicine organizations, the American Academy of Pediatrics (AAP) created the Preparticipation Physical Evaluation, now in its fourth edition. Additionally, free templates for history, physical examination, and clearance forms are available on the website of the AAP (https://www.aap.org/en-us/about-the-aap/Committees-Councils-Sections/Council-on-sports-medicine-and-fitness/Pages/PPE.aspx). Mandatory components include evaluating for exertional symptoms, family history of premature or sudden cardiac death, and presence of a heart murmur.

Digital stethoscopes, point-of-care ultrasonography, smart phone applications, and other technological advances are gradually becoming more commonplace in the physical examination. However, it is unclear whether these tools improve diagnosis or contribute to overdiagnosis.

KEY POINT

- The periodic health examination may improve surrogate outcomes, such as reduction in cardiovascular risk factors and increased receipt of preventive services; however, the periodic health examination has not been shown to reduce mortality or other patient-important outcomes. **HVC**

Screening
Principles of Screening

Levels of prevention have traditionally been categorized as primary, secondary, and tertiary. Primary prevention is preventing disease or injury before it occurs (for example, through immunization). Secondary prevention is early detection and treatment of disease in asymptomatic patients to slow or stop disease progression. Most screening tests, such as those for colorectal and breast cancers, are secondary prevention measures. Tertiary prevention involves reducing morbidity and mortality due to established disease, such as cardiac rehabilitation after myocardial infarction.

Screening is appropriate for common conditions for which (1) early intervention can decrease morbidity and mortality and (2) safe, acceptable, widely available, and reasonably priced screening tests exist. Screening tests must also have adequate sensitivity and specificity to minimize false-positive and false-negative results.

The effectiveness of screening tests in reducing morbidity and mortality is evaluated through clinical trials; however, studies of screening tests are problematic and subject to three types of bias. Lead-time bias occurs when early detection artificially leads to an increase in measured survival. The time between early detection and clinical diagnosis is mistakenly counted as survival time; however, only the measured time with diagnosed disease, not survival time, has increased (**Figure 2**). Using disease-specific mortality rates rather than survival time as the primary outcome in studies of screening tests can help minimize lead-time bias. Length-time bias occurs when screening detects more cases of disease with a prolonged asymptomatic phase than cases of disease with a short asymptomatic phase. Slowly progressive disease is more likely than aggressive disease to be detected with screening, leading to an overestimation of survival benefit in those with screen-detected disease. Overdiagnosis, or finding and treating illness that otherwise would not have become clinically apparent or caused harm in the patient's lifetime, is an extreme example of length-time bias. Overdiagnosis is an increasingly recognized harm of breast and prostate cancer screening and may also occur with incidental detection of thyroid and kidney

cancers on imaging studies. Selection bias, also referred to as volunteer, referral, or compliance bias, occurs when patients who undergo screening tests are healthier and more interested in their health than nonadherent patients or the general population. Intention-to-treat analyses, in which patients are analyzed according to their original group assignment in randomized clinical trials regardless of intervention received, reduce selection bias.

Screening Recommendations for Adults

The USPSTF and many specialty societies routinely aggregate and review available evidence to inform clinical practice guidelines for screening, counseling, and use of preventive medications. The American College of Physicians (ACP) has developed several different types of clinical recommendations, including clinical practice guidelines, clinical guidance statements, best practice advice, and recommendations regarding high value care, all of which are available at https://www.acponline.org/clinical-information/guidelines. Although there is much agreement among screening recommendations, guidelines often disagree when (1) sufficient evidence is lacking and expert opinion plays a larger role or (2) potential benefits and harms both exist and the balance depends on a person's risk, preferences, and values.

An additional resource to help clinicians identify appropriate screening tests and preventive services is the electronic Preventive Services Selector (ePSS) created by the Agency for Healthcare Research and Quality (available at epss.ahrq.gov in web-based or mobile application–based formats). With this tool, users can select USPSTF-recommended practices based

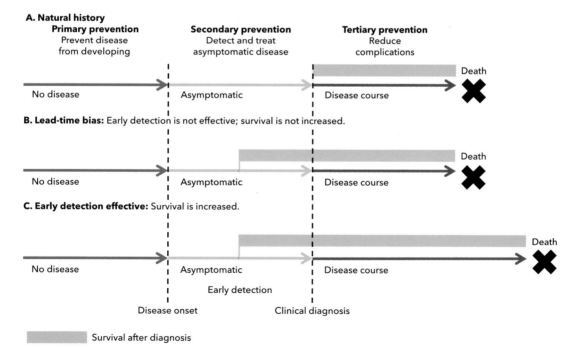

FIGURE 2. The effect of early detection (screening) on survival after diagnosis. (*A*) Screening is not implemented, and the disease takes its normal course. (*B*) Lead-time bias occurs when survival time appears to be lengthened because the screened patient is diagnosed earlier during the preclinical phase but does not live longer in actuality. (*C*) Screening effectively detects disease during the asymptomatic phase, and survival time is lengthened.

on patient age, sex, and other characteristics (such as tobacco use or pregnancy).

Screening recommendations frequently change as supportive evidence emerges. It is important to be aware of changes in recommendations as they occur, to reflect on the rationale and implications of the changes, to contemplate how to best help patients understand new recommendations, and to incorporate these changes appropriately into practice.

Specific Screening Tests

The following section describes screening recommendations from the USPSTF and other organizations. The grading system of the USPSTF (A, B, C, D, and I) is explained in **Table 7**.

TABLE 7. U.S. Preventive Services Task Force Grading and Suggestions for Practice

Grade	Definition	Suggestions for Practice
A	The USPSTF recommends the service. There is high certainty that the net benefit is substantial.	Offer or provide this service.
B	The USPSTF recommends the service. There is high certainty that the net benefit is moderate or there is moderate certainty that the net benefit is moderate to substantial.	Offer or provide this service.
C	The USPSTF recommends selectively offering or providing this service to individual patients based on professional judgment and patient preferences. There is at least moderate certainty that the net benefit is small.	Offer or provide this service for selected patients depending on individual circumstances.
D	The USPSTF recommends against the service. There is moderate or high certainty that the service has no net benefit or that the harms outweigh the benefits.	Discourage the use of this service.
I statement	The USPSTF concludes that the current evidence is insufficient to assess the balance of benefits and harms of the service. Evidence is lacking, of poor quality, or conflicting, and the balance of benefits and harms cannot be determined.	Read the Clinical Considerations section of USPSTF Recommendation Statement. If the service is offered, patients should understand the uncertainty about the balance of benefits and harms.

USPSTF = U.S. Preventive Services Task Force.

Reproduced from U.S. Preventive Services Task Force. Procedure Manual. https://www.uspreventiveservicestaskforce.org/Page/Name/procedure-manual. November 2017. Accessed June 27, 2018.

Screening for Chronic Diseases
Abdominal Aortic Aneurysm
The USPSTF recommends one-time abdominal ultrasonography to screen for abdominal aortic aneurysm (AAA) in all men aged 65 to 75 years who have ever smoked (grade B). Ever-smokers are commonly defined as persons who have smoked more than 100 cigarettes in their lifetime. The number needed to screen (NNS) to prevent one death from AAA in this population is 667. The number needed to treat (NNT) with surgery to prevent one death is 1.5, owing to the high mortality rate associated with AAA rupture. In men aged 65 to 75 years who have never smoked, selective screening is recommended (grade C), especially in those with a first-degree relative with a history of treated or ruptured AAA. The USPSTF makes no recommendation regarding screening for AAA in women who have smoked and specifically recommends against routine screening in women who have never smoked (grade D).

Cardiovascular and Cerebrovascular Disease
Cardiovascular risk assessment is performed in asymptomatic adults to evaluate a patient's risk for future cardiac events; it does not identify pre-existing disease and is therefore considered separate from screening (see MKSAP 18 Cardiovascular Medicine).

The USPSTF does not recommend screening for coronary artery disease with either resting or exercise electrocardiography (ECG) in asymptomatic patients at low risk, defined by the USPSTF as a 10-year cardiovascular event risk of less than 10% using the Pooled Cohort Equations (grade D). In patients at intermediate or high risk for such events, there was inadequate evidence to assess the relative benefits and harms of screening. Similarly, the ACP recommends against screening low-risk and asymptomatic adults with resting ECG or stress testing. No specialty organization recommends screening these populations with resting or exercise ECG, coronary calcium scoring, or coronary angiography.

The USPSTF also does not recommend screening for carotid artery stenosis in the general adult population (grade D).

Depression
The USPSTF suggests that all adults, including pregnant and postpartum women, be screened for depression, with adequate systems in place for assessment, treatment, and follow-up (grade B). Most adults can be screened with the brief PHQ-2, which consists of two questions: "During the past 2 weeks, how often have you been bothered by feeling down, depressed, or hopeless?" and "During the past 2 weeks, have you often been bothered by having little interest or pleasure in doing things?" Answers are graded on a scale of 0 to 6, with a score of 3 indicating a positive screen. The PHQ-2 has a sensitivity of 83% and specificity of 90% for detecting depression; longer screening instruments, such as the PHQ-9, do not have a clear advantage over the PHQ-2. Patients with a positive screening result should complete the PHQ-9, which can be used for diagnosis and monitoring of depression.

Other screening instruments may be more accurate in specific patient populations, such as the Geriatric Depression Scale in older adults and the Edinburgh Postnatal Depression Scale in postpartum and pregnant women.

Diabetes Mellitus

The USPSTF recommends screening for diabetes mellitus in adults aged 40 to 70 years who are overweight or obese (grade B). Screening can be accomplished by measuring levels of fasting plasma glucose or hemoglobin A_{1c}. Those with a positive screening result should undergo intensive behavioral counseling to promote a healthful diet and physical activity. Earlier screening should be considered in persons at increased risk, including individuals who belong to certain racial or ethnic groups (blacks, American Indians, Asian Americans, Hispanics or Latinos, Native Hawaiians, Pacific Islanders), and those with a family history of diabetes or a personal history of gestational diabetes or polycystic ovary syndrome.

In contrast to the USPSTF, the American Diabetes Association (ADA) recommends that screening be performed in obese or overweight patients of any age with one or more risk factors for diabetes (**Table 8**). The ADA also recommends screening all adults beginning at age 45 years, regardless of risk factors, and repeating screening at 3-year intervals. Patients with prediabetes (hemoglobin $A_{1c} \geq 5.7\%$, impaired glucose tolerance, or impaired fasting glucose) should be screened annually.

Dyslipidemia

The USPSTF recommends lipid screening for adults aged 40 to 75 years for the purposes of calculating 10-year risk for atherosclerotic cardiovascular disease (ASCVD) and guiding initiation of statin therapy for primary prevention (see Dyslipidemia chapter on p. 79). Measuring lipid levels every 5 years is reasonable. If lipid levels are close to those that require therapy, testing may be performed at shorter intervals, whereas longer intervals can be considered for persons without cardiovascular risk factors who have repeatedly normal levels. For adults aged 21 to 39 years, the USPSTF recommends that clinicians use their clinical judgment regarding screening for and treating dyslipidemia due to a lack of supportive data.

The American Heart Association recommends assessing traditional cardiovascular risk factors, including total and HDL cholesterol levels, starting at age 20 years. Risk factor assessment should be performed every 4 to 6 years if the patient is at low 10-year risk (<7.5%). Patients with a family history of premature coronary artery disease or patients with a family history of or evidence on examination of familial hypercholesterolemia should also be screened at a younger age.

Hypertension

The USPSTF supports screening all adults for hypertension (grade A). Screening should occur annually in adults aged 40 years and older and in younger adults at increased risk (including patients with high-normal blood pressure [130 to 139/85 to 89 mm Hg], patients who are overweight or obese, and black patients). Screening should otherwise occur every 3 to 5 years. Before treatment is initiated, the diagnosis should be confirmed with blood pressure measurements outside of the clinical setting, such as ambulatory or home blood pressure monitoring.

The American Heart Association/American College of Cardiology recommend evaluating patients with a normal blood pressure (<120/<80 mm Hg) annually and patients with elevated blood pressure (120-129/<80 mm Hg) whose 10-year estimated ASCVD risk is less than 10% every 3 to 6 months.

Obesity

The USPSTF suggests that all adults should be screened for obesity by calculating BMI (grade B), without specifically delineating how frequently screening should be repeated. The American College of Cardiology, American Heart Association, and The Obesity Society recommend annual screening with BMI and waist circumference measurements. Adults with a BMI of 30 or higher should be offered or referred for intensive behavioral interventions, according to the USPSTF.

Obstructive Sleep Apnea

According to the USPSTF, there is insufficient evidence to assess the balance of benefits and harms of screening for obstructive sleep apnea in asymptomatic adults with the currently available tools. Because obstructive sleep apnea is widely underrecognized, clinicians should have a low threshold for investigating for sleep apnea in patients with symptoms consistent with the disease (see MKSAP 18 Pulmonary and Critical Care Medicine).

Osteoporosis

The USPSTF recommends screening for osteoporosis in women aged 65 years and older and in postmenopausal

TABLE 8.	Risk Factors for Diabetes Mellitus
First-degree relative with diabetes	
High-risk race/ethnicity (e.g., African American, Latino, Native American, Asian American, Pacific Islander)	
History of cardiovascular disease	
Hypertension (≥140/90 mm Hg or on therapy for hypertension)	
HDL cholesterol level <35 mg/dL (0.90 mmol/L) and/or a triglyceride level >250 mg/dL (2.82 mmol/L)	
Women with polycystic ovary syndrome	
Physical inactivity	
Other clinical conditions associated with insulin resistance (e.g., severe obesity, acanthosis nigricans)	
History of gestational diabetes	

Information from American Diabetes Association. 2. Classification and diagnosis of diabetes: Standards of Medical Care in Diabetes—2018. Diabetes Care. 2018;41:S13-S27. [PMID: 29222373] doi:10.2337/dc18-S002

women younger than 65 years at increased risk for osteoporosis, as determined by a formal clinical risk assessment tool. One commonly used clinical risk assessment tool is the Fracture Risk Assessment (FRAX), available at www.shef. ac.uk/FRAX. Women who have a 10-year FRAX risk for major osteoporotic fracture equal to or higher than that of a 65-year-old white woman without additional risk factors (10-year risk of 8.4%) should undergo screening for osteoporosis. Screening can be accomplished with bone mineral density measurement, most commonly with dual-energy x-ray absorptiometry (DEXA) of the hip and lumbar spine.

The USPSTF concludes that there is insufficient evidence to recommend routine screening for osteoporosis in men (I statement); however, the National Osteoporosis Foundation recommends osteoporosis screening in men aged 70 years or older. Screening may be considered in men at high risk for osteoporosis on the basis of risk factors, such as low body weight, recent weight loss, physical inactivity, use of oral glucocorticoids, previous fragility fracture, alcohol use, and androgen deprivation through pharmacologic agents or orchiectomy.

Risk assessment and screening for osteoporosis are further discussed in MKSAP 18 Endocrinology and Metabolism.

Thyroid Disease

The USPSTF concludes that there is insufficient evidence to recommend for or against screening for thyroid disease (I statement). The American Thyroid Association and the American Association of Clinical Endocrinologists, however, recommend measuring thyroid-stimulating hormone in individuals at risk for hypothyroidism (for example, personal history of autoimmune disease, neck radiation, or thyroid surgery); they additionally recommend considering screening in adults aged 60 years and older.

Screening for Infectious Diseases

Screening for infectious diseases is primarily recommended for individuals at increased risk (**Table 9** and **Table 10**), although there are several diseases for which average-risk patients should be screened.

According to the USPSTF, screening for chlamydia and gonorrhea should be performed in all sexually active women aged 24 years or younger because of increased prevalence in this population.

One-time hepatitis C screening is recommended for adults born between 1945 and 1965 and those who received

TABLE 9. U.S. Preventive Services Task Force Recommendations on Screening for Infectious Diseases

Infectious Disease	Screening Recommendation	Screening Test	Populations at Risk
Chlamydia and gonorrhea	Screen all sexually active women aged ≤24 y and women aged >24 y who are at increased risk for infection	Nucleic acid amplification test	Persons with a history of STIs, persons with new or multiple sexual partners, those who use condoms inconsistently, persons who exchange sex for money or drugs
HIV	Perform one-time screening for all adults aged 15-65 y; repeat screening for adults at high risk	Combination HIV antibody immunoassay/p24 antigen test	Men who have sex with men, active injection drug users, persons who engage in risky behaviors (unprotected vaginal or anal intercourse; sexual partners who are HIV infected, bisexual, or injection drug users; exchanging sex for drugs or money), persons with other STIs, persons who live and receive care in a high-prevalence setting (HIV seroprevalence of ≥1%)
HBV	Screen all adults at high risk	Hepatitis B surface antigen test; obtain antibodies (anti-HBs, anti-HBc) to differentiate between immunity and infection	Persons born in countries with ≥2% prevalence of HBV infection, persons receiving dialysis or cytotoxic or immunosuppressive treatments, persons with HIV infection, injection drug users, men who have sex with men, household contacts or sexual partners of persons with HBV infection
HCV	Screen all adults at high risk and perform one-time screening in adults born between 1945 and 1965	Anti-HCV antibody test, followed by PCR viral load test if result is positive	Injection/intranasal drug users, persons who received a blood transfusion before 1992, persons receiving long-term hemodialysis, prisoners, and persons who received unregulated tattoos
Syphilis	Screen all adults at increased risk	VDRL or RPR test	Persons with HIV infection, prisoners, men who have sex with men, persons who exchange sex for money or drugs
Latent TB	Screen populations at increased risk	Tuberculin skin test or interferon-γ release assay	Persons born in or former residents of countries with high TB prevalence, close contacts of persons with known or suspected TB, persons who live or work in high-risk settings

Anti-HBc = hepatitis B core antibody; Anti-HBs = hepatitis B surface antibody; HBV = hepatitis B virus; HCV = hepatitis C virus; PCR = polymerase chain reaction; RPR = rapid plasma reagin; STIs = sexually transmitted infections; TB = tuberculosis; VDRL = Venereal Disease Research Laboratory.

TABLE 10. Screening for Infectious Diseases in High-Risk Populations

Specific Populations	Recommended Screening
Pregnant women	Chlamydia and gonorrhea, hepatitis B, HIV, syphilis
Persons engaging in high-risk sexual behavior	Hepatitis B and C, HIV, syphilis
Men who have sex with men	Chlamydia and gonorrhea[a], hepatitis B, HIV, syphilis
Injection drug users	Hepatitis B and C, HIV
Prisoners	Hepatitis C, syphilis, tuberculosis
Persons receiving hemodialysis	Hepatitis B and C, tuberculosis
Persons born in or living in certain countries[b]	Hepatitis B and tuberculosis depending on prevalence of disease
Health care workers	Tuberculosis (annually); pre-employment verification of immunity to hepatitis B virus, measles, mumps, rubella, and varicella

[a]The Centers for Disease Control and Prevention recommends screening for chlamydia and gonorrhea in men who have sex with men; however, the U.S. Preventive Services Task Force has found insufficient evidence to recommend screening for these diseases in men.

[b]Countries with ≥2% hepatitis B virus prevalence, including most of sub-Saharan Africa, central and southeast Asia, and parts of South America. See https://wwwnc.cdc.gov/travel/yellowbook/2018/infectious-diseases-related-to-travel/hepatitis-b for further details.

a blood transfusion before 1992. Screening is accomplished by testing for antibodies to the disease, followed by polymerase chain reaction viral load testing if results of initial testing are positive (see MKSAP 18 Gastroenterology and Hepatology).

The USPSTF recommends that all persons aged 15 to 65 years receive one-time HIV screening regardless of risk, and the Centers for Disease Control and Prevention (CDC) recommends routine HIV screening for all persons aged 13 to 64 years. The USPSTF suggests screening persons at very high risk for HIV (men who have sex with men and active injection drug users) at least annually. The CDC recommends at least annual screening for men who have sex with men. Combination HIV antibody immunoassay/p24 antigen testing is recommended for screening. Diagnosis of HIV is discussed in MKSAP 18 Infectious Disease.

Screening for Substance Use Disorders

The USPSTF recommends that clinicians ask all adults about tobacco use, advise them to stop using tobacco, and provide behavioral intervention and pharmacotherapy for tobacco cessation (grade A) (see Mental and Behavioral Health).

The USPSTF supports asking all adults about alcohol misuse and providing persons engaged in risky or hazardous drinking with brief behavioral counseling interventions to reduce alcohol misuse (grade B). Screening instruments to identify harmful drinking include the Alcohol Use Disorders Identification Test (AUDIT), the AUDIT-Consumption (AUDIT-C),

and single-item screening. The AUDIT (https://pubs.niaaa.nih.gov/publications/Audit.pdf) is a validated 10-item screening test that takes approximately 2 to 3 minutes to administer; the AUDIT-C is a briefer (three-item) version of the AUDIT. With single-item screening, the clinician asks, "How many times in the past year have you had five [four for women] or more drinks in 1 day?" A positive test result, defined as any answer other than zero, has a sensitivity and specificity of approximately 80% for unhealthy alcohol use.

The USPSTF concluded that there is insufficient evidence to assess the balance of benefits and harms of routine screening for illicit drug use. Screening tools include the Drug Abuse Screening Test (DAST-10) (https://www.integration.samhsa.gov/clinical-practice/DAST_-_10.pdf) and the CAGE questionnaire expanded to include drugs (CAGE-AID) (https://www.integration.samhsa.gov/images/res/CAGEAID.pdf). Prescription opioids are the most commonly abused opioids and are the leading cause of opioid overdoses in the United States. Clinicians must be aware of the potential for opioid abuse. The opioid risk tool can be useful to assess risk for abuse of opioid medications; however, this tool needs further validation in clinical practice.

Screening for Abuse

The USPSTF recommends screening for intimate partner violence in all women of child-bearing age (grade B). Available screening tools include the Hurt, Insult, Threaten, Scream (HITS); Ongoing Abuse Screen/Ongoing Violence Assessment Tool (OAS/OVAT); Slapped, Threatened, and Throw (STaT); Humiliation, Afraid, Rape, Kick (HARK); Modified Childhood Trauma Questionnaire–Short Form (CTQ-SF); and Woman Abuse Screen Tool (WAST).

Screening for abuse in elderly and vulnerable adults may be considered, although there is currently insufficient evidence to recommend universal screening (I statement) (see Geriatric Medicine).

Screening for Cancer

This section discusses cancer screening in asymptomatic, average-risk persons. Screening for cancer in patients at high risk is covered in the respective specialty books of MKSAP 18.

Breast Cancer

The balance of benefits and harms of screening mammography has shifted with the advent of increasingly effective breast cancer treatments, which reduce the benefits of early detection, as well as emerging information about overdiagnosis. In women aged 50 to 74 years, there is a clear benefit to screening mammography, and all breast cancer guidelines recommend screening mammography in this age group. Biennial screening mammography imparts most of the benefits of annual screening mammography with fewer harms, although the recommended screening frequency differs between guidelines. In women younger than 50 years or aged 75 years and older, the balance of benefits and harms is less clear, and screening recommendations vary widely (**Table 11**).

TABLE 11. Recommendations for Breast Cancer Screening in Women at Average Risk

Expert Group	Recommendation
American Cancer Society (2015)	Age 40-44 y: Provide women with the opportunity to begin annual screening mammography
	Age 45-54 y: Perform annual screening mammography
	Age ≥55 y: Perform biennial screening mammography with the opportunity to continue annual screening
	Do not perform CBE for breast cancer screening
American College of Obstetricians and Gynecologists (2017)	Age 25-39 y: May offer CBE every 1-3 y
	Age 40-49 y: Offer screening mammography and engage women in a shared decision-making process. May offer annual CBE
	Age 50-75 y: Perform annual or biennial screening mammography based on a shared decision-making process
	Age >75 y: Engage women in a shared decision-making process about discontinuing screening
American College of Physicians (2015)	Age <40 y: Do not perform screening
	Age 40-49 y: Discuss the benefits and harms of screening mammography and order biennial mammography screening if an informed woman requests it
	Age 50-74 y: Encourage biennial mammography screening
	Age >75 y: Do not perform screening
American College of Radiology (2017)	Age 40 y: Begin annual screening mammography
National Comprehensive Cancer Network (2016)	Age 25-39 y: Perform CBE every 1-3 y
	Age 40 y: Begin annual screening mammography and perform annual CBE
U.S. Preventive Services Task Force (2016)	Age 40-49 y: Decision to begin screening should be individualized (grade C)
	Age 50-74 y: Perform biennial screening mammography (grade B)
	Age ≥75 y: Insufficient evidence to assess the balance of benefits and harms of screening mammography (grade I)

CBE = clinical breast examination.

When recommendations differ, shared decision making with consideration of the patient's level of risk, values, and preferences guides the screening decision. The benefit of screening is largest in those aged 60 to 69 years but is substantially lower for younger and older women (**Table 12**). Potential harms of screening include false-positive results and overdiagnosis. For patients starting mammography at age 40 or 50 years, the 10-year cumulative false-positive rates are 42% with biennial screening and 61% with annual screening. Such

TABLE 12. Breast Cancer Deaths Averted per 10,000 Women Screened Over 10 Years

Variable	Patient Age			
	40-49 Years	50-59 Years	60-69 Years	70-74 Years
Breast cancer deaths averted (95% CI)	3 (0-9)	8 (2-17)	21 (11-32)	13 (0-32)
NNS	3333	1250	476	769

NNS = number needed to screen for 10 years to avoid one breast cancer death.

Data from Nelson HD, Fu R, Cantor A, Pappas M, Daeges M, Humphrey L. Effectiveness of breast cancer screening: systematic review and meta-analysis to update the 2009 U.S. Preventive Services Task Force recommendation. Ann Intern Med. 2016;164:244-55. [PMID: 26756588] doi:10.7326/M15-0969

results may cause unnecessary biopsies and substantial patient anxiety. Overdiagnosis accounts for roughly 30% of all breast cancers diagnosed.

Approximately 50% of women have dense breasts on mammography. Increased breast density is associated with an increased breast cancer risk but decreased sensitivity of mammography (more so with film than digital mammography). As a result, legislation in many states requires that breast density be included on mammogram reports (**Table 13**). In women in whom increased breast density is the sole breast cancer risk factor, there is no evidence that adding MRI or ultrasonography to mammography affects breast cancer mortality, and most guidelines conclude that there is insufficient evidence to recommend adjunctive screening when dense breasts are present. The American College of Radiology, however, notes that ultrasonography may be considered in this circumstance. Women with dense breasts should undergo further risk stratification; for those at high risk, additional screening may be considered (see MKSAP 18 Hematology and Oncology).

Prostate Cancer

Screening for prostate cancer in asymptomatic, average-risk men has been controversial, and recommendations among professional organizations continue to evolve (**Table 14**). For men aged 55 to 69 years, the USPSTF recommends that the decision to undergo periodic prostate-specific antigen (PSA)-based screening should be an individual one and should include discussion of the potential benefits and harms of screening with their clinician. The USPSTF recommends that clinicians should not screen men who do not express a preference for screening and recommends against PSA-based screening for prostate cancer in men aged 70 years and older.

Benefits of screening for men aged 55 to 69 years include prevention of one prostate cancer–related death for every 1000 men screened for 10 years (NNS, 1000). Risks include overdiagnosis, overtreatment, and false-positive results that trigger unnecessary biopsies and patient anxiety. Estimated rates of overdiagnosis and overtreatment vary widely.

If the decision is made to proceed with screening, the American Urological Association (AUA) recommends

TABLE 13. Breast Imaging Reporting and Data System (BI-RADS) Breast Composition Categories

a.	The breasts are almost entirely fatty
b.	There are scattered areas of fibroglandular density
c.	The breasts are heterogeneously dense, which may obscure small masses
d.	The breasts are extremely dense, which lowers the sensitivity of mammography

Reproduced with permission of the American College of Radiology (ACR) from D'Orsi CJ, Sickles EA, Mendelson EB, et al. ACR BI-RADS® Atlas, Breast Imaging Reporting and Data System. Reston, VA, American College of Radiology; 2013. No other representation of this material is authorized without expressed, written permission from the ACR. Refer to the ACR website at https://www.acr.org/Clinical-Resources/Reporting-and-Data-Systems/Bi-Rads for the most current and complete version of the BI-RADS® Atlas.

TABLE 14. Recommendations for Prostate Cancer Screening

Expert Group	Recommendation
American Cancer Society (2010)	Age 40-44 y: Engage men at higher risk (≥2 first-degree relatives with prostate cancer before age 65 y) in shared decision making
	Age 45-49 y: Engage men at high risk (African American race or first-degree relative with prostate cancer before age 65 y) in shared decision making
	Age ≥50 y with life expectancy >10 y: Engage in shared decision making
American College of Physicians (2013)	Age 50-69 y: Inform men about the limited potential benefits and substantial harms of screening for prostate cancer; test only men who request screening after informed discussion
	Age <50 y, >69 y, or with a life expectancy <10 y: Recommend against screening
American Urological Association (2013, reviewed and confirmed 2015)	Men at higher risk (African American race or with positive family history): Individualize screening decisions
	Age <40 y: Recommend against screening
	Age 40-54 y: Do not recommend routine screening
	Age 55-69 y: Engage men considering PSA-based screening in shared decision making; proceed based on patient values and preferences. If proceeding with screening, consider PSA testing every 2 years or longer
	Age ≥70 y or with life expectancy <10-15 y: Do not recommend routine screening
U.S. Preventive Services Task Force (2018)	Age 55-69: Discuss potential benefits and harms of PSA-based screening for prostate cancer and individualize decision making by incorporating the patient's values and preferences
	Age ≥70 y: Recommend against PSA-based screening

PSA = prostate-specific antigen.

choosing less frequent screening intervals (≥2 years), which may reduce overdiagnosis and the number of false-positive results while preserving most of the screening benefit. The AUA also recommends that the interval for rescreening may be based on the baseline PSA level. Screening is not recommended for men with less than a 10- to 15-year life expectancy.

Methods to better use PSA testing, including one-time PSA measurement at prespecified ages, adjusted-threshold testing, or PSA velocity and doubling time, are being investigated. However, there is currently insufficient evidence to support these methods.

Colorectal Cancer

The USPSTF recommends screening for colorectal cancer in asymptomatic adults aged 50 to 75 years (grade A). In contrast, the American Cancer Society makes a qualified recommendation to initiate screening for colorectal cancer at age 45 years. According to the USPSTF, screening decisions in patients aged 76 to 85 years should be individualized according to life expectancy and ability to tolerate treatment of colorectal cancer if diagnosed. Screening history should also be considered because patients who have not undergone screening are the most likely to benefit (grade C). The USPSTF suggests that screening may be discontinued in patients older than 85 years; most other guidelines recommend stopping screening if life expectancy is less than 10 years.

There is little head-to-head comparative evidence that any one recommended screening modality provides a greater benefit than the others. In addition, despite unequivocal evidence that colon cancer screening reduces mortality, an estimated one in three U.S. adults who are eligible for colon cancer screening has not been screened. Therefore, the USPSTF supports using the test that is most likely to result in completion of screening. Understanding a patient's values and preferences and selecting a test to which the patient is most likely to adhere may improve screening rates. Clinicians should be familiar with the characteristics of each screening strategy to facilitate effective discussion with patients (**Table 15**).

The U.S. Multi-Society Task Force on Colorectal Cancer (MSTF), an initiative of U.S. gastroenterology societies, has ranked colorectal cancer screening tests in tiers based on the available evidence, cost-effectiveness, test availability, and several other factors. The MSTF recommends colonoscopy every 10 years or annual fecal immunochemical testing (FIT) as first-tier tests; CT colonography every 5 years, FIT–fecal DNA testing every 3 years, or flexible sigmoidoscopy every 5 to 10 years as second-tier tests; and capsule colonography every 5 years as a third-tier test. The serum circulating methylated *SEPT9* DNA test is an FDA-approved screening strategy that holds promise because blood tests may result in increased adherence. However, this test's sensitivity for detecting colorectal cancer is only 48%, and the MSTF does not recommend its use.

TABLE 15. Characteristics of Colorectal Cancer Screening Strategies

Screening Strategy	Frequency	Reduction in Mortality Rate	Notes
Stool-based Tests (Cancer Detection)			
gFOBT	Every year	32%	High-sensitivity gFOBT has superior test performance characteristics than older tests Requires dietary restrictions; does not require bowel preparation, anesthesia, or transportation to and from the screening examination
FIT	Every year	Unknown	Improved accuracy compared with gFOBT Does not require bowel preparation, anesthesia, or transportation to and from the screening examination
FIT-DNA	Every 1 to 3 y	Unknown	Higher sensitivity but lower specificity than FIT, resulting in more false-positive results
Direct Visualization Tests (Cancer Prevention)			
Colonoscopy	Every 10 y	68%	Requires full bowel preparation Usually requires sedation and a patient escort ACG/MSTF recommend split-dose preparation[a]
CT colonography	Every 5 y	Unknown	Requires bowel preparation Imaging only (cannot remove polyps or biopsy) Extracolonic findings are common
Flexible sigmoidoscopy	Every 5 y	27%	Limited bowel preparation compared with colonoscopy
Flexible sigmoidoscopy with FIT	Flexible sigmoidoscopy every 10 y with FIT every year	38%	

ACG = American College of Gastroenterology; FIT = fecal immunochemical test; gFOBT = guaiac fecal occult blood test; MSTF = U.S. Multisociety Task Force on Colorectal Cancer.

[a]Split-dose preparation has been shown to increase detection rates for sessile polyps and possibly adenomas. It involves taking half of the preparation the evening before and half of the preparation on the day of colonoscopy, starting 4 to 5 hours before the procedure start and finishing 3 hours before the procedure start.

Adapted from U.S. Preventive Services Task Force. Final recommendation statement: colorectal cancer: screening. June 2017. https://www.uspreventiveservicestaskforce.org/Page/Document/RecommendationStatementFinal/colorectal-cancer-screening2. Accessed June 28, 2018. The Agency for Healthcare Research and Quality and the U.S. Department of Health and Human Services do not endorse derivative or excerpted materials and cannot be held liable for this content.

Cervical Cancer

Cervical cancer incidence and mortality have steadily decreased over the last half-century, largely because of the implementation of widespread screening. The USPSTF, in a 2018 recommendation statement, recommends screening women aged 21 to 65 years every 3 years with cytology (Pap test). In women aged 30 to 65 years who want to lengthen the screening interval, high-risk human papillomavirus (HPV) testing (preferred) or cytology combined with high-risk HPV testing can be performed every 5 years. The USPSTF recommends against screening women younger than 21 years regardless of sexual history because screening has not been shown to reduce cervical cancer incidence or mortality compared with starting screening at age 21 years.

Screening can be discontinued at age 65 years in non-high-risk women with adequate prior screening, commonly defined as three consecutive negative cytology results or two consecutive negative cytology plus HPV test results within the last 10 years, with the most recent test occurring within 5 years. In women older than 65 years with life expectancy of at least 10 years and risk factors for cervical cancer (history of abnormal Pap smears, history of a high-grade precancerous lesion, in utero exposure to diethylstilbestrol, immunocompromise, previous HPV infection), continued screening should be considered.

Women who have never been screened have the highest incidence of and mortality from cervical cancer. The mortality reduction from screening in women who have not been previously screened may be as high as 74%. Women older than 65 years who have never been screened or in whom adequacy of prior screening cannot be confirmed should undergo screening with cytology every 3 years, high-risk HPV testing every 5 years, or combined high-risk HPV testing and cytology every 5 years.

Screening should not be performed in women who have had a hysterectomy with removal of the cervix unless a high-grade precancerous lesion (cervical intraepithelial neoplasia 2 or 3) was present, in which case screening should be continued for at least 20 years after hysterectomy.

Additional Cancer Screening Tests

The USPSTF, Society of Gynecologic Oncology, and the American College of Obstetricians and Gynecologists all recommend against screening for ovarian cancer with serum CA-125 testing or ultrasonography in women at average risk. Women with a family history indicating a hereditary cancer syndrome should be referred to a genetic counselor for consideration of genetic testing (see MKSAP 18 Hematology and Oncology).

According to the USPSTF, evidence is insufficient to determine the balance of benefits and harms of screening for skin cancer with a visual skin examination. However, the USPSTF recommends that persons younger than 24 years who have fair skin receive counseling to minimize exposure to ultraviolet radiation to reduce risk for skin cancer (grade B) and recommends offering selective counseling to adults older than 24 years with fair skin types (grade C).

The USPSTF recommends against screening for pancreatic cancer in asymptomatic adults. Because up to 15% of pancreatic ductal adenocarcinomas are attributable to genetic factors, patients with a family history suggestive of a genetic syndrome associated with pancreatic cancer (*BRCA1/2* mutations, Peutz-Jeghers syndrome, Lynch syndrome) should be referred for genetic counseling and possible genetic testing.

There is insufficient evidence to recommend routine anal cancer screening in average-risk populations, but such screening may be considered in high-risk populations. The Infectious Diseases Society of America suggests screening patients with genital warts, men who have sex with men, and women who have a history of abnormal cervical cytology or participate in receptive anal intercourse.

Lung cancer screening with annual low-dose CT is recommended for persons aged 55 years to 74-80 years (guidelines vary) with a 30-pack-year smoking history, including former smokers who have quit in the last 15 years (see MKSAP 18 Pulmonary and Critical Care Medicine).

The USPSTF recommends against screening for testicular cancer and thyroid cancer in asymptomatic adults. Routine screening for bladder cancer is not recommended by any expert group, including the USPSTF.

KEY POINTS

- The U.S. Preventive Services Task Force supports routine screening for depression, hypertension, obesity, tobacco use, and alcohol misuse in asymptomatic, average-risk adults.
- Lipid screening is indicated in adults aged 40 to 75 years for the purposes of calculating 10-year risk for atherosclerotic cardiovascular disease and guiding initiation of statin therapy for primary prevention.

(Continued)

KEY POINTS (continued)

- Adults aged 40 to 70 years who are overweight or obese should be screened for diabetes mellitus, according to the U.S. Preventive Services Task Force.
- The U.S. Preventive Services Task Force recommends that all persons aged 15 to 65 years receive one-time HIV screening regardless of risk.
- All women aged 50 to 74 years should undergo screening mammography; the recommended screening interval varies by expert group.
- Evidence has not demonstrated that any one recommended screening test for colorectal cancer provides a greater benefit than the others; therefore, the U.S. Preventive Services Task Force supports using the test that is most likely to result in screening completion.

Genetics and Genetic Testing

Taking a Family History

Obtaining a family history is an inexpensive and important risk assessment tool that allows clinicians to identify persons at increased risk for certain conditions. Up to 40% of genetic risk factors that would have otherwise been missed can be detected with a family history. Features that suggest the presence of a genetically inherited condition include earlier age of onset than expected for a common disease; two or more relatives with the same disorder, especially if the disorder is uncommon or known to be caused by a single gene mutation; and the presence of a disease in the less-often-afflicted sex, such as breast cancer in a man.

Agreement on the essential components of a family history is lacking; however, obtaining a complete three-generation family history is a reasonable approach. Although time consuming, documenting the history in the form of a family pedigree provides a helpful pictorial representation of the relationship between family members and the presence of medical conditions (**Figure 3**). Several easy-to-use family history tools are also available. The My Family Health Portrait tool (https://familyhistory.hhs.gov) can be self-administered and updated over time by patients.

Genetic Tests and Testing Strategies

Understanding different types of genetic tests and testing strategies is helpful in ensuring that genetic testing is used effectively (**Table 16**). Prenatal genetic testing is performed during pregnancy to identify conditions in utero, such as Down syndrome. In adults, genetic testing is most commonly performed in persons with a family history suggestive of a genetically inherited condition. Presymptomatic or predictive genetic testing is performed to detect the presence of a genetic mutation before the onset of symptoms. The presence of some genetic mutations, such as the *HD* gene for Huntington disease, will invariably lead to disease development. With other

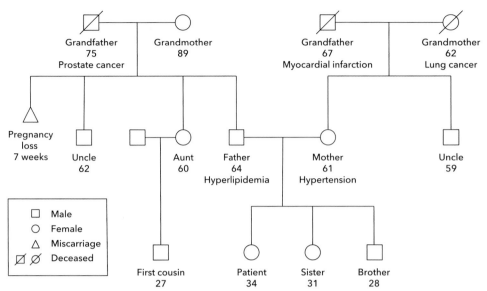

FIGURE 3. Example of a family history.

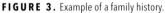

TABLE 16.	Commonly Used Genetic Tests
Type of Testing	**Description**
Cytogenetic testing or karyotyping (Giemsa staining, in situ hybridization, microarray analysis)	Permits analysis of chromosomal structure
	Giemsa staining produces banding pattern, allowing for gross structural analysis
	In situ hybridization and microarray analysis allow for detection of more subtle abnormalities
Direct DNA testing (polymerase chain reaction analysis, Southern blot analysis)	Permits detection of specific genetic mutations
Indirect DNA testing (linkage analysis)	Useful when the genetic location for a condition is known but the genetic mutation is unknown
Biochemical testing	Involves measurement of metabolite levels to assess enzymatic activity
Whole exome sequencing	Useful when there is a clear family history of a genetic disorder based on pedigree but the affected gene is unknown

genetic mutations, such as those involving the breast cancer susceptibility genes *BRCA1* and *BRCA2*, the risk for the disease is significantly increased, but not everyone with the mutation will develop disease. Diagnostic testing refers to genetic testing performed in those with a suspected genetic condition based on clinical features.

All patients for whom genetic testing is being considered should undergo genetic counseling. The basic components of genetic counseling are education on the condition being tested, including the natural history, possible treatments, and preventive measures; the risks and benefits of genetic testing;

alternatives to testing, including the option to forgo testing; and the implications for the patient and family members. Patients should be informed that the Genetic Information Nondiscrimination Act of 2008 protects against discrimination from obtaining employment and health insurance; however, this protection does not extend to discrimination involving other types of insurance, such as disability and life insurance. Clinicians can use a searchable database provided by the American College of Medical Genetics and Genomics (www. acmg.net/GIS) to locate a genetic counselor in their area.

Pharmacogenetics

Pharmacogenetics is the study of how genetic differences lead to varying drug responses. Genetic testing for several common enzymes that affect drug metabolism, such as CYP2C19 and CYP2D6, are increasingly available. The CYP2C19 enzyme is involved in metabolizing the antiplatelet agent clopidogrel to its active form. Patients who have one or two copies of the reduced-function *CYP2C19* gene have an attenuated antiplatelet effect when taking clopidogrel, which may be associated with an increased risk for cardiovascular events. The CYP2D6 enzyme is responsible for converting codeine to its active metabolite, morphine. The presence of *CYP2D6* polymorphisms leads to variation in enzyme activity between individuals. Patients with high CYP2D6 activity may be subject to serious side effects of codeine, including respiratory depression and death, whereas patients with low CYP2D6 activity are unlikely to achieve adequate analgesia with codeine. The role of pharmacogenetic testing is unclear, and routine testing is not widespread at present.

Direct-to-Consumer Genetic Testing

Direct-to-consumer (DTC) genomic testing is a commercial service that allows patients to obtain genetic information for a low cost. The FDA has approved DTC genetic testing for 10 disorders, including Parkinson disease and hemochromatosis, and physicians may be asked to provide guidance to persons who have undergone testing. DTC genomic testing typically estimates the risk for many common medical conditions by genotyping polymorphic nucleotides. Single-nucleotide polymorphisms (SNPs) that are disproportionately found in affected individuals are identified, and odds ratios for each SNP are determined. The SNPs are usually common but have low penetrance (that is, most people with an SNP do not develop disease). Individually, SNPs contribute very little to overall disease risk; most SNPs have an odds ratio of less than 1.5. As an example, if a condition has a general population prevalence of 8%, possessing an associated SNP with an odds ratio of 1.3 would increase one's risk for the condition to approximately 10%. Advocates of these services argue that they promote patient autonomy because patients can directly access information on genetic predispositions without physician referral. Critics counter that DTC testing is not usually accompanied by pre- or posttest genetic counseling, potentially leading to patient harms.

KEY POINTS

- Obtaining a three-generation family history is an inexpensive and important risk assessment tool that allows clinicians to identify persons at increased risk for certain conditions.

- Presymptomatic or predictive genetic testing is performed to detect the presence of a genetic mutation before the onset of symptoms, such as identification of the breast cancer susceptibility genes *BRCA1/2*; all patients for whom genetic testing is being considered should undergo genetic counseling.

- **HVC** • Direct-to-consumer genomic testing estimates the risk for many common medical conditions by genotyping polymorphic nucleotides; however, the identified single-nucleotide polymorphisms contribute very little to overall disease risk.

Immunization

Immunization is a safe and cost-effective preventive health measure that is often underused in adult patients. In the United States, annual immunization recommendations are issued by the Advisory Committee on Immunization Practices (ACIP). ACIP recommendations can be accessed at https://www.cdc.gov/vaccines/acip.

It is important to adhere to recommended vaccine schedules as closely as possible. Administering doses at longer-than-recommended intervals does not appear to reduce immunologic response; however, doses should not be given at shorter-than-recommended intervals in order to allow for a complete immunologic response. If a vaccination series is interrupted, the series can be resumed at the point of interruption. Whenever possible, multiple vaccines should be given simultaneously to improve vaccination rates.

Vaccines can be safely administered to patients with mild acute febrile illness, during illness convalescence, and to patients who have previously developed low- or moderate-grade fever or local reactions with vaccination. Vaccines should be avoided if there is a history of anaphylaxis to the vaccine or the vaccine components. Contraindications to live vaccines are listed in **Table 17**.

Vaccinations Recommended for All Adults
Influenza
Influenza revaccination is necessary each year, owing to ongoing genetic changes in the influenza virus (antigenic drift). Annual vaccination is recommended for all individuals aged 6 months and older. The influenza vaccine should be administered as soon as it becomes available, preferably by October. The ACIP makes no preferential recommendation for one formulation over another, although use of the quadrivalent live attenuated influenza vaccine (LAIV4) was not recommended for the 2016 to 2018 influenza seasons as a result of poor efficacy against the H1N1 strain. A reformulated LAIV has received approval and a weak recommendation by the ACIP for the 2018 to 2019 influenza season. A high-dose, trivalent, inactivated formulation (IIV3-HD) is available for patients aged 65 years and older and is 24% more effective in preventing laboratory-confirmed influenza compared with its standard-dose counterpart.

Persons with a history of egg allergy of any severity can receive any influenza vaccine formulation; however, in persons who have had an egg-related reaction that caused symptoms other than hives, such as angioedema or respiratory distress, the vaccine should be administered by a provider trained in recognizing and managing severe allergic reactions.

Tetanus, Diphtheria, and Pertussis
Primary vaccination against tetanus, diphtheria, and acellular pertussis consists of a five-dose vaccine series administered during childhood. Persons aged 11 to 18 years who have completed the primary series should receive a single dose of the tetanus toxoid, reduced diphtheria toxoid, and acellular pertussis (Tdap) vaccine. Adults aged 19 years and older should receive a tetanus and diphtheria toxoids (Td) booster every

TABLE 17. Contraindications to Administration of Live Vaccines
Pregnancy or probable pregnancy within 4 weeks
HIV with CD4 count ≤200/µL or CD4% ≤15% of total lymphocytes
Immunosuppressant therapy, including high-dose glucocorticoids (≥20 mg/d of prednisone or equivalent for ≥2 wk)
Leukemia, lymphoma, or other bone marrow and lymphatic system malignancies
Cellular immunodeficiency
Solid organ transplant recipient
Recent hematopoietic stem cell transplantation

10 years. In adults who did not receive Tdap during adolescence, one of the 10-year Td booster doses should be replaced with a dose of the Tdap vaccine.

Unvaccinated adults should receive a three-dose series consisting of Td doses and at least one Tdap dose. Adults who have received fewer than three doses of the primary series should complete the series with the Td or Tdap (if not previously administered) vaccine.

Pregnant women should receive one dose of the Tdap vaccine between 27 weeks' and 36 weeks' gestation with every pregnancy, regardless of when the Td or Tdap vaccine was last administered.

Vaccinations Recommended for Some Adults

Varicella and Herpes Zoster

All immunocompetent adults without evidence of varicella immunity should receive two varicella vaccine doses. Evidence of varicella immunity includes laboratory-confirmed disease or immunity, diagnosis or verification of varicella or zoster by a provider, or documentation of age-appropriate varicella vaccination. U.S. birth before 1980 is also considered to be evidence of immunity, except in pregnant women and immunocompromised persons (who are at risk for severe disease) and health care workers (who are at risk for repeated varicella exposure and spreading the disease to those at high risk for severe disease). These patient groups must meet the other criteria for varicella immunity.

All adults aged 50 years and older, including those with a previous episode of zoster, should receive the recombinant (inactivated) herpes zoster vaccine to reduce the incidence of zoster and postherpetic neuralgia. The recombinant vaccine has demonstrated 97% efficacy in persons aged 50 to 69 years and 91% efficacy in those aged 70 years and older. It is recommended in preference to the live attenuated zoster vaccine, and adults who have been previously vaccinated with the live attenuated zoster vaccine should be revaccinated with the recombinant zoster vaccine after at least 8 weeks. The recombinant vaccine is administered intramuscularly in two doses, with an interval of 2 to 6 months between doses. The safety of the vaccine in pregnant women and patients with significant immunosuppression has not been determined. Healthy adults aged 60 years or older may receive either the recombinant vaccine (preferred) or the live attenuated vaccine. The live attenuated vaccine is administered subcutaneously in one dose.

Pneumococcal Disease

Pneumococcal vaccination is recommended in all adults aged 65 years and older and adults aged 19 to 64 years with certain high-risk conditions (**Table 18**). Two pneumococcal vaccines are available: the 13-valent conjugate vaccine (PCV13) and the 23-valent polysaccharide vaccine (PPSV23). In a randomized controlled trial involving more than 80,000 persons aged 65 years and older, the efficacy of PCV13 was 75% against vaccine-type invasive disease and 46% against vaccine-type pneumonia. PPSV23 is 60% to 70% effective in preventing vaccine-type invasive disease, although its effect on noninvasive disease is unclear.

All adults aged 65 years and older who have not previously been vaccinated should receive PCV13, followed by a dose of PPSV23 1 year later. In immunocompetent adults aged 65 years and older who have already received a dose of PPSV23, PCV13 should be administered no sooner than 1 year later. In adults aged 19 to 64 years with high-risk conditions who require vaccination with both PCV13 and PPSV23 but who have not yet received either vaccine, a single dose of PCV13 should be given first, followed by a single dose of PPSV23 given at least 8 weeks later. Adults aged 19 to 64 years with high-risk conditions who require vaccination with both PCV13 and PPSV23 and who have already received PPSV23 should be administered a single dose of PCV13 no sooner than 1 year after receiving the most recent PPSV23. A second dose of PPSV23 should also be administered 5 years after the first PPSV23 dose in adults aged 19 to 64 years with certain immunocompromising conditions (see Table 18).

Human Papillomavirus

HPV vaccination prevents persistent HPV infection, which can lead to cervical, anogenital, and nasopharyngeal cancers. Bivalent, quadrivalent, and nine-valent HPV vaccines are approved for use in females; quadrivalent and nine-valent vaccines are approved for use in males. Females should be administered the vaccine series at age 11 or 12 years or between the ages of 13 and 26 years if not given previously. In males, the series should be administered at age 11 or 12 years, between the ages of 13 and 21 years if not previously administered, or through age 26 years for immunocompromised men (including those with HIV infection) and men who have sex with men. If administered before the age of 15 years, a two-dose series is recommended, whereas a three-dose series is recommended in older individuals. Vaccination is not recommended during pregnancy, although no harmful effects have been noted when inadvertently given to pregnant women.

Measles, Mumps, and Rubella

All U.S. adults born before 1957 are considered to be immune to measles and mumps. Adults born in 1957 or later without documented evidence of receiving one or more doses of the measles, mumps, and rubella (MMR) vaccine or laboratory-confirmed immunity against all three diseases should receive at least one MMR dose. A second MMR dose should be administered to postsecondary students, health care workers, and international travelers. For persons who have been previously vaccinated with two doses of a mumps virus-containing vaccine but are at increased risk because of an outbreak, the ACIP recommends administering a third dose of mumps virus-containing vaccine to improve protection.

In women of childbearing age, it is necessary to determine rubella immunity. Nonpregnant women who lack immunity should be vaccinated. Pregnant women who lack

TABLE 18. Pneumococcal Vaccination Recommendations for Adults Aged 19 Years and Older With Underlying Medical Conditions

Risk Group	Underlying Medical Condition	PCV13 Recommended	PPSV23 Recommended	PPSV23 Revaccination at 5 Years After First Dose
Immunocompetent persons	Chronic heart disease[a]		X	
	Chronic lung disease[b]		X	
	Diabetes mellitus		X	
	CSF leaks	X	X	
	Cochlear implants	X	X	
	Alcoholism		X	
	Chronic liver disease		X	
	Cigarette smoking		X	
Persons with functional or anatomic asplenia	Sickle cell disease/other hemoglobinopathies	X	X	X
	Congenital or acquired asplenia	X	X	X
Immunocompromised persons	Congenital or acquired immunodeficiencies[c]	X	X	X
	HIV infection	X	X	X
	Chronic kidney failure	X	X	X
	Nephrotic syndrome	X	X	X
	Leukemia	X	X	X
	Lymphoma	X	X	X
	Hodgkin lymphoma	X	X	X
	Generalized malignancy	X	X	X
	Iatrogenic immunosuppression[d]	X	X	X
	Solid-organ transplant	X	X	X
	Multiple myeloma	X	X	X

CSF = cerebrospinal fluid; PCV13 = 13-valent pneumococcal conjugate vaccine; PPSV23 = 23-valent pneumococcal polysaccharide vaccine.

[a]Including heart failure and cardiomyopathies.

[b]Including COPD, emphysema, and asthma.

[c]Including B- (humoral) or T-lymphocyte deficiency, complement deficiencies (particularly C1, C2, C3, and C4 deficiencies), and phagocytic disorders (excluding chronic granulomatous disease).

[d]Diseases requiring treatment with immunosuppressive drugs, including long-term systemic glucocorticoids and radiation therapy.

Adapted from Centers for Disease Control and Prevention (CDC). Use of 13-valent pneumococcal conjugate vaccine and 23-valent pneumococcal polysaccharide vaccine for adults with immunocompromising conditions: recommendations of the Advisory Committee on Immunization Practices (ACIP). MMWR Morb Mortal Wkly Rep. 2012 Oct 12;61(40):816-9. [PMID: 23051612]

immunity should be vaccinated at the time of delivery before leaving the hospital or at the time of pregnancy termination.

The MMR vaccine is a live virus vaccine and should not be administered to immunocompromised individuals.

Meningococcal Disease
Meningococcal vaccines used in the adult population include the quadrivalent meningococcal conjugate vaccine (MenACWY), which protects against serogroups A, C, W135, and Y, and the MenB vaccine, which protects against serogroup B disease. The quadrivalent conjugate vaccine is used in most patients, whereas the MenB vaccine is reserved for specific high-risk situations.

Indications for meningococcal vaccination in adults are summarized in **Table 19**.

Hepatitis A
Vaccination against hepatitis A is recommended for all persons who desire vaccination and for persons who are at increased risk for infection or complications of infection. Persons at increased risk include those who work in or travel to endemic areas, men who have sex with men, individuals with chronic liver disease, illicit drug users, persons with clotting disorders, persons who conduct hepatitis A–related research, and household or close contacts of children adopted from endemic areas.

TABLE 19. Indications for Meningococcal Vaccination in Adults	
Vaccine	**Indicated Populations**
Quadrivalent meningococcal conjugate vaccine (MenACWY)	
Single dose[a]	First-year college students living in a dormitory
	Travelers to endemic areas
	Microbiologists exposed to *Neisseria meningitidis*
	Military recruits
	Adults at increased risk because of serogroup A, C, W, or Y meningococcal outbreak
Two-dose primary series[b]	Adults with anatomic or functional asplenia
	Adults with persistent complement component deficiencies (C5-C9, factor H, factor D, properdin, or patients taking eculizumab)
	Adults with HIV infection
Serogroup B meningococcal vaccine (MenB)[c,d]	Adults with persistent complement component deficiencies (C5-C9, factor H, factor D, properdin, or patients taking eculizumab)
	Adults with functional or anatomic asplenia
	Microbiologists exposed to *Neisseria meningitidis*
	Adults at increased risk because of serogroup B meningococcal outbreak
	May be administered to patients aged 16-23 years for short-term protection, preferably between age 16 and 18 years

[a]A single dose should be administered unless the patient has been vaccinated with MenACWY within the past 5 years. If exposure is ongoing, revaccination is indicated every 5 years.

[b]Doses should be administered 8-12 weeks apart, followed by a booster dose every 5 years.

[c]MenB vaccine is approved for use in persons aged ≥10 years.

[d]Persons who are considered to be at increased risk for infection should be given three separate doses at 0, 1-2, and 6 months. If the second dose is administered at >6 months, a third dose is not necessary.

Hepatitis B

Hepatitis B vaccination is recommended for any nonimmune adult who desires vaccination or who is considered to be at high risk for infection (**Table 20**). The typical hepatitis B vaccination series is a three-dose series, with doses administered at 0, 1, and 6 months. In adults aged 40 years and younger, 30% to 55% of patients will mount a protective antibody response after being administered one dose, 75% after the second dose, and more than 90% after the third dose. Older adults and patients undergoing hemodialysis have lower protective antibody response rates. A newer vaccine with a novel adjuvant, which was released in 2017 and endorsed by the ACIP in 2018, requires only two doses over a 1-month period and appears to be more immunogenic than previous vaccines.

Checking serum antibodies is not typically recommended after routine vaccination but is indicated in persons in whom subsequent clinical management is dependent upon knowledge of serologic response (chronic hemodialysis patients, persons with HIV, health care and public safety workers, and needle-sharing partners of persons with positive hepatitis B surface antigen).

Vaccinations Recommended for Specific Populations

Health care workers (HCWs) are at increased risk for acquiring and transmitting hepatitis B, influenza, measles, mumps,

TABLE 20. Populations With an Indication for Hepatitis B Vaccination
Any nonimmune adult desiring vaccination
Sexually active persons who are not in a monogamous relationship (any person with more than one sexual partner within the past 6 months)
Sexual partners of persons who are HBsAg positive
Persons seeking evaluation or treatment for sexually transmitted infection
Men who have sex with men
Household contacts of persons who are HBsAg positive
Residents and staff members of institutions for persons who are developmentally disabled
Current or recent injection drug users
Health care and public safety workers with anticipated risk for exposure
Persons with end-stage kidney disease, including those receiving hemodialysis and peritoneal dialysis
International travelers to regions with intermediate or high levels of endemic hepatitis B infection
Persons with chronic liver disease
Persons with HIV infection

HBsAg = hepatitis B surface antigen.

ella viruses. All HCWs, regardless
eive the influenza vaccine annu-
ty should be vaccinated against
ps, and rubella; and varicella.
have not previously received the
one dose, irrespective of when
ine.

or functional asplenia are at
from encapsulated organisms,
zae type B, meningococcus, and
appropriately vaccinated.

itions for international travelers
ation. Trip-specific recommen-
accessed at https://wwwnc.cdc.
ion on vaccination in travelers,
ise, Travel Medicine.

ion is recommended for all
and older.

ceive one dose of the tetanus
toxoid, and acellular pertus-
ich pregnancy between
_station.

HVC
- All adults aged 50 years and older should receive the recombinant (inactivated) herpes zoster vaccine, regardless of previous immunization or clinical infection, to reduce the incidence of zoster and postherpetic neuralgia.

- Pneumococcal vaccination is recommended in all adults aged 65 years and older and adults aged 19 to 64 years with certain high-risk conditions.

- Patients with anatomic or functional asplenia should be vaccinated against *Haemophilus influenzae* type B, meningococcal, and pneumococcal diseases.

Aspirin as Primary Prevention

Aspirin therapy for primary prevention is a continually debated and constantly evolving topic. The decision to initiate low-dose aspirin for primary prevention of ASCVD and colorectal cancer is predominantly based on weighing the benefits of prevention with the harms of increased bleeding. Factors that increase bleeding risk include concurrent anticoagulant or NSAID use, history of gastrointestinal ulcer, upper gastrointestinal pain, uncontrolled hypertension, male sex, and increasing age. Other factors, such as patient preferences on taking aspirin, may also shift the balance.

Aspirin has been found to reduce nonfatal myocardial infarction (relative risk [RR], 0.78; 95% CI, 0.71-0.87) but not nonfatal stroke, cardiovascular mortality, or all-cause mortality. The benefits of ASCVD prevention are apparent within the first 5 years of therapy and continue for as long as aspirin is taken. The evidence for cancer prevention is stronger, with a 34% to 40% reduction in colorectal cancer mortality with at least 5 to 10 years of aspirin therapy. The benefit is not apparent until 10 to 20 years after initiation of aspirin; no mortality benefit was observed in the first 10 years of follow-up. Therefore, adults older than 60 years are less likely to experience these benefits.

The USPSTF recommends low-dose aspirin for the primary prevention of ASCVD and colorectal cancer in adults aged 50 to 59 years with a 10-year ASCVD risk of 10% or higher who do not have an increased risk for bleeding, have a life expectancy of at least 10 years, and are willing to take low-dose aspirin daily for at least 10 years (grade B). ASCVD risk can be calculated by using the American College of Cardiology/American Heart Association risk calculator based on the Pooled Cohort Equations, available at http://tools.acc.org/ASCVD-Risk-Estimator/. In those aged 60 to 69 years with a 10-year ASCVD risk of 10% or higher, the benefits of aspirin use for primary prevention are smaller but still outweigh the risk for bleeding; the decision to initiate low-dose aspirin in this population should be individualized (grade C). Owing to limited evidence, the USPSTF does not make a recommendation on aspirin use for primary prevention in persons younger than 50 years and older than 70 years (I statement).

In contrast to the USPSTF, the American Diabetes Association and American Heart Association suggest low-dose aspirin for primary prevention in adults with diabetes with a 10-year ASCVD risk greater than 10% who are not at increased risk for bleeding. Low-dose aspirin therapy may be considered in patients with diabetes and intermediate risk for ASCVD (10-year risk, 5%-10%). Notably, the European Society of Cardiology does not recommend any antiplatelet therapy for individuals without ASCVD because of the increased risk for bleeding and lack of convincing data on cardiovascular mortality benefit.

For patients in whom the balance of benefits and harms is unclear, the Aspirin Guide, a clinical decision making support tool available online (www.aspiringuide.com) and as a mobile application, may offer guidance. The Aspirin Guide uses internal algorithms to calculate the patient's ASCVD risk and bleeding risk as well as the NNT with aspirin to prevent one ASCVD event and the number needed to harm (NNH) to cause one excess bleeding event due to aspirin. The tool has not yet been validated in clinical trials and does not include NNT for cancer prevention. In general, the Aspirin Guide advises initiating low-dose aspirin if the NNT is less than the NNH; however, clinical judgment is warranted.

KEY POINT

- The U.S. Preventive Services Task Force recommends aspirin for primary prevention of atherosclerotic cardiovascular disease (ASCVD) and colorectal cancer in adults aged 50 to 59 years with a 10-year ASCVD risk of 10% or greater who do not have an increased risk for bleeding, have a life expectancy of at least 10 years, and are willing to take low-dose aspirin daily for at least 10 years.

Healthy Lifestyle Counseling

Healthy lifestyle counseling is directed at the leading preventable causes of death. More than one third of preventable deaths are attributable to tobacco use and obesity and the resulting increased risks for cancer and cardiovascular disease. Other preventable causes of death include alcohol use, infectious diseases, toxins, accidents, deaths from firearms, and drug use.

Tobacco cessation is a high priority health intervention from a health and cost-effectiveness standpoint. Smokers should be offered pharmacologic therapy and behavioral interventions (see Mental and Behavioral Health).

All overweight and obese patients should undergo counseling on the benefits of a healthy weight, regular exercise, and a healthy diet (see Behavioral Counseling).

Injury prevention, including seat belt use, use of safety helmets for motorcycles and bicycles, and home safety measures (such as weapons safety), should be emphasized. Patients should be counseled to use smoke alarms in the home and to set water heaters to lower than 49 °C (120 °F). The "5 Ls" may be used for firearm safety counseling; they involve asking the following questions regarding a firearm in the home:

- Is it Locked?
- Is it Loaded?
- Are there Little children present?
- Anyone feeling Low in the house?
- Is the operator Learned about firearm safety?

Sleep and stress reduction are also components of a healthy lifestyle. The American Heart Association and the American Academy of Sleep Medicine recommend that adults obtain at least 7 hours of sleep per night for optimal health. Stress reduction, development of strong social ties, and community involvement are also associated with better health outcomes.

Even small changes at the population level, such as improving social determinants of health, can create large preventive benefits. Healthy People 2020 is a CDC initiative with the goal of creating social and physical environments that promote good health. Using strategies from behavioral economics, such as making healthy choices the default option or nudging (gently steering people in a certain direction), may help improve health outcomes. Pricing and taxation strategies and food stamp programs can help promote the purchase of fruits and vegetables and inhibit the purchase of unhealthy processed foods. Making neighborhoods and cities safer and improving bicycle lanes, walking paths, and stairs may encourage physical activity and reduce inequalities in health.

Climate change could cause numerous deleterious effects on human health, including higher rates of respiratory and heat-related illness, increased prevalence of vector-borne (malaria, chikungunya, dengue fever) and waterborne (cholera) diseases, food and water insecurity, and malnutrition. The ACP advises that physicians become educated about climate change, its effect on human health, and how to respond to future challenges.

Behavioral Counseling

For adults who are overweight or obese and have additional risk factors for cardiovascular disease (hypertension, dyslipidemia, impaired fasting glucose/diabetes), the USPSTF recommends offering or referral to intensive behavioral counseling interventions to promote a healthful diet and physical activity (grade B). Because the benefit of behavioral counseling is small in adults who do not meet these criteria, the USPSTF recommends an individualized approach to offering or referring these patients to behavioral counseling to promote a healthy lifestyle (grade C). Strategies such as motivational interviewing and setting specific and attainable goals can help facilitate lifestyle changes. Using a multidisciplinary team of health care professionals (dieticians, nurses, and psychologists) can be helpful when available.

Behavioral counseling does not need to be complex or time consuming. An analysis of more than 5000 patients who participated in the National Health and Nutritional Examination Survey found that patients who were informed that they were overweight by their physicians were more likely to report significant weight loss, although it has been shown that overweight and obesity are commonly unmentioned and undiagnosed. Advising patients to maintain a healthy weight and adopt healthy practices, including eliminating sugar-containing beverages, implementing a reduced-calorie diet, avoiding processed foods, and practicing mindful eating can be beneficial. Providers may also help patients by modeling healthy behaviors; evidence shows that doctors who improve their health habits may be better able to counsel their patients regarding preventive and healthful behaviors.

Diet and Physical Activity

Adults who adhere to a healthful diet and engage in regular physical activity have lower cardiovascular mortality and may have improved cognitive function and decreased disability. Dietary guidelines from the U.S. Department of Health and Human Services recommend following a healthy eating pattern that consists of vegetables, whole fruits, whole grains, low-fat dairy, protein (poultry, fish, legumes), and oils (including nuts), while limiting consumption of added sugars, saturated and *trans* fats, and sodium. Adults of legal drinking age should be advised to limit consumption of alcohol to no more than one drink per day for women and two drinks per day for men.

Adults should perform at least 150 minutes of moderate-intensity physical activity per week or 75 minutes of vigorous-intensity physical activity per week. For increased benefit, 300 minutes of moderate-intensity activity or 150 minutes of vigorous-intensity activity is recommended. Muscle-strengthening activities (resistance training and weight lifting) are also beneficial, and adults should perform moderate- or high-intensity muscle-strengthening activities that involve all major muscle groups 2 or more days per week. It is important to note that any physical activity is better than no activity. Physical activity need not be formal exercise; incorporating natural movement into the day offers some health benefits.

KEY POINTS

- For adults who are overweight or obese and have additional risk factors for cardiovascular disease, the U.S. Preventive Services Task Force recommends offering or referral to intensive behavioral counseling interventions to promote healthful diet and physical activity.
- Dietary guidelines from the U.S. Department of Health and Human Services recommend following a healthy eating pattern that consists of vegetables, whole fruits, whole grains, low-fat dairy, protein, and oils, while limiting consumption of added sugars, saturated and *trans* fats, and sodium.

Supplements and Herbal Therapies

Dietary supplements, including vitamins, minerals, botanicals, herbals, metabolites, and amino acids, are categorized as foods by the FDA and are therefore not subject to the same regulations as over-the-counter and prescription drugs. Manufacturers are not required to demonstrate efficacy or safety unless the supplement includes ingredients that were introduced after 1994. Manufacturers are also not allowed to make specific medical claims; however, the product's purported effect on body structure or function may be described.

Patients take dietary supplements for various reasons, such as to prevent illness, enhance health, and correct perceived deficiencies. In the United States, approximately 50% of adults report using vitamins or dietary supplements, with total consumer spending of more than $20 billion each year.

Despite their prevalent use, the USPSTF does not recommend multivitamins or herbal supplements for the prevention of cardiovascular disease or cancer. The USPSTF also concludes that there is insufficient evidence for use of vitamin D and calcium to prevent fractures. Evidence has shown that supplementation with vitamin D and calcium together increases the incidence of kidney stones. Multivitamins should not be used in the absence of a specific indication and are not effective in compensating for a poor diet. Smokers should avoid β-carotene altogether, as evidence has linked β-carotene with increased risk for lung cancer.

There are several populations for which vitamin or supplement use is strongly recommended. Women of childbearing age are advised to take 0.4 to 0.8 mg (400 to 800 μg) of folic acid daily to prevent fetal neural tube defects. Vegans and older adults may consider vitamin B_{12} supplementation to address dietary deficiency.

In addition to questionable efficacy, supplement use is associated with risk for both direct and indirect harms. Direct harms include side effects, interactions with other drugs, and harms related to inclusion of unadvertised additives, compounds, or

toxins. Many supplements, such as St. John's wort, affect the cytochrome P450 system, which may affect warfarin and antidepressant metabolism. *Ginkgo biloba*, ginseng, garlic, vitamin E, and fish oil may interact with anticoagulant or antiplatelet medications, potentially causing increased risk for bleeding or inadequate anticoagulation. Harms may also occur indirectly when herbal supplement use replaces or delays standard treatments.

Despite these risks, many patients strongly believe in supplement use, and the role of the physician is to inform these patients of harmful supplements and suggest safer alternatives (**Table 21**). The National Institute of Health's MedlinePlus directory of herbs and supplements (https://medlineplus.gov/druginfo/herb_All.html) and Nutrition.gov (https://www.nutrition.gov/dietary-supplements) are useful resources.

KEY POINTS

- Manufacturers of dietary supplements are not required to demonstrate efficacy or safety unless the supplement includes ingredients that were introduced after 1994.
- The U.S. Preventive Services Task Force does not recommend multivitamins or herbal supplements for the prevention of cardiovascular disease or cancer. **HVC**

Patient Safety and Quality Improvement

Introduction

Patient safety is defined by the World Health Organization as the prevention of errors and adverse events related to medical care. Although it is a necessary component of high-quality health care, integrating safety into medical practice is a complex process that requires involvement and action at both the clinician and systems levels. Importantly, health care systems must be built on a culture of safety and structured to prevent errors, empower individuals to promote safety, and recognize and respond to errors that occur.

Quality in health care refers to the extent to which the clinician or organization meets or exceeds the needs and expectations of patients. Quality improvement involves the systematic and continuous implementation of changes that measurably improve patient care. Because quality improvement is based on the understanding that it is easier to improve that which can be measured, quality improvement usually entails ongoing monitoring and assessment.

Patient Safety and Quality Issues at the Clinician Level

Common patient safety and quality issues that occur at the clinician level include diagnostic errors, medication errors, and errors occurring during transitions of care.

TABLE 21.	Common Herbal Supplements			
Name	**Common Uses**	**Effectiveness**	**Adverse Effects**	**Important Drug Interactions**
Black cohosh	Treatment of menopausal hot flashes	Likely effective, low-quality evidence	Possible estrogenic effect on breast Avoid in women with estrogen receptor–positive breast cancer Reports of hepatotoxicity	
Cranberry	Prevention of urinary tract infections	Likely ineffective, low-quality evidence	Increased glucose intake with juice, GI upset	
Echinacea	Prevention of common colds	Small effect	GI upset, nausea, allergic reactions	
	Treatment of common colds	Not effective		
Evening primrose oil	Treatment of breast pain	Mixed data on effectiveness	GI upset, headache May increase risk for pregnancy complications	May increase bleeding if used with warfarin
	Treatment of eczema	Not effective		
	Treatment of diabetic neuropathy	Possibly effective		
Garlic	Treatment of high cholesterol	Not effective	Increased bleeding risk, breath and body odor, heartburn	May decrease effectiveness of isoniazid and saquinavir May increase bleeding if used with warfarin, likely due to antiplatelet effect
	Treatment of hypertension	Possibly effective, weak evidence		
Ginger	Treatment of nausea	Likely effective for pregnancy-related and chemotherapy-related nausea	Increased bleeding	May increase risk for bleeding when used with anticoagulants
	Treatment of inflammation	Possibly effective		
Ginkgo biloba	Treatment and prevention of cognitive decline	Not effective	Headache, GI upset, allergic skin reactions, increased risk for bleeding	May increase risk for bleeding when used with anticoagulants and NSAIDs; potentiates MAOIs
	Treatment of claudication	Not effective		
Kava	Treatment of anxiety	Likely effective	Hepatotoxicity Use with caution in patients with liver disease or at risk for liver disease	
Milk thistle	Reduction in liver inflammation	Not effective	Nausea, indigestion, diarrhea	May interact with medications metabolized by CYP2C9
Red yeast rice (contains monacolin K, identical active ingredient to lovastatin)	Treatment of hyperlipidemia	Likely effective; risks likely outweigh benefits	Myalgia, liver function abnormalities Some may contain citrinin (a harmful contaminant), which can cause kidney failure	May interact with medications metabolized by CYP3A4 enzymes
Saw palmetto	Treatment of benign prostatic hyperplasia	Likely not effective	Headache, nausea, dizziness Contraindicated in pregnancy and lactation	
Soy (isoflavones)	Treatment of menopausal symptoms	Likely effective, low-quality evidence	GI upset, allergic reaction Avoid high doses in patients with breast cancer	

(Continued on the next page)

TABLE 21.	Common Herbal Supplements *(Continued)*			
Name	**Common Uses**	**Effectiveness**	**Adverse Effects**	**Important Drug Interactions**
St. John's wort	Treatment of depression	Mixed data on effectiveness	GI upset, fatigue, headache, dizziness	Inducer of CYP3A4 and CYP2C9 enzymes Many interactions Do not use with antidepressants
Valerian	Treatment of anxiety Treatment of sleep disorders, insomnia	Not effective Inconclusive	Tremor, headache, sedation, hepatotoxicity	

CYP2C9 = cytochrome P-450 2C9; CYP3A4 = cytochrome P-450 3A4; GI = gastrointestinal; MAOIs = monoamine oxidase inhibitors.

Diagnostic Errors

A diagnostic error occurs when a patient is not provided with a timely and correct diagnosis or the diagnosis is not communicated to the patient. More specifically, a diagnostic error is present when there was a missed opportunity to make the correct diagnosis in a timely manner. The rate of diagnostic error is approximately 10%, and most patients will be subject to a diagnostic error at some point in their lifetime. Diagnostic errors are also the leading cause of malpractice claims against internists.

Diagnostic errors are usually multifactorial in etiology, with flawed cognitive processes on the part of the clinician and issues at the systems level contributing to most errors. Examples of cognitive errors include premature closure, diagnostic momentum, confirmation bias, and faulty knowledge or knowledge application. Premature closure involves accepting a diagnosis and discontinuing the diagnostic process before the data necessary to establish the diagnosis have been obtained. Diagnostic momentum is a similar phenomenon in which a diagnosis is suggested early in the diagnostic process, and the diagnostic evaluation continues to move toward this diagnosis even if the data do not support it. Confirmation bias, the predisposition to seek evidence to confirm a suspected diagnosis without looking for evidence that disproves it, is a common feature of premature closure and diagnostic momentum. Faulty application of knowledge occurs when the clinician does not possess the underlying knowledge necessary to make the diagnosis or does not apply the knowledge properly.

Systems factors common to diagnostic error include poor communication, lack of test availability, and productivity pressures. Poor communication of crucial laboratory and imaging results (for example, the incidental finding of a pulmonary nodule) may result in delayed diagnosis and patient harm. Similarly, lack of test availability (such as advanced imaging in resource-poor environments) may result in delayed diagnoses. Productivity pressures and their effect on clinician time with patients may also contribute to diagnostic errors. **Table 22** provides techniques for avoiding some common diagnostic errors.

Medication Errors

Medication errors can occur from the time of prescription to the time of administration and may or may not result in patient harm. Medication errors are often caused by prescribing faults (inappropriate prescribing, underprescribing, or overprescribing) or prescription errors (errors in drug dose, route of administration, frequency of use, or duration of therapy; duplicative orders; prescription of drugs that interact; or prescription to the incorrect patient). In contrast, an adverse drug event is harm experienced by a patient as a result of exposure to a medication. Adverse drug events, which account for 100,000 hospitalizations in the United States each year, may be secondary to an accepted risk of a medication or may be the result of a medication error.

There are several known risk factors for medication errors. Polypharmacy, advanced patient age, and impaired kidney or liver function are patient-specific factors that increase the risk for medication errors. Clinician-specific risk factors include illegible handwriting and use of nonstandard abbreviations. Errors are also more likely to occur with the use of specific drugs, including those with look-alike or sound-alike names.

Measures to reduce medication errors include computerized physician order entry (CPOE) systems, medication reconciliation, improved labeling for medications with similar names, and barcode-assisted medication administration. The Institute for Healthcare Improvement (www.ihi.org) and the Institute for Safe Medication Practices (www.ismp.org/tools) have issued tools and resources to reduce harms related to medications. In addition, the Agency for Healthcare Research and Quality (AHRQ) has developed several strategies to prevent adverse drug events (**Table 23**).

Transitions of Care

Patient transitions between inpatient and outpatient settings, institutions, or hospital units present unique challenges to patient safety. A medication error occurs in almost 50% of patients at the time of hospital admission and is the most common form of postdischarge adverse event. The risk for diagnostic error at the time of hospital discharge is similarly high, as almost 40% of patients have test results pending or require

TABLE 22. Twelve Tips for Avoiding Diagnostic Errors

Technique	Comments
1. Understand heuristics[a]	Availability heuristic: Diagnosing based on what is most easily available in the physician's memory (e.g., because of a patient recently seen) rather than what is most probable
	Anchoring heuristic: Settling on a diagnosis early in the diagnostic process despite data that refute the diagnosis or support another diagnosis (premature closure)
	Representativeness heuristic: Application of pattern recognition (a patient's presentation fits a "typical" case; therefore, it must be that case)
2. Use "diagnostic timeouts"	Taking time to periodically review a case based on data but without assuming that the diagnosis is that which was previously reached
3. Practice "worst-case scenario medicine"	Consider the most life-threatening diagnoses first: • Lessens chance of missing these diagnoses • Does not mandate testing for them
4. Use systematic approach to common problems	For example, anatomic approach to abdominal pain beginning from exterior to interior
5. Ask why	For example, when a patient presents with diabetic ketoacidosis or a COPD exacerbation, ask what prompted this acute exacerbation of a chronic condition
6. Use the clinical examination	Decreases reliance on a single test and decreases chance of premature closure
7. Use Bayes theorem	Use pre- and posttest probabilities • Helps avert premature closure based on a single test result
8. Acknowledge the effect of the patient	How does the patient make the physician feel? • Physicians may avoid making unfavorable diagnoses in patients with whom they identify • Physicians may discount important data in patients with whom they have difficult encounters
9. Look for clinical findings that do not fit the diagnosis	Encourages a comprehensive approach and incorporates healthy skepticism
10. Consider "zebras"	Resist temptation to lock onto common diagnoses at risk of missing the uncommon
11. Slow down and reflect	Difficult to do in most health care systems, which stress the economy of "getting it right the first time"
12. Admit mistakes	Awareness of one's own fallibility may lead to fewer diagnostic errors later

[a]Heuristics are shortcuts in reasoning used in discovery, learning, or problem solving.

Information from Trowbridge RL. Twelve tips for teaching avoidance of diagnostic errors. Med Teach. 2008;30:496-500. [PMID: 18576188] doi:10.1080/01421590801965137

CONT. completion of a diagnostic evaluation as an outpatient. Furthermore, almost one fifth of discharged Medicare patients are rehospitalized within 30 days of discharge; at least 25% of these readmissions are potentially preventable.

Medication reconciliation, predischarge patient education, and timely scheduling of posthospitalization appointments can improve safety during care transitions. Medication reconciliation entails creating an accurate, comprehensive list of the patient's prescription and nonprescription medications (including the dosage, frequency, and route of administration) and comparing the list to medication orders (at admission, transfer, or discharge) to resolve inconsistencies. Completion of medication reconciliation has been shown to decrease adverse drug events, and although the effect on hospital readmissions is less clear, medication reconciliation should occur at all care transitions to prevent medication errors. The Institute for Healthcare Improvement has published a guide to implementing medication reconciliation and measuring improvement, available at www.ihi.org/Topics/ADEsMedicationReconciliation.

Detailed communication between the hospital discharge and receiving teams is also recommended to promote patient safety. A discharge summary that includes the evaluations performed, medication reconciliation, pending test results, required follow-up tests, and follow-up appointments is an important tool in the communication between the hospital and the follow-up physician. A meta-analysis, however, revealed that crucial information on pending test results and required follow-up testing is omitted from up to two thirds of discharge summaries, and only one third of summaries are received by the accepting outpatient clinician by the time of the initial posthospitalization visit.

KEY POINTS

- Diagnostic error is a common cause of patient harm and is usually the result of a combination of cognitive and systems errors.
- Measures to reduce medication errors include computerized physician order entry systems, medication reconciliation, improved labeling for medications with similar names, and barcode-assisted medication administration.

HVC

(Continued)

TABLE 23.	Strategies to Prevent Adverse Drug Events
Stage	**Safety Strategy**
Prescribing	Avoid unnecessary medications by adhering to conservative prescribing principles
	Use computerized provider order entry, especially when paired with clinical decision support systems
	Perform medication reconciliation at times of transitions in care
Transcribing	Use computerized provider order entry to eliminate handwriting errors
Dispensing	Have clinical pharmacists oversee the medication dispensing process
	Use "tall man" lettering and other strategies to minimize confusion between look-alike, sound-alike medications (for example, **DOP**amine and **DOBUT**amine)
Administration	Adhere to the "five rights" of medication safety (administering the right medication, in the right dose, at the right time, by the right route, to the right patient)
	Use barcode medication administration to ensure medications are given to the correct patient
	Minimize interruptions to allow nurses to administer medications safely
	Use smart infusion pumps for intravenous infusions
	Use patient education and revised medication labels to improve patient comprehension of administration instructions

Adapted from Agency for Healthcare Research and Quality. Patient safety primer: medication errors. https://psnet.ahrq.gov/primers/primer/23/medication-errors. Updated June 2017. Accessed June 27, 2018.

KEY POINTS (continued)

HVC
- A discharge summary that includes the evaluations performed, medication reconciliation, pending test results, required follow-up tests, and follow-up appointments is an important tool in the communication between the hospital and the follow-up physician.

Patient Safety and Quality Issues at the Systems Level

Diagnostic errors, medication errors, and communication errors (especially errors associated with care transitions) are among the many patient safety issues that require systems-level interventions to effect improvement. Similarly, improvement of many quality measures (such as readmission rates, health care–associated infections, and appropriate treatment) largely depends on systems-level changes. Individual clinicians play an important role in systems-level quality and safety programs by identifying areas in need of improvement and participating in improvement activities.

Quality Improvement Models

Successful quality improvement programs include the following components: (1) a health care delivery system with resources (people, information, technology), processes (what is done and how it is done), and outcomes (change in health behavior, patient satisfaction); (2) the objective of meeting the needs and expectations of the patient; (3) a team-based interprofessional approach; and (4) outcome assessment using both qualitative and quantitative data. Several different quality improvement models are used in the health care setting; these models focus on identifying, measuring, and correcting areas that need improvement.

Model for Improvement

The Model for Improvement focuses on achieving specific and measurable results in a specified population. This model relies on identifying a goal to be accomplished with a change, determining how the results of a change will be measured, and deciding on the changes that will bring about an improvement. These changes are tested and implemented by using a Plan-Do-Study-Act (PDSA) cycle. PDSA cycles are rapid tests of improvement, and additional PDSA cycles are completed until the desired results are achieved. A medical center, for example, may set the specific goal of decreasing central line–associated bloodstream infections and use a PDSA cycle to rapidly implement and assess the impact of changes, such as using a central line bundle.

Lean

The Lean model aims to maximize value and minimize waste by closely examining a system's processes and eliminating non–value-added activities within the system. Value stream mapping can be used to graphically display the steps of a process and the time required for each step, thereby highlighting process inefficiencies or areas of waste and allowing for their improvement. Lean also uses a 5S strategy (Sort, Shine, Straighten, Systematize, and Sustain) to create an organized workplace. Lean, for example, may be used to improve the time used to obtain, submit, analyze, and report the results of a laboratory test.

Six Sigma

Six Sigma is a quality improvement model that improves processes by identifying and removing causes of error and minimizing variability in patient care. The term Six Sigma is derived from statistical quality control measures in manufacturing processes and refers to a process that delivers nearly perfect production quality. The Six Sigma model achieves quality improvement by implementing several methods, including the stepwise DMAIC (Define, Measure, Analyze, Improve, and Control) process. The Define step of DMAIC involves developing the objectives of the project. In the Measure step, baseline data on the number and types of defects within the system are measured. The Analyze stage uses the data collected to determine the magnitude of the effects. The Improve step involves implementation of tools to improve the process. Finally, in the Control phase, future processes are controlled to sustain the gains. Six Sigma may be applied to complex, multistep health care processes, such as the ordering and administration of high-risk medications like chemotherapy, to decrease medication errors.

Operational Excellence

As its name suggests, Operational Excellence is a management system that focuses on the consistent and reliable operation of an institutional strategy. It also involves building and sustaining a culture in which each person is empowered and engaged, often by using aspects of Lean, Six Sigma, and other improvement methods. Operational Excellence can be used to improve quality by focusing key performance indicators on quality and safety metrics, such as timely completion of medication reconciliation.

KEY POINTS

HVC
- Successful quality improvement programs include a health care delivery system, the objective of meeting the needs and expectations of the patient, a team-based approach, and outcome assessment using both qualitative and quantitative data.

HVC
- The Model for Improvement, Lean, Six Sigma, and Operational Excellence are examples of quality improvement models that can be used in the health care setting.

Measurement of Quality Improvement

Multiple organizations and payers now assess quality of care as a condition of accreditation or participation. For example, quality of care and patient safety are important elements in the Joint Commission accreditation process. The Joint Commission assesses a wide variety of quality metrics, such as timely provision of reperfusion therapy in acute myocardial infarction, the incidence of potentially preventable venous thromboembolic disease cases, and rates of immunization.

Medicare also has a significant impact on measurement of health care quality. The Medicare Access and CHIP Reauthorization Act of 2015 (MACRA) includes a new payment structure, the Merit-based Incentive Payment System (MIPS). MIPS consolidates previous quality-based programs and includes elements of the Physicians Quality Reporting System and Meaningful Use programs. More specifically, MIPS includes payment incentives and penalties related to quality and safety, value-based care, improvement activities, and meaningful use of the electronic health record (EHR). Clinicians will be required to report clinical quality metrics, participate in improvement activities (such as the patient-centered medical home), and continue to implement the EHR.

Medicare will adjust reimbursement, with bonuses and penalties based on overall performance, as determined by these measures. For American College of Physicians (ACP) resources on MACRA, see https://www.acponline.org/practice-resources/business-resources/payment/medicare/macra. **H**

Patient Safety and Quality Improvement Initiatives
Patient-Centered Medical Home

The patient-centered medical home is a model of providing health care in which the patient's care is coordinated by a primary provider in a team-based practice. The functions of the patient-centered medical home include providing comprehensive care (including preventive, acute, and chronic care), supporting and partnering with patients to make care patient centered, coordinating care across settings with a specific focus on care transitions, delivering accessible services with extended clinician availability, and engaging in quality and safety improvement programs. Further information about the patient-centered medical home is available from AHRQ (www.pcmh.ahrq.gov/page/defining-pcmh).

The concept of the patient-centered medical home has been expanded in the patient-centered medical neighborhood, which includes other clinicians and institutions involved in an individual patient's care (such as specialists and hospitals).

High Value Care

The ACP High Value Care initiative aims to improve health, avoid harms, and eliminate wasteful practices. This initiative addresses high value care broadly, offering learning resources for clinicians and medical educators, curricula, clinical guidelines, best practice advice, case studies, and patient resources on a wide variety of related topics (https://www.acponline.org/clinical-information/high-value-care). Some learning opportunities offer free Continuing Medical Education credits and Maintenance of Certification points. Components of the High Value Care initiative that are evident in MKSAP 18 include the identification of High Value Care key points in the text and a list of high value care recommendations assembled for each MKSAP section.

Choosing Wisely

The Choosing Wisely initiative was developed by the American Board of Internal Medicine Foundation in collaboration with *Consumer Reports* to encourage discussions between clinicians and patients on selecting tests, treatments, and procedures that are evidence based and truly necessary, thereby avoiding unnecessary evaluations and treatments. More than 80 specialist organizations have participated to create lists of overused tests and treatments in their specialties (www.choosingwisely.org/clinician-lists), and *Consumer Reports* has generated patient education materials based on these lists to engage and empower patients to participate in care discussions.

National Patient Safety Goals

The Joint Commission establishes annual National Patient Safety Goals to address important issues in health care safety (https://www.jointcommission.org/standards_information/npsgs.aspx). The National Patient Safety Goals are recommended by a panel of patient safety experts and apply to a variety of patient care settings. The Joint Commission focuses on goals that will have the highest impact on both quality and safety and provides specific metrics for each goal to facilitate implementation. The 2018 National Patient Safety Goals for the hospital setting emphasize improving the accuracy of patient identification, improving staff communication, using medications safely, reducing harms associated with alarm systems, preventing infection, identifying patient safety risks, and preventing surgical mistakes.

Health Information Technology and Patient Safety

Health information technology (HIT) is the use of an electronic environment to share patient health information. The EHR, CPOE, and clinical decision support (CDS) are some common examples of HIT.

The EHR is a compilation of all health data for a specific patient, including medical notes and test results, in a digital format. The EHR enables the timely sharing of patient information by multiple users, including those spread across several geographic sites, resulting in improved communication and care efficiency.

CPOE is a system by which clinicians electronically enter medication, radiology, and laboratory orders, thereby eliminating errors related to illegible handwriting, improving efficiency by reducing delays between order entry and receipt, and ensuring that directions for use are shared exactly as ordered.

CDS refers to the use of information technology to facilitate clinical decision making. When integrated into a CPOE system, for example, CDS can highlight potential contraindications to diagnostic tests, specify dose recommendations, identify potential drug interactions, and suggest modifications to drug dosage in patients with kidney or liver dysfunction. When integrated into EHR systems, CDS can promote protocols to improve care and provide ready access to clinical guidelines.

Limitations of HIT include the expense associated with system implementation and maintenance as well as concerns related to protection of patient privacy. Although useful for preventing many types of errors, HIT does not provide a fail-safe against errors and may facilitate errors itself, such as those resulting from charting templates and use of the copy-and-paste function in composing notes.

For more information on how to incorporate HIT in practice, useful resources are available from ACP (https://www.acponline.org/practice-resources/business-resources/health-information-technology) and AHRQ (https://www.ahrq.gov/professionals/prevention-chronic-care/improve/health-it).

Health Literacy

As defined by AHRQ, health literacy is the degree to which individuals have the capacity to obtain, process, and understand the information required to make informed health decisions. Low health literacy is more common among older adults, minority populations, persons with lower socioeconomic status, and medically underserved groups. Low health literacy may hinder patients' ability to describe their health concerns, complete health forms accurately, understand medical information, and manage their health conditions. Furthermore, evidence shows that low health literacy is associated with poorer health outcomes as well as decreased utilization of care.

Clinicians need to be aware of the health literacy of their patients and identify those who may need assistance. Tools to assess health literacy in specific populations are available at the Health Literacy Tool Shed (http://healthliteracy.bu.edu). Steps the clinician can take to improve patient understanding include using simple sentences, repeating information, providing an opportunity for the patient to ask questions, and supplying the patient with educational materials written in plain language. ACP offers a collection of patient education materials developed to help patients and their families understand health conditions and facilitate communication between patients and the health care team at https://www.acponline.org/practice-resources/patient-education-resources-and-tools.

Professionalism and Ethics
Professionalism

Professionalism is the foundation of medicine's relationship with society and governs the conduct of the physician community. Professionalism in medicine is specifically characterized by the placement of the patient's interests above the physician's self-interests (the fiduciary relationship); acquisition, maintenance, and expansion of specialized medical knowledge; adherence to ethical principles; and self-regulation of members and responsibilities. The Charter on Medical Professionalism from the American Board of Internal Medicine Foundation, the American College of Physicians–American Society of Internal Medicine Foundation, and the European Federation of Internal Medicine sets forth three fundamental principles along with 10 professional commitments that form the ideals and values to be pursued by all physicians (Table 24).

Primacy of Patient Welfare

The principle of primacy of patient welfare is rooted in the importance of placing the patient's interests at the heart of the clinical enterprise. The patient's welfare must supersede all economic, personal, societal, and administrative forces. Under this principle, the physician has a duty to act for the benefit of the patient (beneficence) and to minimize patient harm

TABLE 24.	Principles and Commitments of Professionalism
Principle or Commitment	**Comment**
Fundamental Principle	
Primacy of patient welfare	Altruism is a central trust factor in the physician-patient relationship. Market forces, societal pressures, and administrative exigencies must not compromise this principle.
Patient autonomy	Patients' decisions about their care must be paramount, as long as those decisions are in keeping with ethical practice and do not lead to demands for inappropriate care.
Social justice	Physicians should work actively to eliminate discrimination in health care, whether based on race, gender, socioeconomic status, ethnicity, religion, or any other social category.
Professional Commitment	
Competence	Physicians must be committed to lifelong learning and to maintaining the medical knowledge and clinical and team skills necessary for the provision of quality care.
Honesty with patients	Obtain informed consent for treatment or research. Report and analyze medical errors in order to maintain trust, improve care, and provide appropriate compensation to injured parties.
Patient confidentiality	Privacy of information is essential to patient trust and even more pressing with electronic health records.
Appropriate patient relations	Given the inherent vulnerability and dependency of patients, physicians should never exploit patients for any sexual advantage, personal financial gain, or other private purpose.
Improve quality of care	Work collaboratively with other professionals to reduce medical errors, increase patient safety, minimize overuse of health care resources, and optimize the outcomes of care.
Improve access to care	Work to eliminate barriers to access based on education, laws, finances, geography, and social discrimination. Equity requires the promotion of public health and preventive medicine, as well as public advocacy, without concern for the self-interest of the physician or the profession.
Just distribution of resources	Work with other physicians, hospitals, and payers to develop guidelines for cost-effective care. Providing unnecessary services not only exposes one's patients to avoidable harm and expense but also diminishes the resources available for others.
Scientific knowledge	Uphold scientific standards, promote research, create new knowledge, and ensure its appropriate use.
Manage conflicts of interest	Medical professionals and their organizations have many opportunities to compromise their professional responsibilities by pursuing private gain or personal advantage. Such compromises are especially threatening with for-profit industries, including medical equipment manufacturers, insurance companies, and pharmaceutical firms. Physicians have an obligation to recognize, disclose to the general public, and deal with conflicts of interest that arise.
Professional responsibilities	Undergo self-assessment and external scrutiny of all aspects of one's performance. Participate in the processes of self-regulation, including remediation and discipline of members who have failed to meet professional standards.

Adapted with permission from ABIM Foundation; American Board of Internal Medicine; ACP-ASIM Foundation; American College of Physicians–American Society of Internal Medicine; European Federation of Internal Medicine. Medical professionalism in the new millennium: a physician charter. Ann Intern Med. 2002;136:243-6. [PMID: 11827500] Copyright 2002, American College of Physicians.

(nonmaleficence). This is especially important in the context of the physician-patient relationship, given the inherent vulnerability of many patients. The altruism of serving the patient's interests before the physician's interests creates the trust that is essential to the physician-patient relationship.

Physicians must perform their duties irrespective of the health care setting or the patient's characteristics, including age, religion, gender, sexual orientation, decision-making capacity, insurance status, or immigration status. Care should be provided with respect, competence, compassion, and attention to the uniqueness of the patient and his or her circumstances.

Appropriate Patient Relationships

The physician-patient relationship should be based on mutual agreement. Once this relationship has been established, the physician should strive to understand the patient's health concerns, values, goals, and expectations to guide the provision of care.

Appropriate boundaries between the physician and patient must always be maintained. It is unethical for a physician to become sexually involved with a current patient, and sexual relationships with former patients should be avoided owing to concerns of continued vulnerability and transference (unconscious redirection of the feelings a person has about a second person to feelings that person has about a third person). Physicians must also maintain boundaries during the history, physical examination, and treatment maneuvers by communicating the planned actions in advance and effectively conveying the purpose of these actions (for example, "I will now lift the gown to examine your abdomen more closely"). During the examination of intimate areas, a chaperone should be present.

Physicians may be asked to care for persons with whom they have an existing nonprofessional relationship, including close friends and family members. Caring for these persons may be associated with impaired objectivity, insufficient history taking (for example, failure to obtain an adequate sexual history), incomplete examination, and incomplete or biased assessment. Physicians should weigh these considerations carefully and encourage alternative sources of care whenever feasible.

When communicating with patients online, physicians should conduct themselves according to the usual standards for professional interactions, including treating the patient with respect and maintaining privacy and confidentiality. Social media can lead to confusion over the boundaries between personal and professional interactions, and physicians should keep these spheres separate and behave professionally in both because their behavior reflects upon themselves and upon the profession as a whole. Importantly, all electronic physician-patient communications should be maintained in a secure electronic health record. Benefits, pitfalls, and recommended safeguards for online physician activities are described in **Table 25**.

Physician-patient relationships should generally be established based on an in-person professional encounter. Telemedicine, or the use of electronic communication and technologies to provide health care to patients at a distance, may improve physician-patient collaboration, access to care, and reduce costs. The American College of Physicians holds the position that a valid patient-physician relationship must be established for professionally responsible telemedicine services to occur; however, the patient-physician relationship may be formed during a telemedicine encounter through real-time audiovisual technology.

TABLE 25. Online Physician Activities: Benefits, Pitfalls, and Recommended Safeguards

Activity	Potential Benefits	Potential Pitfalls	Recommended Safeguards
Communications with patients using e-mail, text, and instant messaging	Greater accessibility Immediate answers to nonurgent issues	Confidentiality concerns Replacement of face-to-face or telephone interaction Ambiguity or misinterpretation of digital interactions	Establish guidelines for types of issues appropriate for digital communication Reserve digital communication only for patients who maintain face-to-face follow-up
Use of social media sites to gather information about patients	Observe and counsel patients on risk-taking or health-averse behaviors Intervene in emergency	Sensitivity to source of information Threaten trust in patient-physician relationship	Consider intent of search and application of findings Consider implications for ongoing care
Use of online educational resources and related information with patients	Encourage patient empowerment through self-education Supplement resource-poor environments	Non-peer-reviewed materials may provide inaccurate information Scam "patient" sites that misrepresent therapies and outcomes	Vet information to ensure accuracy of content Refer patients only to reputable sites and sources
Physician-produced blogs, microblogs, and physician posting of comments by others	Advocacy and public health enhancement Introduction of physician "voice" into such conversations	Negative online content, such as "venting" or ranting, that disparages patients and colleagues	"Pause before posting" Consider the content and the message it sends about a physician as an individual and the profession
Physician posting of physician personal information on public social media sites	Networking and communications	Blurring of professional and personal boundaries Impact on representation of the individual and the profession	Maintain separate personas, personal and professional, for online social behavior Scrutinize material available for public consumption
Physician use of digital venues (e.g., text and Web) for communicating with colleagues about patient care	Ease of communication with colleagues	Confidentiality concerns Unsecured networks and accessibility of protected health information	Implement health information technology solutions for secure messaging and information sharing Follow institutional practice and policy for remote and mobile access of protected health information

Reproduced with permission from Farnan JM, Snyder Sulmasy L, Worster BK, Chaudhry HJ, Rhyne JA, Arora VM; American College of Physicians Ethics, Professionalism and Human Rights Committee; American College of Physicians Council of Associates; Federation of State Medical Boards Special Committee on Ethics and Professionalism. Online medical professionalism: patient and public relationships: policy statement from the American College of Physicians and the Federation of State Medical Boards. Ann Intern Med. 2013;158:621. [PMID: 23579867] doi: 10.7326/0003-4819-158-8-201304160-00100. Copyright 2013, American College of Physicians.

Challenging Physician-Patient Relationships

Conflicts between the physician and patient can arise for many reasons. Common causes of conflict include patient requests for inappropriate or nonindicated tests or treatments and patient refusal of a recommended course of treatment. Patients may disagree with the physician's recommendation because of a lack of understanding of the appropriate diagnostic or therapeutic approach, which can be exacerbated by a lack of trust or low health literacy. Other factors include financial or socioeconomic status, which can hinder patient participation in the recommended plan, and cultural considerations, which may lead to a divergent understanding of the cause of the health problem or appropriate approaches to treatment. In response to these conflicts, the physician should offer the rationale for the proposed intervention and explore the patient's reasoning. Physicians also should work to understand the social determinants of health for local communities and how these forces may affect the intersection of health and health care delivery. Furthermore, physicians have a responsibility to develop cultural responsiveness and to sensitively inquire and learn about how a patient's belief system can affect his or her understanding of the health condition. Physicians should consider cultural traditions, the specific social context, and communication standards when discussing care with patients and their families. A deeper understanding of the patient's background and rationale for decision making may allow for conflict resolution or prompt a search for more appropriate alternatives.

There are circumstances in which the physician–patient relationship becomes irreparably compromised because of lack of trust, lack of mutual goals, or failure to maintain an effective working relationship despite efforts to resolve differences. In these cases, the patient and physician can mutually terminate the relationship so long as the patient's health is stable enough for such a transition. The physician should provide formal, written documentation of the termination and provide the patient with information on obtaining a new provider. Patient abandonment (withdrawing from an established relationship without giving reasonable notice or providing a competent replacement) is unethical and may be a cause for legal action.

Requests for Interventions

Patients and their family members may request specific diagnostic or therapeutic interventions that challenge the physician's sense of what is best for the patient. Examples include requests for antibiotic therapy for a suspected viral infection and demands for aggressive chemotherapy in a debilitated patient with cancer. Although the physician needs to respect patient autonomy, this duty must be weighed against the physician's professional judgment and integrity, the potential harms of inappropriate interventions, possible secondary effects (for example, antimicrobial resistance caused by inappropriate antibiotic prescribing), and responsible stewardship of medical resources. When there is no evidence that the desired diagnostic or therapeutic intervention will provide clinical benefit, physicians are not obligated to provide these treatments.

Particularly difficult requests may occur in the setting of ambiguous or conflicting goals of care. For example, a physician may perceive that a patient with multiorgan failure will not achieve the goal of returning to his or her previous level of functioning and therefore conclude that continued intensive care is inappropriate. However, family members may have the goal of extending their loved one's life for as long as possible, regardless of the incurred risk and costs.

Effective communication regarding the preferences and goals of the patient and family members can often help adjudicate conflicts of values, clarify prognosis and uncertainties, and lead to conflict resolution. When resolution cannot be achieved, ethics consultation can be beneficial. Prompt transfer of care to a physician who concurs with the patient's or family's plan and is willing to provide the requested intervention may be necessary when resolution is not possible.

Conflicts of Interest

Conflicts of interest are financial, professional, or other personal concerns that have the potential to compromise the physician's objectivity. Real or potential conflicts threaten the physician's ability to ensure that the patient's welfare is the primary motivating factor in patient care and may undermine trust in the profession. Conflicts of interest may also exist in research and medical education.

Physicians should recognize, disclose, and manage all conflicts of interest. Researchers should disclose sources of funding and minimize opportunities for bias, and medical educators should disclose pertinent conflicts to learners. Disclosure of conflicts, however, may not be an adequate safeguard against bias in decision making, and potential conflicts should be removed if at all possible.

Physician acceptance of gifts, hospitality, and other items and services of value is also strongly discouraged, as even small and seemingly inconsequential gestures may lead to bias. To help guide decision making, physicians can consider whether they think it would be appropriate for their own physician to accept such an inducement and what the public or patient perception of the inducement might be. Other strategies for controlling conflicts of interest are listed in **Table 26**. Physicians should also recognize that the Physician Payments Sunshine Act requires medical product and pharmaceutical manufacturers to disclose payments and gifts to physicians and teaching hospitals, a list of which is published annually in a searchable database. **H**

KEY POINTS

- Patient abandonment, or withdrawing from an established relationship without giving reasonable notice or providing a competent replacement, is unethical and may be a cause for legal action.

(Continued)

TABLE 26. A Selection of Institute of Medicine Recommendations for Individual Physicians to Control Conflicts of Interest

Do not accept items of material value from pharmaceutical, medical device, and biotechnology companies, except when a transaction involves payment at fair market value for a legitimate service.

Do not make educational presentations or publish scientific articles that are controlled by industry or contain substantial portions written by someone who is not identified as an author or who is not properly acknowledged.

Do not enter into consulting arrangements unless they are based on written contracts for expert services to be paid for at fair market value.

Do not meet with pharmaceutical and medical device sales representatives except by documented appointment and at the physician's express invitation.

Do not accept drug samples except in certain situations for patients who lack financial access to medications.

Reproduced with permission from Institute of Medicine. Conflict of Interest in Medical Research, Education, and Practice. Washington, DC: National Academies Press, 2009. https://www.ncbi.nlm.nih.gov/books/NBK22942/. Accessed June 28, 2018. Copyright 2009, The National Academy of Sciences.

KEY POINTS *(continued)*

HVC
- If a patient requests diagnostic or therapeutic interventions for which there is no evidence of clinical benefit, physicians are not obligated to provide these interventions.
- Conflicts of interest threaten the physician's objectivity and the public's trust in the profession; physicians must avoid acceptance of financial, professional, or other personal inducements from health care companies and manufacturers.

Respecting Patient Autonomy

Confidentiality

Physicians are required to protect the privacy and confidentiality of a patient's medical information. The promise of confidentiality fosters trust and encourages honest disclosure of sensitive personal details, thereby improving patient care.

Physicians must recognize that disclosure of medical information outside of the physician–patient relationship requires patient consent and that there is real risk for inadvertent disclosure. Physicians should be vigilant about protecting patient confidentiality in the era of electronic health records, e-mail, patient portals, and social media. Communication with and regarding patients should involve secure communication systems and storage, and physicians should follow best practices. Discussing patients outside of a clinical or educational setting, such as in a hospital cafeteria, violates confidentiality and may compromise trust in the physician and profession. Physicians must also be knowledgeable in the relevant state and federal statutes regarding confidentiality, including the Health Insurance Portability and Accountability Act of 1996 (HIPAA).

There are circumstances in which competing interests may conflict with the need for confidentiality, and disclosure becomes necessary to minimize a greater harm. For example, physicians may be required to breach confidentiality in situations of child or elder abuse, on behalf of public health concerns (for example, sexually transmitted infections), or when patients may be a threat to themselves or others. In these situations, the duty to the public good and other patients overrides the duty to maintain patient confidentiality.

Informed Consent and Refusal

Informed consent and refusal is the process of engaging the patient in meaningful dialogue about his or her health conditions, assessing the patient's understanding, and respecting the patient's autonomy to accept or refuse care. Informed consent requires that a patient be provided with all of the information necessary to determine the individual acceptability and appropriateness of the proposed treatment or intervention. Pertinent information includes the nature of the underlying condition; the goals of treatment; and the risks, benefits, and alternatives to treatment (including the option to forgo treatment). Information should be communicated in ways that are sensitive, appropriate for the patient's literacy level, and attentive to the cultural context. For informed consent to be considered valid, the patient must have decision-making capacity and be free from coercion. An exception to informed consent is a medical emergency in which a patient is unable to participate in the decision-making process; in these instances, consent for life-saving therapies should be presumed unless available information or directives suggest otherwise.

Therapeutic privilege, or the withholding of information due to concern that the disclosure will cause the patient harm, bypasses the process of informed consent and should rarely, if ever, be used. Therapeutic privilege may be used only after consultation with a colleague and a thorough weighing of the risks and benefits of the disclosure.

Advance Care Planning

Advance care planning is the process by which a patient articulates preferences, goals, and values regarding his or her future medical care. Advance care planning should consist of ongoing conversations between the patient, the physician, and loved ones to inform decisions and direct medical care in the event that the patient loses decision-making capacity. These conversations should be a routine component of care and ideally occur before an acute event or medical crisis. Advance care planning should include written documentation of the patient's preferences (advance directives) and be documented in the medical record.

Advance directives may include a living will or durable power of attorney for health care. In a living will, a patient can outline specific preferences for treatment decisions (for example, use of dialysis or mechanical ventilation). A durable power of attorney allows the patient to designate a surrogate to be the primary medical decision maker when the patient cannot make his or her own decisions.

The legal requirements for and implementation of advance directives vary by state, and physicians should be familiar with the laws pertaining to advance directives in the state in which they practice. State laws regarding the withdrawal of artificial nutrition and hydration may be particularly variable, and patients who have preferences regarding these interventions should clearly document these preferences in a living will.

Decision-Making Capacity

All adult patients should be presumed legally competent to make medical decisions unless found otherwise by judicial determination. However, in routine clinical care, physicians must frequently determine the patient's decision-making capacity, including the patient's ability to understand the relevant information, appreciate the medical consequences of the situation, consider various treatment options, and communicate a choice. Decision-making capacity should be evaluated for each decision to be made, and frequent reassessment is necessary to confirm previous determinations of capacity (**Table 27**). The presence of depression or early dementia may complicate the evaluation but

TABLE 27. Legally Relevant Criteria for Decision-Making Capacity and Approaches to Assessment of the Patient

Criterion	Patient's Task	Physician's Assessment Approach	Questions for Clinical Assessment[a]	Comments
Communicate a choice	Clearly indicate preferred treatment option	Ask patient to indicate a treatment choice	Have you decided whether to follow your doctor's (or my) recommendation for treatment? Can you tell me what the decision is? (If no decision) What is making it hard for you to decide?	Frequent reversals of choice because psychiatric or neurologic conditions may indicate lack of capacity
Understand the relevant information	Grasp the fundamental meaning of information communicated by the physician	Encourage patient to paraphrase disclosed information regarding medical condition and treatment	Please tell me in your own words what your doctor (or I) told you about: • The problem with your health now • The recommended treatment • The possible benefits and risks (or discomforts) of the treatment • Any alternative treatments and their risks and benefits • The risks and benefits of no treatment	Information to be understood includes nature of patient's condition, nature and purpose of proposed treatment, possible benefits and risks of that treatment, and alternating approaches (including no treatment) and their benefits and risks
Appreciate the situation and its consequences	Acknowledge medical condition and likely consequences of treatment options	Ask patient to describe views of medical condition, proposed treatment, and likely outcomes	What do you believe is wrong with your health now? Do you believe that you need some kind of treatment? What is treatment likely to do for you? What makes you believe it will have that effect? What do you believe will happen if you are not treated? Why do you think your doctor has (or I have) recommended this treatment?	Courts have recognized that patients who do not acknowledge their illnesses (often referred to as "lack of insight") cannot make valid decisions about treatment. Delusions or pathologic levels of distortion or denial are the most common cause of impairment
Reason about treatment options	Engage in a rational process of manipulating the relevant information	Ask patient to compare treatment options and consequences and to offer reasons for selection of option	How did you decide to accept or reject the recommended treatment? What makes (chosen option) better than (alternative option)?	This criterion focuses on the process by which a decision is reached, not the outcome of the patient's choice, because patients have the right to make "unreasonable" choices

[a]Questions are adapted from Grisso T, Appelbaum PS. Assessing Competence to Consent to Treatment: A Guide for Physicians and Other Health Professionals. New York: Oxford University Press; 1998. Patients' responses to these questions need not be verbal.

Reproduced with permission from Appelbaum PS. Clinical practice. Assessment of patients' competence to consent to treatment. N Engl J Med. 2007;357:1836. [PMID: 17978292] Copyright 2007, Massachusetts Medical Society.

CONT. does not necessarily preclude the presence of decision-making capacity, highlighting the importance of an appropriate assessment. When a decision may result in serious consequences, determination of capacity is of even greater importance. Decisions are likely more valid when consistent with previously stated values, beliefs, and choices. Decisions that run counter to previously expressed preferences may be equally valid; however, when such changes occur, it must be clear that the patient maintains capacity and understands the ramifications of the decisions.

Surrogate Decision Making

In the absence of patient decision-making capacity, a surrogate is required to make health care decisions. The most appropriate surrogate is the person who has been legally appointed by the patient as a health care proxy. If the patient has not designated a surrogate, a person who is knowledgeable about the patient's preferences should serve as decision maker. Many states have laws that provide a hierarchy of preferred surrogates based upon relationship to the patient (typically in the sequence of spouse, adult child, parent, and adult sibling).

The surrogate should adhere to the instructions described in the living will, and physicians should assist surrogate decision makers in fulfilling these duties. If there is no living will, the surrogate should make decisions based on knowledge of the patient's preferences and values, also known as substituted judgment. If the surrogate does not have first-hand knowledge of the patient's preferences or values, he or she should make decisions based on what he or she perceives to be the patient's best interests.

Withholding or Withdrawing Treatment

When a patient with decision-making capacity refuses further treatment, even life-saving care, patient autonomy must be respected, and treatment should be stopped. If the patient lacks decision-making capacity but has articulated future wishes through an advance directive or surrogate, those preferences should guide the treatment decision. Ethically and legally, there is no distinction between withholding (not initiating) or withdrawing (removing) treatment. The decision to withdraw care can be fraught with guilt or concerns about suffering for some family members, and the physician can play an important role in explaining the process and ameliorating these concerns. An ethics committee or ethics consultation can also be helpful in assisting family members. If the patient or surrogate decides to withhold or withdraw life-sustaining treatment, other care (including symptom management and palliative care) should be continued.

Physician-Assisted Suicide

Physician-assisted suicide, or physician-assisted death, occurs when a physician provides a lethal prescription to a competent patient who has requested a means to end his or her life. The patient self-administers the drug with the intent to cause death. Physician-assisted suicide must be distinguished from euthanasia, in which a physician directly and intentionally administers an agent to cause death, and from interventions that are administered with the intent of relieving suffering but unintentionally hasten the patient's death.

Physician-assisted suicide raises profound legal, clinical, and social concerns. It may erode trust in the profession, cause harm to the most vulnerable, and hinder progress in improving end-of-life care. The American College of Physicians does not support legalization of physician-assisted suicide or euthanasia and instead emphasizes the need to provide palliative care, relief from suffering, and emotional support to the patient and family members during the end of life. Several states, however, have legalized physician-assisted suicide, and physicians may be asked to participate in discussions regarding the practice. **H**

KEY POINTS

- Physicians may be required to breach confidentiality in situations of child or elder abuse, on behalf of public health concerns, or when patients may be a threat to themselves or others.

- Informed consent requires that the patient be informed of the nature of the underlying condition; the goals of treatment; and the risks, benefits, and alternatives to treatment (including the option to forgo treatment).

- The presence of depression or early dementia does not necessarily preclude the presence of decision-making capacity, but these conditions increase the importance of an appropriate assessment.

- Surrogates and physicians are required to act in accordance with the patient's expressed preferences for medical care, and if these are not available, they should serve the patient's best interests.

- The American College of Physicians does not support legalization of physician-assisted suicide or euthanasia and instead emphasizes the need to provide palliative care, relief from suffering, and emotional support to the patient and family members during the end of life.

Justice

The principle of justice is predicated on fairness. Physicians have an obligation to promote and respect patients' rights and to justly allocate health care resources. Physicians should work to reduce disparities in the allocation of such resources based on patient characteristics, including sex, race, ethnicity, socioeconomic status, sexual orientation, or gender identify. However, resource allocation or rationing decisions should not be made at the bedside. Rather, these decisions are best made on the societal and policy levels; physicians should work at these levels (for example, through professional societies) to reduce disparities.

Physicians also have the responsibility to provide effective and efficient health care that uses health care resources responsibly (that is, high value care). At times, attention to just distribution of societal resources may seem contradictory to the principles of primacy of patient welfare and patient autonomy; however, physicians must weigh each of these considerations in a particular context to determine the appropriate course of action. By practicing high value care, physicians can ensure excellent care while also using resources wisely and ensuring that resources are equitably available.

Medical Error Disclosure

In the 1999 report *To Err Is Human: Building a Safer Health System*, the Institute of Medicine (now called the National Academy of Medicine) defined a medical error as "the failure of a planned action to be completed as intended or the use of a wrong plan to achieve an aim." Full disclosure of medical errors is recommended practice, and several states mandate such disclosures. Disclosure of errors is necessary to respect the patient's autonomy, promote trust through honesty, and promote justice through appropriate compensation. Disclosure may also benefit physicians by alleviating distress, improving physician-patient communication, and reducing litigation. Strategies that focus on early communication and response after an error have been associated with fewer malpractice lawsuits and lower litigation costs, although these outcomes are not the primary drivers of such initiatives.

The process of error disclosure should include an explanation of the course of events and how the error occurred, an apology by the physician, a description of how the effects of the error will be minimized or rectified, and steps the physician or system will take to reduce recurrences. Disclosure should be performed thoughtfully and sensitively, accounting for the emotional effect on both the patient and provider. ⊞

KEY POINT

- Medical error disclosure should include an explanation of the course of events and how the error occurred, an apology by the physician, a description of how the effects of the error will be minimized or rectified, and steps the physician or system will take to reduce recurrences.

⊞ Colleague Responsibility

Physicians have the responsibility to maintain professional competence, create and share new knowledge with colleagues and trainees, and work collaboratively to optimize patient care. These behaviors must be governed by self-regulation and mutual respect for the members of the health care team.

In accordance with these tenets of professionalism, physicians also have the responsibility to safeguard patients from impaired physicians and to assist impaired colleagues by identifying appropriate sources of help. Physicians have an individual obligation to report an impaired physician to the appropriate authorities and should also work collectively with institutions to develop methods for reporting, treating, and remediating impaired or disruptive colleagues.

Approaching Ethical Dilemmas

Clinical ethical dilemmas can often be resolved by analyzing (1) the patient's medical indications, including the medical condition, problems, and treatment options; (2) patient preferences, including a consideration of decision-making capacity and need for a surrogate; (3) patient quality of life, including the likelihood of restoring the patient to his or her previous state, possible harms to the patient with treatment, and patient and physician impressions of these considerations; and (4) contextual factors, including family, social, legal, religious, and other issues that might affect the decision. When ethical dilemmas are difficult to resolve, physicians may obtain assistance through an ethics consultation.

Providing Care as a Physician Bystander

Physicians' specialized knowledge creates a unique opportunity to intervene and benefit other citizens in emergency situations, and in this context, physicians may provide care outside of the clinical setting to persons who are not their patients. When physicians assist in emergency situations, patient consent to receive treatment is usually presumed or implied. If the treatment is provided in good faith, Good Samaritan laws usually protect the physician from liability, except in cases of gross negligence. Providing medical care as a bystander is typically voluntary; however, state laws vary on this point, and several states have "failure to act" laws that are not specific to physicians. ⊞

Palliative Medicine
Introduction
⊞

Palliative medicine improves quality of life for patients with a serious illness and their caregivers. It focuses on reducing pain, nonpain symptoms, and psychosocial stress associated with advanced disease. All physicians practice some degree of palliative medicine and should learn and use basic palliative medicine skills in patient care (**Table 28**). Specialty palliative medicine, which is palliative medicine delivered in conjunction with specialists in this field, involves an interdisciplinary team that coordinates with referring clinicians to align care with the patient's goals, preferences, and values. Notably, a palliative medicine team does not replace the primary care clinician, hospitalist, or specialist; rather, the team acts as an added layer of support, integrating key information from the referring clinician into goal-concordant care plans and attending to symptoms that affect quality of life.

Evidence has shown that specialty palliative medicine improves overall quality of life, physical symptom burden, mood, and caregiver satisfaction with patient care in the setting of serious or life-threatening illness. Although referral to palliative care historically occurred at the end of life, an

TABLE 28. Representative Skill Sets for Primary and Specialty Palliative Care

Primary Palliative Care
Basic management of pain and symptoms
Basic management of depression and anxiety
Basic discussions about:
Prognosis
Goals of treatment
Suffering
Code status

Specialty Palliative Care
Management of refractory pain or other symptoms
Management of more complex depression, anxiety, grief, and existential distress
Assistance with conflict resolution regarding goals or methods of treatment
Within families
Between staff and families
Among treatment teams
Assistance in addressing cases of near futility

Reproduced with permission from Quill TE, Abernethy AP. Generalist plus specialist palliative care—creating a more sustainable model. N Engl J Med. 2013;368:1174. [PMID: 23465068] doi:10.1056/NEJMp1215620. Copyright 2013, Massachusetts Medical Society.

CONT.

emerging consensus of research indicates that early initiation during a serious or life-threating illness is associated with substantial advantages. Much of the evidence on the benefits of subspecialty palliative care has involved patients with incurable cancer; however, numerous guidelines highlight the need for early palliative care in patients with advanced cardiac, pulmonary, or kidney disease; patients with advanced dementia; critically ill patients; and patients undergoing potentially curative interventions, such as hematopoietic stem cell transplantation.

KEY POINT

HVC
- Specialty palliative medicine improves overall quality of life, physical symptom burden, mood, and caregiver satisfaction with patient care in the setting of serious or life-threatening illness.

Communicating with Patients with Serious Illness

For patients with serious illness, there are considerable disparities between the care that patients report they want and the care that they receive. Patients report a strong desire to have serious illness and end-of-life conversations and wish to have them with the clinicians they view as their primary physician contacts. Timely and skillful communication with patients, family members, and caregivers is essential to align care with patients' wishes. However, many clinicians report that they do not have the training for conversations about end-of-life care, and many conversations occur too late, with poor quality, and outside of the patient's primary clinician-patient relationship. Even among clinicians caring for populations for whom consistent advance care and end-of-life planning are considered to be standard care, it may be unclear who should facilitate end-of-life discussions, and such clinicians may feel ill-equipped. One study of clinicians caring for patients with advanced heart failure found that primary care clinicians, cardiologists, and heart failure clinicians all felt unprepared for conversations related to advance care planning, despite guideline recommendations that such conversations should occur yearly.

Structured conversations are associated with improved goal-concordant care and reduced patient anxiety. One model for skilled conversations with patients facing a serious illness is outlined in **Table 29**. The Serious Illness Conversation Guide provides sample phrases that are designed to elicit a patient's goals, preferences, and values after the patient's illness understanding is assessed. In contrast to discussion techniques in which information is shared and patients are subsequently asked to choose from a list of medical interventions, the Serious Illness Conversation Guide encourages shared decision making and enables the physician to help patients understand the illness and prognosis, elicit important patient goals, and make recommendations for care. The output of these conversations should be communicated to the patient's family and surrogate decision maker. Institutional advance directives, commercial advance directive forms or electronic applications, physician orders for life-sustaining treatment (POLST) paradigm forms, and medical orders for life-sustaining treatment (MOLST) forms should be viewed as mechanisms to record the outcomes of these discussions rather than as conversation guides. For further discussion of advance care planning and advance directives, see Professionalism and Ethics.

KEY POINTS

- Patients report a strong desire to have serious illness and end-of-life conversations and wish to have them with the clinicians they view as their primary physician contact. **HVC**

- Structured conversations about serious illness are associated with improved goal-concordant care and reduced patient anxiety. **HVC**

Symptom Management

Effective and proactive symptom management is critical to the success of both basic and specialty palliative care interventions. Management of debilitating and distressing symptoms, such as pain or nausea, can markedly improve a patient's mood, sense of hope, and quality of life.

TABLE 29. Serious Illness Conversation Guide	
Conversation Flow	**Patient-Tested Language**
1. Set up the conversation:	
Introduce the idea and benefits.	"I'm hoping we can talk about where things are with your illness and where they might be going. Is this okay?"
Ask permission.	
2. Assess illness understanding and information preferences.	"What is your understanding now of where you are with your illness?"
	"How much information about what is likely to be ahead with your illness would you like from me?"
3. Share prognosis:	
Tailor information to patient preference.	Prognosis: "I'm worried that time may be short."
	or "This may be as strong as you feel."
Allow silence; explore emotion.	
4. Explore key topics:	
Goals	"What are your most important goals if your health situation worsens?"
Fears and worries	"What are your biggest fears and worries about the future with your health?"
Sources of strength	"What gives you strength as you think about the future with your illness?"
Critical abilities	"What abilities are so critical to your life that you can't imagine living without them?"
Tradeoffs	"If you become sicker, how much are you willing to go through for the possibility of gaining more time?"
Family	"How much does your family know about your priorities and wishes?"
5. Close the conversation:	
Summarize what you've heard.	"It sounds like _____ is very important to you."
Make a recommendation.	"Given your goals and priorities and what we know about your illness at this stage, I recommend...."
Affirm your commitment to the patient.	"We're in this together."
6. Document your conversation.	

Copyright 2015, Ariadne Labs: A Joint Center for Health Systems Innovation (www.ariadnelabs.org) and Dana-Farber Cancer Institute. Licensed under the Creative Commons Attribution-NonCommercial-ShareAlike 4.0 International License (http://creativecommons.org/licenses/by-nc-sa/4.0/). Ariadne Labs licenses the original content as-is and as-available, and makes no representations or warranties of any kind concerning the original content or concerning this material, which Ariadne Labs has not reviewed or endorsed.

Pain

Although pain in advanced illness shares some features with chronic noncancer pain, pain management in palliative care has several unique attributes, which will be discussed in this section. For a discussion of pain mechanisms as well as the evaluation and initial treatment of patients with pain, refer to Common Symptoms.

Pain commonly occurs in patients with serious illness, and recognition and constant evaluation of pain are integral to effective management. Up to 90% of patients with advanced cancer have pain. Unfortunately, cancer pain remains undertreated, with about one third of patients with cancer receiving inadequate analgesia. The incidence of pain in patients with other serious illnesses is also underappreciated. Most patients with advanced COPD, severe heart failure, amyotrophic lateral sclerosis, or end-stage kidney disease undergoing hemodialysis have undertreated pain.

Many patients additionally face complex psychosocial and spiritual issues related to their illness and may experience total pain, defined as physical, social, psychological, and spiritual suffering. Engaging interdisciplinary team members, such as nurses, psychologists, chaplains, and social workers, is important in addressing the nonphysical components of pain.

The pharmacologic management of pain in patients with a serious illness requires a multimodal approach that uses both opioids and nonopioid analgesics, such as acetaminophen, NSAIDs, glucocorticoids, topical therapies, neuropathic agents, and antidepressants with analgesic properties. (See Common Symptoms for a discussion of common coanalgesic agents.) Current approaches eschew the use of opioid-acetaminophen combination medications because of the risk for acetaminophen overdose with titration of the opioid component, particularly when used concurrently with other acetaminophen-containing drugs. Additionally, the so-called "weak opioids" (codeine, tramadol) should be avoided in this population because of significant drug–drug interactions, marginal effectiveness, and wide variations in hepatic metabolism. For patients in whom nonopioid treatment is ineffective or not tolerated, opioids are appropriate, with careful attention paid to dosing, frequency, and side effect profile. **Table 30** outlines the most commonly used opioids in the treatment of pain resulting from a serious illness, as well as specific patient population concerns.

Short-acting opioids should be titrated to achieve symptom relief. In patients using short-acting opioids who require longer-lasting relief, long-acting agents are appropriate; however, long-acting opioids should not be initiated in opioid-naïve patients. Selection of a long-acting opioid should be based on underlying organ function and previous response to the equivalent short-acting formulation (for example, oxycodone immediate-release and controlled-release forms).

Fentanyl patches are commonly used for long-acting pain relief, although they have a more complex pharmacokinetic profile than oral agents and are less easily titrated. Fentanyl patches must be used with caution in patients with a serious illness, especially those who lack adipose tissue or are subject to recurrent infections. Absence of adipose tissue may result in irregular transdermal absorption, whereas fever may cause increased absorption with a greater potential for adverse events.

Orally administered transmucosal immediate-release fentanyl (TIRF) products are approved for the treatment of cancer-related pain. TIRF formulations are rapidly absorbed and offer immediate onset for patients who are not achieving adequate analgesia with high-dose morphine. Management of these medications is challenging because the dosing regimen, escalation, and frequency differ among brands. Additionally, clinicians require specialized education and certification (TIRF Risk Evaluation and Mitigation Strategy program) to initiate these medications. Methadone is another long-acting agent used to treat pain from a serious illness; however, its complex

dosing and variable half-life restrict its general use. Owing to their complicated management, TIRF formulations and methadone should be prescribed in collaboration with an expert in pain management or a palliative medicine specialist with experience in their use.

Medical cannabis has long been used in the management of symptoms associated with serious illness. It has been studied for numerous clinical indications and is approved in many states for the treatment of cancer symptoms or symptoms associated with other terminal illnesses. Cannabis extracts, predominantly those containing higher concentrations of cannabidiol, have shown a moderate degree of benefit in the treatment of patients with chronic pain and patients with pain symptoms from spasticity in the setting of neurodegenerative disorders. However, given the lack of data on medical cannabis in managing complex cancer pain and the need for multimodal analgesic therapy in seriously ill patients, the role of medical cannabis for this indication remains unclear.

Constipation

Constipation is a common symptom in patients with serious illness and negatively affects quality of life. Causes include opioids, dehydration, immobility, metabolic disturbances, and numerous nonopioid medications. More than 90% of patients with cancer who are receiving opioids experience constipation.

Patients with constipation in the setting of serious illness should be educated on increasing their intake of fluids and dietary fiber. Patients taking opioids, however, should not receive supplemental fiber, owing to concerns for worsening constipation in the setting of opioid-reduced gastrointestinal motility. Pharmacologic therapy for constipation and for all patients taking scheduled opioids should include a stimulant laxative, such as senna or bisacodyl. Osmotic laxatives, such as

TABLE 30.	Opioids Commonly Used in Palliative Care		
Opioid	**Protein Binding**	**Metabolism**	**Comments**
Hydrocodone	Low	Liver enzyme CYP2D6	Variable efficacy; combination with acetaminophen limits use
			Increased time to analgesic onset in liver failure
Hydromorphone	Low	Liver (glucuronidation)	Better choice if kidney disease is present
			Reduce dose and frequency in liver failure/cirrhosis
Tramadol	Low/moderate	Liver enzymes CYP2D6/CYP3A4	Variable time to onset and analgesic efficacy in liver failure
			Interactions with other serotonergic medications, potentially leading to serotonin syndrome (agitation, clonus, muscle rigidity, hyperreflexia)
Oxycodone	Moderate/high	Liver enzymes CYP2D6/CYP3A4	Increased half-life and variable onset in liver failure; if used, reduce dose and frequency
Morphine	Moderate/high	Liver (glucuronidation)	Avoid in liver failure/cirrhosis, kidney failure
			Increased bioavailability with liver failure
			Increased toxic metabolites with kidney failure
Fentanyl	High	Liver enzyme CYP3A4	Safest long-acting drug in kidney and liver failure
			Increased bioavailability with liver failure; start lower-dose patch in liver failure

CYP2D6 = cytochrome P-450 2D6; CYP3A4 = cytochrome P-450 3A4.

polyethylene glycol, are often added to achieve a regular bowel pattern. Docusate, alone or in combination, is no more effective than placebo for constipation in patients with a serious illness. Third-line therapy consists of rectal suppositories and/or enema preparations. Phosphate- or magnesium-containing enema preparations are contraindicated in seriously ill patients because of the potential for dangerous electrolyte shifts. If maximal medical therapy has failed to achieve laxation in patients taking opioids, peripheral opioid antagonists (such as methylnaltrexone) should be considered; these medications do not cross the blood-brain barrier and therefore do not affect analgesia.

Nausea

Nausea and vomiting are common and debilitating symptoms in patients with a serious illness, with many patients rating nausea as more distressing than unrelieved pain. Management of nausea should be tailored to address the underlying mechanism and associated neurotransmitter pathway (**Table 31**). More than one agent is frequently required for symptom relief. In hospitalized patients, parenteral forms should be administered on a scheduled basis to achieve symptom control and not just reduce the number of emesis events. ◼

Other Symptoms

Anorexia and weight loss frequently occur in patients at the end of life. Clinicians should identify and treat any reversible conditions that may contribute to anorexia to ease patient and family distress. Although some medications are marketed for patients with anorexia and weight loss, they are marginally effective in a minority of terminally ill patients and often have unacceptable side effects. The use of enteral or parenteral artificial nutritional support at the end of life does not improve survival, is invasive, and can cause side effects, including increased terminal secretions and painful edema. Discussing the dying process, including the common presence of weight loss and anorexia and the lack of effective treatment for these expected changes, can prepare patients and their family members and set realistic expectations.

Audible oropharyngeal secretions at the end of life ("death rattle") are often distressing for families and clinicians alike and may occur in up to 50% of dying patients. However, these secretions rarely affect respiratory status or cause patient distress, and educating family members on the normal process of dying can ease concerns. Treatment is often initiated in anticipation of family distress but is generally ineffective. Current literature does not support the routine use of antimuscarinic drugs in the treatment of death rattle. There is also no evidence that scopolamine, glycopyrronium, hyoscine butylbromide, atropine, or octreotide are superior to no treatment. The use of anticholinergic agents in patients who are awake can lead to undesirable symptoms, such as dry mouth and urinary retention. Suctioning by catheter should be avoided unless secretions are causing obvious respiratory distress.

Although symptoms of anticipatory grief are common at the end of life, clinical depression is not experienced by most patients and should not be expected. Clinical depression worsens quality of life and should be aggressively treated if present. In contrast to neurovegetative symptoms that accompany terminal illness (such as poor appetite and low energy), symptoms of unrelenting helplessness, hopelessness, and lack of pleasure should raise concerns for clinical depression. If depression is diagnosed, pharmacotherapy consists of antidepressant agents that are appropriate for the patient's estimated prognosis. Selective serotonin reuptake inhibitors are effective and safe in patients with end-organ dysfunction; however, their therapeutic effects may not be reached for several weeks. In patients with an estimated life expectancy of less than 6 weeks, psychostimulants, such as methylphenidate, are favored.

Delirium is a common symptom in patients at the end of life. It can result from many potentially reversible causes (medication side effects, inadequate analgesia, urinary retention, constipation), although a cause is often not identified.

TABLE 31. Treatment of Nausea in the Palliative Care Patient		
Cause of Nausea	**Mediating Receptor Pathway**	**Treatment**
Gut wall stretching or dilatation (constipation, bowel obstruction, ileus)	Dopamine type 2 (D_2) receptors in the gastrointestinal tract	Antidopaminergic antiemetics (metoclopramide, prochlorperazine, haloperidol)
Gut mucosal injury (radiation, chemotherapy, infection, inflammation, direct tumor invasion)	Serotonin (5-hydroxytryptamine-3 [5-HT_3]) receptors in the gastrointestinal tract	Serotonin antagonists (ondansetron, granisetron)
Drugs, metabolic by-products, bacterial toxins	D_2 receptors, 5-HT_3 receptors, and neurokinin type 1 receptors in the chemoreceptor trigger zone	Antidopaminergic antiemetics and serotonin antagonists
Motion sickness, labyrinthine disorders	Histamine type 1 (H_1) receptors and muscarinic acetylcholine receptors in the vestibular system	Anticholinergic antiemetics (scopolamine, diphenhydramine, promethazine)
Anticipatory nausea	Unknown, presumed cerebral cortex	Benzodiazepines
Increased intracranial pressure	Unknown	Glucocorticoids

Nonpharmacologic interventions remain standard care; however, for some patients, medications may be required to maintain patient and caregiver safety and to ensure relief from suffering. First-generation antipsychotics, such as haloperidol or chlorpromazine, are effective and have not been shown to be inferior to newer-generation antipsychotics. The combination of benzodiazepines and antipsychotics may be more effective than antipsychotics alone in the treatment of delirium at the end of life.

Dyspnea can be a prominent and distressing symptom in patients with advanced illness and those at the end of life. The patient's subjective sensation of difficulty breathing should be measured on an iterative basis during evaluation and treatment. Although the initial goal of treatment is to address the underlying cause of dyspnea, many patients with advanced illness will have persistent dyspnea despite maximal medical management. In these patients, opioids are the treatment of choice. Opioids reduce the sensation of dyspnea and, when appropriately selected and dosed, do not cause respiratory depression. Refer to Common Symptoms for further discussion of the evaluation and management of dyspnea. ◨

KEY POINTS

- The pharmacologic management of pain in patients with serious illness requires a multimodal approach that uses opioids and nonopioid analgesics such as acetaminophen, NSAIDs, glucocorticoids, topical therapies, neuropathic agents, and antidepressants with analgesic properties.

- For patients in whom nonopioid analgesic agents are ineffective or not tolerated, opioids are appropriate, with careful attention paid to dosing, frequency, and side effect profile.

- Pharmacologic therapy for patients with constipation and for all patients taking opioids should include a scheduled stimulant laxative, such as senna or bisacodyl.

- **HVC** Enteral or parenteral artificial nutritional support at the end of life does not improve survival, is invasive, and can cause side effects, such as increased terminal secretions and painful edema.

- Clinical depression should not be expected in patients at the end of life; if present, it should be aggressively treated.

◨ Hospice

Hospice is a form of palliative medicine that delivers specialized interdisciplinary care to patients with an expected prognosis of 6 months or less. Hospice care can be provided to patients in multiple settings, including the home, skilled nursing facilities, and residential hospice homes. Hospice teams are skilled in managing the symptoms of advanced and terminal illness and improve overall satisfaction with care. ◨

Common Symptoms

Introduction

Specific symptom concerns account for nearly half of all outpatient visits. Although most symptoms resolve in several weeks, they sometimes present clinicians with the challenge of how to best determine their significance and the role of testing in the diagnostic approach. Unnecessary testing accounts for nearly 30% of health care costs. Hence, when evaluating symptoms, physicians have a responsibility to use testing strategies that offer the highest value. Fortunately, a thorough history alone generates the highest diagnostic yield, up to 75% in some studies, with the physical examination contributing an additional 10% to 15%. In contrast, testing results in less than 10% of diagnoses. Although diagnostic testing may provide crucial information and justify the costs incurred, physicians should consider the value of diagnostic testing and the effects of test results on patient management.

This chapter focuses on high-value approaches to the diagnosis and treatment of commonly encountered symptoms, including chronic noncancer pain, medically unexplained symptoms, dyspnea, cough, fatigue, dizziness, syncope, insomnia, and lower extremity edema. In addition, in-flight emergencies, a common event encountered by physicians, are reviewed.

Chronic Noncancer Pain

The classification, assessment, and management of chronic noncancer pain are discussed in this section. For a discussion of cancer-related pain and pain in the setting of advanced illness, refer to Palliative Medicine.

Chronic pain is defined as a painful sensation lasting for more than 3 months or beyond the time frame expected for normal healing. Chronic pain has substantial negative effects on patient quality of life and physical, social, financial, and functional status. More than 10% of the U.S. population has symptoms consistent with chronic pain.

The approach to the patient with chronic pain is guided by the type of pain the patient experiences. Classification of chronic pain as nociceptive or neuropathic can be helpful in designing a tailored therapeutic approach; however, many patients with chronic noncancer pain syndromes will experience both nociceptive and neuropathic pain from multiple sources.

Nociceptive pain syndromes are caused by involvement of either visceral or somatic nociceptors. Visceral pain syndromes classically result from injury to or abnormal firing of visceral pain fibers; patients typically report poorly localized cramping or aching. In contrast, somatic pain syndromes are more commonly associated with injury to somatic pain fibers that convey signals from muscles, bones, and joints. Types of somatic pain include musculoskeletal pain (see Musculoskeletal Pain) and inflammatory pain. Often described by patients as sharp and stabbing pain, somatic nociception is easier to localize than visceral pain.

Neuropathic pain syndromes result from injury to peripheral nerve structures or central nervous system damage. Peripheral nerve syndromes, such as postherpetic neuralgia, are common and can be diagnosed by identifying sensory symptoms within the distribution of the affected peripheral nerve or nerves. Central neuropathic pain syndromes, such as those caused by cerebrovascular accidents or spinal cord injuries, often have widely varying presentations and symptom expression and can evade initial diagnostic approaches. A high index of suspicion is required because pain is often vaguely localized. Clinicians should look for key features, such as hyperalgesia (oversensitivity to a normally painful stimulus) or allodynia (pain from a normally nonpainful stimulus) occurring in the setting of underlying central nervous system injury.

In addition to nociceptive and neuropathic pain, pain induced by opioid therapy can occur paradoxically. Opioid-induced hyperalgesia is thought to result from repeated exposure to systemic opioids. Patients with this pain syndrome may experience a change in the character of their pain during the course of opioid therapy, a worsening of pain with increased opioid dosages, and a reduction in pain when opioid dosages are decreased.

Assessment

The first step in the assessment of chronic pain is a thorough history and physical examination. Determination of pain location, duration, severity, temporal nature, and responsiveness to treatment is crucial in identifying the pain generator and tailoring the diagnostic and therapeutic approaches. In most cases of chronic pain, additional testing and imaging are unlikely to produce further diagnostic yield.

A key component of the assessment is a thorough review of the patient's functional status, including physical functioning, ability to perform basic activities of daily living, and psycho-social-spiritual functioning. Psychological comorbidities influence and are influenced by experiences of chronic pain, and they affect response and adherence to a multimodal treatment strategy. Patients should be screened for mental health disorders, and if present, these disorders should be treated in conjunction with the patient's chronic pain whenever possible. Depending on severity, treatment of concomitant mental health conditions may take precedence over interventions targeting chronic pain.

Patients with chronic pain are up to four times more likely to have concomitant depression. Depression increases as pain symptoms magnify, and depression may also manifest as pain. Aggressive treatment of depression, with both pharmacologic and nonpharmacologic behaviorally based therapies, can lead to substantial improvement in both chronic pain and depressive symptoms. Iterative evaluation of depressive symptoms during chronic pain treatment is critical to ensuring that patients are able to sustain improvements.

Substance abuse screening is another essential part of the assessment of patients with chronic pain (see Routine Care of the Healthy Patient). Substance use disorders are more common in patients with chronic pain syndromes and increase the risk for opioid misuse.

In the setting of chronic pain without a treatable underlying cause, clinicians should monitor for significant changes in pain experience, new acute pain syndromes superimposed on chronic pain, and development of "red flag" symptoms. Red flags include pain occurring with constitutional symptoms (such as fever and involuntary weight loss), change in bowel or bladder function, and weakness or sensory deficits. These signs and symptoms should trigger further investigation.

Management

Management is determined by the cause of the patient's pain; the pain severity (as it relates to functional status); medical and psychosocial comorbid conditions; and barriers to treatment, such as health care access and concomitant mental health disorders. Developing a therapeutic relationship in which patients feel that their physician takes their pain seriously and in which patients, as well as family, friends, or other social supports, are active participants in the treatment strategy are important for success over time. Physical activity, engagement in work activities, and behavioral interventions should be encouraged regardless of pain score. Pharmacologic therapy should be viewed as adjunctive to nonpharmacologic therapy in the treatment of chronic pain. Patients receiving treatment should undergo periodic evaluation of pain, functional status, response to interventions, and quality of life.

Nonpharmacologic Therapy

All patients with chronic pain should be referred to a structured physical therapy program for evaluation and treatment. Physical therapy teaches patients safe, self-guided exercises to improve functional status. High-quality evidence suggests that physical therapy programs improve both pain and function in patients with debilitation due to pain symptoms. Continuation of physical therapy beyond 12 weeks should be based on iterative clinical assessments and documented gains. Like physical therapy, exercise programs improve pain and function in patients with chronic pain, although no specific regimen has proved superior. Low- to moderate-quality evidence supports the use of complementary and integrative therapies, such as massage and acupuncture, to manage chronic pain.

Cognitive behavioral techniques, including cognitive behavioral therapy (CBT), mindfulness practices, and biofeedback, have been associated with reduced pain and improved overall function and mood. Referral to practices or specialized pain centers that provide these therapies should be explored when available.

Interventional approaches may be appropriate for patients with pain syndromes that can be anatomically targeted with injection-based therapy. In addition, advanced therapies, such as high-frequency neurostimulation, hold promise for appropriately selected patients. Patients may be referred to a pain specialist for consideration of these therapies.

Pharmacologic Therapy

Pharmacologic therapy should be used as adjunctive treatment for chronic pain when nonpharmacologic therapies have not achieved their desired effect. Clinicians should emphasize that pharmacologic therapies have limited efficacy in the long-term management of chronic pain and are intended to improve function and quality of life, not pain scores. Patients should be informed that adjuvant pharmacologic therapies may take weeks to be effective and that a combination of medications with differing mechanisms may be necessary to provide optimal benefit. When selecting pharmacologic therapies to add to a multimodal treatment regimen, attention to comorbid illness (particularly organ dysfunction) and concurrent medications is critical to limit side effects.

For chronic musculoskeletal or inflammatory nociceptive pain, trials of acetaminophen (≤3 g/d) or NSAIDs can be considered as initial pharmacologic therapy in patients without contraindications to their use. In cases of inflammatory nociceptive pain, NSAIDs can be given both orally and topically. NSAIDs are typically used for periodic pain flares or potentially while opioid therapy is being down-titrated but not for long-term therapy. Topical NSAIDs, such as topical diclofenac, have few systemic side effects, are generally well tolerated, and are effective for short-term treatment of musculoskeletal nociceptive conditions. Although short courses of muscle relaxants may be beneficial in some patients with acute pain, long-term use should be avoided because of the potential for side effects and drug-drug interactions.

In chronic neuropathic pain syndromes, gabapentinoids (such as gabapentin and pregabalin) and serotonin-norepinephrine reuptake inhibitors (such as duloxetine) are first-line therapy. When pain generators are topically located, capsaicin and topical lidocaine can be considered. Tricyclic antidepressants, such as nortriptyline and desipramine, are also effective for neuropathic pain syndromes, although titration to effective dosages is often limited by side effects and drug-drug interactions.

Medical cannabis is increasingly available for use in patients with chronic pain. Many states have passed laws legalizing the use of cannabis or allowing its use for medical conditions, although it is still classified by the U.S. Drug Enforcement Administration as a schedule I agent. Current data on the effectiveness of medical cannabis for chronic pain are characterized by significant heterogeneity in both patient populations and cannabis preparations, although recent systematic reviews have demonstrated that cannabis has some efficacy in the treatment of chronic noncancer pain. The most robust data originate from studies of compounds available outside the United States (such as nabiximols), which contain higher ratios of cannabidiol to tetrahydrocannabinol (THC) than the existing FDA-approved synthetic THC (dronabinol). Little is known about the comparative efficacy of cannabis preparations in states where medical cannabis is available.

Opioids

Patients who present to physicians' offices with chronic pain are frequently provided with prescriptions for opioids. Despite high prescribing rates, no evidence supports the use of long-term opioid therapy in patients with chronic noncancer pain. In fact, evidence demonstrates that long-term opioid use is associated with poorer overall functional status, worse quality of life, and worse pain (possibly mediated through opioid tolerance and hyperalgesic mechanisms). In addition, although often well intentioned, these prescribing patterns lead to substantial morbidity and mortality. From 1999 to 2015, more than 183,000 Americans died from overdose related to prescription opioids, and in 2011, an estimated 400,000 emergency department visits were attributable to opioid misuse or abuse. Importantly, most opioid-related overdoses occurred in patients taking opioids as prescribed. Opioids should not be considered first-line therapy in any patient with a chronic noncancer pain syndrome.

In patients in whom multimodal analgesic therapy has not improved function and quality of life or in patients already receiving opioids, the decision to initiate or continue opioids should include a thorough assessment of the benefits and burdens of therapy. In 2016, the Centers for Disease Control and Prevention (CDC) released a comprehensive guideline for prescribing opioids in patients with chronic pain syndromes, not including patients with active cancer, patients receiving palliative care, and patients at the end of life. Central to these guidelines are a robust discussion of risks and benefits, close monitoring, and use of risk-mitigation strategies (**Table 32**). The CDC provides a checklist to assist clinicians in the prescribing of opioids in the setting of chronic noncancer pain, available at https://stacks.cdc.gov/view/cdc/38025.

When discussing opioid therapy with patients, it is important to emphasize the lack of evidence for long-term opioid therapy in chronic pain syndromes and the substantial risks associated with long-term use of these medications. **Table 33** summarizes some of the important risks associated with long-term opioid therapy.

Clear treatment goals based on functional improvement and quality-of-life considerations should be established to manage patient expectations and provide a means for measuring the success or failure of treatment. These goals can be incorporated into a patient-physician prescribing agreement, which can also be used to communicate expectations for follow-up, monitoring, and risk mitigation.

The CDC guideline recommends that before starting and periodically during continuation of opioid therapy, clinicians should evaluate risk factors for opioid-related harms. A commonly used risk assessment instrument, the Opioid Risk Tool, is available at https://www.drugabuse.gov/sites/default/files/files/OpioidRiskTool.pdf. Urine drug screening and surveillance of state prescription monitoring databases are important

TABLE 32. Centers for Disease Control and Prevention Recommendations for Prescribing Opioids for Chronic Pain Outside of Active Cancer, Palliative, and End-of-Life Care[a]

Determining When to Initiate or Continue Opioids for Chronic Pain

1. Nonpharmacologic therapy and nonopioid pharmacologic therapy are preferred for chronic pain. Clinicians should consider opioid therapy only if expected benefits for both pain and function are anticipated to outweigh risks to the patient. If opioids are used, they should be combined with nonpharmacologic therapy and nonopioid pharmacologic therapy, as appropriate.

2. Before starting opioid therapy for chronic pain, clinicians should establish treatment goals with all patients, including realistic goals for pain and function, and should consider how therapy will be discontinued if benefits do not outweigh risks. Clinicians should continue opioid therapy only if there is clinically meaningful improvement in pain and function that outweighs risks to patient safety.

3. Before starting and periodically during opioid therapy, clinicians should discuss with patients known risks and realistic benefits of opioid therapy and patient and clinician responsibilities for managing therapy.

Opioid Selection, Dosage, Duration, Follow-up, and Discontinuation

4. When starting opioid therapy for chronic pain, clinicians should prescribe immediate-release opioids instead of extended-release/long-acting (ER/LA) opioids.

5. When opioids are started, clinicians should prescribe the lowest effective dosage. Clinicians should use caution when prescribing opioids at any dosage, should carefully reassess evidence of individual benefits and risks when increasing dosage to ≥50 morphine milligram equivalents (MME)/day, and should avoid increasing dosage to ≥90 MME/day or carefully justify a decision to titrate dosage to ≥90 MME/day.

6. Long-term opioid use often begins with treatment of acute pain. When opioids are used for acute pain, clinicians should prescribe the lowest effective dosage of immediate-release opioids and should prescribe no greater quantity than needed for the expected duration of pain severe enough to require opioids. Three days or less will often be sufficient; more than 7 days will rarely be needed.

7. Clinicians should evaluate benefits and harms with patients within 1 to 4 weeks of starting opioid therapy for chronic pain or of dose escalation. Clinicians should evaluate benefits and harms of continued therapy with patients every 3 months or more frequently. If benefits do not outweigh harms of continued opioid therapy, clinicians should optimize other therapies and work with patients to taper opioids to lower dosages or to taper and discontinue opioids.

Assessing Risk and Addressing Harms of Opioid Use

8. Before starting and periodically during continuation of opioid therapy, clinicians should evaluate risk factors for opioid-related harms. Clinicians should incorporate into the management plan strategies to mitigate risk, including considering offering naloxone when factors that increase risk for opioid overdose, such as history of overdose, history of substance use disorder, higher opioid dosages (≥50 MME/day), or concurrent benzodiazepine use, are present.

9. Clinicians should review the patient's history of controlled substance prescriptions using state prescription drug monitoring program (PDMP) data to determine whether the patient is receiving opioid dosages or dangerous combinations that put him or her at high risk for overdose. Clinicians should review PDMP data when starting opioid therapy for chronic pain and periodically during opioid therapy for chronic pain, ranging from every prescription to every 3 months.

10. When prescribing opioids for chronic pain, clinicians should use urine drug testing before starting opioid therapy and consider urine drug testing at least annually to assess for prescribed medications as well as other controlled prescription drugs and illicit drugs.

11. Clinicians should avoid prescribing opioid pain medication and benzodiazepines concurrently whenever possible.

12. Clinicians should offer or arrange evidence-based treatment (usually medication-assisted treatment with buprenorphine or methadone in combination with behavioral therapies) for patients with opioid use disorder.

[a]All recommendations are category A (apply to all patients outside of active cancer treatment, palliative care, and end-of-life care) except recommendation 10 (designated category B, with individual decision making required); see full guideline at https://www.cdc.gov/mmwr/volumes/65/rr/rr6501e1.htm for evidence ratings.

Reproduced from Dowell D, Haegerich TM, Chou R. CDC guideline for prescribing opioids for chronic pain—United States, 2016. MMWR Recomm Rep. 2016;65:16. [PMID: 26987082] doi:10.15585/mmwr.rr6501e1

TABLE 33. Risks of Long-Term Opioid Therapy

Endocrinopathies (e.g., osteoporosis, hypogonadism)

Increased risk for opioid addiction

Increased risk for overdose and death

Increasing pain through mechanisms of opioid-induced hyperalgesia

Opioid tolerance resulting from adaptive central nervous system mechanisms

risk-mitigation strategies for patients receiving opioids in the setting of chronic pain. Although the optimal frequency of urine drug screening is unclear, patients taking long-term opioid therapy should undergo urine screening at least yearly to assess for adherence to the prescribed agent and for the presence of substances that could increase the risk for opioid overdose. More frequent screening may be recommended based on individual patient characteristics. State prescription monitoring databases (where available) should also be reviewed on a regular basis for adherence to the terms of the prescribing agreement.

The CDC guideline also provides recommendations on safe dosing. The risk for opioid-related overdose is dose dependent, with significantly increased risk for overdose in patients receiving dosages higher than 90 morphine milligram equivalents per day. The lowest possible dosage should be used to achieve the functional and quality-of-life goals established by the patient and prescriber. Given the risks and limited efficacy of opioid therapy in treating chronic noncancer pain, these dosages should not typically exceed more than 50 morphine milligram equivalents per day. Follow-up evaluation should occur at frequent intervals after therapy initiation or dosage changes and at least every 3 months. Dosages exceeding 50 morphine milligram equivalents per day should prompt re-evaluation and closer follow-up intervals. Dosages higher than 90 morphine milligram equivalents per day are considered high risk and should be prescribed only in consultation with pain specialists. Co-prescription of opioids and benzodiazepines is associated with an increased risk for death from overdose and should be avoided.

Evidence shows that naloxone, an opioid antagonist that reverses life-threatening respiratory depression, is effective in preventing opioid-related overdose death at the community level through community-based distribution. Primary care clinicians should consider offering naloxone kits and associated overdose prevention education to patients at increased risk for overdose, such as those receiving daily doses of 50 morphine milligram equivalents per day or more, concurrently taking a benzodiazepine, or with a history of substance use disorder, as well as to the patient's family members or caregivers.

For patients who previously received prescriptions for opioids in the setting of chronic pain and present to a physician for referral or as a new patient, a discussion on opioid prescribing best practices should be framed by the CDC guideline recommendations. Discussions on tapering opioid therapy, incorporating a nonopioid multimodal pain strategy as the cornerstone of pain management, and setting appropriate goals are fundamental to these prescribing relationships.

For a discussion on the treatment of opioid use disorder, see Mental and Behavioral Health.

KEY POINTS

- **HVC** In patients with chronic pain, determining the pain location, duration, severity, temporal nature, and responsiveness to treatment is crucial in identifying the pain generator and tailoring the diagnostic and therapeutic approaches; in most cases of chronic pain, additional testing and imaging is unlikely to produce further diagnostic yield.
- In the setting of chronic pain without a treatable underlying cause, clinicians should monitor for significant changes in pain experience, new acute pain syndromes superimposed on chronic pain, and the development of red flag symptoms.

(Continued)

KEY POINTS *(continued)*

- Physical therapy improves both pain and function in patients with debilitation due to chronic pain. **HVC**
- Cognitive behavioral techniques, including cognitive behavioral therapy, mindfulness practices, and biofeedback, have been associated with reduced pain and improved overall function and mood in patients with chronic pain. **HVC**
- For chronic musculoskeletal or inflammatory nociceptive pain, trials of acetaminophen (≤3 g/d) or NSAIDs can be considered as initial pharmacologic therapy in patients without contraindications to their use. **HVC**
- In chronic neuropathic pain syndromes, gabapentinoids and serotonin-norepinephrine reuptake inhibitors are first-line therapy.
- No evidence supports long-term opioid therapy in patients with chronic noncancer pain, and evidence demonstrates that long-term opioid use is associated with poorer overall functional status, worse quality of life, and worse pain. **HVC**
- The decision to initiate opioid therapy in patients with chronic pain should involve a robust discussion of risks and benefits, close monitoring for benefits and harms, avoidance of long-acting opioid formulations, and use of risk-mitigation strategies.
- Primary care clinicians should consider offering naloxone kits and associated overdose prevention education to patients at increased risk for overdose, such as those receiving daily doses of 50 morphine milligram equivalents per day or more, concurrently taking a benzodiazepine, or with a history of substance use disorder.

Medically Unexplained Symptoms

Medically unexplained symptoms (MUS) are symptoms that cannot be attributed to a specific medical cause after a thorough medical evaluation. The prevalence of MUS is high; a recent systematic review of 32 studies involving 70,085 patients determined that the prevalence of patients with at least one unexplained symptom ranges from 40% to 49%. Patients with MUS are frequently seen in both primary and subspecialty clinics, resulting in significantly increased health care utilization. The costs associated with MUS are estimated at more than $250 billion annually. Unsurprisingly, the high prevalence, increased resource utilization and frequency of visits, ongoing inexplicable symptoms, and looming fear of a missed diagnosis all contribute to patient and clinician dissatisfaction.

Many terms have been incorrectly and interchangeably used to describe and diagnose MUS, further complicating an already challenging scenario. Patients with MUS must be distinguished from those with somatic symptom and related disorders, which are psychiatric conditions with specific diagnostic criteria (see Mental and Behavioral Health). Although many somatic symptom and related disorders involve MUS, most patients with MUS do not meet the diagnostic criteria for these disorders.

Clinical Presentation and Evaluation

Symptoms that are common in patients with MUS include fatigue, headache, abdominal pain, musculoskeletal pain (back pain, myalgia, and arthralgia), dizziness, paresthesia, generalized weakness, transient edema, insomnia, dyspnea, chest pain, chronic facial pain, chronic pelvic pain, and chemical sensitivities. MUS appear more frequently in women, persons with lower levels of education, and those with lower socioeconomic status.

There is no formal approach to the diagnostic evaluation of MUS; however, the initial evaluation should involve a thorough history and physical examination related to each symptom. Clinicians must approach each symptom in a focused manner and diligently review any previous diagnostic evaluations. Laboratory and radiographic studies should be guided by the findings on the history and physical examination, and subspecialty referrals should be used judiciously. Given the high comorbidity of mood disturbances in patients with MUS, patients with features concerning for an underlying mood disorder should be evaluated accordingly.

If an underlying medical cause cannot be identified after an appropriately thorough evaluation, it is imperative that clinicians have an open and honest discussion of the results with the patient, being mindful to acknowledge the patient's concerns and frustrations. Frequently, patients will request, or even demand, additional testing and consultations that may not be clinically indicated. Although doing so may be challenging, clinicians should limit additional evaluations to those deemed medically necessary, as unnecessary studies provide negligible reassurance, pose iatrogenic risks, and result in additional patient anxiety.

Management

The foundation of management of patients with MUS is an open, honest, and effective therapeutic relationship. Patients should be treated respectfully and cared for in a nonjudgmental manner. It is important to not only expect but to accept the patient's feelings of frustration; acknowledging these feelings early in the patient's management course can help to build and strengthen the therapeutic alliance.

Management of MUS requires a patient-focused, holistic, and multimodal approach. The goals of management are functional restoration, decreased symptom focus, and acquisition of coping mechanisms rather than abatement of symptoms. Office visits should be scheduled at regular intervals, allowing for additional discussion, educational opportunities, and longitudinal reassessment. Frequency of appointments can gradually be decreased over time as tolerated by the patient. It should be made clear to patients that the treatment of MUS will not likely be curative and that symptoms may persist.

Patients should be encouraged to develop short-term and long-term goals with the recognition that many goals will change from a physical symptom focus to a psychosocial focus. If additional symptoms arise, clinicians should respond empathically and perform an appropriately thorough investigation.

Interventions that may benefit patients with MUS include CBT, physical therapy, occupational therapy, individual or group psychotherapy, social support, biofeedback therapy, graded exercise therapy, stress management activities, and training in coping mechanisms. Patients with comorbid mood conditions should be considered for a trial of antidepressant therapy and referral to a psychiatrist or psychologist. Given the wide-ranging effects of MUS, treatment should be focused on both physical and psychosocial aspects (**Table 34**).

Knowledge of barriers to the treatment of patients with MUS can help clinicians prevent unnecessary missteps and provide ongoing value-based care. Common barriers include a poor physician-patient relationship, the heterogeneity of symptoms, varying diagnostic labels, and ongoing changes in the health care system (insurance coverage, access to care, and value-based metrics).

KEY POINTS

- In patients with medically unexplained symptoms, clinicians should limit diagnostic tests to those deemed medically necessary because unrevealing studies provide negligible reassurance, pose iatrogenic risks, and result in additional patient anxiety. **HVC**
- The goals of management in patients with medically unexplained symptoms are functional restoration, decreased symptom focus, and acquisition of coping mechanisms rather than abatement of symptoms. **HVC**

Dyspnea

Dyspnea is a common symptom with a diverse pathophysiologic basis and substantial variation in patient experience. The American Thoracic Society defines dyspnea as "a subjective experience of breathing discomfort that consists of qualitatively distinct sensations that vary in intensity." Patients may describe this symptom as breathlessness or tightness, an inability to catch their breath, or a feeling of drowning. The prevalence of dyspnea increases with age, with more than one third of those older than 70 years reporting sensations of dyspnea in an ambulatory setting. Dyspnea affects up to half of hospitalized patients and is a common reason for patients to seek care in urgent and emergent care settings.

Dyspnea results from multiple underlying neurophysiologic mechanisms, including greater work of breathing, air hunger, and airway irritation or damage. These mechanisms may be triggered by poor functional status, organ-specific pathology, medication effects, or physiologic stimuli (including hypoxia and hypercapnia).

TABLE 34. Follow-up Management of the Patient With Medically Unexplained Symptoms

Category	Issue	How?	How Often?	Notes
Nonpharmacologic therapy	Maintaining an effective relationship with the patient	Elicit and address the patient's emotional concerns; use a negotiated rather than a prescriptive approach; tailor care to patient's personality; address your own negative reactions to the patient.	Each visit	Monitor the provider-patient relationship regularly as you would, for example, monitor blood pressure in a patient with hypertension. Ask, "So how is all this going; how are you and I working together?" Examples of indicators of an effective relationship are adherence to the treatment plan, friendliness, improved eye contact, positive statements about the provider and the treatment.
	Dissociating treatment regimen from symptoms	Schedule regular, consistent, time-contingent visits rather than ad hoc (as-needed) visits; give all medications on a scheduled rather than on an as-needed basis.	Each visit	Titrate number of scheduled visits and amount of treatment to patient's needs and progress.
Pharmacologic therapy	MUS symptoms	Consider lowest effective dose of antidepressant and nonopioid analgesics.	Each visit	Minimize or avoid use of opioids and tranquilizers.
	Comorbid depression and anxiety	Treat depression as indicated.	As needed	
Patient education	Overall management	Review patient's diary and facilitate understanding of how his or her thoughts, emotions, and behaviors are related to symptoms.	Ongoing	
	Education and treatment plan	Educate the patient so that the patient understands the plan of care and its purpose.	Each visit	
	Reinforcing patient commitment to treatment	Give appropriate praise for commitment behavior, such as completing homework; address noncommittal behavior, such as not keeping appointments or visiting an acute care facility without prior discussion.	Each visit	
	Reviewing and revising patient goals	Reinforce previous short-term goals or negotiate new ones to operationalize patient's long-term goals.	Each visit	Help patient to identify solutions to roadblocks.
	Negotiating new plans	Negotiate plans to adjust physical activity; recommend relaxation techniques; refer for physical therapy.	Each visit	Continuously encourage the patient to add new healthy behaviors and to progress in what he or she is already doing.

MUS = medically unexplained symptoms.

Adapted with permission from Dwamena FC, Fortin AH, Smith RC. Medically unexplained symptoms. In ACP Smart Medicine (online database). Philadelphia: American College of Physicians, 2015. Accessed June 25, 2015.

Evaluation

The history and physical examination are the most important components of the evaluation of dyspnea. A crucial aspect of the history is determining whether the patient's dyspnea is new in onset or an acute-on-chronic exacerbation of a known disease. Evaluation of the patient with acute-on-chronic symptoms should include an investigation for a potentially new generator of dyspnea (such as pleural effusion in the setting of existing lung malignancy) or progression of the underlying cause.

Dyspnea has many causes (**Table 35**). A cardiac or respiratory origin is most common, although some patients will have a mixed presentation. In the absence of an obvious cause, the initial evaluation in most patients will include measurement of oxygen saturation and hemoglobin, as well as electrocardiography and chest radiography. Depending on the results of these tests, further evaluation may entail measurement of B-type natriuretic peptide, D-dimer assay, pulmonary function testing, and advanced imaging of the cardiac or pulmonary systems. Such testing, however, should be pursued only when the

TABLE 35.	Common Causes of Dyspnea
Acute Dyspnea	
Decreased cardiac output/function	
Ischemic heart disease	
Pulmonary infection	
Pneumothorax	
Pleural effusion	
Bronchospasm	
Pulmonary vascular disease (e.g., pulmonary embolism or hemorrhage)	
Chronic Dyspnea	
Airflow obstruction (e.g., COPD)	
Restrictive lung diseases	
Decreased cardiac output/function	
Deconditioning	

initial evaluation reveals a reasonable likelihood of disease; scattershot testing should be avoided. Referral to a cardiologist or pulmonologist may be appropriate when the diagnosis remains elusive or when conditions require subspecialty input.

Dyspnea should be assessed on an iterative basis during the patient's care. Many validated dyspnea scoring systems are available; however, these instruments are lengthy, take significant time to complete, and may not account for contributing factors in the patient's experience of dyspnea. Standard measurement with a numeric scale akin to a pain-rating scale is advantageous for its ease of use, but it must be paired with a functional assessment of quality of life and dyspnea-related impairment.

Management

Initial treatment strategies are aimed at treating or modifying the patient's dyspnea generator and the underlying disease state responsible for causing the symptom. In patients with chronic conditions, the first step in reducing dyspnea is to maximize standard therapies, with regular assessment of symptomatic response.

In patients with persistent debilitating symptoms despite maximal medical therapy, there are nonpharmacologic and pharmacologic strategies to reduce dyspnea severity, with varying levels of evidence to support each one. Of these therapies, pursed-lip breathing, handheld fans, and devices that enhance air flow are the least invasive and easiest to administer. Studies examining the efficacy of guided relaxation training and acupuncture/acupressure have yielded mixed results, but these therapies are safe and may be reasonable for appropriately selected patients. Pulmonary rehabilitation can provide significant benefits for patients with chronic lung diseases and has been shown to improve subjective dyspnea in patients with severe COPD.

In patients with hypoxemia and COPD, oxygen therapy offers substantial benefits in survival, quality of life, and dyspnea reduction. However, the role of supplemental oxygen in other patient groups, including those with normoxemic dyspnea, is less clear. Data from a randomized controlled trial of palliative oxygen versus medical air in normoxemic patients demonstrated no improvement in quality of life or scores of subjective dyspnea with palliative oxygen therapy, supporting the hypothesis that movement of air is more important in reducing breathlessness in these patients. In patients with refractory dyspnea despite maximal therapy, a brief trial of supplemental oxygen is reasonable.

Opioids are an effective therapy for patients with dyspnea that is refractory to nonpharmacologic therapies and maximal medical management of the underlying disease. Opioids, both endogenous and exogenous, appear to exert an antidyspneic effect through modulation of central nervous system processing of sensory inputs, similar to their modulation of pain signaling. Although opioids affect respiratory mechanics and may blunt respiratory drive, appropriately dosed opioids should not cause respiratory depression if treatment is directed by symptoms. Patient selection and subsequent opioid selection should be based on symptom burden, underlying disease, comorbid organ dysfunction, and overall risk for respiratory depression. Although systemic opioids have shown clear benefit in treating refractory dyspnea, inhaled opioids have not shown significant efficacy in several placebo-controlled trials.

KEY POINTS

- An important aspect of the evaluation of dyspnea is determining whether the patient's dyspnea is new in onset or an acute-on-chronic exacerbation of a known disease state.
- Pursed-lip breathing, handheld fans, and devices that enhance air flow are easy, noninvasive interventions to reduce dyspnea severity.   **HVC**
- Opioids are an effective therapy for patients with dyspnea that is refractory to nonpharmacologic therapies and maximal medical management of the underlying disease.

Cough

Cough is another common symptom, resulting in roughly 30 million physician office visits and costing billions of dollars annually in the United States. An evidence-based approach to the evaluation of cough that ensures cost-effective care is framed around the duration of cough (acute, subacute, and chronic).

Acute Cough

Acute cough (<3 weeks' duration) is most often caused by viral respiratory tract infections, including upper respiratory tract infections (URIs) and bronchitis. Other conditions that may present with acute cough include allergic rhinosinusitis, pneumonia, medication adverse reactions, and pulmonary edema.

The initial evaluation of the patient with acute cough focuses on identifying potentially life-threatening illnesses. Concomitant fever, dyspnea, chest pain, and abnormalities on lung or cardiovascular examination suggest a serious respiratory or cardiovascular disease as the source of cough, and further evaluation should be completed as appropriate. If signs and symptoms are primarily respiratory and constitutional, a lower respiratory tract infection is most likely, and chest radiography may be warranted. Pneumonia is an unlikely cause of acute cough, and chest radiography is not indicated in the absence of abnormal vital signs (heart rate >100/min, respiration rate >24/min, temperature >38 °C [100.4 °F]) or abnormal lung examination findings, unless there are other concerning clinical features (such as altered mental status).

Acute cough without evidence of lower respiratory tract infection or cardiovascular disease is most often caused by viral rhinosinusitis or acute bronchitis. Coronaviruses and rhinoviruses are the most common causative pathogens, but influenza virus should be highly suspected in patients presenting with fever and myalgia, especially during influenza season (between autumn and early spring). Bacterial infections can also cause acute sinusitis or bronchitis, although sinus imaging is not recommended unless a complication, such as spread of infection into contiguous structures, is suspected.

Another important cause of acute cough is ACE inhibitor therapy. Up to 20% of patients taking an ACE inhibitor develop a dry cough, usually within 1 to 2 weeks of therapy initiation. Onset of cough, however, may be delayed by months in a small percentage of patients, and cough may additionally persist for weeks after discontinuation of the offending agent. All ACE inhibitors may cause this side effect. Angiotensin receptor blockers typically do not cause cough and may be substituted if ACE inhibitor therapy is not tolerated.

Treatment of acute cough is primarily symptomatic and dependent on the underlying etiology. Antibiotics are not recommended in patients with acute bronchitis or URIs without clearly established bacterial infection, although most patients with acute bacterial sinusitis will improve without antibiotics. A meta-analysis of patients with acute rhinosinusitis found that use of intranasal glucocorticoids increased the rate of symptom response compared with placebo; there was a dose-response curve, with higher doses offering greater relief. Analgesics, such as NSAIDs and acetaminophen, may provide pain relief. Only limited evidence supports saline irrigation in the relief of nasal symptoms; careful attention should be paid to the use of sterile or bottled water. Instructions for nasal saline irrigation are available online (https://www.fda.gov/ForConsumers/ConsumerUpdates/ucm316375.htm). First-generation antihistamines may help dry nasal secretions; however, evidence supporting their efficacy is lacking, and sedation is a common side effect. Decongestants are of possible benefit in patients with evidence of eustachian tube dysfunction but should be used with caution in elderly patients and those with cardiovascular disease, hypertension, angle-closure glaucoma, or bladder neck obstruction. Antitussive agents are generally ineffective.

Subacute and Chronic Cough

Subacute cough (3-8 weeks' duration) is most often a postinfectious cough following an acute respiratory tract infection, particularly viral or *Mycoplasma* infection. Postinfectious cough is usually caused by postnasal drip or airway hyperreactivity. If postnasal drip is the primary problem, first-generation antihistamines may be beneficial. In patients with evidence of airway hyperreactivity, such as wheezing, therapies for asthma are usually effective. Patients with postinfectious cough not caused by postnasal drip or airway hyperreactivity may benefit from inhaled ipratropium. *Bordetella pertussis* infection should be considered in patients with subacute cough characterized by paroxysms of severe coughing and posttussive emesis. If infectious causes of subacute cough are excluded, the evaluation shifts to consideration of the causes of chronic cough.

Chronic cough (>8 weeks' duration) is most often caused by upper airway cough syndrome (UACS; formerly postnasal drip syndrome), gastroesophageal reflux disease (GERD), asthma, smoking, and ACE inhibitor use. Nonasthmatic eosinophilic bronchitis is another increasingly documented cause of chronic cough. Important but less common causes include chronic bronchitis, lung neoplasm, bronchiectasis, and chronic aspiration.

Evaluation of chronic cough begins with a thorough history, physical examination, and chest radiography (**Figure 4**). ACE inhibitor therapy and tobacco use should be discontinued. If an etiology is not determined after initial evaluation, a stepwise approach is pursued, beginning with a 2-week trial of empiric treatment for UACS. Allergic rhinitis–associated UACS is optimally treated with intranasal glucocorticoids, whereas UACS resulting from nonallergic rhinitis responds best to first-generation antihistamines (chlorpheniramine, brompheniramine, diphenhydramine) and decongestants (pseudoephedrine).

Asthma should be considered in patients with symptoms that do not respond to empiric treatment for UACS. Cough-variant asthma is diagnosed if spirometry and/or bronchial hyperresponsiveness testing results are abnormal and symptoms improve with standard therapy for asthma, including inhaled glucocorticoids.

In patients with normal findings on evaluation or failed empiric treatment for UACS and asthma, the most reasonable next step is to exclude nonasthmatic eosinophilic bronchitis with sputum analysis for eosinophils or exhaled nitric oxide testing. If test results are abnormal, therapy with inhaled glucocorticoids should be initiated.

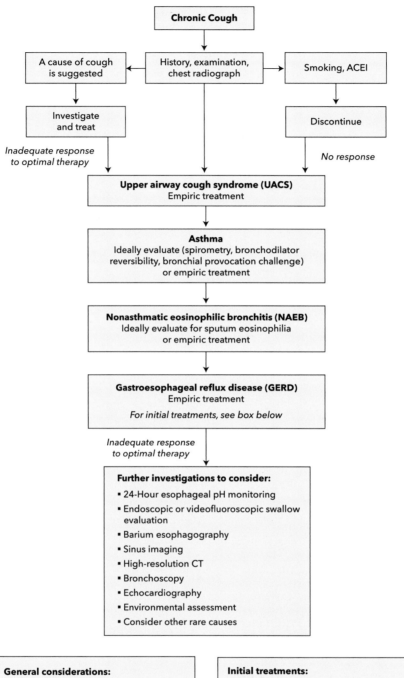

FIGURE 4. Evaluation of chronic cough. ACEI = ACE inhibitor; LTRA = leukotriene receptor antagonist.

Reproduced with permission of the American College of Chest Physicians from Irwin RS, Baumann MH, Bolser DC, et al; American College of Chest Physicians (ACCP). Diagnosis and management of cough executive summary: ACCP evidence-based clinical practice guidelines. Chest. 2006;129(1 suppl):4S. [PMID: 16428686] Copyright 2006, American College of Chest Physicians.

Cough without a clear etiology that does not respond to the aforementioned empiric therapies should be treated with empiric proton pump inhibitor therapy and antireflux lifestyle changes to address possible GERD. Failure of empiric GERD treatment of 8 weeks' duration should prompt an advanced investigation (see Figure 4).

Persistent cough without an identifiable cause despite comprehensive evaluation is termed unexplained chronic cough.

Patients with unexplained chronic cough may benefit from other therapies for symptomatic relief. Antitussives, including dextromethorphan and topical anesthetics (benzonatate), have been shown to reduce cough and improve quality of life. Opioids, such as codeine, may have a similar effect but should be used with caution and only if other measures fail. Gabapentin can also be effective at controlling unexplained chronic cough and should be considered if the risk for adverse effects is acceptable. Protussives, such as guaifenesin, can improve mucus clearance and cough intensity in selected patients with excessive sputum production. Finally, multimodality speech pathology therapy may provide benefit and should be offered to all patients with chronic cough of undetermined cause.

Cough in the Immunocompromised Patient

Immunocompromised patients with cough require heightened suspicion for infections, particularly if immunosuppression is severe. In addition to common pathogens, other causes to consider include fungi, cytomegalovirus, varicella, herpesvirus, and *Pneumocystis jirovecii*. Clinicians should have a low threshold for initiating empiric antibiotic therapy while diagnostic testing is pursued.

Hemoptysis

Hemoptysis is expectoration of blood from the lower respiratory tract with coughing. Causes include bronchitis, bronchiectasis, malignancy, tuberculosis, pulmonary embolism, and left ventricular failure. Rare causes include anti–glomerular basement membrane antibody disease (Goodpasture syndrome) and granulomatosis with polyangiitis. Hemoptysis requires urgent evaluation, which begins with assessment to confirm the lower respiratory tract as the source of bleeding and exclude bleeding from the nasopharynx (nosebleed) or the gastrointestinal tract (hematemesis). Chest radiography should be performed, but most patients additionally require chest CT and/or bronchoscopy to accurately determine the cause.

KEY POINTS

HVC
- In patients with acute cough, chest radiography is not indicated in the absence of abnormal vital signs or abnormal lung examination findings, unless there are other concerning clinical features (such as altered mental status).

HVC
- Treatment of acute cough is primarily symptomatic; antibiotics are not recommended in patients with acute bronchitis or upper respiratory tract infection without a clear bacterial cause.

- Common causes of chronic cough include smoking, ACE inhibitor use, upper airway cough syndrome, gastroesophageal reflux disease, asthma, and nonasthmatic eosinophilic bronchitis.

- Patients with unexplained chronic cough may benefit from antitussives, gabapentin, and multimodality speech pathology therapy.

Fatigue and Systemic Exertion Intolerance Disease

Fatigue is generally defined as tiredness, exhaustion, or lack of energy precipitated by exertion or stress. It is a common symptom, occurring in one quarter to one third of patients in the primary care setting. Despite its high prevalence, the cause of fatigue is often elusive, leading to prolonged delays in diagnosis, substantial functional decline, and high direct and indirect societal costs. Chronic fatigue is defined as fatigue lasting longer than 6 months.

Fatigue is a truly subjective symptom with little to no corroborating objective measures. It can be classified as fatigue secondary to another cause (**Table 36**), secondary to multiple factors (termed chronic multifactorial fatigue [CMF]), or as a primary condition. In the past, the latter condition was termed chronic fatigue syndrome (CFS), myalgic encephalitis (ME), or neurasthenia. Each of these diagnoses had specific diagnostic criteria,

TABLE 36.	Common Causes of Fatigue
Lifestyle	
Alcohol	
Drug dependency (overuse and withdrawal)	
Extremes of activity	
Night shift work	
Sleep deprivation, poor sleep habits	
Work/life imbalance	
Medical	
Anemia	
Cancer	
Chronic liver and kidney disease	
Chronic lung disease, hypoxemia	
Heart failure	
HIV/AIDS	
Hyperglycemia, uncontrolled diabetes mellitus	
Medication side effects	
Antidepressants	
Antihistamines	
Antipsychotics	
β-Blockers	
Benzodiazepines	
Opioids	
Obesity	
Thyroid disorder (hyper- and hypothyroidism)	
Psychological	
Anxiety	
Depression	
Stress	

creating inconsistencies in diagnosis and wide variability in treatment across providers and institutions. In 2015, the Institute of Medicine (IOM), now called the National Academy of Medicine, issued an extensive guideline aimed at developing validated, evidence-based clinical diagnostic criteria for this condition and using consensus-building methods. The IOM recommended using the term systemic exertion intolerance disease (SEID) rather than CFS, ME, or other similar terms. Diagnosis of SEID requires the presence of all of the following three symptoms:

- A substantial reduction or impairment in the ability to engage in preillness levels of occupational, educational, social, or personal activities that persists for more than 6 months and is accompanied by fatigue, which is often profound, is of new or definite onset (not lifelong), is not the result of ongoing excessive exertion, and is not substantially alleviated by rest
- Postexertional malaise
- Unrefreshing sleep

In addition, the patient must have at least one of the following two manifestations:

- Cognitive impairment
- Orthostatic intolerance (symptoms such as lightheadedness, dizziness, and headache that worsen with upright posture and improve with recumbency)

An estimated 836,000 to 2.5 million U.S. adults have SEID; however, 84% to 91% of affected individuals are not yet diagnosed. In 2015, the economic cost associated with SEID was estimated to be between $17 billion and $24 billion annually.

Although the pathophysiology of SEID remains unclear, the phenomenon of central sensitization (the pathophysiologic dysregulation of the thalamus, hypothalamus, and amygdala) is gaining acceptance as a potential cause of SEID as well as of other highly prevalent comorbid conditions, including fibromyalgia, mood disturbances, irritable bowel syndrome, and interstitial cystitis. Central sensitization is often triggered by a prodromal event, such as infection, physical or emotional trauma, a motor vehicle accident, surgery, medical illness, or prolonged stress. Studies on central sensitization and its relationship to SEID and associated comorbid conditions are ongoing.

Evaluation

The diagnostic evaluation of acute or chronic fatigue begins with a careful history and physical examination. Clinicians should note the duration of fatigue, preceding factors, concomitant symptoms, prolonged deleterious lifestyle factors, medication use, and the presence of "red flag" signs or symptoms (fever, involuntary weight loss, persistent lymphadenopathy, muscle atrophy, and synovitis). Patients should also be assessed for an underlying sleep disturbance. Mood disorders are often comorbid in patients with SEID (approximately 70% of patients), and all patients with SEID should be screened for depression and anxiety. Clinicians should additionally ensure that all age-appropriate screenings have been performed.

The history and physical examination should guide the choice of diagnostic tests. In patients with fatigue without a clear cause, it is reasonable to obtain a complete blood count, electrolyte panel, thyroid-stimulating hormone level, fasting glucose level, and kidney and liver chemistry tests. Unnecessary laboratory, imaging, and invasive studies should be avoided because most patients will have unrevealing findings, which usually provide little reassurance.

Management

Treatment of fatigue should focus on correcting any underlying causes. In patients with SEID, the goals of treatment shift to functional rehabilitation and restoration. Patients benefit most from a structured, well-defined, multimodal approach that includes regularly scheduled office visits, which allow for discussion, educational opportunities, and longitudinal reassessment. There is evidence that CBT and graded exercise therapy may decrease fatigue and improve function, and these therapies should be offered to patients. Additionally, all patients should receive instruction on effective sleep hygiene. Other modalities that may be of benefit include physical therapy, occupational therapy, biofeedback therapy, massage therapy, acupuncture, yoga, tai chi, and stress management activities. In patients with comorbid mood conditions, treatment or referral to a psychiatrist or psychologist is reasonable.

There are no FDA-approved medications for the treatment of SEID. Medications play a very limited role in management, except in the treatment of comorbid conditions (such as depression). One small study found that methylphenidate increased concentration and decreased fatigue in 20% of patients, but its use is tempered by its addictive potential and adverse effects. There is no consistent evidence that opioids, glucocorticoids, pharmacologic sleep aids, prolonged antibiotics or antiviral agents, or immunotherapies improve symptoms or prognosis.

The prognosis for chronic fatigue varies and is often a source of frustration for patients and providers. The prognosis depends on many factors, including patient age, formal education level, severity of symptoms, duration of symptoms, decline in functional status relative to premorbid level of function, presence of other somatic (or medically unexplained) symptoms, comorbid mood disorders, availability of resources, and adherence to the treatment recommendations.

KEY POINTS

- In patients with fatigue without a clear cause, it is reasonable to obtain a complete blood count, electrolyte panel, thyroid-stimulating hormone level, fasting glucose level, and kidney and liver chemistry tests. **HVC**

- Patients with systemic exertion intolerance disease benefit most from a structured, well-defined, multimodal approach that includes regularly scheduled office visits; cognitive behavioral therapy and graded exercise therapy may decrease fatigue and improve function and should be offered. **HVC**

(Continued)

KEY POINTS (continued)

- There are no FDA-approved medications for the treatment of systemic exertion intolerance disease, and medications play a very limited role in management, except in the treatment of comorbid conditions.

Dizziness

Approach to the Patient with Dizziness

Dizziness is a common nonspecific symptom seen in inpatient and outpatient settings. Patients often interchangeably use the terms dizzy, lightheaded, woozy, cloudy, faint, or off-balance to describe the perception of dizziness. Owing to its subjective nature, the variability in symptom description, and broad differential diagnosis (which includes stroke and other life-threatening disorders), dizziness is a challenging symptom to assess and treat.

In patients with dizziness, a relevant history and physical examination should be performed to classify the symptom into one of four focused groupings: vertigo, presyncope, disequilibrium, and nonspecific dizziness. This classification facilitates establishing a formal diagnosis and treatment strategy.

Vertigo

Vertigo is the false perception of personal or environmental movement. Patients describe a spinning or whirling sensation, which is often associated with concomitant nausea, vomiting, and sudden-onset fatigue. Symptoms are typically episodic and brief and are usually triggered by positional changes of the head. Vertigo is classified as peripheral or central, depending on the specific etiology.

A thorough history and examination are crucial for differentiating between central and peripheral causes of vertigo, especially in patients with acute vertigo concerning for vertebrobasilar ischemia and other central causes. Examination should include an in-depth neurologic assessment as well as the HINTS (Head Impulse, Nystagmus, and Test of Skew) oculomotor assessment (**Table 37**). An abnormal result on any one of the three HINTS components suggests a central rather than peripheral cause of acute vertigo. Major causes of acute vertigo are presented in **Table 38**.

Peripheral Vertigo

Benign paroxysmal positional vertigo (BPPV) is the most common form of vertigo, with a lifetime prevalence of 2.4%. It is more common in women (female-to-male ratio of 2:1 to 3:1). BPPV is characterized by sudden-onset, recurrent, and brief (usually <1 minute) vertiginous symptoms, which are provoked and worsened with positional changes of the head. Patients report dizziness, imbalance, nausea, and vomiting that occur with positional changes; however, no focal neurologic findings are present. Symptoms lead to increased risk for falls and a decline in functional status. BPPV is caused by displacement and migration of otoconia (calcium carbonate

TABLE 37. HINTS (Head Impulse, Nystagmus, and Test of Skew) Examination

Maneuver	Method	Results
Head impulse test	With the patient focusing on the examiner, the examiner slowly moves the patient's head in either direction about 20 degrees and then rapidly rotates back to midline, while assessing for catch-up saccades	Reassuring: presence of catch-up saccades (consistent with peripheral cause of vertigo) Concerning: absence of catch-up saccades (consistent with central cause of vertigo)
Nystagmus assessment	Examiner observes for the presence and directionality of nystagmus on lateral gaze	Reassuring: unidirectional nystagmus Concerning: bidirectional nystagmus
Test of skew deviation	Examiner alternates covering and uncovering each eye and assesses for vertical adjustment or refixation	Reassuring: absence of vertical skew Concerning: presence of vertical skew

crystals) within the semicircular canals. Up to 90% of all cases of BPPV involve the posterior semicircular canal because it is the most gravity-dependent semicircular canal.

The diagnostic test of choice for BPPV is the Dix-Hallpike maneuver (**Figure 5**), which can help differentiate between peripheral and central causes of vertigo (**Table 39**). In the setting of BPPV, a positive finding includes the presence of a mixed upbeat-torsional nystagmus toward the affected side. Brain imaging is not necessary for diagnosis. First-line therapy for BPPV is canalith repositioning with the Epley maneuver, which is effective in up to 85% of patients (**Figure 6** on p. 58).

Other common causes of peripheral vertigo include vestibular neuronitis, labyrinthitis, Meniere disease, medication effects (toxicity from aminoglycoside or diuretic use), Ramsay Hunt syndrome (herpes zoster involving cranial nerve VII), and vestibular schwannoma (acoustic neuroma). Vestibular neuronitis is most often preceded by a viral infection affecting the vestibular portion of cranial nerve VIII. Symptoms are generally more severe and of longer duration than in BPPV and may take longer to resolve. Labyrinthitis has a presentation similar to that of vestibular neuronitis, with the additional symptom of hearing loss. Meniere disease classically presents with the triad of vertigo, tinnitus, and hearing loss; symptoms are episodic and recurrent and may be severe.

Evidence supports the utility of diuretics in the treatment of Meniere disease, but pharmacologic therapy has not otherwise been shown to be significantly effective for peripheral vertigo. Rather, vestibular suppressants (antihistamines, benzodiazepines, and antiemetics) can be used in conjunction with other forms of therapy for temporary symptomatic relief.

TABLE 38. Differential Diagnosis of Acute Vertigo

Cause	Onset and Course	Nystagmus	Auditory Symptoms	Other Features
BPPV	Recurrent, transient, positional; usually provoked by turning over or getting in and out of bed	Positional, with mixed vertical torsional nystagmus in BPPV involving posterior canal and horizontal nystagmus in BPPV involving horizontal canal	None	Recent inciting event possible (e.g., recumbent position at dentist's office or hair salon, prolonged bed rest, head trauma); history of similar episodes
Stroke	Spontaneous, usually sustained; may be worsened by positional change	Spontaneous, with beating in various or changing directions	Occasional	Neurologic symptoms or signs often occur, but stroke may present as isolated vertigo; results of head impulse test are typically normal[a]
Vestibular neuronitis	Spontaneous, sustained; may be worsened by positional change	Spontaneous, predominantly horizontal	None	May be preceded by viral illness; results of head impulse test are abnormal[a]
Vestibular migraine	Recurrent, spontaneous; duration for minutes to hours; may be positional	Rare, but when present usually positional	Occasional	Migrainous headaches, motion sickness, family history
Meniere disease	Recurrent, spontaneous; typical duration for hours	Spontaneous, horizontal	Fluctuating hearing loss, tinnitus	Ear pain, sensation of fullness in ear

BPPV = benign paroxysmal positional vertigo.

[a]In the head impulse test, the result is considered abnormal when a corrective movement (saccade) is required to maintain straight-ahead fixation after the head has been rotated to the side.

Reproduced with permission from Kim JS, Zee DS. Clinical practice. Benign paroxysmal positional vertigo. N Engl J Med. 2014;370:1140. [PMID: 24645946] doi:10.1056/NEJMcp1309481. Copyright 2014, Massachusetts Medical Society.

If vestibular suppressants are selected, it is imperative to limit the treatment duration because these agents can impede vestibular functioning, vestibular recovery, and centralized compensatory mechanism. Vestibular and balance rehabilitation therapy (VBRT) is also effective in the treatment of various forms of dizziness (vertigo, disequilibrium, and nonspecific dizziness). VBRT focuses on balance training, core stabilization, and desensitization exercises. It is often performed by physical and occupational therapists.

Central Vertigo
Central vertigo is a frequently missed and potentially life-threatening diagnosis. It may be caused by vertebrobasilar stroke (posterior circulation ischemic or hemorrhagic events), migraine, central nervous system infection, trauma (concussion, traumatic brain injury), demyelinating disease (multiple sclerosis), and chronic alcoholism.

Patients with central vertigo secondary to vertebrobasilar stroke frequently display concomitant neurologic findings in addition to vertigo, such as nystagmus, dysphagia, dysarthria, diplopia, ataxia, postural instability, hemiparesis, and mental status changes. A normal result on a head impulse test, direction-changing nystagmus, or skew deviation in the HINTS assessment additionally suggest a central cause of vertigo. Roughly 20% of patients with vertebrobasilar stroke present with isolated vertigo, and studies have shown that up to one third of cases of vertebrobasilar stroke that manifest as isolated vertigo are misclassified as peripheral vertigo. Risk factors for posterior circulation stroke include advanced age, atrial fibrillation, diabetes, peripheral vascular disease, hypertension, and hyperlipidemia. To a lesser extent, neurologic findings may also be present in patients with other central processes, but they are not present in peripherally mediated forms of vertigo.

Advanced imaging should be performed in patients with central vertigo. MRI is more sensitive than CT in detecting ischemic stroke and can detect infarction in the posterior fossa on the first day. CT can provide an effective and expedited evaluation of hemorrhagic stroke, although hemorrhagic vertebrobasilar stroke accounts for a very small minority of cases of centrally mediated vertigo.

Presyncope
Presyncope is a temporary reduction in global cerebral perfusion, leading to symptoms of lightheadedness, dizziness, visual changes (tunnel vision), auditory changes, a sense of impending doom, warmth, nausea, and near loss of consciousness. Patients often report the sensation of "almost blacking out." Postural tone is retained. In contrast, syncope is transient reduction in global cerebral perfusion, leading to a true loss of consciousness and loss of postural tone. Notably, patients with presyncope do not have vertiginous symptoms. The differential diagnosis for presyncope is similar to that of syncope (see Syncope).

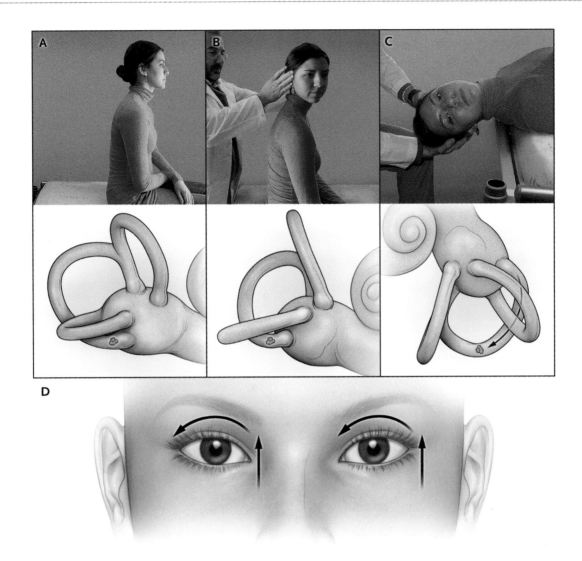

FIGURE 5. Use of the Dix-Hallpike maneuver to induce nystagmus in benign paroxysmal positional vertigo involving the right posterior semicircular canal. With the patient sitting upright (A), the head is turned 45 degrees to the patient's right (B). The patient is then moved from the sitting position to the supine position with the head hanging below the top end of the examination table at an angle of 20 degrees (C). The resulting nystagmus would be upbeat and torsional, with the top poles of the eyes beating toward the lower (right) ear (D).

Reproduced with permission from Kim JS, Zee DS. Clinical practice. Benign paroxysmal positional vertigo. N Engl J Med. 2014;370:1142. [PMID: 24645946] doi:10.1056/NEJMcp1309481. Copyright 2014, Massachusetts Medical Society.

TABLE 39.	Interpretation of the Dix-Hallpike Maneuver	
Findings	**Peripheral Disease**	**Central Disease**
Latency of nystagmus[a]	Delayed	No delay
Duration of nystagmus	<1 min	>1 min
Fatigability of nystagmus[b]	Fatigable	Not fatigable
Direction of nystagmus	Unidirectional or mixed upbeat-torsional	Variable (vertical or horizontal)
Severity of symptoms	More severe	Less severe

[a]Time to onset of nystagmus after positioning the patient.

[b]Decrease in the intensity and duration of nystagmus with repeated maneuvers.

Disequilibrium

Disequilibrium refers to a sensation of imbalance or unsteadiness that is primarily experienced during positional changes, standing, or walking and is relieved with sitting or lying down. Disequilibrium predominantly affects older adults, and its prevalence increases with age. Falls are four times more likely in patients with disequilibrium and are, in turn, associated with significant morbidity, functional decline, and fear of future falls.

The etiology of disequilibrium is thought to be multifactorial, involving visual and auditory impairment; muscle weakness or atrophy; physical deconditioning; pain; and impairment in proprioception, balance, and gait. Brain imaging (MRI) studies of patients with disequilibrium have shown significantly more subcortical white matter lesions and frontal

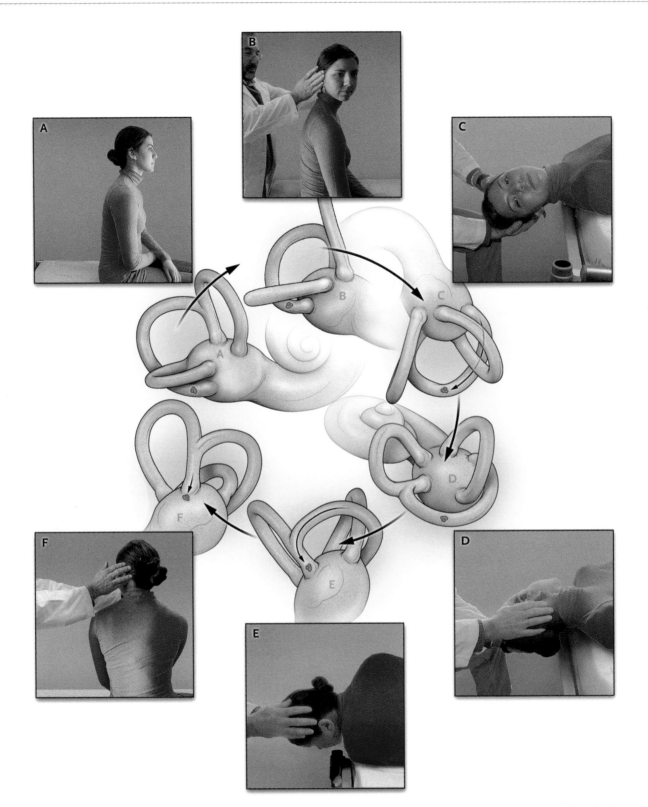

FIGURE 6. Epley canalith-repositioning maneuver for the treatment of benign paroxysmal positional vertigo involving the right posterior semicircular canal. After resolution of the induced nystagmus with the use of the right-sided Dix-Hallpike maneuver (A, B, and C), the head is turned 90 degrees toward the unaffected left side (D), causing the otolithic debris to move closer to the common crus. The induced nystagmus, if present, would be in the same direction as that evoked during the Dix-Hallpike maneuver. The head is then turned another 90 degrees, to a face-down position, and the trunk is turned 90 degrees in the same direction, so that the patient is lying on the unaffected side (E); the otolithic debris migrates in the same direction. The patient is then moved to the sitting position (F), and the otolithic debris falls into the vestibule, through the common crus. Each position should be maintained until the induced nystagmus and vertigo resolve but always for a minimum of 30 seconds.

Reproduced with permission from Kim JS, Zee DS. Clinical practice. Benign paroxysmal positional vertigo. N Engl J Med. 2014;370:1144. [PMID: 24645946] doi:10.1056/NEJMcp1309481. Copyright 2014, Massachusetts Medical Society.

atrophy than in patients without disequilibrium, although the significance of these findings is unclear.

Given the multifactorial nature of disequilibrium, treatment should be multifaceted. Treatment options include visual and auditory corrective measures (such as eye glasses and hearing aids), medication review (assessment of side effect profiles), mobility aids, physical therapy (balance and gait training), weight-bearing and resistive exercises, and fall prevention counseling.

Persistent Postural-Perceptual Dizziness

Dizziness that remains nonspecific despite a thorough history, examination, and evaluation is referred to as persistent postural-perceptual dizziness (PPPD, formerly chronic subjective dizziness). PPPD is described as persistent, nonvertiginous dizziness or imbalance that worsens with personal motion, upright positioning, and movement of objects in the surrounding environment. Symptoms must be present on most days for at least 3 months. It is most often preceded by another vestibular process (BPPV, vestibular neuronitis, vestibular migraine, or stroke), trauma (concussion or traumatic brain injury), infection, or certain psychiatric conditions (anxiety, panic disorder, or major depression). Approximately 75% of patients with PPPD have concomitant anxiety or depressive symptoms.

Treatment options for PPPD include pharmacologic therapies, such as selective serotonin reuptake inhibitors and serotonin-norepinephrine reuptake inhibitors, and ongoing VBRT.

KEY POINTS

- **HVC** • The diagnostic test of choice for benign paroxysmal positional vertigo is the Dix-Hallpike maneuver, which can help differentiate between peripheral and central causes of vertigo; routine imaging is not recommended.

- **HVC** • First-line therapy for benign paroxysmal positional vertigo is canalith repositioning with the Epley maneuver; vestibular and balance rehabilitation therapy is also effective.

- • Patients with central vertigo may display focal neurologic findings; however, approximately 20% of patients with vertebrobasilar stroke present with isolated vertigo.

- • In acute vertigo, the examination should include an in-depth neurologic assessment as well as the HINTS (Head Impulse, Nystagmus, and Test of Skew) oculomotor assessment.

- **HVC** • In patients with central vertigo, MRI is more sensitive than CT in detecting ischemic stroke, whereas CT provides an expedited, cost-effective assessment for hemorrhagic stroke.

- • Treatment options for disequilibrium include visual and auditory corrective measures, medication review, mobility aids, physical therapy, weight-bearing and resistive exercises, and fall prevention counseling.

Syncope

Syncope is complete and transient loss of consciousness and postural tone due to global cerebral hypoperfusion resulting from a decrease in cardiac output or systemic vascular resistance. The onset of syncope is sudden and abrupt, and recovery is rapid, with a complete return to the baseline level of functioning. Syncope is a very common medical condition, with a reported cumulative incidence of 3% to 6% over a 10-year period. Approximately 40% of adults have experienced a syncopal event, and 80% of these patients had a first episode before age 30 years. Although the Framingham Heart Study found that 44% of patients who experienced a syncopal event did not seek medical care, a recent 2014 financial analysis showed that the diagnostic and therapeutic costs associated with syncope exceed $4.1 billion annually in the United States.

Classification

Syncope can be classified according to the specific etiology of the event as neurally mediated (reflex), cardiovascular, orthostatic, neurologic, psychogenic, or idiopathic. These etiologies can be further subdivided according to the specific pathophysiologic mechanism. Approximately 40% of syncopal events are unexplained (idiopathic). Historical characteristics that are associated with increased probability of cardiac and noncardiac causes are detailed in **Table 40**.

Neurally mediated syncope, or reflex syncope, is the most common form of syncope and is seen primarily in younger adults. The underlying syncopal mechanism, termed the neurocardiogenic or vasodepressor reflex, is a response of vasodilation, bradycardia, and systemic hypotension, which leads to transient hypoperfusion of the brain. Neurally mediated syncope includes vasovagal syncope, which may be provoked by noxious stimuli, fear, stress, or heat overexposure; situational syncope, which is triggered by cough, micturition, defecation, or deglutition; and carotid sinus hypersensitivity, which is sometimes experienced during head rotation, shaving, or use of a tight-fitting neck collar. Prodromal symptoms, including nausea and diaphoresis, are classically present before the syncopal event, and fatigue and generalized weakness are typically present afterward.

Cardiovascular syncope is the second most common form of syncope and is associated with increased morbidity, mortality (including sudden death), and direct traumatic injury. Cardiovascular syncopal events often occur suddenly and usually without a significant prodrome, although chest pain and palpitations may be present. Causes of cardiovascular syncope include cardiac arrhythmia; coronary artery disease; and structural and obstructive disease, including aortic and pulmonary valve stenosis, obstructive hypertrophic cardiomyopathy, aortic dissection, and cardiac tamponade. Pulmonary embolism is increasingly appreciated as a cause of syncope, with a prevalence as high as 17% in some studies.

Orthostatic syncope is the third most common form of syncope and predominantly affects older adults. It classically

TABLE 40. Historical Characteristics Associated With Increased Probability of Cardiac and Noncardiac Causes of Syncope

More Often Associated With Cardiac Causes of Syncope

Older age (>60 y)

Male sex

Presence of known ischemic heart disease, structural heart disease, previous arrhythmias, or reduced ventricular function

Brief prodrome, such as palpitations, or sudden loss of consciousness without prodrome

Syncope during exertion

Syncope in the supine position

Low number of syncope episodes (one or two)

Abnormal cardiac examination

Family history of inheritable conditions or premature sudden cardiac death (<50 y of age)

Presence of known congenital heart disease

More Often Associated With Noncardiac Causes of Syncope

Younger age

No known cardiac disease

Syncope only in the standing position

Positional change from supine or sitting to standing

Presence of prodrome: nausea, vomiting, feeling of warmth

Presence of specific triggers: dehydration, pain, distressful stimulus, medical environment

Situational triggers: cough, laugh, micturition, defecation, deglutition

Frequent recurrence and prolonged history of syncope with similar characteristics

Reproduced with permission from Shen WK, Sheldon RS, Benditt DG, Cohen MI, Forman DE, Goldberger ZD, et al. 2017 ACC/AHA/HRS guideline for the evaluation and management of patients with syncope: executive summary: a report of the American College of Cardiology/American Heart Association Task Force on Clinical Practice Guidelines and the Heart Rhythm Society. Circulation. 2017;136:e32. [PMID: 28280232] doi:10.1161/CIR.0000000000000498. Copyright 2017, American Heart Association, Inc.

occurs after changes in position and is typically associated with prodromal symptoms, such as lightheadedness. Orthostatic syncope is most commonly caused by hypovolemia, medications, and alcohol intoxication. Less commonly, primary autonomic failure (Parkinson disease, multiple system atrophy, multiple sclerosis) or secondary autonomic failure (diabetes, amyloidosis, connective tissue disease, spinal cord injury) can lead to neurogenic orthostatic syncope.

Neurologic conditions are a rare cause of syncope. Cerebrovascular events (transient ischemic attack, ischemic or hemorrhagic stroke), seizures, and direct head trauma may lead to transient loss of consciousness but should be distinguished from true syncope. Cerebrovascular events that lead to true syncope primarily involve the posterior (vertebrobasilar) circulation and usually present with concomitant symptoms of dizziness, vertigo, gait changes, and focal neurologic findings. Anterior circulation involvement rarely leads to syncope.

Seizures can be confused with syncope, and bystander information can help distinguish between these two events. A prospective study demonstrated that the features most suggestive of a seizure in patients with loss of consciousness were witnessed abnormal posturing, involuntary head turning, and tongue laceration. Auras, incontinence, and prolonged postepisode confusion also favor a seizure.

Psychogenic syncope, which has also been referred to as pseudosyncope, generally occurs in younger patients with underlying anxiety, panic disorder, or depression.

Evaluation

The American Heart Association (AHA), American College of Cardiology (ACC), and Heart Rhythm Society (HRS) jointly conclude that the history and physical examination are the most important diagnostic tools in determining the underlying cause of a syncopal event. The history should focus on eliciting prodromal or postepisode symptoms, comorbid medical or psychiatric conditions, the psychosocial context of the event, and bystander information. A thorough review of the patient's prescription and over-the-counter medications should also be completed.

The physical examination should include an in-depth cardiovascular evaluation, including orthostatic (postural) blood pressure measurements, as well as a basic neurologic examination to evaluate for focal defects. Carotid hypersensitivity can be assessed in individuals older than 40 years with syncope of unknown cause with the use of carotid sinus massage; however, this technique is contraindicated in patients with known carotid disease or recent transient ischemic attack/stroke within the past 3 months.

The AHA/ACC/HRS syncope guideline recommends that electrocardiography be performed in all patients with syncope to identify an underlying arrhythmia, myocardial ischemia, or QT prolongation. Generally, additional studies have a low diagnostic yield; however, when there is a moderate to high pretest probability of a specific condition, these studies can help to identify or confirm a diagnosis (**Figure 7**). Echocardiography is indicated to detect suspected valvular heart disease, hypertrophic cardiomyopathy, and reduced left ventricular function. An exercise stress test is most likely to be helpful in patients with exercise-related syncope. Electrocardiographic monitoring (with an ambulatory monitor, event monitor, or implantable loop recorder) should be considered in selected patients with a probable arrhythmic cause; the choice of test is based on the frequency and nature of the syncopal event (see MKSAP 18 Cardiovascular Medicine). Targeted laboratory studies are guided by findings in the history and physical examination. Tilt-table testing is most commonly useful in patients suspected of having recurrent vasovagal syncope or when the initial evaluation of delayed orthostatic hypotension is not diagnostic. Cardiac imaging with CT or MRI is most useful when structural or infiltrative heart disease is suspected but initial diagnostic tests are inconclusive. CT angiography is

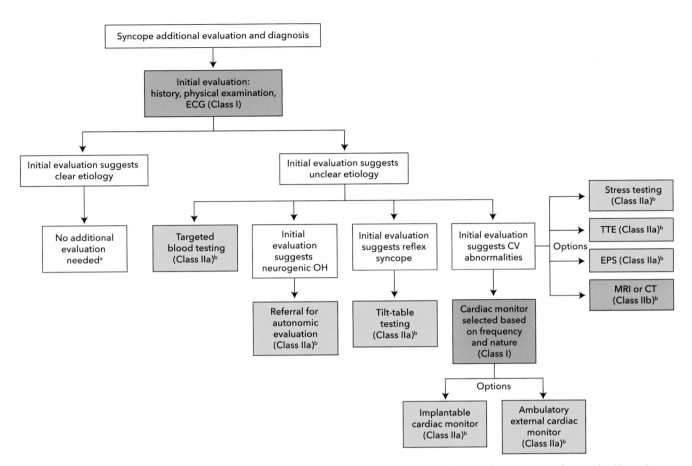

FIGURE 7. Additional evaluation and diagnosis of syncope. Colors correspond to class (strength) of recommendation, with green corresponding to a class I (strong) recommendation, yellow corresponding to a class IIa (moderate) recommendation, and orange corresponding to a class IIb (weak) recommendation. CV = cardiovascular; ECG = electrocardiography; EPS = electrophysiology study; OH = orthostatic hypotension; TTE = transthoracic echocardiography.

[a]Applies to patients after a normal initial evaluation without significant injury or cardiovascular morbidities; patients should be followed up by a primary care physician as needed.

[b]In selected patients.

Reproduced with permission from Shen WK, Sheldon RS, Benditt DG, Cohen MI, Forman DE, Goldberger ZD, et al. 2017 ACC/AHA/HRS guideline for the evaluation and management of patients with syncope: executive summary: a report of the American College of Cardiology/American Heart Association Task Force on Clinical Practice Guidelines and the Heart Rhythm Society. Circulation. 2017;136:e25-e59. [PMID: 28280232] doi:10.1161/CIR.0000000000000498. Copyright 2017, American Heart Association, Inc.

indicated for patients with a high pretest probability of pulmonary embolism. Electrophysiology studies are reserved for patients suspected of having an arrhythmic cause of syncope, and electroencephalography should be based on the specific clinical scenario. The American College of Physicians (ACP) recommends against routinely obtaining brain imaging (CT or MRI) in cases of syncope that do not involve objective focal neurologic findings. Carotid duplex ultrasonography plays no role in the evaluation of a patient with syncope.

Risk Stratification and Decision for Hospital Admission

The AHA/ACC/HRS syncope guideline recommends evaluation to determine the cause of syncope and assessment of the patient's short- and long-term morbidity and mortality risk. Short-term adverse events and deaths are mainly determined by the underlying cause and the effectiveness of the treatment. Risk scores have been developed to assist in risk stratification

and to guide patient disposition; however, they generally do not outperform unstructured clinical judgment. The presence of high-risk clinical characteristics should prompt consideration of hospitalization (**Table 41**). Patients with likely reflex-mediated syncope who do not have serious underlying medical conditions can usually be managed in the outpatient setting.

Management

The management of syncope depends on the underlying cause. In cases of neurally mediated syncope, clinicians should provide reassurance and counsel patients to avoid provoking measures. Physical counterpressure techniques, such as leg crossing, squatting, or handgrip maneuvers, can be beneficial in patients with neurally mediated syncope and a prolonged prodrome. The management of cardiovascular syncope should target the specific underlying cause. Orthostatic syncope may be treated with volume expansion (with salt liberalization, if appropriate), reconsideration of contributing medications, compression

TABLE 41. High-Risk Clinical Characteristics in the Patient With Syncope[a]

Syncope during exertion

Syncope in supine position

Symptoms of chest discomfort or palpitations before syncope

Family history of sudden death

History of heart failure, aortic stenosis, left ventricular outflow tract disease, dilated cardiomyopathy, hypertrophic cardiomyopathy, arrhythmogenic right ventricular cardiomyopathy, ventricular arrhythmia, coronary artery disease, congenital heart disease, pulmonary hypertension, left ventricular ejection fraction <35%, implantable cardioverter-defibrillator placement

New or previously unknown left bundle branch block, bifascicular block, Brugada pattern, findings consistent with acute ischemia, nonsinus rhythm, prolonged QTc interval (>450 ms)

Hemoglobin <9 g/dL (90 g/L)

Systolic blood pressure <90 mm Hg

Sinus bradycardia <40/min

QTc = corrected QT interval.

[a]A patient is considered at high cardiac risk if any of the above risk factors are present.

Information from Costantino G, Sun BC, Barbic F, Bossi I, Casazza G, Dipaola F, et al. Syncope clinical management in the emergency department: a consensus from the first international workshop on syncope risk stratification in the emergency department. Eur Heart J. 2016;37:1493-8. [PMID: 26242712] doi:10.1093/eurheartj/ehv378

CONT.

stockings, and education on postural changes. Initiation of additional vasoactive agents, such as fludrocortisone or midodrine, can be considered; however, available evidence on their efficacy is limited and conflicting. In cases of psychogenic syncope, referral to a mental health specialist is appropriate.

Prognosis

The underlying cause of the syncopal event determines the prognosis. Patients with a syncopal episode are at increased risk for all-cause mortality (hazard ratio [HR], 1.3; 95% CI, 1.1-1.5) and cardiovascular events (HR, 1.3; 95% CI, 1.0-1.6). The risk for death is even greater in cases of cardiac syncope (HR, 2.0; 95% CI, 1.5-2.7). Neurally mediated and orthostatic syncope do not portend increased cardiovascular mortality. Syncope of any cause, especially if recurrent, can severely affect quality of life, functional independence, and self-confidence. Clinicians should assess for any ensuing mood changes, the need for skilled assistance, and the need for possible driving restrictions (which vary per state law).

KEY POINTS

HVC
- The history and physical examination, including orthostatic (postural) blood pressure measurement, are the most important diagnostic tools in determining the underlying cause of a syncopal event.

- All patients with syncope should undergo electrocardiography to identify underlying arrhythmia, ischemia, or QT prolongation.

(Continued)

KEY POINTS *(continued)*

- Echocardiography, ischemia evaluation, electrocardiographic monitoring, chest radiography, tilt-table testing, electroencephalography, and laboratory studies have low diagnostic yield for the cause of syncope and should be performed only when there is a moderate to high pretest probability of a specific underlying condition. **HVC**

- The American College of Physicians recommends against routinely obtaining brain imaging (CT or MRI) in cases of syncope that do not involve objective focal neurologic findings. **HVC**

- Neurally mediated syncope is treated with reassurance and avoidance of provoking measures; physical counterpressure techniques can be useful in patients with a prolonged prodrome. **HVC**

- Orthostatic syncope may be treated with volume expansion (with salt liberalization, if appropriate), reconsideration of contributing medications, compression stockings, and education on postural changes.

Insomnia

Insomnia is a complex health problem that affects many adults. Symptoms of insomnia vary and may include poor sleep quality, frustration with sleep quantity, difficulty initiating sleep, or an inability to return to sleep after awakening. The prevalence of insomnia increases with age, and women tend to be affected more than men. Medical disorders, including cardiopulmonary diseases, neurodegenerative disorders, and psychiatric disorders, are often implicated in sleep disruption. Medications and other substances also commonly contribute to symptoms of insomnia, and clinicians should screen for common culprits (such as caffeine, alcohol, glucocorticoids, diuretics, and antidepressants).

Chronic insomnia is diagnosed by the presence of symptoms that (1) cause substantial functional distress or impairment; (2) occur at least 3 nights per week for at least 3 months; and (3) are not associated with other sleep, medical, or mental disorders. Although 1 in 10 adults meet the diagnostic criteria for chronic insomnia, some studies have shown that up to 50% of adults report experiencing sleep symptoms.

Evaluation

Given the wide range of patients affected and the significant impact insufficient sleep can have on function, all patients should be asked about problems of sleep disruption. In patients with symptoms of insomnia, a thorough history and physical examination may point to potentially reversible causes, such as sleep apnea or restless legs syndrome. Eliciting an accurate medication history, including use of over-the-counter medications, herbal supplements, caffeine, alcohol, tobacco, and illicit drugs, is also an important part of the diagnostic approach. Physicians should obtain information on sleep pattern, including sleep difficulties (sleep initiation, sleep maintenance, sleep quality) and environmental factors (work schedule). There is increasing evidence that screen time, such as smart phone and tablet use, before bed can alter circadian patterns and increase symptoms of insomnia, and use of electronics should be assessed. A sleep diary can facilitate collection of an accurate sleep history, and obtaining a collateral history from the patient's sleep partner may shed light on specific sleep-related disorders.

Diagnostic testing, such as polysomnography, is not a first-line approach unless guided by specific findings on the history and physical examination or directed by a sleep specialist.

Treatment

The goals of treatment of insomnia are to improve overall sleep and quality of life. Effective treatment programs are multimodal in their approach and include cognitive behavioral therapy for insomnia (CBT-I), sleep hygiene techniques, environmental changes, and, in poorly controlled cases, pharmacologic therapy.

Nonpharmacologic Treatments

The ACP recommends CBT-I as first-line therapy for insomnia. This multicomponent therapy includes cognitive therapy (to address maladaptive beliefs and expectations about sleep), educational interventions (such as sleep hygiene), and behavioral interventions (such as sleep restriction therapy, stimulus-control therapy, and relaxation techniques). It may be delivered in various formats, such as individual or group therapy, web-based modules, or written materials. CBT-I provides significant value over pharmacologic-driven approaches and carries little risk for adverse effects.

Sleep hygiene strategies focus on optimizing environmental factors (instituting stable bed times and rising times); reducing stimuli (limiting screen time [television, laptop computers, and cell phones] and creating a dark environment) around bedtime; avoiding caffeine, alcohol, and nicotine before bedtime; reducing daytime naps; and limiting the bedroom activities to intimacy and sleep. Sleep restriction therapy, which entails limiting the amount of time in bed to increase sleep efficiency, may also be used.

Pharmacologic Therapy

The ACP recommends that physicians engage in a thorough shared decision-making process to decide whether to add pharmacologic therapies in patients with insomnia refractory to CBT-I. Several pharmacologic agents have been demonstrated to improve sleep latency and total sleep time (**Table 42**), but few studies have examined their overall impact on function and quality of life. Pharmacologic therapy is also associated with harms, including daytime drowsiness, increased risk for falls and hip fracture, and medication-related hallucinations. Factors that should be considered before initiating pharmacologic therapy for insomnia are included in **Table 43**. Medications ideally should be taken in short-term trials (no more than 4-5 weeks).

Patients frequently use over-the-counter medications, such as sedating antihistamines, for insomnia despite associated anticholinergic side effects and carry-over daytime sleepiness. Because of the risk for side effects, antihistamines are not recommended in the treatment of insomnia, especially in older adults, in whom the risk is magnified. Melatonin may be effective for circadian rhythm disruptions affecting sleep and has a more favorable side effect profile than antihistamines. Although melatonin is often recommended to older adults owing to the lower risk for side effects, there is insufficient evidence to support its use in this population.

Benzodiazepines induce sedation by activating inhibitory γ-aminobutyric acid (GABA) receptors. These drugs decrease sleep latency and have a sleep-promoting effect, although onset and effect differ between agents. The associated risk for rebound insomnia, addiction potential, and side effect profile make benzodiazepines poor candidates for treatment of insomnia, particularly in combination with other sedating agents (including opioids) and in geriatric populations.

Nonbenzodiazepine GABA-receptor agonists are typically more selective in their activity at the GABA receptor and represent a large class of medications for insomnia. These agents (zolpidem, eszopiclone, and zaleplon) have a rapid onset of action and short half-life, making them better choices for patients with difficulty initiating sleep. Long-acting formulations and formulations meant for use with middle-of-the-night awakenings are also available. There is potential for prolonged impaired driving skills and somnolence with their use, and there are few data on the long-term safety or efficacy of these agents.

KEY POINTS

- Diagnostic testing, such as polysomnography, is usually unnecessary in the evaluation of insomnia, unless guided by specific findings on the history and physical examination or directed by a sleep specialist. **HVC**

- First-line therapy for insomnia is cognitive behavioral therapy, which includes cognitive therapy, educational interventions, and behavioral interventions. **HVC**

- Sleep hygiene strategies for insomnia focus on optimizing environmental factors; reducing stimuli around bedtime; avoiding caffeine, alcohol, and nicotine before bedtime; reducing daytime naps; and limiting the bedroom activities to intimacy and sleep. **HVC**

- Pharmacologic therapies for insomnia are associated with adverse effects and should only be initiated in patients with insomnia refractory to nonpharmacologic interventions. **HVC**

Lower Extremity Edema

Lower extremity edema is a common symptom in both the inpatient and outpatient settings. Resulting from accumulation of interstitial fluid in the most dependent part of the body, lower extremity edema may be secondary to several different

TABLE 42.	FDA-Approved Prescription Drug Treatment for Insomnia			
Agent[a]	Usual Dosage	Onset of Action[b]	Duration of Action[c]	Notes
Benzodiazepines (oral)				
Estazolam (generic)	1-2 mg	Slow	Intermediate	
Flurazepam (generic)	15-30 mg	Rapid	Long	
Quazepam (generic)	7.5-15 mg	Slow	Long	
Temazepam (generic)	7.5-30 mg	Slow	Intermediate	
Triazolam (generic)	0.125-0.5 mg	Rapid	Short	Short-acting benzodiazepines have been associated with an increased risk for anterograde amnesia
Nonbenzodiazepines				
Zolpidem				
Oral tablet (generic)	5-10 mg	Rapid	Short	
Extended-release oral tablet (generic)	6.25-12.5 mg	Rapid	Intermediate	
Sublingual				
Intermezzo	1.75-3.5 mg	Rapid	Ultra-short	Indicated for as-needed use for treatment of middle-of-the-night insomnia with ≥4 h of sleep time remaining
Edluar	10 mg	Rapid	Short	
Oral spray (Zolpimist)	10 mg	Rapid	Short	
Eszopiclone (generic)	1-3 mg	Rapid	Intermediate	The recommended initial dosage was reduced to 1 mg because of prolonged impaired driving skills, memory, and coordination at the previously recommended 3-mg dosage
Zaleplon (generic)	10-20 mg	Rapid	Short	
Orexin-Receptor Antagonist				
Suvorexant (Belsomra)	5-20 mg	Slow	Long	The recommended initial dosage is 10 mg; the daily dosage should not exceed 20 mg
Antidepressant				
Doxepin (Silenor)	3-6 mg	Rapid	Intermediate	
Melatonin Agonist				
Ramelteon (Rozerem)	8 mg	Rapid	Short	

[a]All agents classified as schedule C-IV by the Drug Enforcement Agency (DEA) except doxepin and ramelteon, which are not scheduled.

[b]Onset of action: rapid = 15-30 minutes; slow = 30-60 minutes.

[c]Based on elimination half-life and preparation: short = 1-5 hours; intermediate = 5-12 hours; long = >12 hours.

Adapted with permission from Masters PA. In the clinic. Insomnia. Ann Intern Med. 2014;161:ITC9. [PMID: 25285559] doi:10.7326/0003-4819-161-7-201410070-01004. Copyright 2014, American College of Physicians.

pathophysiologic mechanisms, including increased capillary hydrostatic pressure, increased capillary permeability, and decreased plasma oncotic pressure. Obstruction of the lymphatic system is a less common mechanism of edema.

The most common causes of lower extremity edema include venous obstruction or insufficiency, heart failure (including right-sided heart failure secondary to pulmonary disease), cirrhosis, nephrotic syndrome and hypoalbuminemia of other etiologies, and use of certain medications (**Table 44**). If lower extremity edema is unilateral, it is usually the result of a mechanical obstruction to venous or lymphatic flow, such as venous thrombosis or malignancy.

A detailed history and physical examination will suggest the cause of lower extremity edema in most patients. Reasonable initial laboratory testing includes measurement of kidney and liver function, urinalysis (for detection of protein), and albumin measurement. The decision to pursue further testing, including echocardiography, lower extremity Doppler ultrasonography, and advanced imaging should be guided by the findings on the initial evaluation.

Chronic Venous Insufficiency

Chronic venous insufficiency is a condition in which the veins or valves in the lower extremities are incompetent, resulting in

TABLE 43. Factors to Consider When Prescribing Drugs to Treat Insomnia

Use the minimal effective dosage.
Avoid long-half-life medications, including long-half-life metabolites.
Be aware of potential interactions between drugs, including over-the-counter drugs.
Caution patients who are receiving these medications about interaction with alcohol.
Review potential side effects—in particular, daytime sleepiness.
Confer with the patient to determine an appropriate period of use.
Use a γ-aminobutyric acid agonist before other sedative-hypnotics for treatment of acute or short-term insomnia.
Look for rebound insomnia after discontinuation.
Consider intermittent or long-term use of hypnotic medications, depending on the clinical situation.
Consider consulting a sleep specialist before starting long-term therapy with hypnotic medication.

Adapted with permission from Masters PA. In the clinic. Insomnia. Ann Intern Med. 2014;161:ITC1-15; quiz ITC16. [PMID: 25285559] doi:10.7326/0003-4819-161-7-201410070-01004. Copyright 2014, American College of Physicians.

pooling of blood in the legs. It is most commonly caused by venous hypertension, but it may also be congenital. Symptoms include aching, itching, restlessness, leg heaviness, leg swelling, and pain.

A thorough history and physical examination should be performed. The examination may reveal edema, dilated veins (both varicosities and superficial telangiectasias), thin or hyperpigmented skin, and ulceration. Physical findings are best observed in the gravity-dependent upright position. Chronic venous insufficiency is a clinical diagnosis, but venous duplex Doppler ultrasonography can be used if the diagnosis is in doubt and in those considering intervention. Air plethysmography, which uses air displacement in a cuff surrounding the calf to measure venous outflow and filling, can be used when venous duplex ultrasonography is nondiagnostic or to guide therapy.

Conservative measures, including exercise, leg elevation, lifestyle changes (weight loss), and gradient compression stockings (20-50 mm Hg depending on the stage of disease) are first-line therapies. The presence of skin changes or ulceration should prompt at least 30 mm Hg of compression. To increase patient adherence, knee-length stockings are prescribed, and if used daily with an alternate pair, stockings should be replaced every 6 to 9 months. Skin care is also an important part of management, and daily use of topical moisturizers may reduce skin breakdown and prevent infection. Stasis dermatitis may require sparing use of a topical steroid (see MKSAP 18 Dermatology). Wound care, including use of hydrocolloids and foam dressings, is essential to control drainage from ulcers and to prevent maceration of the surrounding skin. Many drugs, including pentoxifylline and horse chestnut

extracts, have been studied for chronic venous insufficiency; however, none are FDA approved for this condition. Patients with bothersome spider veins and small varicose veins can undergo sclerotherapy, thermocoagulation, or laser therapy. Patients with confirmed reflux and persistent symptoms despite conservative therapy may be treated with venous ablation, stripping or excision, or, in the case of stenosis and obstruction, stenting. Surgical options can be considered for those with symptoms refractory to medical and endovenous therapies.

KEY POINTS

- The most common causes of lower extremity edema include venous obstruction or insufficiency, heart failure, cirrhosis, nephrotic syndrome and hypoalbuminemia of other etiologies, and use of certain medications.
- Conservative measures, including exercise, leg elevation, lifestyle changes, and compression stockings, are first-line therapies for chronic venous insufficiency. **HVC**

Common In-Flight Emergencies

In-flight medical emergencies are relatively common during air travel, occurring in an estimated 1 in 600 flights. In the United States, physicians are not legally mandated to assist in the event of an in-flight emergency, although some countries do impose such obligations. The laws of the country in which the aircraft is registered usually prevail. Ethically, physicians should provide assistance as able. The Aviation Medical Assistance Act of 1998 includes a Good Samaritan provision that protects individuals who are medically qualified "from liability for rendering assistance unless that person is engaged in gross negligence or willful misconduct," such as providing care while intoxicated. Providers should practice within their scope of training, be mindful of patient privacy, and document the patient encounter.

Physicians who respond to an in-flight emergency typically have access to several medical resources. Most airlines have contracts with 24-hour call centers, and ground-based physicians trained in emergency or aerospace medicine can assist the on-board physician remotely and help direct care. Additionally, flight crews are required to receive cardiopulmonary resuscitation training, including training on the use of automated external defibrillators, and to be familiar with first-aid equipment. If the patient's condition is critical, the physician can recommend diversion of the flight to the nearest airport, although the ultimate decision rests with the aircraft captain.

Airlines based in the United States are mandated by the Federal Aviation Administration to carry at least one automated external defibrillator, supplemental oxygen, and a medical kit that contains a stethoscope, sphygmomanometer, gloves, airway supplies, intravenous access supplies (needles, syringes, saline), and some basic medications (epinephrine, lidocaine,

TABLE 44. Differential Diagnosis of Lower Extremity Edema

Condition or Cause	Clinical Presentation	Diagnostic Testing
Chronic venous insufficiency	Gradual-onset leg aching/heaviness that is more likely to improve with elevation/recumbency and walking (decreased venous pressure)	Duplex ultrasonography if considering intervention
	Edema (most commonly bilateral but can be unilateral) that usually spares forefoot	
	Hyperpigmentation (hemosiderin deposits); telangiectasias, reticular veins, varicose veins; eczematous dermatitis and lipodermatosclerosis leading to ulceration, especially over the medial malleolus	
Heart failure	Dyspnea, orthopnea, paroxysmal nocturnal dyspnea, elevated jugular venous pressure, lung crackles, ventricular gallop, symmetric pitting edema	Echocardiography
Kidney disease	Symmetric pitting edema	Urinalysis, random urine albumin-creatinine ratio, serum creatinine level
Liver disease	Symmetric pitting edema, ascites, spider angiomas, palmar erythema, jaundice/icterus	Liver chemistry tests, albumin level, INR
Hypothyroidism	Symptoms of hypothyroidism, nonpitting bilateral edema	Thyroid-stimulating hormone level, serum thyroxine
Lymphedema (bilateral)	Brawny induration; pitting edema present initially; nonpitting present late in process; involves feet (square toes)	Can consider CT or the abdomen/pelvis, lymphoscintigraphy
	Kaposi-Stemmer sign (inability to pinch a fold of skin on the dorsal surface of the base of the second toe)	
Lipedema	Fatty tissue accumulation, nonpitting edema that spares the feet	
Pregnancy	Symmetric pitting edema	
Obstructive sleep apnea	Daytime sleepiness, snoring, witnessed apnea, neck circumference >43 cm (17 in), symmetric pitting edema	Polysomnography
Pulmonary hypertension	Exertional dyspnea, elevated jugular venous distention, prominent jugular venous a wave, widened split S_2	Echocardiography
Deep venous thrombosis	Unilateral, painful edema (most commonly) that may be tender on examination; typically pitting edema	D-dimer and/or lower extremity ultrasonography depending on pretest probability
	Should be strongly suspected with acute edema <72 h	
Drugs (vasodilators, NSAIDs, gabapentinoids, hormones, antiestrogens, thiazolidinediones)	Gradual-onset, bilateral pitting edema that usually improves with recumbency; one side may be larger than the other, particularly if there is more pronounced venous disease	No diagnostic testing; symptoms resolve within days of discontinuing the offending agent

atropine, aspirin, nitroglycerin, antihistamines, bronchodilators, and dextrose). Many U.S. airlines augment their kits with additional supplies. The contents of international kits may vary. Other passengers may volunteer their own medical supplies, such as prescription medications, injectable epinephrine pens, or glucometers. The physician must weigh the benefits of using another passenger's glucometer against the potential harms, including transmission of blood-borne pathogens. Passengers may also be able to help with translation, although it is important to respect patient privacy.

In most in-flight medical emergencies, the physician's role involves assessing the patient, establishing a diagnosis when possible, administering basic medical treatments, providing reassurance as appropriate, and recommending flight diversion if necessary. The most common in-flight emergencies include presyncope or syncope (typically vasovagal), gastrointestinal disorders (diarrhea and vomiting), cardiovascular symptoms, and respiratory symptoms (asthma and hyperventilation). In-flight cardiac arrest is rare, accounting for approximately 0.3% of in-flight emergencies; however, it is responsible for 86% of in-flight deaths. In the event of suspected acute myocardial infarction or stroke, immediate flight diversion should be recommended to the crew. Other frequently encountered issues include trauma caused by objects falling from overhead bins, hypoglycemia, psychiatric problems (most commonly anxiety or phobias), allergic reactions, seizures, headaches, and obstetric or gynecologic events. Several in-flight births occur each year.

KEY POINTS

- In the United States, physicians are not legally mandated to assist in the event of an in-flight emergency; however, physicians have an ethical obligation to provide assistance as able.
- The physician's role in in-flight emergencies involves assessing the patient, establishing a diagnosis when possible, administering basic medical treatments, providing reassurance as appropriate, and recommending flight diversion if necessary.

Musculoskeletal Pain
Low Back Pain
Diagnosis and Evaluation
Low back pain can be classified by duration as acute (<4 weeks), subacute (4-12 weeks), or chronic (>12 weeks). Approximately 90% of patients have nonspecific low back pain, in which no specific cause can be determined. The most common identifiable causes of low back pain are spinal stenosis, disk herniation, and compression fractures. Less common identifiable causes include cancer (vertebral metastases) and infection (diskitis, osteomyelitis, epidural abscess); visceral disease, such as nephrolithiasis, pyelonephritis, and abdominal aortic aneurysm, may also cause low back pain.

History and Physical Examination
Evaluation of patients with low back pain includes a detailed history directed toward factors that increase the likelihood of specific causes of pain (**Table 45**). Psychosocial factors may also affect the course of low back pain and should be assessed. Psychosocial distress; comorbid psychiatric conditions; somatization; and maladaptive coping strategies, such as avoiding work, are associated with poor clinical outcomes.

The physical examination should similarly search for evidence of an underlying disorder (see Table 45). Specific attention should be paid to "red flag" findings on examination, including fever and neurologic signs. A thorough neurologic examination, including strength, sensory, and reflex testing of the legs, in addition to performing both the ipsilateral and contralateral straight leg raise test (**Figure 8**), can identify patterns of deficits that point to lesions (most commonly disk herniation) at specific levels (**Table 46**). Similarly, decreased anal sphincter tone and perianal sensation raise concern for

cauda equina syndrome. Many of the examination findings, however, are insensitive or nonspecific for the presence of a specific underlying disorder.

Further Diagnostic Testing
Clinicians should not routinely obtain imaging and other diagnostic tests in patients with nonspecific low back pain. Obtaining imaging studies in these patients is not associated with clinically meaningful outcomes. Notably, imaging abnormalities are commonly present in asymptomatic individuals. They are also common in patients with nonspecific low back pain, and their presence may lead to unhelpful and unnecessary interventions.

In contrast, imaging is recommended when neurologic deficits are present or if serious underlying conditions are suspected. Plain radiography may be considered to evaluate for ankylosing spondylitis or vertebral compression fracture. When malignancy is suspected, the American College of Physicians recommends immediately obtaining plain radiography in addition to measuring the erythrocyte sedimentation rate. If results of these initial tests are negative and significant concern remains, MRI should then be obtained. Immediate MRI should be obtained when there are risk factors for spinal infection or concern for cord compression or cauda equina syndrome. In patients with persistent pain despite conservative measures, symptoms/signs of radiculopathy, or spinal stenosis, MRI or, less preferably, CT may be considered only if the patient is a potential candidate for surgical intervention or epidural glucocorticoid injection.

Treatment
Patient education is a key component in the treatment of low back pain regardless of duration. Education includes providing information on the expected course of the back pain, promoting self-management, addressing misconceptions, and encouraging physical activity as appropriate. In all patients with low back pain, bed rest should be avoided, and depressive features should be appropriately assessed and managed.

In addition to education, treatment modalities for patients with low back pain may include nonpharmacologic and/or pharmacologic therapies and, rarely, surgery. The interventions chosen should be based on the patient's signs, symptoms, and comorbid conditions.

Nonpharmacologic Treatment
Clinical guidelines consistently emphasize nonpharmacologic therapies as a cornerstone of therapy for acute and chronic low back pain. For acute low back pain, potentially useful nonpharmacologic therapies include local heat, massage, acupuncture, and spinal manipulation, although the evidence supporting these approaches is generally weak.

Multiple nonpharmacologic options are available for chronic low back pain, including exercise therapy, manual and massage therapy, acupuncture, yoga, intensive interdisciplinary therapy, and cognitive behavioral therapy, with varying

TABLE 45. History and Examination Features and Suggested Diagnoses in Low Back Pain

Suggested Diagnosis	History Features	Examination Features
Cancer	Personal history of malignancy	Vertebral tenderness
	Unexplained weight loss	
	Failure to improve after 1 mo	
	No relief with bed rest	
Infection	Fever	Fever
	Injection drug abuse	Vertebral tenderness
	Urinary tract infection	
	Skin infection	
Inflammatory/ rheumatologic condition	Onset before age 40 y	
	Gradual onset	
	Presence of morning stiffness	
	Pain not relieved when supine	
	Pain persisting for >3 mo	
	Involvement of other joints	
Nerve root irritation (radiculopathy)	Sciatica (pain that radiates from the back through the buttocks down into the leg[s])	Positive ipsilateral SLR (LR+ of 3.7)
	Increased pain with cough, sneeze, or Valsalva maneuver	Positive contralateral SLR (LR+ of 4.4)
Spinal stenosis	Severe leg pain	
	No pain when seated	
	Improvement in pain when bending forward	
	Pseudoclaudication[a] (worsened pain with walking or standing and relief with sitting)	
Compression fracture	Advanced age	Vertebral tenderness
	Trauma	
	Glucocorticoid use	
	Osteoporosis	
Cauda equina syndrome[b]	Bowel or bladder dysfunction	Decreased anal sphincter tone
	Perineal (saddle) sensory loss	Decreased perineal/perianal sensation
	Rapidly progressive neurologic deficits	

LR+ = positive likelihood ratio; SLR = straight leg raise.

[a]Lower extremity symptoms caused by lumbar spinal stenosis mimicking vascular ischemia; also termed neurogenic claudication.

[b]Compression of the lumbar and sacral nerves below the termination of the spinal cord (conus medullaris). Characterized by back pain; sensory changes in the S3 to S5 dermatomes (saddle anesthesia); bowel, bladder, and sexual dysfunction; and absent Achilles tendon reflexes bilaterally.

levels of predominantly weak evidence supporting these approaches. The 2016 National Institute for Health and Care Excellence (NICE) guidelines endorse self-management, exercise, manual therapy, psychological therapy, and return-to-work programs.

Pharmacologic Treatment

NSAIDs are considered first-line pharmacologic therapy for acute low back pain and should be used at the lowest effective dose for the shortest duration needed. A recent meta-analysis suggests that NSAIDs, compared with placebo, reduce pain and disability in patients with acute low back pain. Notably, another meta-analysis concluded that acetaminophen is ineffective for acute low back pain. Second-line agents include nonbenzodiazepine muscle relaxants. Opioids and tramadol should be avoided in acute low back pain if possible.

A similar approach is appropriate in patients with chronic low back pain. NSAIDs remain first-line pharmacologic therapy, and nonbenzodiazepine muscle relaxants may be used as second-line therapy. The serotonin-norepinephrine reuptake inhibitor duloxetine is approved by the FDA to treat chronic low back pain and may be useful in selected patients.

A 2018 randomized controlled trial demonstrated that opioids were not superior to nonopioid medications for improving pain-related function for chronic back pain or osteoarthritis-related hip or knee pain; pain intensity was

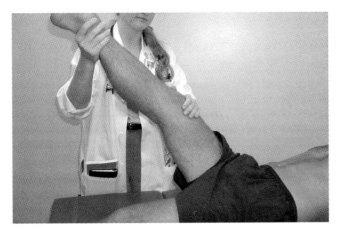

FIGURE 8. Straight leg raise test. With the patient lying supine on his or her back, the patient lifts the leg with the knee fully extended on the affected side (ipsilateral straight leg raise test) and then repeats on the opposite side (contralateral straight leg raise test). The test result is considered positive when pain radiates down the leg past the level of the knee when the hip is flexed between 30 and 70 degrees.

Reproduced with permission from Moore G. Atlas of the Musculoskeletal Examination. Philadelphia, PA: American College of Physicians; 2003:65. Copyright 2003, American College of Physicians.

TABLE 46. Patterns of Neurologic Deficits in Patients With Low Back Pain

Nerve Root Level	Motor Deficit	Sensory Deficit	Involved Reflex
L3	Hip flexion	Anteromedial thigh	Patella
L4	Knee extension	Anterior leg/medial foot	Patella
L5	Great toe dorsiflexion	Lateral leg/dorsal foot	N/A
S1	Plantar flexion of foot	Posterior leg/lateral foot	Achilles

N/A = not applicable.

Adapted with permission from Diagnosis and Treatment of Acute Low Back Pain, February 15, 2012, Vol 85, No 4, American Family Physician. Copyright © 2012 American Academy of Family Physicians. All Rights Reserved.

significantly improved in the nonopioid group. The 2016 NICE guidelines recommend against the use of opioids for chronic back pain, and the 2016 Centers for Disease Control and Prevention guideline for prescribing opioids states that nonpharmacologic and nonopioid therapies are preferred over opioids.

Systemic glucocorticoids, tricyclic antidepressants, and neuromodulators (gabapentin and pregabalin) have not demonstrated effectiveness for chronic low back pain.

Interventional and Surgical Treatment

Most patients with low back pain do not require surgery. Immediate surgery is indicated for most patients with suspected cord compression or cauda equina syndrome. Nonurgent surgery may be considered in patients with neurologic deficits, progressively worsening spinal stenosis, or

chronic pain with corresponding abnormalities on imaging that has been refractory to conservative measures and has the potential to respond to surgery. Typical surgical approaches include diskectomy for disk herniation and posterior decompressive laminectomy for spinal stenosis.

Epidural glucocorticoid injections are frequently performed in patients with radiculopathy; however, available evidence suggests they offer only small, short-term benefits.

KEY POINTS

- Evaluation of patients with low back pain includes a detailed history and physical examination to help distinguish nonspecific low back pain from pain attributable to a specific cause. **HVC**
- Most patients with nonspecific low back pain do not require imaging or other diagnostic testing. **HVC**
- Patient education for low back pain includes providing information on the expected course of the back pain, promoting self-management, addressing misconceptions, and encouraging physical activity as appropriate.
- Nonpharmacologic therapies are considered a cornerstone of treatment for both acute and chronic low back pain. **HVC**
- NSAIDs are considered first-line pharmacologic therapy for low back pain and should be used at the lowest effective dose for the shortest duration needed. **HVC**

Neck Pain
Diagnosis and Evaluation

As with low back pain, a priority in evaluating neck pain is differentiating nonspecific neck pain from other conditions that may result in serious complications or be amenable to specific therapy. Evaluation begins with a thorough history, including circumstances of the onset, presence of antecedent trauma, duration, progression, impact on daily activities, and accompanying symptoms. Examination includes inspection and palpation of the cervical spine and muscles, range of motion testing, and comprehensive neurologic assessment of the arms, including sensory, motor, and reflex testing.

The most common cause of neck pain is cervical sprain (nonspecific or axial neck pain), which is characterized by pain and stiffness in the paraspinal neck muscles frequently accompanied by neck and upper back muscle spasms. Examination findings include decreased cervical range of motion, muscle spasms, and absence of abnormal neurologic findings.

Whiplash-associated neck pain develops after trauma involving abrupt neck flexion or extension. Symptoms and signs are similar to those of cervical sprain.

Cervical radiculopathy is caused by nerve root compression as a result of disk herniation or adjacent bony degeneration. Several conditions can cause symptoms that may be mistaken for cervical radicular pain, including shingles, entrapment syndromes (such as median or ulnar nerve entrapment, thoracic outlet syndrome), complex regional pain syndrome, and cardiac ischemia. Radiculopathy, however, usually causes neck pain accompanied by radiating arm pain and paresthesias that follow a dermatomal distribution. In some cases, pain may be limited to the shoulder girdle. On examination, the patient's symptoms may be reproduced with the Spurling test (sensitivity, 94%; specificity, 30%) **(Figure 9)** and improved by holding the patient's hand above the head (shoulder abduction test: variable sensitivity, 17%-78%; specificity, 75%-92%).

Cervical myelopathy (compression of the cervical spinal cord) can also cause neck pain. Symptoms are typically progressive and include difficulty with manual dexterity, fine object manipulation (buttoning a shirt), and gait disturbance. On examination, there are upper motor neuron signs such as increased muscle tone, hyperreflexia, and clonus.

Involvement of the cervical spine by malignancy should be considered in the presence of a history of malignancy or suggestive systemic symptoms such as weight loss. Infectious causes, such as an epidural abscess or osteomyelitis, should be considered in the presence of fevers and chills, a history of injection drug use, or a history of recent bacteremia.

Most patients with neck pain do not require imaging studies. Plain radiography should be obtained when evaluation suggests fracture, infection, or malignancy and can be considered in patients with cervical sprain that has been unresponsive to 6 to 8 weeks of conservative measures. MRI is recommended when suspicion for malignancy or infection remains high despite normal plain radiographs, when myelopathy is suspected, and in patients with progressive neurologic symptoms. In patients who cannot undergo MRI, CT myelography can be

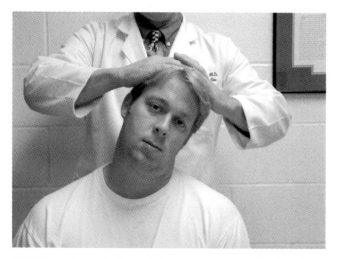

FIGURE 9. Spurling test for cervical nerve root compression. With the patient in a sitting position, the examiner extends the patient's head and then laterally flexes the neck. A downward pressure is then applied to the head in this position. A positive Spurling test reproduces the patient's pain, which radiates into the ipsilateral arm in a dermatomal distribution and supports the diagnosis of cervical radiculopathy (sensitivity, 94%; specificity, 30%).

Reproduced with permission from Davis MF, Davis PF, Ross DS. Expert Guide to Sports Medicine. Philadelphia, PA: American College of Physicians, 2005:271. Copyright 2005, American College of Physicians.

considered. Electrodiagnostic studies may be performed when there is diagnostic uncertainty about a patient's symptoms (for example, to help distinguish peripheral nerve entrapment or peripheral neuropathy from radiculopathy).

Treatment

Most patients with neck pain have resolution or near-resolution of their symptoms within 8 to 12 weeks of onset by using conservative measures. A multimodal approach that is tailored to the individual patient appears to work best and may include mobilization, exercise, physical therapy, and analgesic agents.

Stretching and strengthening exercises appear to provide intermediate-term relief of symptoms. Spinal manipulation, mobilization, and acupuncture may provide short-term pain relief. Although widely used, immobilization with a cervical collar appears to be no more effective than sham interventions. Immobilization for longer than 1 to 2 weeks may lead to atrophy of the neck muscles. The benefit of traction appears limited.

Oral and topical NSAIDs are considered first-line pharmacologic therapy for neck pain. Notably, a recent meta-analysis suggests that NSAIDs, compared with placebo, reduce pain in patients with neck pain. Because of its favorable side-effect profile, acetaminophen is also frequently used, although its effectiveness is not clearly established. Cyclobenzaprine, when used at intermediate or higher doses (≥15 mg/d), is more effective than placebo for treatment of acute neck pain associated with muscle spasm. For patients with chronic radicular symptoms, venlafaxine and neuromodulators, such as gabapentin and tricyclic antidepressants, may provide some pain relief. Because of abuse potential, opioids are generally avoided and, if used, should only be used on a short-term basis and restricted to persons with severe, intractable pain. No evidence supports the use of oral glucocorticoids. Epidural glucocorticoid injections may be considered in patients with cervical radiculopathy and significant symptoms that do not respond to other conservative measures, although the data supporting this practice are unconvincing.

Surgery is generally reserved for patients with structural disorders on imaging along with myelopathic findings and progressive neurologic symptoms, or for those with symptoms that do not respond to 6 months of conservative therapy.

For those with neck pain with a systemic cause, the underlying disorder should be appropriately treated.

KEY POINTS

- Most patients with neck pain do not require imaging studies; plain radiography should be obtained when evaluation suggests fracture, infection, or malignancy and can be considered in patients with cervical sprain that has been unresponsive to 6 to 8 weeks of conservative measures. **HVC**

- Neck pain usually resolves with conservative measures, including mobilization, exercise, physical therapy, and analgesic agents. **HVC**

Upper Extremity Disorders

Thoracic Outlet Syndrome

Diagnosis and Evaluation

The three subtypes of thoracic outlet syndrome (TOS) are differentiated according to the affected structure within the neurovascular bundle between the first rib and the clavicle. Neurogenic TOS, the most common type (>90% of cases), results from compression of the brachial plexus. Symptoms (arm paresthesias, pain, and weakness) worsen with repetitive arm use, especially overhead activities. Venous TOS is caused by axillary vein compression and usually thrombosis within the thoracic outlet. Symptoms (arm pain/fatigue, edema, and cyanosis) occur with repetitive arm use, especially overhead activities. Dilated collateral veins of the chest wall and shoulder may be present. Arterial TOS, due to subclavian artery compression (with or without thrombosis), usually occurs in the presence of an anomalous cervical rib; less commonly, it occurs with frequent and vigorous overhead activities, such as baseball pitching. Symptoms include arm pain (which may be exertional), weakness, paresthesias, coolness, and pallor.

Diagnosis of neurogenic TOS is clinical, although electrodiagnostic testing may be helpful in some patients. Vascular causes require imaging of the affected vessel, with ultrasonography being the most useful initial test.

Treatment

First-line therapy for neurogenic TOS includes improving posture and strengthening shoulder girdle muscles. Surgical decompression is reserved for progressive, disabling, or unresponsive symptoms. Treatment of both arterial and venous TOS involves catheter-directed thrombolysis followed by prompt surgical decompression of the thoracic outlet.

> **KEY POINT**
>
> - Neurogenic thoracic outlet syndrome (TOS), the most common type of TOS, results from compression of the brachial plexus; arm paresthesias, pain, and weakness worsen with repetitive arm use, especially overhead activities.

Shoulder Pain

Diagnosis and Evaluation

Shoulder pain assessment involves a detailed history with attention to the presence of antecedent trauma and relevant occupational or recreational activities. A comprehensive shoulder examination, performed with both shoulders fully exposed, includes inspection, palpation, range of motion assessment, and specialized maneuvers.

The initial step in evaluating shoulder pain is to determine whether the pain is arising from the shoulder (intrinsic) or is referred from another site (extrinsic), such as the cervical spine. Extrinsic pain is suggested by the inability to reproduce pain with shoulder movement, pain extending beyond the elbow, and pain with neck movement.

Rotator Cuff Disease

Rotator cuff disease, the most common cause of shoulder pain, refers to all symptomatic rotator cuff disorders, including rotator cuff tendinitis, rotator cuff tears, and subacromial bursitis. Pain from rotator cuff disease is frequently localized to the upper arm near the deltoid insertion, is worsened with overhead activities, and is often worse at night, particularly with lying on the affected side. Except for acute traumatic rotator cuff tears, onset of symptoms is usually insidious. Risk factors for rotator cuff disease include increasing age and participation in activities that require repetitive overhead arm use.

On examination, shoulder inspection may reveal infraspinatus muscle atrophy (positive likelihood ratio of 2.0 for rotator cuff disease). Many examination maneuvers are available for rotator cuff disease assessment; however, each is limited by test characteristics, and they are most useful in combination (**Table 47**). The combination of positive results on painful arc and drop arm tests in the setting of weakness in external rotation is particularly suggestive of a rotator cuff tear.

Most patients with rotator cuff disease do not require imaging studies. Ultrasonography or MRI should be reserved for patients with acute or progressive functional loss and for those who are unresponsive to conservative measures.

Patients with acute full-thickness tears should be referred for consideration of immediate repair. Treatment of other rotator cuff disorders should include education about the expected course, avoidance or modification of aggravating activities, and physical therapy. Immobilization with a sling should be avoided to prevent development of adhesive capsulitis. Pharmacologic treatment should begin with acetaminophen and, if ineffective, progress to oral or topical NSAIDs. Subacromial glucocorticoid injections may provide short-term pain relief in patients with subacromial bursitis in whom other measures have failed but should be limited to one or two courses to limit complications. Surgery is reserved for patients in whom 3 to 6 months of conservative therapy has failed or in physically active patients with functionally significant tears.

Adhesive Capsulitis

Adhesive capsulitis (frozen shoulder) usually occurs in patients aged 40 to 70 years. The cause is unclear but appears to involve glenohumeral joint capsular thickening and fibrosis. Adhesive capsulitis can be idiopathic but is also associated with prolonged immobilization, antecedent shoulder surgery or injury, diabetes mellitus, hypothyroidism, and autoimmune disorders. Patients describe shoulder pain that is often constant but is worse at night and in cold weather; shoulder stiffness is common. Both the degree of pain and stiffness may vary in an individual patient over time. On examination, patients have limited passive and active range of motion in all directions.

Treatment of adhesive capsulitis focuses on pain control and improved range of motion. Intra-articular glucocorticoid injections appear more effective than physical therapy alone, although evidence supports combining modalities. Acetaminophen and NSAIDs can be used as an adjunct for analgesia. Surgery is

TABLE 47. Physical Examination Maneuvers in Rotator Cuff Disease

Maneuver	Technique	Positive LR[a] (95% CI)	Negative LR[a] (95% CI)	Notes
Painful arc test	During full passive abduction of the affected arm, pain occurs between 60° and 120°.	3.7 (1.9-7.0)	0.36 (0.23-0.54)	Highest LR+ of all special RC maneuvers.
Drop arm test	The affected arm is fully passively abducted, and the patient is asked to slowly lower the arm. A sudden drop of the arm with reproduction of the patient's pain is a positive result.	3.3 (1.0-11)	0.82 (0.7-0.97)	An uncontrolled drop of the arm suggests a full tear of the supraspinatus.
Hawkins test	The arm is passively flexed to 90° with the elbow in 90° flexion. The examiner then internally rotates the shoulder. Reproduction of pain during internal rotation is a positive result.	1.5 (1.1-2.0)	0.51 (0.39-0.66)	Believed to maximize impingement of the supraspinatus tendon; if the painful arc test, Hawkins test, and resisted external rotation are positive, the LR+ for a full-thickness RC tear is 16.4.
Empty can test	The extended arm is passively abducted to 90° in the plane of the supraspinatus (30° anterior to the coronal plane) and internally rotated (as though pouring a glass of water onto the floor). The patient is asked to maintain the position while the examiner exerts downward force on the arm. Weakness or reproduction of pain is a positive result.	1.3 (0.97-1.6)	0.64 (0.33-1.3)	Inability to maintain the position before resistance is applied suggests a full tear of the supraspinatus.
Resisted external rotation	The arm is abducted to 0° with the elbow flexed to 90° and the thumb pointing upward. The examiner exerts an internal rotation force proximal to the wrist, which the patient is asked to resist. Weakness or reproduction of pain is a positive result.	2.6 (1.8-3.6)	0.49 (0.33-0.72)	Pain or weakness suggests infraspinatus pathology. Limitation in external rotation range of motion suggests glenohumeral disease or adhesive capsulitis.
Internal rotation lag sign	The patient places the dorsum of the hand on the lower back with the elbow flexed to 90°. The examiner lifts the hand off the back, further internally rotating the shoulder. Inability to maintain the hand away from the back is a positive result.	6.2 (1.9-12)	0.04 (0.0-0.58)	Subscapularis is the primary muscle of internal rotation; LRs are for a full tear of the subscapularis.

LR+ = positive likelihood ratio; RC = rotator cuff.

[a]LRs relate to the diagnosis of rotator cuff disease unless otherwise indicated.

Reproduced with permission from Whittle S, Buchbinder R. In the clinic. Rotator cuff disease. Ann Intern Med. 2015;162:ITC1. [PMID: 25560729]. Copyright 2015, American College of Physicians.

reserved for patients who do not respond to 12 weeks of conservative measures.

Acromioclavicular Joint Degeneration

Acromioclavicular joint degeneration is typically characterized by poorly localized pain on the superior shoulder, although pain may be throughout the shoulder region. On examination, pain may be elicited with palpation of the acromioclavicular joint. The crossed-arm adduction test often reproduces the pain, as does shoulder abduction beyond 120 degrees, but neither test is specific for acromioclavicular joint disease. Plain radiography is often completed to assess for other structural disease and usually reveals degenerative changes of the acromioclavicular joint.

First-line therapy consists of NSAIDs and activity modification. Glucocorticoid injections may provide short-term pain relief.

KEY POINTS

- Rotator cuff disease pain is frequently localized to the upper arm near the deltoid insertion, is worsened with overhead activities, and is often worse at night, particularly with lying on the affected side.

- Most patients with rotator cuff disease do not require imaging studies; treatment may include education, avoidance/modification of aggravating activities, physical therapy, and acetaminophen or NSAIDs.

HVC

(Continued)

KEY POINTS (continued)

- Treatment of adhesive capsulitis focuses on pain control and improved range of motion; intra-articular gluco-corticoid injections appear more effective than physical therapy alone, although evidence supports combining both modalities.

- First-line therapy for acromioclavicular joint degeneration consists of NSAIDs and activity modification; glucocorticoid injections may provide short-term pain relief.

Elbow Pain
Diagnosis and Evaluation
Elbow pain may be caused by pathology within the elbow joint, surrounding tissues, or nerves. Diseases within the neck, shoulder, and wrist may also cause pain radiating to the elbow. Evaluation focuses on patient history and physical examination.

Epicondylitis
Epicondylitis (epicondylosis) refers to noninflammatory conditions of the tendons surrounding the elbow. Lateral epicondylitis (tennis elbow) is induced by activities with repetitive use of extensor tendons, such as computer use or tennis. Pain and tenderness are located over the lateral epicondyle and increase with resisted wrist extension. Medial epicondylitis (golfer's elbow) is less common and is caused by repetitive flexion of the wrist. Pain occurs over the medial elbow and ventral forearm and worsens with resisted wrist flexion. Diagnostic imaging is unnecessary if the clinical picture is consistent with medial or lateral epicondylitis.

There is little strong evidence regarding the optimal means of treatment. Initial management includes avoidance of pain-inducing activities and NSAIDs for analgesia. Physical therapy and counterforce braces may improve symptoms and prevent future exacerbations. Glucocorticoid injections may reduce pain in the short term, but they provide no long-term benefit and are used only as a temporizing measure. Surgery is rarely indicated for recalcitrant pain.

Olecranon Bursitis
Several conditions cause inflammation of the olecranon bursa, including trauma, gout, and infection. Posterior elbow swelling and tenderness with normal elbow range of motion are typical (**Figure 10**); swelling and pain on elbow extension suggest elbow joint effusion and an alternate cause. Aspiration with culture and fluid analysis should be performed for severe pain or suspicion of infection.

Noninfectious bursitis is treated by avoidance of bursal trauma and short-term use of NSAIDs. Glucocorticoid injections may provide short-term benefit but are associated with complications and should be considered only when conservative treatment fails. Surgery may be necessary for infectious or refractory bursitis.

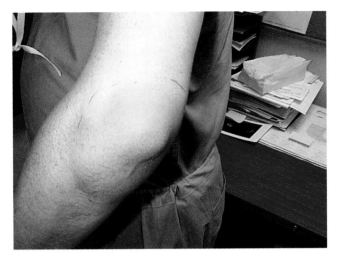

FIGURE 10. Olecranon bursitis is characterized by warmth, redness, and swelling. The ability to extend and flex the elbow generally excludes an intra-articular process.

Reproduced with permission from Moore G. Atlas of the Musculoskeletal Examination. Philadelphia, PA: American College of Physicians; 2003:24. Copyright 2003, American College of Physicians.

Ulnar Nerve Entrapment
Ulnar nerve entrapment (cubital tunnel syndrome) results from ulnar nerve impingement at the elbow by fibrous scar tissue, ulnar nerve subluxation, ganglion cysts, or bone spurs. Characteristics include pain at the elbow that worsens with flexion, paresthesias and numbness of the fourth and fifth fingers, and weakness of the interosseous muscles. The diagnosis is usually clinical, but electromyography is often used for diagnostic confirmation; MRI or ultrasonography may be useful in some situations.

Initial treatment consists of avoidance of elbow trauma and nocturnal splinting. NSAIDs are beneficial for short-term pain relief. Surgery is an option when conservative measures fail in the setting of significant or progressive symptoms.

KEY POINTS

- Olecranon bursitis is characterized by posterior elbow swelling and tenderness with normal elbow range of motion; swelling and pain on elbow extension suggest elbow joint effusion and an alternate cause.

- Elbow pain is generally managed with avoidance of trauma and pain-inducing activities; NSAIDs may be effective for analgesia. **HVC**

Wrist and Hand Pain
Carpal Tunnel Syndrome
Carpal tunnel syndrome develops from increased pressure within the carpal tunnel causing median nerve compression. Diagnosis is usually established based on history. The syndrome presents with wrist pain that may radiate to the forearm and hand; paresthesias and weakness of the first three fingers and thenar eminence (median nerve distribution) may be present. Symptoms are often worse at night and with

repetitive wrist motion. Risk factors include obesity, female sex, hypothyroidism, pregnancy, and connective tissue disorders. Although keyboard use has been suggested as a risk factor, it has not been confirmed by studies.

Examination findings may include decreased sensation over the median nerve distribution, thenar muscle atrophy, and weakened thumb abduction. Examination is often normal early in the disease, and provocative testing with the Phalen maneuver (flexion of hands at wrists) or Tinel test (percussion of the median nerve on top of the carpal tunnel) is rarely useful. Electrodiagnostic testing is beneficial when the diagnosis is unclear, especially when cervical radiculopathy is possible.

Initial treatment includes activity modification and wrist splinting. Methylprednisolone injection or short-term oral glucocorticoids may also provide benefit as second-line therapy. Surgical treatment is necessary for patients who do not respond to conservative therapy or who have evidence of significant neurologic dysfunction.

Other Causes

Acute wrist or hand pain associated with trauma suggests fracture or dislocation and requires plain radiography for evaluation. Although multiple injuries are possible, special consideration for hamate and scaphoid fractures is necessary. Hamate hook fractures can occur from a fall onto an outstretched hand or activities with repetitive impact at the palm base (baseball hitting). Plain radiographs usually reveal the fracture. Scaphoid fractures are also commonly associated with falling onto an extended hand and are characterized by pain and tenderness in the anatomic snuffbox. Initial radiographs are normal in up to 20% of patients. If clinical suspicion is high and radiographs are normal, thumb splinting and repeat radiography in 1 to 2 weeks or immediate advanced imaging (MRI or CT) are recommended.

Wrist or hand pain lasting more than 2 weeks also has a wide differential diagnosis. De Quervain tendinopathy results from noninflammatory thickening of the thumb tendons. Pain occurs at the thumb base, radiates to the distal radius, and is elicited with making a fist over the thumb and ulnar deviation of the wrist (Finkelstein test). Initial management includes rest, NSAIDs, and splinting. When conservative measures fail, glucocorticoid injections provide symptomatic relief. Surgery may benefit patients with symptoms that do not respond to glucocorticoid injections.

Ganglion cysts are caused by herniated synovial tissue surrounding tendon sheaths or joints; they are often palpable on the ventral aspect of the wrist. Asymptomatic cysts require no treatment. Ganglion cysts causing pain may be treated with aspiration. The benefit of glucocorticoid or hyaluronidase injections is questionable; they are not indicated given the potential for complications. If cysts recur after aspiration, surgical resection is effective.

Ulnar neuropathy from ulnar nerve entrapment at the wrist presents with wrist pain and decreased hand strength and sensation. This condition can result from prolonged ulnar nerve compression in the Guyton canal, such as may occur with bicycling.

Osteoarthritis and inflammatory arthritis may affect the interphalangeal and carpometacarpal joints and cause hand and wrist pain (see MKSAP 18 Rheumatology).

> **KEY POINT**
>
> - Initial treatment of carpal tunnel syndrome includes   **HVC** activity modification, wrist splinting, and methylprednisolone injection or short-term oral glucocorticoid therapy if needed; surgical treatment is necessary for patients in whom conservative therapy fails or who have significant neurologic dysfunction.

Lower Extremity Disorders

Hip Pain

Diagnosis and Evaluation

Evaluation of hip pain should be guided by location of the pain. Anterior hip and groin pain is caused by both intra- and extra-articular factors. Lateral hip pain is most commonly due to greater trochanteric pain syndrome (GTPS; formerly known as trochanteric bursitis) or meralgia paresthetica. Posterior hip pain is caused by sacroiliac joint dysfunction, lumbar radiculopathy, or vascular claudication.

Anterior hip pain that starts insidiously and worsens with standing and activity in older patients suggests osteoarthritis. The same pain characteristics in a younger person raise concern for a labral tear, especially when accompanied by painful clicking or catching. Gradual onset of anterior hip pain can also occur with avascular necrosis (or osteonecrosis), which should be considered in the presence of alcohol abuse, glucocorticoid use, systemic lupus erythematosus, or sickle cell anemia. Acute-onset, anteriorly located hip pain that interferes with weight bearing and is accompanied by fevers raises suspicion for infectious arthritis, whereas acute pain after a fall suggests fracture.

Lateral hip pain that worsens with lying on the affected side suggests GTPS; this pain may also radiate to the buttock or knee. Meralgia paresthetica is characterized by distal anterolateral thigh paresthesias associated with tight-fitting clothes and obesity.

Posterior or buttock pain associated with radiation down the leg suggests lumbar radiculopathy, whereas concomitant exertional leg pain or peripheral vascular disease suggests vascular claudication. Posterior pain without other features may be secondary to sacroiliac joint dysfunction.

Examination of patients with hip pain includes evaluation of the hip, abdomen, and back; neurologic and vascular assessments of the legs; and gait assessment. Pain with both passive and active hip movement suggests an intra-articular cause. The FABER (Flexion, ABduction, and External Rotation) test may cause posterior hip pain in the presence of sacroiliac joint dysfunction, groin pain with an intra-articular cause, and lateral hip pain with GTPS (**Figure 11**). The

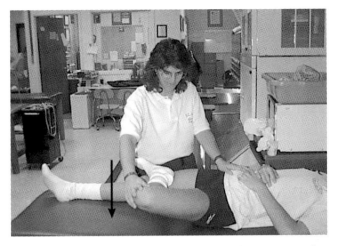

FIGURE 11. The FABER (Flexion, ABduction, and External Rotation) test. With the patient supine, the leg on the tested side is placed in the "figure 4" position (the knee of the tested side is flexed 90 degrees, and the lateral malleolus is placed on top of the opposite leg). The examiner then applies a posteriorly directed force with one hand while using the other hand to stabilize the patient's other hip. A positive test result occurs if groin pain or buttock pain is produced. Buttock pain suggests sacroiliac joint dysfunction, and groin pain suggests an intra-articular cause of pain.

Reproduced with permission from Davis MF, Davis PF, Ross DS. Expert Guide to Sports Medicine. Philadelphia, PA: American College of Physicians, 2005:360. Copyright 2005, American College of Physicians.

most common examination finding in GTPS is tenderness to palpation of the greater trochanter. A normal hip examination in a patient with groin pain suggests an extra-articular cause, such as an inguinal hernia. Pain reproduction on straight leg raise test (see Figure 8) supports lumbar radiculopathy.

Plain radiography (anteroposterior pelvic view and frog-leg lateral view) should be performed if intra-articular pathology, fracture, or dislocation is suspected. In patients with persistent anterior pain and normal plain radiographs, MRI of the hip can be performed; however, if suspicion is high for a labral tear, MR arthrography should be performed. Hip aspiration should be performed if infectious arthritis is suspected.

Treatment

Initial management of labral tears includes muscle strengthening and activity modification, with arthroscopic surgery reserved for those in whom conservative measures fail. Patients with advanced avascular necrosis often require total hip arthroplasty.

Initial GTPS management includes activity modification and analgesia with acetaminophen or NSAIDs. Glucocorticoid injection can be considered for persistently symptomatic GTPS, with surgery limited to recalcitrant cases. Primary treatment of meralgia paresthetica consists of reassurance, avoiding tight-fitting clothes, and weight loss. First-line therapy for sacroiliac joint dysfunction is physical therapy, with limited evidence existing for local glucocorticoid injection.

Management of osteoarthritis is discussed in MKSAP 18 Rheumatology.

KEY POINTS

- The FABER (Flexion, ABduction, and External Rotation) test may cause posterior hip pain in the presence of sacroiliac joint dysfunction, groin pain from an intra-articular cause, and lateral hip pain from greater trochanteric pain syndrome.
- Plain hip radiography (anteroposterior pelvic view and frog-leg lateral view) should be performed if an intra-articular pathology, fracture, or dislocation is suspected.

HVC

Knee Pain

Diagnosis and Evaluation

The history obtained from patients with knee pain should focus on pain characteristics as well as history of knee injury or surgery, osteoarthritis, gout, and acute calcium pyrophosphate crystal arthritis (pseudogout).

Knee examination, performed with both knees fully exposed, includes inspection, palpation, range of motion testing, and special maneuvers (**Table 48**).

Plain radiography should be performed if fracture, bony pathology, or osteoarthritis is suspected. MRI can be performed if there is concern for meniscal or ligamentous injury and surgical therapy is being considered. Joint aspiration should be performed for suspicion of inflammatory or infectious arthritis.

Knee osteoarthritis is discussed in MKSAP 18 Rheumatology.

Ligament and Meniscal Tears

Acute, traumatic onset of knee pain, especially when associated with swelling, should raise concern for ligamentous and/or meniscal tears. Anterior cruciate ligament (ACL) tears usually involve noncontact twisting injuries. Patients may report a popping sound and frequently cannot immediately bear weight. Large effusions due to hemarthrosis frequently develop within 2 hours and may make initial examination challenging. The anterior drawer and Lachman tests frequently demonstrate increased ligamentous laxity, although the Lachman test may be most useful in the acute setting (see Table 48). Plain radiography should be obtained to evaluate for possible accompanying tibial avulsion fractures. ACL tears usually require surgical reconstruction, especially in active patients or those with an unstable knee. A nonoperative approach may be appropriate in older and less active patients. Medial collateral ligament (MCL) tears typically involve a lateral blow to the knee causing valgus stress, whereas posterior collateral ligament (PCL) tears involve a posteriorly directed force applied to the proximal anterior tibia with the knee flexed. Increased MCL laxity suggesting a tear may be detected by applying a medially directed force with the knee flexed at 30 degrees (valgus stress test), whereas increased PCL laxity may be detected by applying a posteriorly directed force to the proximal tibia with the knee flexed at 90 degrees. Most MCL and PCL tears can be managed conservatively.

TABLE 48. Knee Examination Maneuvers

Maneuver	Purpose	Description	Likelihood Ratios[a]
Anterior drawer	ACL integrity	Patient is supine with hip flexed to 45° and knee flexed to 90°. Examiner sits on dorsum of foot and places hands on proximal calf and then pulls anteriorly while assessing movement of tibia relative to femur. Positive result: Increased laxity with lack of firm end point (suggests ACL tear)	Positive likelihood ratio: 3.8[a] Negative likelihood ratio: 0.30[a]
Lachman	ACL integrity	Patient is supine with leg in slight external rotation and knee flexed 20° to 30° at examiner's side. Examiner stabilizes femur with one hand and grasps proximal calf with other. Calf is pulled forward while assessing movement of tibia relative to femur. Positive result: Increased laxity with lack of firm end point (suggests ACL tear)	Positive likelihood ratio: 42.0[b] Negative likelihood ratio: 0.1[b]
Posterior drawer	PCL integrity	Patient is supine with hip flexed to 45° and knee flexed to 90°. Examiner sits on dorsum of foot and places hands on proximal calf and then pushes posteriorly while assessing movement of tibia relative to femur. Positive result: Increased laxity with lack of firm end point (suggests PCL tear)	Positive likelihood ratio: 50.11[c] Negative likelihood ratio: 0.11[c]
Valgus stress	MCL integrity	Patient is supine with knee flexed to 30° and leg slightly abducted. Examiner places one hand on lateral knee and other hand on medial distal tibia and applies valgus force. Positive result: Increased laxity and pain (suggests MCL tear)	Positive likelihood ratio: 7.7 Negative likelihood ratio: 0.2
Varus stress	LCL integrity	Patient is supine with knee flexed to 30° and leg slightly abducted. Examiner places one hand on medial knee and other hand on lateral distal tibia and applies varus force. Positive result: Increased laxity and pain (suggests LCL tear)	Positive likelihood ratio: 16.2
Thessaly	Meniscal integrity	Examiner holds patient's outstretched hands while patient stands on one leg with knee flexed to 5° and with other knee flexed to 90° with foot off of floor. Patient rotates body internally and externally three times. Repeat with knee flexed to 20°. Always perform on uninvolved knee first. Positive result: Medial or lateral joint line pain (suggests meniscal tear)	Positive likelihood ratio: 1.37[d] Negative likelihood ratio: 0.68[d]
Medial-lateral grind	Meniscal integrity	With patient supine, examiner places calf in one hand and thumb and index finger of opposite hand over joint line and applies varus and valgus stress to tibia during extension and flexion. Positive result: Grinding sensation palpable over joint line (suggests meniscal injury)	Positive likelihood ratio: 4.8[b] Negative likelihood ratio: 0.4[b]
McMurray	Meniscal integrity	With patient supine, the examiner fully flexes the knee and rotates the tibia externally. The knee is then extended with the hand over the medial joint line. The maneuver is then repeated with the tibia internally rotated and the hand over the lateral joint line. Positive result: Snapping is detected over the joint line with extension on the knee	Positive likelihood ratio: 1.3[b] Negative likelihood ratio: 0.8[b]
Noble	Iliotibial band integrity	With patient supine, examiner repeatedly flexes and extends knee with examiner's thumb placed on lateral femoral epicondyle. Positive result: Reproduces patient's pain (suggests iliotibial band syndrome)	

ACL = anterior cruciate ligament; LCL = lateral collateral ligament; MCL = medial collateral ligament; PCL = posterior cruciate ligament.

[a]Data used to derive these values are of limited quality.

[b]Data from Solomon DH, Simel DL, Bates DW, Katz JN, Schaffer JL. The rational clinical examination. Does this patient have a torn meniscus or ligament of the knee? Value of the physical examination. JAMA. 2001;286:1610-20. [PMID: 11585485]

[c]Data from Rubinstein RA Jr, Shelbourne KD, McCarroll JR, VanMeter CD, Rettig AC. The accuracy of the clinical examination in the setting of posterior cruciate ligament injuries. Am J Sports Med. 1994;22:550-7. [PMID: 7943523]

[d]Data from Goossens P, Keijsers E, van Geenen RJ, Zijta A, van den Broek M, Verhagen AP, et al. Validity of the Thessaly test in evaluating meniscal tears compared with arthroscopy: a diagnostic accuracy study. J Orthop Sports Phys Ther. 2015;45:18-24, B1. [PMID: 25420009] doi:10.2519/jospt.2015.5215

Meniscal tears usually result from an acute twisting knee injury or can develop more insidiously as a result of chronic degeneration. Symptoms include pain, locking, catching, and grinding. Patients with acute meniscal tears are usually able to immediately bear weight. On examination, effusions, if present, are generally small to moderate in size. Results of specialized tests, such as the medial-lateral grind and Thessaly tests, are frequently positive (see Table 48). Initial management of both acute and chronic meniscal tears is conservative and consists of rest, ice, and strengthening the quadriceps and hamstring muscles. Surgery is reserved for patients with persistent (>4 weeks) mechanical symptoms.

Patellofemoral Pain Syndrome

Patellofemoral pain syndrome is caused by disordered patellar tracking with knee movement. It is characterized by anterior knee pain and/or stiffness with prolonged sitting, climbing, or descending stairs, and with running or squatting. On examination, applying pressure to the patella may reproduce pain. Patellar mobility can be assessed by medially and laterally displacing the patella, and abrupt patellar deviation may be noted during squatting and standing, although the utility of these findings is unclear.

Treatment is focused on identifying the underlying cause; activity modification, such as relative rest; cryotherapy (ice or cold water immersion); and physical therapy. NSAIDs, acetaminophen, and patellar taping and bracing are frequently used, although evidence for the effectiveness of these measures is limited.

KEY POINTS

HVC
- In patients with knee pain, plain radiography should be obtained if fracture, bony pathology, or osteoarthritis is suspected.
- Anterior cruciate ligament tears often require surgical reconstruction, whereas most medial collateral ligament and posterior collateral ligament tears can be managed conservatively.
- Patellofemoral pain syndrome is characterized by anterior knee pain and/or stiffness with prolonged sitting, climbing, or descending stairs, and with running or squatting; treatment may include activity modification, cryotherapy, and physical therapy.

Bursitis

Prepatellar bursitis presents as acute or chronic swelling anterior to the patella. Acute cases are often associated with tenderness, warmth, and erythema. Most cases of acute prepatellar bursitis are caused by infection with skin bacteria and less commonly by trauma and gout. Chronic prepatellar bursitis is usually caused by trauma, although gout and infection are possible. All patients with prepatellar bursitis regardless of duration should undergo fluid aspiration and analysis. Septic bursitis is managed with knee immobilization, systemic antibiotics, and re-aspiration if needed. Gouty bursitis is managed with appropriate gout therapy (see MKSAP 18 Rheumatology). Traumatic bursitis is managed by activity modification (avoidance of kneeling) and NSAIDs.

Pes anserine bursitis (pes anserine pain syndrome) classically presents with localized pain and swelling of the region overlying the proximal medial tibia several centimeters distal to the knee (**Figure 12**). It commonly occurs in athletes (especially runners) and in patients with knee osteoarthritis. First-line therapy includes quadriceps strengthening, local cryotherapy, activity modification, and NSAIDs.

Iliotibial Band Syndrome

Patients with iliotibial band syndrome (ITBS) report diffuse, poorly localized lateral knee and distal thigh pain. Pain is initially present at the end of exercise involving knee flexion and extension but may progress to occur earlier in exercise or with rest. Running outdoors or downhill may worsen symptoms. On examination, there is often tenderness approximately 2 to 3 cm proximal to the lateral femoral condyle. Patients also frequently have a positive result on a Noble test and weakness with hip abduction (see Table 48). Imaging is not usually required.

Initial treatment of ITBS centers on abstinence from inciting activity and use of ice, followed by gradual return to activity, stretching, strengthening, and local massage. NSAIDs appear effective when used as part of a multimodal approach. Local glucocorticoid injections may provide at least short-term relief.

Popliteal Cysts

A popliteal (Baker) cyst is a benign swelling of the synovial bursa behind the knee joint; synovial fluid fills the cyst. Popliteal cysts most commonly develop in the setting of knee trauma, osteoarthritis, or inflammatory arthritis. They are frequently asymptomatic but can present with posterior knee pain and swelling.

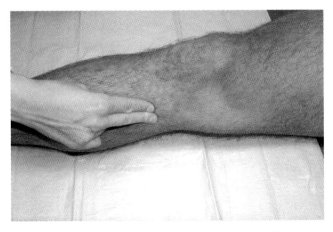

FIGURE 12. Location of the anserine bursa and pain associated with pes anserine bursitis.

Reproduced with permission from Moore G. Atlas of the Musculoskeletal Examination. Philadelphia, PA: American College of Physicians; 2003:87. Copyright 2003, American College of Physicians.

Ruptured cysts may mimic deep venous thromboses (pseudo-thrombophlebitis) and may be associated with ecchymosis from the popliteal fossa to the ankle. The "crescent sign" may be present, recognized as an ecchymotic area below the medial malleolus. In rare instances, cysts may cause compression of adjacent structures, leading to compression syndrome, posterior tibial nerve entrapment, or popliteal artery occlusion. In patients with asymptomatic popliteal cysts, no treatment is necessary. Symptomatic patients often experience relief with joint aspiration and intra-articular glucocorticoid injection. Pseudothrombophlebitis can be treated with rest, elevation, and NSAIDs. Surgical excision is reserved for severely symptomatic and functionally limited patients in whom conservative measures fail or who develop serious complications.

KEY POINTS

- All patients with prepatellar bursitis regardless of duration should undergo fluid aspiration and analysis.

- Iliotibial band syndrome is characterized by pain at the end of exercise involving knee flexion and extension but may progress to occur earlier in exercise or with rest; treatment is typically nonsurgical.

HVC • In patients with asymptomatic popliteal (Baker) cysts, no treatment is necessary; joint aspiration and intra-articular glucocorticoid injection may provide relief for those with symptoms.

Ankle and Foot Pain
Ankle Sprains
Acute ankle sprains are usually caused by excessive ankle inversion; ankle eversion injuries are rare. Common examination findings include overlying ecchymosis and swelling with tenderness of involved ankle ligaments. Weight-bearing ability and bony tenderness are components of Ottawa ankle rules, which help to determine the necessity of obtaining plain radiography to exclude fracture (**Figure 13**). Treatment includes

intermittent cryotherapy and a lace-up support or air stirrup brace combined with elastic compression wrapping. Early mobilization should be encouraged with weight bearing as tolerated. Acetaminophen and oral or topical NSAIDs can be used for pain control. Patients with persistent ligamentous laxity 4 to 6 weeks after injury should be referred for proprioceptive training and strengthening therapy.

High ankle sprains (distal tibiofibular syndesmosis ligament injuries) occur when an externally rotated force is applied to a dorsiflexed ankle. Pain may be elicited by squeezing the leg at mid-calf (squeeze test) and by dorsiflexing and externally rotating the foot with the knee flexed (dorsiflexion-external rotation test). Treatment is similar to other ankle sprains, although recovery is usually delayed.

Hindfoot Pain
Achilles tendinopathy typically develops in persons who initiate or abruptly increase activity. Patients report activity-related posterior heel pain and stiffness that improves with rest. On examination, there is usually tenderness of the Achilles tendon approximately 2 to 6 cm above the calcaneal insertion. Treatment includes activity modification, eccentric exercises (muscle lengthening in response to external resistance), and use of appropriate footwear. NSAIDs can be used for pain control.

Achilles tendon rupture commonly occurs during strenuous activities, although it may occur spontaneously in the elderly or with fluoroquinolone use. Patients usually have heel pain and may report hearing a "pop." On examination, a tendon defect may be palpable; a lack of plantar flexion with calf squeezing (Thompson test) suggests complete rupture (sensitivity, 93%; specificity, 96%) (**Figure 14**). Treatment is controversial and consists of surgery with immobilization or immobilization alone.

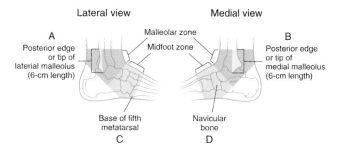

FIGURE 13. Ottawa ankle and foot rules. An ankle radiographic series is indicated if a patient has pain in the malleolar zone and any of the following findings: bone tenderness at *A*, bone tenderness at *B*, or inability to bear weight immediately and in the emergency department (or physician's office). A foot radiographic series is indicated if a patient has pain in the midfoot zone and any of the following findings: bone tenderness at *C*, bone tenderness at *D*, or inability to bear weight immediately and in the emergency department (or physician's office).

Reproduced with permission from Davis MF, Davis PF, Ross DS. Expert Guide to Sports Medicine. Philadelphia, PA: American College of Physicians, 2005:404. Copyright 2005, American College of Physicians.

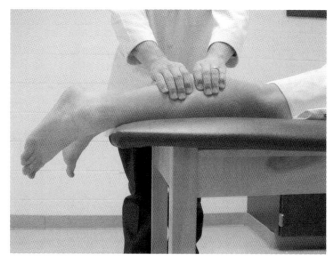

FIGURE 14. Thompson test. The patient is positioned in the prone position. The examiner squeezes mid-calf and observes for plantar flexion of the foot. When the patient has an intact Achilles tendon, plantar flexion will occur. When there is a complete Achilles tendon rupture, no plantar flexion is observed.

Reproduced with permission from Davis MF, Davis PF, Ross DS. Expert Guide to Sports Medicine. Philadelphia, PA: American College of Physicians; 2005:401. Copyright 2005, American College of Physicians.

Plantar fasciitis classically causes sharp, medial-inferior heel pain with the first morning steps and after prolonged rest. Pain usually improves with further walking but may persist in severe cases. On examination, the medial calcaneal tubercle is frequently tender. Passive toe dorsiflexion with standing (weight-bearing windlass test) may reproduce pain (sensitivity, 32%; specificity, 100%). Treatment includes weight loss, rest, calf/heel stretching, and arch supports (if pes planus is present). Because the underlying pathology is thought to be degenerative, use of NSAIDs is primarily for pain control. Patients should be educated that eventual resolution is expected but may take months. For recalcitrant cases, ultrasonography, extracorporeal shockwave therapy, night splints, and glucocorticoid injections can be considered. Surgery is reserved for patients who do not respond to these measures.

Heel pad syndrome causes inferior heel pain when walking barefoot and on hard surfaces. On examination, palpation may reproduce pain. Treatment consists of heel cushioning, rest, ice, and NSAIDs.

Midfoot Pain

Tarsal tunnel syndrome (posterior tibial nerve compression as it passes through the tarsal tunnel) causes posteromedial heel paresthesias that radiate distally into the plantar foot surface. On examination, pain may be reproduced with nerve tapping (Tinel sign) and with provocative measures that compress the nerve (plantar flexion-inversion and dorsiflexion-eversion tests). First-line treatment consists of activity modification, orthotics, NSAIDs, and neuromodulators.

Forefoot Pain

Morton neuromas (interdigital nerve injury) cause pain between the metatarsal heads and the sensation of walking on a pebble. First-line therapy consists of footwear modification and padding. Glucocorticoid injections may provide temporary relief. Interdigital nerve resection is reserved for those who do not respond to conservative measures.

Hammertoe deformities (proximal interphalangeal joint flexion deformity with distal interphalangeal joint extension and extended or neutral position of metatarsophalangeal [MTP] joint) occur with constricting footwear and increasing age. Treatment includes footwear modification, padding, and possibly surgery.

Hallux or bunion deformity (lateral deviation of great toe with medial bony deformity) can lead to pain, first MTP joint osteoarthritis, and overlying bursitis. Treatment includes orthotic devices, NSAIDs, and possibly surgery.

KEY POINTS

- Acute ankle sprains are usually caused by excessive ankle inversion; treatment includes intermittent cryotherapy, a lace-up support or air stirrup brace combined with elastic compression wrapping, early mobilization with weight bearing as tolerated, and acetaminophen and oral or topical NSAIDs.

(Continued)

KEY POINTS (continued)

- Achilles tendon rupture commonly occurs during strenuous activities, although it may occur spontaneously in the elderly or with fluoroquinolone use.

- Plantar fasciitis classically causes sharp, medial-inferior heel pain with the first morning steps and after prolonged rest; the medial calcaneal tubercle is frequently tender.

- Morton neuromas (interdigital nerve injury) cause pain between the metatarsal heads and the sensation of walking on pebbles.

Dyslipidemia

Evaluation of Lipid Levels

The U.S. Preventive Services Task Force (USPSTF) recommends universal lipid screening in adults aged 40 to 75 years to calculate risk for atherosclerotic cardiovascular disease (ASCVD) using the American College of Cardiology (ACC)/American Heart Association (AHA) Pooled Cohort Equations (see MKSAP 18 Cardiovascular Medicine). Lipid measurement may also be indicated to investigate for familial hypercholesterolemia; to determine therapy adherence and effectiveness; and to evaluate for complications of dyslipidemia, such as pancreatitis.

LDL Cholesterol

The association between high LDL cholesterol levels and increased risk for ASCVD is widely accepted. Historically, cholesterol treatment targeted specific LDL cholesterol goals, as LDL cholesterol is the most atherogenic lipoprotein. The 2013 ACC/AHA cholesterol treatment guideline recommends fixed statin dosing to reduce ASCVD risk and consideration of non-statin drugs in patients who do not achieve adequate lipid lowering. Therefore, based on this guideline, the primary utility of LDL cholesterol measurement is to identify patients who will benefit from treatment with statin therapy and to assess response to therapy.

In patients with elevated LDL cholesterol levels, secondary causes, including hypothyroidism, poorly controlled diabetes mellitus, nephrotic syndrome, and medications (such as glucocorticoids, diuretics, and amiodarone), should be considered. Familial hypercholesterolemia should be considered in patients with an LDL cholesterol level of 190 mg/dL (4.92 mmol/L) or higher.

Triglycerides

Elevated triglyceride levels (>150 mg/dL [1.69 mmol/L]) are independently associated with increased ASCVD risk; however, it is uncertain whether reducing triglyceride levels decreases risk. Causes of hypertriglyceridemia include diabetes; excessive alcohol intake; hypothyroidism; and medications such as glucocorticoids, protease inhibitors, and estrogens. Lifestyle factors, including obesity and concentrated sugar intake, are also implicated causes. Patients with triglyceride levels of 500 mg/dL (5.65 mmol/L) or more without an identifiable cause should be evaluated for familial hypertriglyceridemia.

Acute pancreatitis can be induced by triglyceride levels in excess of 1000 mg/dL (11.3 mmol/L), and triglyceride levels should be measured in selected patients with pancreatitis, especially in cases of pancreatitis without a clear cause (such as alcohol use or biliary disease).

HDL Cholesterol

HDL cholesterol is a protective factor against the development of ASCVD and is an important component in ASCVD risk assessment. However, a causative link between low HDL cholesterol levels and ASCVD has not been established, and pharmacologic treatment to raise HDL cholesterol levels is not recommended.

KEY POINTS

- The U.S. Preventive Services Task Force recommends universal lipid screening in adults aged 40 to 75 years to calculate risk for atherosclerotic cardiovascular disease.
- **HVC** The primary utility of LDL cholesterol measurement is to identify patients who will benefit from treatment with statin therapy and to assess response to therapy.
- Secondary causes of LDL cholesterol elevation include hypothyroidism, poorly controlled diabetes mellitus, nephrotic syndrome, and medication use (such as glucocorticoids, diuretics, and amiodarone).

Management of Dyslipidemia

Following assessment of ASCVD risk, treatment with therapeutic lifestyle changes and statin therapy may be indicated.

Therapeutic Lifestyle Changes

All patients at increased cardiovascular risk should be counseled regarding therapeutic lifestyle changes, including dietary modification, regular physical activity, weight loss, and smoking cessation.

Patients should be encouraged to adhere to a dietary pattern that focuses on consumption of fruits, vegetables, fiber, and monounsaturated fats and minimizes intake of saturated and *trans* fats, simple carbohydrates, and red meats. Replacing saturated fats with polyunsaturated fats has been shown to reduce LDL cholesterol levels and cardiovascular mortality. Examples of heart-healthy diets include the DASH (Dietary Approaches to Stop Hypertension) and Mediterranean diets. The DASH diet provides a suggested number of servings for each food group, with few servings of saturated fats, sweets, and red meat and a higher number of servings of grains, fruits, and vegetables; adherence to the DASH diet has been shown to decrease adverse cardiovascular events. The Mediterranean diet comprises high amounts of unsaturated fats, with ample intake of fruits, vegetables, fiber, seeds, nuts, and fatty fish and low consumption of red meat and dairy products. The ACC/AHA additionally recommend reducing the percentage of calories from saturated fat (<7% of calories from saturated fat; <6% of calories from saturated fat in patients at high cardiovascular risk) and the percentage of calories from *trans* fat. To facilitate these changes, clinicians should provide patients with educational resources and, when appropriate, refer them to a dietician.

Patients should also engage in 40 minutes of moderate to vigorous activity 3 to 4 days per week or 30 minutes on most days of the week. Small incremental changes to reduce sedentary behavior, such as increasing walking and time standing, are beneficial.

Drug Therapy

Statin therapy is the mainstay of pharmacotherapy for dyslipidemia. The ACC/AHA cholesterol treatment guideline defines four patient groups that benefit from statin therapy for primary or secondary prevention of ASCVD:

1. Patients aged 21 years and older with clinical ASCVD, defined as acute coronary syndrome, or a history of myocardial infarction, stable or unstable angina, coronary or other arterial revascularization, stroke/transient ischemic attack, or peripheral artery disease attributable to atherosclerosis (high-intensity statin therapy if aged ≤75 years; moderate-intensity statin therapy if aged >75 years)
2. Patients aged 21 years and older with an LDL cholesterol level of 190 mg/dL (4.92 mmol/L) or higher (high-intensity statin therapy)
3. Patients aged 40 to 75 years with diabetes and an LDL cholesterol level of 70 mg/dL to 189 mg/dL (1.81-4.90 mmol/L) (high-intensity statin therapy if 10-year ASCVD risk ≥7.5%; moderate-intensity statin therapy if 10-year ASCVD risk <7.5%)
4. Patients aged 40 to 75 years with no ASCVD or diabetes and a 10-year ASCVD risk of 7.5% or higher (moderate- or high-intensity statin therapy based on patient preferences, adverse effects, and expected ASCVD risk reduction)

These recommendations are summarized in **Figure 15**. Statin dosages for high- and moderate-intensity therapy are presented in **Table 49**.

A lipid panel should be obtained 4 to 12 weeks after initiation of therapy to determine treatment adherence and response. According to the 2013 ACC/AHA guideline, high-intensity statin therapy should decrease LDL cholesterol levels by at least 50% from baseline levels, whereas moderate-intensity statin therapy should decrease LDL cholesterol levels by 30% to 50%. All patients who do not achieve adequate reduction in LDL cholesterol levels should be assessed for medication adherence and should intensify lifestyle modifications. Additional medical therapy should be considered if the target effect is not realized. Once therapy goals have been achieved,

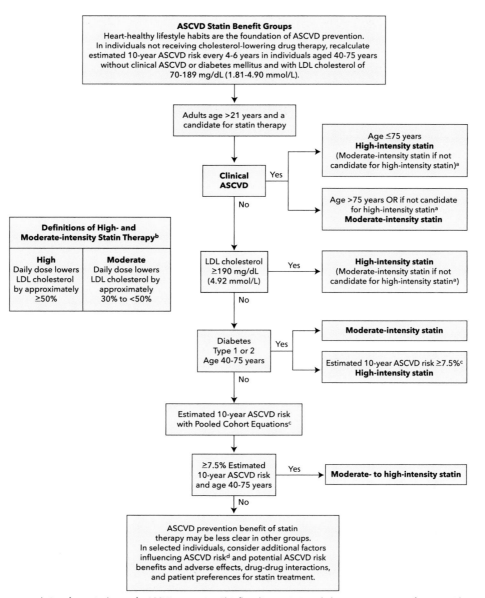

FIGURE 15. Major recommendations for statin therapy for ASCVD prevention. This flow diagram is intended to serve as an easy reference guide summarizing recommendations for ASCVD risk assessment and treatment. Assessment of the potential for benefit and risk from statin therapy for ASCVD prevention provides the framework for clinical decision making incorporating patient preferences. ASCVD = atherosclerotic cardiovascular disease.

[a]Moderate-intensity statin therapy should be used in individuals in whom high-intensity statin therapy would otherwise be recommended when high-intensity statin therapy is contraindicated or when characteristics predisposing them to statin-associated adverse effects are present.

Characteristics predisposing individuals to statin adverse effects include, but are not limited to:

- Multiple or serious comorbidities, including impaired kidney or liver function
- History of previous statin intolerance or muscle disorders
- Unexplained alanine aminotransferase elevations >3 times upper limit of normal
- Patient characteristics or concomitant use of drugs affecting statin metabolism
- >75 years of age

Additional characteristics that may modify the decision to use higher statin intensities may include, but are not limited to:

- History of hemorrhagic stroke
- Asian ancestry

[b]Percent reduction in LDL cholesterol can be used as an indication of response and adherence to therapy but is not in itself a treatment goal.

[c]The Pooled Cohort Equations can be used to estimate 10-year ASCVD risk in individuals with and without diabetes mellitus. A downloadable spreadsheet enabling estimation of 10-year and lifetime risk for ASCVD and a web-based calculator are available at http://my.americanheart.org/cvriskcalculator.

[d]Primary LDL cholesterol level ≥160 mg/dL (4.14 mmol/L) or other evidence of genetic hyperlipidemias; family history of premature ASCVD with onset <55 years of age in a first-degree male relative or <65 years of age in a first-degree female relative; high-sensitivity C-reactive protein ≥2 mg/L; coronary artery calcium score ≥300 Agatston units or ≥75th percentile for age, sex, and ethnicity; ankle-brachial index <0.90; or elevated lifetime risk of ASCVD.

Reproduced with permission from Stone NJ, Robinson JG, Lichtenstein AH, et al; American College of Cardiology/American Heart Association Task Force on Practice Guidelines. 2013 ACC/AHA guideline on the treatment of blood cholesterol to reduce atherosclerotic cardiovascular risk in adults: a report of the American College of Cardiology/American Heart Association Task Force on Practice Guidelines. Circulation. 2013; Epub 2013 Nov 12. Copyright 2013, American Heart Association, Inc.

TABLE 49.	High- and Moderate-Intensity Statin Therapy
Therapy Intensity	**Drug and Dosage**
High intensity	Atorvastatin, 40-80 mg/d
	Rosuvastatin, 20-40 mg/d
Moderate intensity	Atorvastatin, 10-20 mg/d
	Rosuvastatin, 5-10 mg/d
	Simvastatin, 20-40 mg/d
	Pravastatin, 40-80 mg/d
	Lovastatin, 40 mg/d
	Fluvastatin, 40 mg twice daily

lipid levels should be measured every 3 to 12 months as indicated.

The USPSTF recommendations for primary prevention statin therapy differ from those of the ACC/AHA in considering risk factors other than diabetes and the suggested intensity of statin therapy. In asymptomatic adults aged 40 to 75 years without ASCVD who have at least one ASCVD risk factor (dyslipidemia, diabetes, hypertension, or smoking), the USPSTF recommends low- to moderate-intensity statin therapy in those with a calculated 10-year ASCVD event risk of 10% or higher (grade B recommendation) and selective consideration of low- to moderate-intensity statin therapy in those with a calculated 10-year ASCVD event risk of 7.5% to 10% (grade C recommendation).

In contrast to the ACC/AHA guideline and USPSTF recommendations, the 2017 American Association of Clinical Endocrinologists (AACE) and American College of Endocrinology (ACE) guidelines for management of dyslipidemia and prevention of cardiovascular disease recommend treating LDL cholesterol, non-HDL cholesterol, and apolipoprotein B levels to specific targets. On the basis of risk factors and calculated 10-year risk of ASCVD using the Framingham, MESA, Reynolds, or United Kingdom Prospective Diabetes Study risk scores, the AACE/ACE guideline classifies patients as low, moderate, high, very high, or extreme risk. Treatment goals are individualized according to the patient's level of risk, with LDL cholesterol targets of less than 130 mg/dL (3.37 mmol/L) for low-risk patients, less than 100 mg/dL (2.59 mmol/L) for moderate- and high-risk patients, less than 70 mg/dL (1.81 mmol/L) for very-high-risk patients, and less than 55 mg/dL (1.42 mmol/L) for extreme-risk patients. The category of extreme risk represents a new classification for dyslipidemia guidelines and includes patients with progressive ASCVD that persists after achieving an LDL cholesterol level below 70 mg/dL (1.81 mmol/L); patients with established ASCVD with concomitant diabetes mellitus, stage 3 or 4 chronic kidney disease, or hereditary heterozygous familial hypercholesterolemia; and patients with a history of premature ASCVD. The complete guideline, which provides 87 recommendations, is available at https://www.aace.com/files/lipid-guidelines.pdf.

Statins may infrequently cause liver dysfunction or myopathy. Liver chemistry tests should be obtained at baseline, but neither liver chemistry tests nor muscle enzyme studies should be routinely performed in the absence of suggestive symptoms. Statins may also cause memory problems in some patients, but this effect is reversible; evidence suggests that statins do not cause dementia. In patients with statin intolerance, switching to another statin is reasonable, as a patient's response to different statins can vary. Other options include decreasing the statin intensity (decreasing the dosage and/or dosing frequency) and, less preferably, discontinuing statin therapy and initiating nonstatin drugs.

Combination and Nonstatin Drug Therapy

Nonstatin drugs should be considered alone or in combination with statins in patients who do not achieve adequate LDL cholesterol reduction with statin therapy, especially in high-risk patients (those with clinical ASCVD, baseline LDL cholesterol level >190 mg/dL [4.92 mmol/L], or diabetes). Before nonstatin drugs are initiated, patient preferences as well as anticipated ASCVD risk reduction and adverse effects should be discussed. The most commonly used nonstatin drugs and their characteristics are described in **Table 50**.

Ezetimibe and the proprotein convertase subtilisin/kexin type 9 (PCSK9) inhibitors are the preferred nonstatin drugs for high-risk patients who do not achieve goal LDL cholesterol reduction. The PCSK9 inhibitors are a relatively new class of lipid-lowering drugs. These monoclonal antibodies bind to serine protease PCSK9, a liver enzyme that degrades hepatocyte LDL receptors. Treatment with PCSK9 inhibitors produces a 50% to 60% reduction in LDL cholesterol. Barriers to the use of PCSK9 inhibitors include high cost and subcutaneous administration. Additional nonstatin options include bile acid sequestrants, fibrates, and phytosterols. Because of a lack of efficacy and potential harms, niacin is no longer routinely recommended.

In 2017, the ACC published a focused update on nonstatin therapies for LDL cholesterol lowering. Ezetimibe is the preferred nonstatin agent in patients with or without diabetes who have an LDL cholesterol level between 70 mg/dL (1.81 mmol/L) and 189 mg/dL (4.90 mmol/L) and are taking maximally tolerated statin therapy for primary prevention. Likewise, ezetimibe is preferred in patients with stable clinical ASCVD without comorbid conditions who require additional LDL cholesterol lowering. Ezetimibe or a PCSK9 inhibitor may be used in high-risk patients taking maximally tolerated statin therapy, including patients with LDL cholesterol levels greater than 190 mg/dL (4.92 mmol/L) and patients with clinical ASCVD with comorbidities. Factors that favor ezetimibe for these high-risk patients include the need for less than 25% LDL cholesterol reduction, recent myocardial infarction (within the last 3 months), present and future cost savings, and preference for oral administration.

Management of Hypertriglyceridemia

Therapeutic lifestyle changes are the cornerstone of management of elevated triglyceride levels. Patients should be counseled to lose weight (if appropriate); exercise regularly;

TABLE 50. Characteristics of Nonstatin Drugs

Medication	LDL-Cholesterol Lowering	ASCVD Risk Reduction	Adverse Effects	Approximate Cost
PCSK9 inhibitors	↓↓↓↓	↓↓↓	Nasopharyngitis, injection-site reactions, possible cognitive effects	$$$$
Ezetimibe	↓↓	↓↓↓	Diarrhea, arthralgia, abdominal pain, myositis, elevated liver aminotransferase levels when combined with statins	$$-$$$
Bile acid sequestrants	↓↓	↓ (cholestyramine)	Constipation, bloating, nausea, elevated liver aminotransferase levels, interference with drug absorption Increase triglyceride levels only if baseline levels are elevated	$$
Fibrates	↓	Not well determined	Myositis (especially if combined with statins), nausea, abdominal pain	$$
Phytosterols	↓	Not well determined	Mild bloating, diarrhea or constipation	$-$$

ASCVD = atherosclerotic cardiovascular disease; PCSK9 = proprotein convertase subtilisin/kexin type 9.

and avoid consumption of saturated fats, *trans* fats, and concentrated sugars. Although *trans* fats have been eliminated from many commercially prepared foods, some foods (such as creamers, margarine, and baked goods) may still contain *trans* fats, also called partially hydrogenated oil. The use of medications that increase triglyceride levels, such as estrogens, β-blockers, and glucocorticoids, should be avoided if possible.

Omega-3 fatty acids, which are found in many types of fish, reduce triglyceride levels and should be incorporated into the diet. Fibrates are the most effective pharmacotherapy for hypertriglyceridemia, resulting in a 30% to 50% reduction in triglyceride levels; these agents are indicated in patients with triglyceride levels of 500 mg/dL (5.65 mmol/L) or higher. Niacin and prescription omega-3 fatty acid supplements also lower triglyceride levels; however, omega-3 fatty acid supplements do not reduce heart disease, stroke, or death. According to the 2013 ACC/AHA guideline, baseline liver aminotransferase, hemoglobin A_{1c} or fasting plasma glucose, and uric acid levels should be obtained before and during niacin treatment. Niacin therapy should not be used in patients receiving statin therapy who have achieved adequate LDL cholesterol reduction.

Management of Dyslipidemia in Special Populations

In patients aged 75 years and older, there is insufficient evidence to guide the use of statin therapy for primary prevention; however, the ACC/AHA guideline suggests that it is reasonable to engage these patients in a discussion of the potential for ASCVD risk-reduction benefits, adverse effects, and drug-drug interactions, and to consider patient preferences for treatment. For secondary prevention of ASCVD in patients aged 75 years and older, it is reasonable to continue statins in patients who are already tolerating therapy; moderate-intensity therapy is beneficial and preferable to high-intensity therapy in these patients.

Owing to insufficient evidence, the ACC/AHA make no recommendations on the initiation or discontinuation of statin therapy in patients with heart failure (New York Heart Association functional class II-IV symptoms) or patients undergoing hemodialysis.

KEY POINTS

- All patients with elevated LDL cholesterol levels should be counseled regarding therapeutic lifestyle changes, including dietary modification, regular physical activity, weight loss, and smoking cessation. **HVC**

- The American College of Cardiology and American Heart Association recommend initiating statin therapy for primary or secondary prevention of atherosclerotic cardiovascular disease (ASCVD) in (1) patients with clinical ASCVD; (2) patients with an LDL cholesterol level of 190 mg/dL (4.92 mmol/L) or higher; (3) patients aged 40 to 75 years with diabetes mellitus, an LDL cholesterol level of 70 to 189 mg/dL (1.81-4.90 mmol/L), and no clinical ASCVD; and (4) patients aged 40 to 75 years with no ASCVD or diabetes and a 10-year ASCVD risk of 7.5% or higher.

- A lipid panel should be obtained 4 to 12 weeks after statin therapy initiation to determine treatment adherence and response to therapy.

- In patients treated with statin therapy, liver chemistry tests and muscle enzyme studies should not be routinely obtained in the absence of symptoms of liver dysfunction or myopathy. **HVC**

- Nonstatin drugs, such as ezetimibe and proprotein convertase subtilisin/kexin type 9 (PCSK9) inhibitors, should be considered alone or in combination with statins in high-risk patients who do not achieve adequate LDL cholesterol reduction with statin therapy.

Metabolic Syndrome
Epidemiology and Pathophysiology
Metabolic syndrome, also referred to as insulin resistance syndrome, comprises a constellation of risk factors for cardiovascular disease and type 2 diabetes. It is a common condition, occurring in 20% to 35% of U.S. adults.

Although there are several definitions for metabolic syndrome, the diagnostic criteria proposed by the National Cholesterol Education Program Adult Treatment Panel III (with minor modifications by the AHA/National Heart, Lung, and Blood Institute) are the most widely used (**Table 51**). The presence of a pathophysiologic link between the components

TABLE 51. Diagnostic Criteria for the Metabolic Syndrome	
Measure (Any Three of Five Constitute Diagnosis of Metabolic Syndrome)	**Categorical Cutpoints**
Elevated waist circumference[a,b]	≥102 cm [40 in] in men; ≥88 cm [35 in] in women
Elevated triglycerides	≥150 mg/dL (1.7 mmol/L) or On drug treatment for elevated triglycerides
Reduced HDL cholesterol	<40 mg/dL (1.03 mmol/L) in men; <50 mg/dL (1.30 mmol/L) in women or On drug treatment for reduced HDL cholesterol[c]
Elevated blood pressure	≥130 mm Hg systolic blood pressure or ≥85 mm Hg diastolic blood pressure or On antihypertensive drug treatment in a patient with a history of hypertension
Elevated fasting glucose	≥100 mg/dL (5.6 mmol/L) or On drug treatment for elevated glucose

[a]To measure waist circumference, locate top of right iliac crest. Place a measuring tape in a horizontal plane around abdomen at level of iliac crest. Before reading tape measure, ensure that tape is snug but does not compress the skin and is parallel to floor. Measurement is made at the end of a normal expiration.

[b]Some U.S. adults of non-Asian origin (e.g., white, black, Hispanic) with marginally increased waist circumference (e.g., 94-101 cm [37-39 inches] in men and 80-87 cm [31-34 inches] in women) may have strong genetic contribution to insulin resistance and should benefit from changes in lifestyle habits, similar to men with categorical increases in waist circumference. Lower waist circumference cutpoint (e.g., ≥90 cm [35 inches] in men and ≥80 cm [31 inches] in women) appears to be appropriate for Asian Americans.

[c]Fibrates and nicotinic acid are the most commonly used drugs for elevated triglycerides and reduced HDL cholesterol. Patients taking one of these drugs are presumed to have high triglycerides and low HDL cholesterol.

Reproduced with permission from Grundy SM, Cleeman JI, Daniels SR, Donato KA, Eckel RH, Franklin BA at al. Diagnosis and management of the metabolic syndrome: an American Heart Association/National Heart, Lung, and Blood Institute scientific statement. Circulation. 2005;112(17):2735. [PMID: 16157765]

of the metabolic syndrome is controversial; however, insulin resistance and adipocyte cytokines associated with metabolic syndrome appear to play a central role in inducing inflammatory changes that contribute to ASCVD.

Management
Treatment of metabolic syndrome focuses on addressing each of the component risk factors. Lifestyle modifications, particularly weight loss and exercise, are the most important treatment interventions. Routine pharmacotherapy is not recommended in patients who do not meet treatment criteria for the individual risk factors. Aspirin is indicated for patients with metabolic syndrome and a 10-year ASCVD risk of 10% or greater, assuming there is not increased bleeding risk. In some studies, metformin has been shown to prevent progression to diabetes; however, it is inferior to lifestyle modifications, and its role in treating metabolic syndrome has not been established.

Obesity
Definition and Epidemiology
Obesity, defined as a BMI of 30 or greater, is associated with increased risk for type 2 diabetes mellitus, hypertension, dyslipidemia, cardiovascular disease, stroke, obstructive sleep apnea, osteoarthritis, and some cancers; risks for these conditions increase with increasing BMI. Waist circumference of 102 cm (40 in) or greater in men and 88 cm (35 in) or greater in women is additionally associated with increased risk for diabetes mellitus, cardiovascular disease, and all-cause mortality (**Table 52**).

Prevalence of obesity and extreme obesity (BMI ≥40) among adults in the United States increased from 35.1% to 37.7% and 6.5% to 7.7%, respectively, between 2011-2012 and 2013-2014. Prevalence of obesity varies by gender, ethnicity, education, and age, with the highest prevalence among women, non-Hispanic black persons, those with less education, and those aged 40 to 59 years.

The costs associated with providing care to patients with severe obesity are high (more than $69 billion in 2013).

KEY POINTS
- The prevalence of obesity (BMI >30) and extreme obesity (BMI ≥40) is increasing.
- Waist circumference of 102 cm (40 in) inches or greater in men and 88 cm (35 in) or greater in women is associated with increased risk for diabetes mellitus, cardiovascular disease, and all-cause mortality.

Screening and Evaluation
The U.S. Preventive Services Task Force recommends screening adults for obesity by measuring height and weight and

TABLE 52. Classification of Overweight and Obesity by BMI

| Category | BMI | Obesity Class | Disease Risk[a] Relative to Normal Weight and Waist Circumference | |
			Men: ≤102 cm (40 in) Women: ≤88 cm (35 in)	Men: >102 cm (40 in) Women: >88 cm (35 in)
Underweight	<18.5		—	—
Normal	18.5-24.9		—	—
Overweight	25.0-29.9		Increased	High
Obesity	30.0-34.9	I	High	Very high
	35.0-39.9	II	Very high	Very high
Extreme obesity	≥40	III	Extremely high	Extremely high

[a]Disease risk for type 2 diabetes mellitus, hypertension, and cardiovascular disease. Increased waist circumference also can be a marker for increased risk, even in persons of normal weight.

Reproduced from National Heart, Lung, and Blood Institute. Aim for a healthy weight. https://www.nhlbi.nih.gov/health/educational/lose_wt/BMI/bmi_dis.htm. Accessed June 25, 2018.

calculating BMI. Online BMI calculators are available (https://www.nhlbi.nih.gov/guidelines/obesity/BMI/bmicalc.htm). Clinicians should ask patients with obesity about their weight history, previous weight loss attempts, diet and physical activity patterns, social and emotional factors, and family history of obesity. A thorough medication history is recommended to identify medications that may contribute to weight gain (**Table 53**). Physicians should inquire about symptoms of obesity-related conditions, such as heart disease, obstructive sleep apnea, osteoarthritis, and erectile dysfunction.

Physical examination should include measurements of height, weight, waist circumference, and blood pressure. Examining patients with obesity is sometimes challenging and adaptations may be necessary, such as using a scale with an adequate weight limit, using an appropriately sized blood pressure cuff (bladder encircles 80% of the arm), and repositioning patients to optimize hearing of heart sounds. Many patients with obesity are deconditioned, and allowing the patient to sit quietly for 5 minutes after walking from the waiting area to the examination room before measuring heart rate and blood pressure may improve the reliability of these measurements.

TABLE 53. Medications That Promote Weight Gain

α-Blockers
β-Blockers
Glucocorticoids
Progestins (especially depot injections)
Antidiabetic drugs (insulin, sulfonylureas [especially glyburide and glipizide], thiazolidinediones)
Anticonvulsant drugs (carbamazepine, gabapentin, valproic acid)
Antidepressant drugs (amitriptyline, imipramine, doxepin, paroxetine, mirtazapine)
Antipsychotic drugs (clozapine, olanzapine, quetiapine, risperidone)

Laboratory evaluation should include fasting blood glucose and lipid levels. Requests for other laboratory tests should be based on patient-specific signs, symptoms, and risk factors. Although obesity is associated with higher risk for certain cancers, recommendations for cancer screening are the same as for patients without obesity. Screening for cardiovascular disease in asymptomatic patients with obesity is not indicated; testing is reserved for symptomatic patients.

KEY POINT

- The U.S. Preventive Services Task Force recommends screening all adults for obesity by calculating BMI. **HVC**

Treatment

Treatment options for obesity include lifestyle modification, pharmacotherapy, and bariatric surgery. Guidelines published by the American College of Cardiology/American Heart Association/The Obesity Society on the management of obesity recommend lifestyle modification that includes reduced calorie intake, increased physical activity, and behavioral therapy in all patients. Similarly, the U.S. Preventive Services Task Force recommends offering or referring obese patients to intensive, multicomponent behavioral interventions. For patients at highest risk who have tried lifestyle modification measures without success, pharmacotherapy or surgical intervention may be considered. Patients should be advised that weight loss is beneficial even without attaining a normal weight; loss of 3% to 5% of initial body weight is associated with improvement in glycemic control, blood pressure, and lipid levels.

Lifestyle Modification

Readiness to make lifestyle changes should be assessed. Engaging family members and other social supports may increase adherence to lifestyle change. Given the expected slow pace of weight loss, patients may benefit from encouragement to focus on other changes resulting from lifestyle modification, such as improved exercise tolerance.

Reduced Dietary Energy Intake

Typical dietary calorie intake ranges required to produce weight loss are 1200 to 1500 kcal/d for women and 1500 to 1800 kcal/d for men; the calorie intake required to achieve a calorie deficit for a given person varies. Clinicians can estimate basal energy expenditure in calories using the Harris-Benedict Equation (http://www.bmi-calculator.net/bmr-calculator/harris-benedict-equation/).

Any diet that achieves a calorie deficit will produce weight loss; this is true for low-calorie, low-fat, low-carbohydrate, moderate/high-protein, low-glycemic-index, vegan (with or without a low-fat component), and Mediterranean-style diets, as well as commercial diet plans. Patients should be advised to use the diet to which they will most likely adhere.

Very-low-calorie diets (<800 kcal/d) produce accelerated weight loss but require medical supervision. They should be reserved for situations requiring rapid weight loss.

Exercise

Lifestyle interventions should include moderate- to vigorous-intensity physical activity (such as brisk walking) for at least 150 minutes per week. The main contribution of increased physical activity is to minimize the reduction in calories required to achieve a caloric deficit. Because patients are often initially deconditioned, gradual progression may be required. Long-term continuance of a similar program of physical activity is important for maintaining weight loss and improving cardiovascular fitness.

Behavioral Therapy

The Centers for Medicare & Medicaid Services have approved payment for "intensive behavioral weight loss counseling" by primary care providers. Content of this counseling in practice varies widely, as does its effectiveness. Specific components associated with increased effectiveness include a calorie deficit of at least 500 kcal/d, at least 150 minutes of moderate to vigorous physical activity per week, and the use of trained interventionists (nutritionists, behavioral therapists, or exercise therapists). Interventions should incorporate regular self-monitoring of weight and calorie intake as well as education on controlling or altering the environment to avoid excess calorie intake. Examples include removing calorie-dense snacks and beverages from the home or workplace, replacing them with lower-calorie options, and engaging in other behaviors (walking, chewing gum) for situations during which the patient might be tempted to eat for pleasure, for emotional solace, or because of boredom. Programs of high intensity (≥14 sessions over at least 6 months) delivered by trained interventionists are associated with successful weight loss. Comprehensive programs lasting longer than 1 year with at least monthly contact are associated with greater likelihood of maintaining lifestyle change.

Face-to-face interventions most reliably result in weight loss, but interventions delivered electronically or by telephone have also shown success.

Pharmacologic Therapy

Patients who do not achieve weight loss with lifestyle change alone should be considered for pharmacotherapy, especially patients at higher risk for complications (those with BMI ≥30, or with BMI ≥27 and at least one obesity-associated comorbid condition). Weight loss pharmacotherapy is effective but incurs risk for adverse events as well as increased cost, and these factors should be balanced against potential weight-loss benefit.

Table 54 describes the mechanism of action, expected weight loss, and side effects of commonly used agents; all have

TABLE 54.	Medications for Weight Loss		
Medication	**Mechanism of Action**	**Weight Loss Versus Placebo at 52 Weeks in Meta-analysis of Randomized Controlled Trials**	**Common Side Effects (Odds Ratio for Discontinuation Versus Placebo)**
Liraglutide	GLP-1 receptor activator, delays gastric emptying	5.2 kg (11.6 lb)	Gastrointestinal upset, headache, nasopharyngitis (2.82)
Lorcaserin	Selective serotonergic 5HT2C receptor agonist, suppresses appetite	3.3 kg (7.2 lb)	Headache, dizziness, fatigue, nausea, dry mouth, cough, constipation May cause hypoglycemia in patients with diabetes mellitus (1.40)
Naltrexone-bupropion	Opioid antagonist plus norepinephrine/dopamine uptake inhibitor, suppresses appetite	5 kg (10.9 lb)	Gastrointestinal upset, headache, dizziness, insomnia, dry mouth, tachycardia, hypertension, anxiety, tremor (2.60)
Orlistat	Lipase inhibitor, decreases triglyceride absorption	2.6 kg (5.8 lb)	Oily stools, increased defecation, fecal urgency/incontinence (1.84)
Phentermine-topiramate	Noradrenergic/GABA receptor activator plus AMPA glutamate receptor inhibitor, suppresses appetite	8.8 kg (19.4 lb)	Paresthesias, dizziness, taste alterations, insomnia, constipation, dry mouth, tachycardia, cognitive changes (2.32)

5HT2C = 5-hydroxytryptamine2C; AMPA = α-amino-3-hydroxy-5-methyl-4-isoxazole propionic acid; GABA = γ-aminobutyric acid; GLP-1 = glucagon-like peptide-1.

Data from Khera R, Murad MH, Chandar AK, Dulai PS, Wang Z, Prokop LJ, et al. Association of pharmacological treatments for obesity with weight loss and adverse events: a systematic review and meta-analysis. JAMA. 2016;315:2424-34. [PMID: 27299618] doi:10.1001/jama.2016.7602

demonstrated higher rates of achieving 5% to 10% weight loss and larger amounts of weight lost compared with placebo. Orlistat and lorcaserin had the lowest rates of discontinuation due to side effects. Orlistat also has long-term safety data. Liraglutide and phentermine-topiramate produced the greatest weight loss but had higher rates of discontinuation due to side effects.

Patients are inundated with advertisements for over-the-counter weight loss supplements, which often claim the supplements are safer and more effective than prescription medications. These claims and easy access have led to widespread use of weight loss supplements, but systematic reviews show little evidence that any over-the-counter weight loss supplements are effective. Moreover, some supplements, such as ma huang/ephedra and bitter orange, may also be associated with significant adverse effects. Physicians should be prepared to discuss the lack of effectiveness and potential for side effects of these supplements during weight loss counseling. Comprehensive information on supplements is available at https://medlineplus.gov/druginfo/herb_All.html.

As with all other comprehensive weight loss interventions, patients should be monitored regularly. Patients who do not show improved success with weight reduction after 12 weeks of therapy should not continue pharmacotherapy.

Bariatric Surgery

For patients at highest risk for obesity-related complications and for whom other measures have not resulted in the desired clinical end points, bariatric surgery should be considered. Guidelines recommend reserving surgery for patients with a BMI of 40 or greater or for those with a BMI of 35 or greater who have obesity-associated comorbid conditions.

The risks associated with bariatric surgery exceed those associated with nonsurgical treatments. Therefore, candidates for bariatric surgery should be selected carefully on the basis of harm-benefit analysis. Patients should have acceptable operative risk, understand the necessity of lifelong dietary and lifestyle measures for sustained weight loss, and be willing to adhere to lifelong follow-up. Candidates should not have psychological or psychiatric conditions that impede adherence to these requirements. Careful selection of patients in preparation for surgery and adherence to follow-up visits predict successful weight loss and maintenance, as well as avoidance of complications.

Techniques

The three most commonly performed bariatric surgical procedures include Roux-en-Y gastric bypass, sleeve gastrectomy, and gastric banding. Roux-en-Y gastric bypass involves detaching the proximal stomach and creating a small pouch, which is reattached to the Roux limb of the small intestine. Weight loss results from decrease in caloric intake because of the small stomach pouch, malabsorption due to bypassing much of the stomach and proximal small intestines, and

appetite suppression due to changes in glucagon-like peptide-1 (GLP-1) and related hormones.

Sleeve gastrectomy is accomplished by excising the part of the stomach along the greater curvature, creating an approximately 85% reduction in size; similar to gastric bypass, it results in restriction of calorie intake via a smaller stomach and hormonal (GLP-1 and related hormones) appetite suppression. The smaller gastric surface area also results in less production of ghrelin, an appetite stimulant.

Gastric banding involves placement of a silicon fluid-filled band around the proximal stomach, creating a small stomach pouch with subsequent reduction in calorie intake by increasing satiety.

All procedures result in loss of excess weight in the short term, up to 70% with Roux-en-Y, 50% with sleeve gastrectomy, and 30% with gastric banding. Long-term (5-year) data are less robust but suggest sustained weight loss.

More recently, other alternative surgical and nonsurgical procedures have been developed. These include

TABLE 55. Nutrient Deficiencies and Replacement After Bariatric Surgery

Nutrient Deficiency	Replacement Therapy
Iron	MVI with iron, or elemental iron 40-80 mg/d orally
	If deficient, ferrous sulfate 325 mg/d orally
Vitamin B_{12}	Vitamin B_{12} 500-1000 µg/d orally, or 1000 µg IM monthly
Folic acid	MVI with folate
	If deficient, 400 µg/d orally
	For women of childbearing age, folate 1 mg/d orally
Calcium	Calcium citrate 1200 mg/d orally
Vitamin D	Vitamin D 400-1000 U/d orally
	If deficient, 50,000 U weekly orally for 3 mo, then reassess
Thiamine	25-50 mg/d orally
Vitamin A	MVI daily
	If deficient, 5000-10,000 U/d orally with ongoing monitoring
Vitamin E	MVI daily
	If deficient, 400 U/d orally
Vitamin K	MVI daily
	If deficient, 5-10 mg/d orally
Copper	MVI with minerals daily
	If deficient, 2-4 mg/d orally
Zinc	MVI with minerals daily
	If deficient, 220 mg/d orally

IM = intramuscularly; MVI = multivitamin.

Data from Marcotte E, Chand B. Management and prevention of surgical and nutritional complications after bariatric surgery. Surg Clin North Am. 2016;96:843-56. [PMID: 27473805] doi:10.1016/j.suc.2016.03.006

restrictive procedures (endoscopic suturing or stapling in a manner that replicates sleeve gastrectomy) or placement of space-occupying devices (intragastric balloons) or devices intended to decrease caloric absorption (duodenal-jejunal liners). These and other related techniques are less invasive and may carry less risk than surgical procedures, but more experience and data on long-term outcomes are needed.

Postoperative Care

Rates of 30-day postoperative complications are low, ranging from 1.3% to 8.7%. Early complications include bleeding or leakage at the anastomosis (bypass procedures) or staple line (sleeve gastrectomy) and bowel obstruction. Later complications include anastomotic or marginal ulceration, leaks, bowel obstruction and slippage, or excessive tightness of gastric bands. Initial evaluation and management for bleeding or ulceration can be performed endoscopically. Leakage is evaluated with an upper gastrointestinal series or contrast CT scan and managed by laparoscopy. Symptoms of obstruction in patients with gastric band procedures are evaluated with an upper gastrointestinal series and managed by removing fluid from the band device. **H**

Weight should be monitored closely in the early postoperative period. As patients lose weight, frequent reassessment of prescription medications is required (for example, insulin dosage reduction).

Long-term postsurgical care focuses on preventing nutritional deficiencies, managing adherence to lifestyle modifications, and monitoring for behaviors that lead to weight regain. **Table 55** lists the anticipated nutritional deficiencies and recommended replacement strategies. **Table 56** describes post–bariatric surgery syndromes and their management.

TABLE 56. Post–Bariatric Surgery Syndromes		
Syndrome	**Cause**	**Monitoring/Therapy**
Dumping syndrome/postprandial hypoglycemia (tachycardia, sweating, abdominal pain, nausea, vomiting, diarrhea)	Rapid transit of undigested food into small intestines Early symptoms (1 hour postprandial) caused by fluid shift into the GI tract (no hypoglycemia) Late symptoms (2-3 hours postprandial) hypoglycemia caused by insulin surge in response to hyperglycemia	Avoid foods high in simple sugar; replace with higher-fiber/high-protein foods Avoid sweetened beverages (including alcohol)
Chronic loose stool	May relate to rapid transit of food to small intestines, similar to dumping syndrome Consider small intestine bacterial overgrowth	Adherence to dietary modifications to avoid dumping syndrome Rifaximin if bacterial overgrowth is suspected
Kidney stones	Increased urinary oxalic acid related to fat malabsorption	Diet low in fat and oxalate, calcium supplementation, increased hydration
Gallstones	Bile stasis, increased biliary cholesterol saturation with rapid weight loss	Ultrasonography if symptomatic Cholecystectomy is definitive treatment Ursodeoxycholic acid shown to be effective prophylactically in meta-analysis of RCTs
Gastric or marginal ulceration	Often associated with NSAID use	Endoscopy to confirm Avoidance of NSAIDs
Hypotension, hypoglycemia	Improved blood pressure and insulin sensitivity with weight loss	Adjust medications as indicated; consider proactive reduction in dose (especially antidiabetic medications)
Chronic abdominal pain/nausea	Various, including nonadherence to diet recommendations, device slippage (gastric band procedures), bowel obstruction	Evaluate with endoscopy or CT Re-educate patient on diet modifications if no other cause is identified Consider low-dose antidepressant therapy
Gastroesophageal reflux	Incidence usually decreases after diversion procedures but may increase after sleeve gastrectomy	Evaluate with endoscopy PPI therapy, lifestyle modification
Regain of weight lost	Disordered eating, excess intake of high-calorie liquid/semisolid foods or supplements	Re-educate patient on diet modifications Refer to psychiatric care or counseling if indicated

GI = gastrointestinal; PPI = proton pump inhibitor; RCT = randomized controlled trial.

KEY POINTS

HVC
- Lifestyle modifications that are effective for the treatment of obesity include a calorie deficit of at least 500 kcal/d, at least 150 minutes of moderate to vigorous physical activity per week, and the use of trained interventionists (nutritionists, behavioral therapists, or exercise therapists).

- Pharmacologic therapy may be used as an adjunct to lifestyle modifications in patients with a BMI of 30 or greater or in patients with a BMI of 27 or greater who have overweight- or obesity-associated comorbid conditions.

HVC
- Systematic reviews show little evidence that over-the-counter weight loss supplements are effective.

- Bariatric surgery should be reserved for patients with a BMI of 40 or greater or for those with a BMI of 35 or greater who have obesity-associated comorbid conditions.

- Long-term postsurgical care focuses on preventing nutritional deficiencies, managing adherence to lifestyle modifications, and monitoring for behaviors that lead to weight regain.

Men's Health

Male Sexual Dysfunction

Erectile Dysfunction

The American Urological Association (AUA) defines erectile dysfunction as the "inability to achieve or maintain an erection sufficient for satisfactory sexual performance." Erectile dysfunction is a common medical condition, and prevalence increases with age between 18 and 69 years; up to 33% of men older than age 50 years are affected.

Numerous risk factors and conditions are associated with erectile dysfunction, including coronary artery disease, peripheral vascular disease, diabetes mellitus, hypertension, hyperlipidemia, metabolic syndrome, obesity, tobacco use, obstructive sleep apnea, hypothyroidism, hypogonadism (androgen deficiency), benign prostatic hyperplasia, neuropathy, central neurologic conditions (Parkinson disease, Alzheimer disease, and stroke), trauma, surgery, drug and alcohol abuse, depression, and anxiety. Furthermore, numerous medications have been linked to erectile dysfunction, particularly thiazide diuretics and selective serotonin reuptake inhibitors (**Table 57**).

Erectile dysfunction can be an isolated and independent presentation, or it can be an indication of another underlying condition. Erectile dysfunction, as compared with traditional cardiovascular risk factors, portends a similar, if not greater, predictive risk for a future cardiovascular event. As such, the evaluation of erectile dysfunction must include a thorough history and physical examination directed toward identifying any potentially treatable causative factors, including those associated

TABLE 57. Drugs Commonly Associated With Erectile Dysfunction

Antidepressants (monoamine oxidase inhibitors, selective serotonin reuptake inhibitors, tricyclic antidepressants)
Benzodiazepines
Opioids, nicotine, alcohol, amphetamines, barbiturates, cocaine, marijuana, methadone
Anticonvulsants (phenytoin, phenobarbital)
Antihypertensives and diuretics (thiazide diuretics, loop diuretics, clonidine, spironolactone; possibly α-blockers, β-blockers, calcium channel blockers, ACE inhibitors)
5α-Reductase inhibitors (dutasteride, finasteride)
Antihistamines and H_2 blockers (dimenhydrinate, diphenhydramine, hydroxyzine, meclizine, promethazine, cimetidine, nizatidine, ranitidine)
NSAIDs (naproxen, indomethacin)
Parkinson disease medications (levodopa, bromocriptine, biperiden, trihexyphenidyl, benztropine, procyclidine)

with cardiovascular disease. The history should include medical, psychosocial, and sexual components and should focus on the timing of symptoms (whether gradual or sudden in onset) as well as the presence of early-morning and nocturnal spontaneous erections. It is also helpful to interview the patient's partner regarding sexual function and the relationship. Patients should be assessed for other concomitant disorders of sexual function, such as premature ejaculation and decreased libido.

Physical examination should include cardiovascular, genital, digital rectal, peripheral vascular, and neurologic evaluations. Clinicians should pay close attention for any alterations in secondary sexual characteristics suggestive of hypogonadism (reduced testicular volume, loss of normal body hair distribution, gynecomastia).

Laboratory assessment involves obtaining a fasting blood glucose level, lipid panel, 8:00 AM total testosterone level, and thyroid-stimulating hormone level. Additional testing is usually not warranted unless the history or physical examination suggests a separate process.

The treatment of erectile dysfunction has been shown to improve sexual performance, quality of life, and self-esteem and to strengthen interpersonal relationships. Before implementing any treatment strategies for erectile dysfunction, however, it is imperative for clinicians to fully evaluate patients in terms of cardiac risk associated with sexual activity (to determine whether it is safe for a patient to engage in sexual activities). The Princeton III Consensus recommendations provide specific guidelines on the safety of sexual activity based on the patient's cardiac risk level (**Table 58**).

Treatment options include lifestyle modifications, oral phosphodiesterase-5 inhibitor therapies, injectable and intraurethral prostaglandin E_1 therapies, penile device therapies, testosterone therapy, and psychotherapy (**Table 59**). All patients should undergo lifestyle modification as appropriate, including weight loss and tobacco cessation; the use of

TABLE 58. Third Princeton Consensus Conference Guidelines for Treatment of Erectile Dysfunction in Patients With Cardiovascular Disease or Cardiac Risk Factors

Risk Level	Treatment Recommendation
Low Risk	
Patients who are able to do moderate-intensity exercise without symptoms	Can initiate or resume sexual activity or treat for ED with PDE-5 inhibitor (if not using nitrates)
Successfully revascularized patients (e.g., coronary artery bypass grafting, coronary stenting, or angioplasty)	
Asymptomatic controlled hypertension	
Mild valvular disease	
Mild left ventricular dysfunction (NYHA functional class I or II) who can achieve 5 METs without ischemia as determined by recent exercise testing	
Intermediate/Indeterminate Risk	
Mild to moderate stable angina	Further cardiac evaluation and restratification before resumption of sexual activity or treatment for ED
Recent MI (2-8 weeks) without intervention awaiting exercise ECG	
Heart failure (NYHA functional class III)	If the patient can complete 4 minutes of the standard Bruce treadmill protocol without symptoms, arrhythmias, or a decrease in blood pressure, treatment for ED can be safely initiated
Noncardiac atherosclerotic disease (clinically evident PAD, history of stroke/TIA)	
High Risk	
Unstable or refractory angina	Defer sexual activity or ED treatment until cardiac condition is stabilized and reassessed
Uncontrolled hypertension	
Moderate to severe heart failure (NYHA functional class IV)	
Recent MI (<2 weeks) without intervention	
High-risk arrhythmia (exercise-induced ventricular tachycardia, ICD with frequent shocks, poorly controlled atrial fibrillation)	
Obstructive hypertrophic cardiomyopathy with severe symptoms	
Moderate to severe valvular disease (particularly aortic stenosis)	

ECG = electrocardiography; ED = erectile dysfunction; ICD = implantable cardioverter-defibrillator; METs = metabolic equivalents; MI = myocardial infarction; NYHA = New York Heart Association; PAD = peripheral artery disease; PDE = phosphodiesterase; TIA = transient ischemic attack.

Recommendations from Nehra A, Jackson G, Miner M, Billups KL, Burnett AL, Buvat J, et al. The Princeton III Consensus recommendations for the management of erectile dysfunction and cardiovascular disease. Mayo Clin Proc. 2012;87:766-78. [PMID: 22862865] doi:10.1016/j.mayocp.2012.06.015

medications that may contribute to erectile dysfunction should be reconsidered.

Oral phosphodiesterase-5 inhibitors are first-line medical therapy and are safe and effective in most patients. Their use is contraindicated in patients taking nitrates because of the risk for hypotension. Similarly, they should be used with caution in the setting of concomitant α-blocker therapy. Second-line medical therapy includes alprostadil (prostaglandin E₁), which has a mechanism of action similar to that of oral phosphodiesterase-5 inhibitors. Although efficacious, it is administered locally by intracavernous injection, transurethral injection, or transurethral suppository, making it inconvenient and less well tolerated. Testosterone therapy is indicated only in cases of confirmed androgen deficiency and has multiple contraindications.

Premature Ejaculation

The AUA defines premature ejaculation as ejaculation that occurs sooner than desired and is distressful to either or both partners. The diagnosis of premature ejaculation is solely based on history. Clinicians should obtain a thorough sexual history (frequency of premature ejaculation, antecedent sexual activities, aggravating and alleviating factors, the impact of premature ejaculation, and any concomitant erectile dysfunction). Assessment for an underlying mood condition is also imperative given the association between premature ejaculation and quality of life.

Treatment of premature ejaculation consists primarily of counseling and pharmacotherapy. According to the AUA, medication options include selective serotonin reuptake inhibitors (paroxetine, fluoxetine, sertraline) and tricyclic antidepressants (clomipramine) to delay ejaculation, as well as topical anesthetics (lidocaine, prilocaine) to reduce tactile stimulation.

Decreased Libido

Decreased libido is a common symptom and is defined as a reduced desire or inclination to engage in sexual activities, sexual thoughts, or fantasies. When associated with concomitant marked personal or interpersonal distress, the condition

TABLE 59. Treatment Strategies for Erectile Dysfunction

Treatment Option	Additional Information
Lifestyle modification	Recommended for all patients
	Weight loss, smoking cessation, exercise, stress management
Oral phosphodiesterase-5 inhibitor	Increases cGMP → vascular smooth muscle relaxation → increased penile blood flow
Sildenafil	Equally efficacious
Tadalafil	Side effects: headache, flushing, dizziness, hypotension, presyncope/syncope
Vardenafil	Visual disturbances: "blue haze," a benign finding due to inhibition of retinal phosphodiesterase-6; association with anterior ischemic optic neuropathy
	Use with care with drugs that inhibit cytochrome P-450 3A4 pathway (fluconazole, verapamil, erythromycin)
Injectable and intraurethral prostaglandin E$_1$	Increases cAMP → vascular smooth muscle relaxation → increased penile blood flow
Alprostadil	Initial trial dose should be performed by or supervised by a clinician
Testosterone supplementation	Avoid in patients with breast or prostate cancer; prostate nodule; prostate-specific antigen >4 ng/mL (4 µg/L) or >3 ng/mL (3 µg/L) in patients with a first-degree relative with prostate cancer as well as black patients; poorly controlled heart failure; untreated severe obstructive sleep apnea; elevated hematocrit (>50%); severe lower urinary tract symptoms; and desire for future fertility
Psychotherapy	Management of potential underlying mood disorder and psychosocial/interpersonal aspects of erectile dysfunction via cognitive behavioral therapy, biofeedback therapy, and sensory awareness exercises
Penile devices and surgical interventions	Consider in patients with no response to oral/injectable agents
	Options include vacuum constriction devices, rings, and penile prostheses (malleable and inflatable)
	Penile venous reconstructive surgery (to limit venous outflow) is not recommended
	Penile arterial reconstructive surgery is appropriate only in otherwise healthy patients with recent focal occlusion of penile artery without concomitant peripheral vascular disease
Herbal and supplemental therapy	Not recommended given their lack of efficacy, potential side effects, and medication interactions

cAMP = cyclic adenosine monophosphate; cGMP = cyclic guanosine monophosphate.

is termed hypoactive sexual desire disorder. Although decreased libido is commonly experienced as part of normal aging, numerous medical and psychiatric conditions can cause decreased libido directly or indirectly. Common causes include alcohol use, mood disorders, and significant underlying systemic illness. Medications associated with erectile dysfunction similarly can induce decreased libido. Treatment involves addressing the underlying causative factor(s). Testosterone supplementation has no role in the absence of androgen deficiency.

KEY POINTS

- Before implementing any treatment strategies for erectile dysfunction, clinicians must fully evaluate patients in terms of cardiac risk associated with sexual activity (to determine whether it is safe for a patient to engage in sexual activities).

- Oral phosphodiesterase-5 inhibitors are first-line medical therapy for erectile dysfunction and are both safe and effective in most patients; however, they are contraindicated in patients taking nitrates.

Androgen Deficiency

Male hypogonadism is defined as the inability of the testes to produce physiologic levels of testosterone, ultimately leading to signs and symptoms suggestive of androgen deficiency (**Table 60**). Many of these signs and symptoms are nonspecific and can be manifestations of various other common medical conditions. Thus, it is imperative to obtain a thorough history, including medical comorbidities, recent illness, eating disorders, mood disorders, and medication use (including glucocorticoids and opioids).

The Endocrine Society recommends against screening for androgen deficiency in the general population. In patients with clinical features suggestive of androgen deficiency, a morning (ideally, 8:00 AM to 9:00 AM) serum total testosterone level should be measured as an initial diagnostic test, which should not take place during times of acute illness. If low, the total testosterone level should be confirmed with a repeat morning measurement. Hypogonadism should be diagnosed only in men with consistent findings and unequivocally and consistently low serum total testosterone levels. Free and bioavailable testosterone measurements should be reserved for patients with total testosterone

TABLE 60.	Symptoms and Signs Suggestive of Androgen Deficiency in Men

More Specific Symptoms and Signs

Incomplete or delayed sexual development, eunuchoidism

Reduced sexual desire (libido) and activity

Decreased spontaneous erections

Breast discomfort, gynecomastia

Loss of body (axillary and pubic) hair, reduced shaving

Very small (especially <5 mL) or shrinking testes

Inability to father children, low or zero sperm count

Height loss, low-trauma fracture, low bone mineral density

Hot flushes, sweats

Other Less Specific Symptoms and Signs

Decreased energy, motivation, initiative, and self-confidence

Feeling sad or blue, depressed mood, dysthymia

Poor concentration and memory

Sleep disturbance, increased sleepiness

Mild anemia (normochromic, normocytic, in the female range)

Reduced muscle bulk and strength

Increased body fat, BMI

Diminished physical or work performance

Reproduced from Bhasin S, Cunningham GR, Hayes FJ, et al; Task Force, Endocrine Society. Testosterone therapy in men with androgen deficiency syndromes: an Endocrine Society clinical practice guideline. J Clin Endocrinol Metab. 2010;95(6):2537. [PMID: 20525905] Copyright 2010, The Endocrine Society. Licensed under the Creative Commons Attribution-NonCommercial-NoDerivatives 4.0 International License (https://creativecommons.org/licenses/by-nc-nd/4.0/).

KEY POINTS

- In patients with clinical features suggestive of androgen deficiency, morning serum total testosterone level should be measured as an initial diagnostic test, and if low, confirmed with a repeat measurement.
- A careful screening for the multiple contraindications to testosterone therapy must be completed before testosterone supplementation is initiated.
- Treatment is not indicated in patients with low testosterone levels only; it should be reserved for patients with a low testosterone level associated with symptoms.

HVC

levels in the low-normal range and for patients suspected of having alterations in sex hormone–binding globulin (SHBG) levels. Total testosterone levels may be unreliable in patients with increased SHBG levels (advanced age, liver disease) and decreased SHBG levels (obesity, diabetes/insulin resistance, glucocorticoid use), necessitating measurement of free and bioavailable testosterone in these patient populations.

The decision to treat for androgen deficiency is complex and should be individualized after a thorough discussion of the risks (cardiovascular disease, prostate cancer, benign prostatic hyperplasia) and benefits (improvements in sexual function, sense of well-being, bone health, and male sexual characteristics). A careful assessment for contraindications to testosterone must be completed. Treatment is not indicated in patients with low testosterone levels only; it should be reserved for patients with a low testosterone level associated with symptoms. Furthermore, randomized, double-blind, placebo-controlled trials aimed at determining the benefit of testosterone supplementation in men aged 65 years and older showed that testosterone supplementation improved sexual function (sexual activity, desire, and erectile function) but did not improve physical function or vitality.

See MKSAP 18 Endocrinology and Metabolism for details on the evaluation of hypogonadism and testosterone treatment.

Benign Prostatic Hyperplasia

Benign prostatic hyperplasia (BPH) is a very common condition and the most common cause of lower urinary tract symptoms (LUTS) in men. LUTS can be divided into obstructive (hesitancy, weakened stream, straining, incomplete emptying, urinary retention, overflow incontinence) and irritative (frequency, urgency, nocturia) symptoms. The AUA estimates that 90% of men aged 45 to 80 years experience some form of LUTS. The prevalence of BPH and the reported severity of LUTS both increase with age.

From an anatomic perspective, BPH generally begins at the central transition zone of the prostate, running adjacent to the course of the prostatic urethra. LUTS occur as a combined result of direct bladder outlet obstruction with increased resistance to urinary flow and increased smooth muscle tone within the prostate gland. In time, detrusor muscle dysfunction can also develop.

Clinicians should be mindful of the many potential causes of LUTS (Table 61). A thorough history should be taken to assess for any "red flag" symptoms (fever, hematuria, weight loss), recent urinary tract infection, and recent or distant pelvic trauma or surgery, and to assess for the presence of other causes. BPH symptoms can be classified as mild, moderate, or severe by using the AUA Symptom Index (AUA-SI), a validated clinical survey that quantifies and stratifies patients based on their symptoms (available at https://www.hiv.va.gov/provider/manual-primary-care/urology-tool1.asp). A digital rectal examination may be performed to assess for prostate size, symmetry, and nodularity. Physical examination should also assess for bladder distention, reduction in perineal sensation, and adequacy of rectal tone. Although recommended by the AUA, digital rectal examination has a low sensitivity (59%) and low positive predictive value (28%) for BPH and is subject to significant interexaminer variability.

The AUA recommends obtaining a serum prostate-specific antigen (PSA) level in all patients with LUTS and a life expectancy greater than 10 years. An elevated PSA level commonly occurs in BPH, and the finding is less specific for prostate cancer in this population. The decision to obtain a serum PSA level should be individualized to each patient, after an in-depth discussion of risks and benefits. Urinalysis is recommended for all patients to assess for the presence of infection

TABLE 61. Causes of Lower Urinary Tract Symptoms in Men

Benign prostatic hyperplasia

Medications (diuretics, anticholinergics, sympathomimetics, antihistamines, opioids)

Bladder irritants (caffeine, alcohol, spicy and acid-rich foods, carbonated beverages)

Overactive bladder/detrusor dysfunction

Urethral strictures

Bladder stones

Urinary tract infections

Urethritis

Prostatitis

Prostate cancer

Bladder cancer

Polydipsia

Diabetes mellitus

Hypercalcemia

Spinal cord injury

Parkinson disease

Neurogenic bladder

Obstructive sleep apnea

and hematuria. A postvoid residual study is reserved for patients with a history suggesting urinary retention, whereas a uroflow/urodynamic study can be used in ambiguous cases. Other studies, such as serum creatinine measurement, ultrasonography, and endoscopy, are not recommended in the absence of other symptoms.

Treatment of BPH should be guided by the severity of symptoms (by using the AUA-SI) and is aimed at improving quality of life. The AUA suggests that if a patient has mild symptoms (AUA-SI score of 0 to 7) or moderate (AUA-SI score of 8 to 19) to severe (AUA-SI score of 20 to 35) symptoms that are not bothersome, no specific treatment is required beyond reassurance. Conversely, if a patient has bothersome moderate to severe symptoms, treatment should be considered. Treatment options include lifestyle modifications, medications, and surgical interventions.

Lifestyle modifications should be offered to patients as first-line therapy with or without medications. Helpful measures may include weight loss, decreasing nocturnal fluid intake, and timed voiding. The diuretic effects of caffeine and alcohol may worsen symptoms, and intake should be limited.

Medical therapies for BPH should be offered in a systematic approach. The most commonly used classes of medications for BPH include α-blockers, 5α-reductase inhibitors, and anticholinergic agents.

α-Blockers (tamsulosin, terazosin, doxazosin, alfuzosin, silodosin) work by blocking α-receptors in the prostatic urethra and bladder neck, thereby decreasing smooth muscle tone within the gland and leading to reduction in LUTS. Effects are usually reported in approximately 4 weeks, with studies demonstrating roughly equal efficacy among different α-blockers. Patients should be counseled on potential side effects, including hypotension (especially with terazosin and doxazosin), orthostasis, and sexual dysfunction. α-Blockers should also be avoided or discontinued in patients undergoing cataract surgery because of the risk for floppy iris syndrome (intractable intraoperative iris prolapse). In patients taking a phosphodiesterase-5 inhibitor for erectile dysfunction, α-blockers can lead to significant hypotension. Tadalafil, a phosphodiesterase-5 inhibitor useful in the treatment of erectile dysfunction, improves LUTS and may be a reasonable option in patients with concomitant BPH and erectile dysfunction.

5α-Reductase inhibitors (finasteride and dutasteride) block the conversion of testosterone to dihydrotestosterone; this leads to a reduction in prostatic size and thus improvement in LUTS. The AUA recommends the addition of 5α-reductase inhibitors in patients with BPH refractory to α-blocker monotherapy who have an enlarged prostate on examination. Unlike α-blockers, which work relatively quickly, 5α-reductase inhibitors take approximately 6 months to improve symptoms. Side effects include erectile and ejaculatory dysfunction and decreased libido. The reduction in prostatic size causes a reduction in serum PSA levels (up to 50%); knowledge of this effect is important for patients undergoing routine monitoring of serum PSA levels.

Anticholinergic agents (oxybutynin, tolterodine, solifenacin) can be offered to patients with significant irritative symptoms. Studies have shown that combination anticholinergic and α-blocker therapy is more effective than α-blocker monotherapy. Patients should be counseled on potential side effects, including urinary retention, constipation, dry mouth, and dry eyes.

Various herbs, supplements (including saw palmetto), and alternative therapies (such as acupuncture) have been studied to assess for efficacy in improving LUTS associated with BPH but are not recommended because of a lack of clear benefit.

Referral to a urologist for a potential surgical intervention (transurethral resection of the prostate, transurethral needle ablation, transurethral vaporization, transurethral microwave thermotherapy, and various laser techniques) is warranted in patients with medically refractory symptoms or with BPH-mediated complications. BPH-related complications include recurrent urinary tract infection, bladder stone, obstructive nephropathy, persistent hematuria, and urinary retention.

KEY POINTS

- Lifestyle modifications such as weight loss, decreasing nocturnal fluid intake, timed voiding, and avoidance of common diuretics (for example, caffeine and alcohol) is first-line therapy for benign prostatic hyperplasia. **HVC**

- The most commonly used classes of medications for benign prostatic hyperplasia include α-blockers, 5α-reductase inhibitors, and anticholinergic agents (for irritative symptoms).

Acute Testicular and Scrotal Pain

Acute testicular and scrotal pain are common concerns; overall, they account for approximately 1% of all emergency department visits. Causes of acute testicular and scrotal pain include testicular torsion, epididymitis, and orchitis. Several other conditions, including inguinal hernia, nephrolithiasis, and spinal nerve root impingement, can lead to referred pain to the scrotum.

Epididymitis (and epididymo-orchitis when a testicle is also involved) is the most common cause of acute scrotal pain in adults. Noninfectious causes include trauma and connective tissue diseases, but infection is the most frequent cause. In younger patients, gonorrhea and chlamydia are the most likely causes, whereas gram-negative rods are the most likely cause in older patients and in patients engaging in insertive anal intercourse. Epididymitis presents as acute to subacute unilateral pain and swelling in the superolateral aspect of the testicle, sometimes with LUTS (dysuria, urgency, frequency) and fever. Pain relief with lifting of the affected testicle may be present (Prehn sign). Increased blood flow on Doppler ultrasound and an elevated C-reactive protein level (>0.24 mg/dL [2.4 mg/L]) are typically present. Supportive care, including scrotal support, ice, and pain control, is sufficient treatment for noninfectious causes. For infectious epididymitis in patients younger than 35 years, ceftriaxone and doxycycline (or azithromycin) are indicated; ceftriaxone and a fluoroquinolone are recommended in older patients and those engaging in insertive anal intercourse.

Testicular torsion results from a twisting of the testicle on the spermatic cord, eventually leading to ischemia and testicular infarction. It is most common in children and young adults and presents as acute, unilateral, severe scrotal pain and swelling. Examination reveals a "high-riding hemiscrotum" and an absent cremasteric reflex (failure of the testis to pull up when the ipsilateral inner thigh is stroked). Decreased blood flow on Doppler ultrasound is typical, and because this is a mechanical rather than inflammatory process, the C-reactive protein level is normal (<0.24 mg/dL [24 mg/L]). Testicular torsion is a surgical emergency; if repaired within 6 hours, testicular salvage rate is 80% to 100%.

KEY POINTS

- For infectious epididymitis in patients younger than 35 years, ceftriaxone and doxycycline (or azithromycin) are indicated; ceftriaxone and a fluoroquinolone are recommended in older patients and those engaging in insertive anal intercourse.
- Testicular torsion presents as acute, unilateral, severe scrotal pain and swelling with a "high-riding hemiscrotum" on examination and absent cremasteric reflex; it is a surgical emergency with high testicular salvage rates if decompressed within 6 hours.

Hydrocele, Varicocele, and Epididymal Cyst

Hydrocele, varicocele, epididymal cyst/spermatocele, and testicular malignancy most frequently present with chronic symptoms such as scrotal discomfort or swelling. They may also be noted incidentally by the patient. The key differences in the presentation, examination, appropriate diagnostic measures, and indications for treatment are presented in **Table 62**.

KEY POINT

- Hydroceles, varicoceles, and epididymal cysts (spermatoceles) present with scrotal discomfort or swelling and are all treated conservatively, with surgery reserved for worsening pain or enlarging size.

HVC

Acute and Chronic Prostatitis and Pelvic Pain

Prostatitis encompasses several disparate disorders, including acute bacterial prostatitis, chronic bacterial prostatitis, chronic pelvic pain syndrome, and asymptomatic prostatitis. It is a common problem with a reported prevalence of approximately 8%, accounting for approximately 8% of all urology visits and 1% of all primary care visits.

Acute bacterial prostatitis is characterized by irritative voiding symptoms; perineal pain; systemic symptoms of fever, chills, myalgia, and malaise; and potentially features of sepsis. Chronic bacterial prostatitis causes irritative voiding symptoms and perineal pain, but patients are not systemically ill. Bacterial prostatitis is most commonly caused by *Escherichia coli*, *Klebsiella*, *Proteus*, *Pseudomonas*, *Enterococci*, *Neisseria*, and *Chlamydia*. Chronic pelvic pain syndrome is associated with chronic pelvic pain and intermittent voiding symptoms without evidence of infection. It may be inflammatory or noninflammatory and may be idiopathic or associated with trauma, surgery, lumbosacral neuropathy, and pelvic floor dysfunction. Asymptomatic prostatitis is usually discovered incidentally.

When encountering a patient with signs and symptoms concerning for prostatitis, it is imperative to exclude other causes, including testicular, epididymal, urethral, rectal, or urinary tract conditions. The history and physical examination should attempt to address each of these potential causative sources. Evaluation should include examination of the prostate, which often is tender, enlarged, boggy, and edematous in acute bacterial prostatitis; mild tenderness or a normal prostate examination may be present with the other causes of prostatitis. Additional diagnostic measures should include a urinalysis with Gram stain and culture, as well as expressed prostatic secretion culture (by prostatic massage). However, prostatic massage is contraindicated in acute bacterial prostatitis, given concern for possible abscess, bacteremia, and sepsis. Tests such as semen analysis, PSA level, prostatic imaging (ultrasonography or CT), and prostate biopsy are not routinely performed.

TABLE 62. Causes of Chronic Testicular and Scrotal Pain or Swelling

Cause	Presentation	Diagnosis	Treatment	Additional Information
Epididymal cyst/ spermatocele	Small, benign, nontender mass along the epididymis and spermatic cord Asymptomatic; usually an incidental finding	Examination Ultrasonography	Reassurance Surgery (rarely; only if painful or enlarging)	Cysts >2 cm in diameter are referred to as spermatocele
Hydrocele	Asymptomatic to painful swelling Small to large tense, smooth scrotal mass	Examination Transillumination Ultrasonography	Conservative (pain control [analgesics]; scrotal support) Surgery (worsening pain or enlarging size)	Fluid collection between the layers of the tunica vaginalis Common (1% of men)
Varicocele	Asymptomatic to dull ache with scrotal fullness Increased fullness/pain with standing and Valsalva maneuver; improves with support and while supine	Examination ("bag of worms") No transillumination Ultrasonography	Conservative (pain control [analgesics]; scrotal support) Surgery (worsening pain, refractory to conservative methods, infertility)	Dilated testicular vein/ pampiniform plexus Common (15% of men) Left-sided (90%) Associated infertility Consider obstruction of inferior vena cava with right-sided varicocele
Testicular malignancy	Firm, unilateral mass/ nodule adherent to the testicle	Examination Ultrasonography Tumor markers (α-fetoprotein, β-human chorionic gonadotropin, lactate dehydrogenase)	Surgery/chemotherapy	Approximately 15% of testicular cancers present with pain; most are asymptomatic Patients often younger than those with hydrocele, spermatocele, or varicocele

In acute bacterial prostatitis, mild to moderately ill patients are treated with an antimicrobial agent with good prostate tissue penetration, such as ciprofloxacin or trimethoprim-sulfamethoxazole, for approximately 6 weeks. In severely ill patients, hospitalization and parenteral antibiotics may be necessary.

Chronic bacterial prostatitis is treated similarly with an antimicrobial agent for approximately 6 weeks. First-line therapy is a fluoroquinolone or trimethoprim-sulfamethoxazole; second-line therapy is doxycycline or azithromycin. Some patients might require a prolonged antibiotic course of up to 12 weeks to minimize the risk for recurrent episodes.

Chronic pelvic pain syndrome is best managed with a multimodal approach that includes an antimicrobial agent (6 weeks' duration) and an α-blocker such as tamsulosin. Other treatment options include 5α-reductase inhibitors, anti-inflammatory analgesics, neuromodulating agents (pregabalin, gabapentin, nortriptyline), and nonpharmacologic strategies such as cognitive behavioral therapy, biofeedback therapy, and physical therapy. Asymptomatic prostatitis requires no specific treatment.

KEY POINTS

- In acute bacterial prostatitis, mild to moderately ill patients are treated with an antimicrobial agent with good prostate tissue penetration, such as ciprofloxacin or trimethoprim-sulfamethoxazole, for approximately 6 weeks; severely ill patients may require hospitalization and parenteral antibiotics.

(Continued)

KEY POINTS *(continued)*

- Prostatic massage is contraindicated in acute bacterial prostatitis, given concern for possible abscess, bacteremia, and sepsis.
- Chronic pelvic pain syndrome is best managed with a multimodal approach including an antimicrobial agent (6 weeks' duration) and an α-blocker such as tamsulosin.

Hernia

Hernia is defined as a condition in which a portion of an organ protrudes through the wall of the cavity that contains it. This usually occurs at a weakened muscular or connective tissue site and can be congenital or acquired. Hernias most commonly occur in the abdominopelvic region, including ventral (protrusion through the anterior abdominal wall), umbilical (protrusion through the umbilicus), incisional (protrusion through previous surgical scars), femoral (protrusion inferior to inguinal ligament, near the femoral vessels at the femoral canal), and inguinal hernias. Hernias are typically noticeable during times of increased intra-abdominal pressure, such as coughing, sneezing, laughing, heavy lifting, and straining.

Inguinal hernias can be divided into direct or indirect based on their anatomic characteristics. A direct hernia is an intra-abdominal protrusion that occurs outside of the inguinal canal, between the abdominal musculature and the inguinal ligament. It does not involve the internal or external inguinal rings and does not traverse the inguinal canal. Conversely, an indirect inguinal hernia is an intra-abdominal protrusion through the internal inguinal ring that can traverse (partly or entirely) the inguinal canal potentially through the external inguinal ring and into the scrotum. Indirect inguinal hernias are far more common than direct inguinal hernias.

Symptoms from hernias can range from an asymptomatic bulge, to a mildly dull aching sensation, to acute severe pain with concomitant nausea and vomiting. Asymptomatic to mildly symptomatic hernias are generally spontaneously or self-reducible. Conversely, acute and severe symptoms usually occur in the setting of bowel or omental incarceration and strangulation, which if not treated expeditiously could lead to tissue ischemia and necrosis. All patients should be educated on the variability of symptoms and when to seek emergent medical care (signs of bowel incarceration).

Diagnosis is usually made solely based on history and physical examination with provocative maneuvers (Valsalva). Treatment depends on the severity of symptoms and location of the hernia. Whereas surgical repair is recommended for most femoral hernias, given the high incidence of complications, asymptomatic inguinal and umbilical hernias can often be monitored. Symptomatic inguinal hernias usually require surgical repair (options include laparoscopic or open repair techniques with or without mesh). In the case of a strangulated or incarcerated hernia, immediate surgical repair is of critical importance.

KEY POINTS

HVC
- Most asymptomatic hernias can be monitored; symptomatic hernias may require surgical consultation and possible repair.
- Surgical repair is recommended for most femoral hernias given the high incidence of complications.

Women's Health

Breast Symptoms

Breast Mass

A palpable breast mass that differs from the surrounding breast tissue and the corresponding area in the contralateral breast and persists throughout the menstrual cycle warrants evaluation. Although breast cancer should be considered in all patients, most breast masses are benign conditions, such as cysts, fibroadenomas, fat necrosis, or lipomas.

Evaluation requires consideration of breast cancer risk factors, including family history of breast or ovarian cancer and a detailed history of the mass, including onset, changes with the menstrual cycle, associated symptoms, and overlying skin/nipple changes. Examination of the breast includes assessment of the features of the mass, which can be well-defined with smooth margins (cyst or fibroadenoma) or ill-defined (malignancy). The axilla and supraclavicular regions should be examined to assess for lymphadenopathy. Although a detailed history and examination provide useful information, the determination of whether a discrete mass is benign or malignant often requires further evaluation with breast imaging and/or biopsy.

Imaging of a breast mass may include diagnostic mammography and/or targeted ultrasonography of the mass. Mammography is the first test performed in most patients aged 30 years or older with a breast mass. The sensitivity of mammography is lower in women with dense breasts. The mammogram may demonstrate a mass, asymmetric density, and abnormal/pleomorphic calcifications potentially indicating breast cancer. For patients with a focal abnormality noted on clinical examination or mammogram, targeted ultrasonography can clarify the size of the mass, determine whether the mass is solid or cystic, and identify the margins as smooth or irregular. Ultrasonography is the preferred method of evaluation for women younger than 30 years, in whom mammography has low sensitivity due to dense breasts. It is also the test of choice in pregnant patients. When breast imaging is completed, results are categorized by using BI-RADS (Breast Imaging Reporting and Data System) (**Table 63**). Biopsy is recommended for category 4 and 5 breast findings. About one fifth of palpable breast masses are not identified on mammogram or ultrasound, and a normal mammogram in a patient with a discrete breast mass does not rule out malignancy; therefore, a suspicious breast mass should be evaluated with a biopsy even if the mammogram and ultrasound findings are negative.

TABLE 63. Breast Imaging Reporting and Data System (BI-RADS) Assessment Categories	
Category 0	Mammography: Incomplete—Need additional imaging evaluation and/or prior mammograms for comparison
	Ultrasound and MRI: Incomplete—Need additional imaging evaluation
Category 1	Negative
Category 2	Benign
Category 3	Probably benign
Category 4	Suspicious
	Mammography and ultrasound:
	Category 4A: Low suspicion for malignancy
	Category 4B: Moderate suspicion for malignancy
	Category 4C: High suspicion for malignancy
Category 5	Highly suggestive of malignancy
Category 6	Known biopsy-proven malignancy

Reproduced with permission of the American College of Radiology (ACR) from D'Orsi CJ, Sickles EA, Mendelson EB, et al. ACR BI-RADS® Atlas, Breast Imaging Reporting and Data System. Reston, VA, American College of Radiology; 2013. No other representation of this material is authorized without expressed, written permission from the ACR. Refer to the ACR website at https://www.acr.org/Clinical-Resources/Reporting-and-Data-Systems/Bi-Rads for the most current and complete version of the BI-RADS® Atlas.

Breast biopsy can be performed with fine-needle aspiration, image-guided core-needle biopsy, or surgical/excisional biopsy. Fine-needle aspiration is done for cystic lesions; benign cysts that completely resolve with aspiration require no further work-up. Image-guided core-needle biopsy can be a stereotactic biopsy when the lesion is seen only on mammogram, ultrasound-guided biopsy when the lesion can be seen on ultrasound, or an MRI-guided biopsy when the mass is seen only on a breast MRI. Management of an abnormal finding requires a consultation with a breast surgeon. A surgical biopsy is performed when the core-needle biopsy is technically challenging due to location of the lesion, when atypical hyperplasia is seen on core-needle biopsy specimens, or when the pathology report and breast imaging findings are discordant.

Breast Pain

Breast pain (mastalgia) is common and may be cyclic or noncyclic in relation to the menstrual cycle. Cyclic breast pain often occurs in the premenstrual phase, tends to be bilateral, and resolves with onset of menstruation; it is usually associated with hormonal changes and is typically benign. Noncyclic breast pain is usually related to underlying breast conditions, such as fibrocystic breasts, hormone therapy, and stretching of Cooper ligaments (connective tissue that maintains breast structural integrity) with large breast size. Noncyclic breast pain may also result from breast infection or mastitis, breast trauma, or thrombophlebitis of the thoracoepigastric vein (Mondor disease). Non-breast causes of breast pain include costochondritis, coronary artery disease, gastroesophageal reflux disease, and intercostal nerve pain.

Evaluation includes a detailed history of breast pain to identify characteristics of the pain and relationship to menses, along with a careful physical examination to rule out palpable masses or anatomic causes. Women evaluated for breast pain with no obvious abnormal findings should be up to date with routine age- and risk-appropriate breast screening. Patients with noncyclic mastalgia with focal breast pain and no palpable mass should undergo targeted breast ultrasonography because approximately 1% of such patients may have breast cancer at the site of pain. Any palpable breast masses should be evaluated with diagnostic imaging (see Breast Mass).

For women with cyclic breast pain and negative clinical findings, conservative management (education, reassurance of the absence of malignancy, and advice regarding adequate breast support) is recommended as cyclic pain usually resolves spontaneously. There is a lack of evidence to support limiting caffeine intake or using vitamin E as a means of mitigating the pain. Medical management may be offered for patients with severe pain that persists despite conservative management. Danazol is the only FDA-approved agent for cyclic breast pain, but its use is limited because of side effects, including amenorrhea, hirsutism, and adverse changes in lipid profile. Low-dose tamoxifen, although not FDA approved for this indication, has been shown to have benefit with fewer side effects; however,

hot flushes, menstrual irregularities, and the need for contraception must be considered. Treatment of noncyclic breast pain depends on the underlying cause.

KEY POINTS

- Mammography is the first test performed in most women aged 30 years or older with a breast mass; the sensitivity of mammography is lower in women with dense breasts.

- Ultrasonography is the preferred method of evaluation **HVC** of a breast mass in women younger than 30 years, in whom mammography has low sensitivity due to dense breasts.

- A suspicious breast mass should be evaluated with a biopsy even if the mammogram and ultrasound results are negative.

- Cyclic breast pain often occurs in the premenstrual **HVC** phase, tends to be bilateral, and resolves with onset of menstruation and conservative management (education, reassurance of the absence of malignancy, and advice regarding adequate breast support).

- Noncyclic breast pain is usually related to underlying breast conditions; patients with noncyclic focal breast pain and no palpable mass should undergo targeted breast ultrasonography to exclude breast cancer.

Reproductive Health

The Centers for Disease Control and Prevention provides information and recommendations on reproductive health (https://www.cdc.gov/reproductivehealth/index.html).

Contraception

Approximately 50% of pregnancies in the United States are unintended, with a higher prevalence in women with low socioeconomic status, younger women, and those who cohabit. Contraception counseling to reduce unintended pregnancy involves an understanding of the risk for pregnancy, assessing contraceptive options, identifying the appropriate agent based on benefits and risks, and educating the patient on appropriate use of the contraceptive. Contraceptive options include hormonal contraception, barrier methods, sterilization, and emergency contraception (**Table 64**).

Hormonal Contraception

Hormonal contraceptive options include oral contraceptive pills (combination estrogen-progesterone or progesterone-only pills), long-acting reversible contraceptives, transdermal patches, and vaginal rings. Patient factors influencing choice include hypertension, history of breast cancer, obesity, thrombotic disorders, migraines, and tobacco use. Before initiation of hormonal contraception, a negative pregnancy test result must be documented if 7 days have passed since the first day of the patient's last menstrual period.

TABLE 64.	Comparison of Contraceptive Options			
	Women Experiencing Unintended Pregnancy Within the First Year of Use (%)			
Agent	**Typical Use[a]**	**Perfect Use[a]**	**Advantages**	**Disadvantages**
Hormonal Agents				
Oral contraceptives				
Combination estrogen-progestin preparations	9	0.3	Easy to use Rapidly reversible Decreased risk for endometrial and ovarian cancers Decreased dysmenorrhea, menorrhagia, symptomatic ovarian cysts Less iron deficiency anemia	Daily use may affect adherence Increased risk for myocardial infarction, ischemic stroke, VTE, hypertension Increased risk for cancers of the cervix, liver, and breast Breakthrough bleeding May exacerbate migraine
Progestin-only preparations ("mini-pill")	9	0.3	Use when estrogen is contraindicated	Irregular bleeding, breakthrough bleeding; must maintain precise daily dosing schedule
Long-acting reversible preparations				
Depot medroxyproges-terone acetate (IM or SQ)	6	0.2	Administered every 3 months Decreased risk for endometrial cancer, PID Improves endometriosis Decreased menstrual frequency	Delayed return to ovulation (6-10 months) Irregular bleeding, amenorrhea, decreased bone mineral density (especially in adolescents)
Progestin implants	0.05	0.05	Effective up to 3 years	
Intrauterine devices				
Copper	0.8	0.6	Nonhormonal Effective up to 10 years	Bleeding, pain Requires placement and removal in office Expulsion rates up to 5% in first year No protection from STIs
Levonorgestrel	6	0.2	Decreased menstrual flow Effective up to 3-5 years, depending on formulation	
Other hormonal agents				
Patch (combination estrogen-progestin)	9	0.3	Easier adherence Change weekly	Local skin reaction Increased estrogen dose, thus higher VTE risk
Vaginal ring (combination estrogen-progestin)	9	0.3	Easier adherence Change monthly Lowest level of systemic estrogen	Requires self-insertion
Barrier Methods				
Cervical cap	16-32	9-26	-	User dependent, requires spermicide
Diaphragm	12	6	-	Requires spermicide
Male condom	18	2	Protection from STIs	-
Female condom	21	5	Protection from STIs	-
Vaginal sponge	12-24	9-20	-	-
Sterilization				
Female (tubal ligation)	0.5	0.5	May reduce ovarian cancer risk	Surgical complications (rare) Regret Increased risk for ectopic pregnancy
Male (vasectomy)	0.15	0.10	Lower costs, fewer complications, and more effective than tubal ligation	Surgical complications (rare)

IM = intramuscular; PID = pelvic inflammatory disease; SQ = subcutaneous; STI = sexually transmitted infection; VTE = venous thromboembolism.

[a]Perfect use implies correct and consistent use exactly as directed/intended. Typical use reflects rates in actual practice with patients.

Oral Contraceptive Pills

Oral contraceptive pills include combination estrogen-progesterone pills and progesterone-only pills. The combination pills vary in the type and strength of estrogen and the type of progestin. They inhibit ovulation, alter the cervical mucus to prevent migration of the sperm, inhibit endometrial thickening, and prevent implantation. Although all agents are equivalent in terms of the contraceptive efficacy, they vary in terms of side effects. Contraindications to combination pills include breast cancer, venous thromboembolism, uncontrolled hypertension, liver disease, and migraine with aura.

Women who smoke more than 15 cigarettes per day and are older than 35 years should not use estrogen-containing preparations because of the increased risk for thrombotic disorders. Progesterone-only pills can be used for women with a contraindication to estrogen.

Long-Acting Reversible Contraception

Long-acting reversible contraceptives are progestin-only forms of contraception that include depot medroxyprogesterone acetate injections, progestin implants, and intrauterine devices (IUDs). Patients can receive these contraceptives in the outpatient office setting.

An IUD is a small, T-shaped device (copper or levonorgestrel) that is placed inside the uterus. The copper IUD induces a local reaction that impairs implantation of the fertilized ovum, whereas the levonorgestrel IUD releases a low dose of progestin that leads to endometrial atrophy and also prevents implantation. Complications include uterine perforation with approximately 1 per 1000 insertions. Risk factors for perforation include breastfeeding at the time of insertion or insertion within 36 weeks after the last childbirth. Risk for pelvic infection with IUD placement is low, and prophylactic antibiotics are not recommended during the procedure. If a woman with a sexually transmitted infection (STI) has an IUD in place, she should be treated with antibiotics, and the IUD does not need to be removed. Contraindications to IUD placement include pregnancy; anatomic uterine abnormalities with distortion of the uterine cavity; and acute untreated pelvic infection, gonorrhea, or chlamydia.

Barrier Contraception

Barrier contraceptive methods such as diaphragms and condoms are among the least effective of all the modes of contraception. Their efficacy is improved when combined with a spermicidal agent. Use of condoms reduces the risk for STIs.

Sterilization

Female sterilization is a safe and permanent form of sterilization that is associated with a low complication rate. The fallopian tube lumen may be occluded by techniques such as clip or cautery. Preprocedure counseling includes a detailed discussion of the permanence of the procedure, the risk for regret after surgery, the complex nature and poor success rates of reversal procedures, and the availability of alternative long-acting contraceptive methods.

Emergency Contraception

Emergency contraception refers to postcoital contraception using a device or medication to prevent pregnancy after unprotected or inadequately protected intercourse. The most effective form of emergency contraception is the placement of a copper IUD within 5 days of intercourse. The IUD is also the preferred option in obese women because they experience higher failure rates with oral emergency contraception.

FDA-approved medications include levonorgestrel, which is most effective within 3 days of intercourse, and ulipristal, which has a 5-day window.

Preconception Care

Preconception counseling refers to education provided before pregnancy, aimed at reducing the risk for preterm birth and congenital anomalies. Optimizing health before pregnancy reduces exposures to factors that can potentially compromise a healthy pregnancy, as organogenesis starts as early as the third to fifth week of gestation. This differs from prenatal counseling, which occurs after pregnancy is diagnosed.

Any primary care visit for a woman of reproductive age is an opportunity to routinely ask if she could become pregnant or is considering pregnancy. For women who are not interested in pregnancy, contraception should be discussed to reduce the risk for unintended pregnancy. For women considering pregnancy, a comprehensive risk assessment should be completed (**Table 65**). An obstetric history of pregnancy-induced hypertension, preeclampsia, or gestational diabetes is particularly predictive of future risk.

All medications should be reviewed to reduce or avoid exposure to potential teratogens (**Table 66**). The pregnancy letter categories that have been used by the FDA to characterize the safety of drugs in pregnancy are provided in **Table 67**. In 2015, the FDA published changes in pregnancy and lactation labeling for prescription drugs (https://www.fda.gov/Drugs/DevelopmentApprovalProcess/DevelopmentResources/Labeling/ucm093307.htm). The pregnancy letter categories will be discontinued with the new labeling requirements; however, for prescription drugs that were previously approved, these changes will be phased in gradually. Labeling will include information relevant to the use of the drug in pregnant women (such as dosing and potential risks to the developing fetus), information about using the drug while breastfeeding (such as the amount of drug in breast milk and potential effects on the breastfed infant), and information regarding potential risks to females and males of reproductive potential who take the drug.

Physical examination includes assessment of blood pressure and BMI. Pelvic examination may include screening cervical cytology. Testing for STIs and hepatitis is indicated in high-risk patients. HIV counseling and screening are recommended for all women planning pregnancy.

Intervention to prevent complications depends on the results of the risk assessment. All women should be encouraged to follow a healthy lifestyle, with emphasis on complete

TABLE 65. Preconception Risk Assessment

Risk Category	Specific Items to Assess
Reproductive awareness	Desire for pregnancy, number and timing of desired pregnancies, age-related changes in fertility, sexuality, contraception
Environmental hazards and toxins	Exposure to radiation, lead, and mercury
Nutrition and folic acid consumption	Healthy diet; daily consumption of folic acid; low-dose iron supplementation; restricting consumption of shark, swordfish, king mackerel, and tilefish to <2 servings weekly (owing to high mercury content)
Genetics	Family history of genetic disorders
Substance use	Use of tobacco, alcohol, and illicit drugs
Medical conditions	Seizure disorder, diabetes mellitus, hypertension, thyroid disease, asthma, HIV infection, systemic lupus erythematosus
Obstetric history	Pregnancy-induced hypertension, preeclampsia, gestational diabetes
Medications	Over-the-counter and prescription medications, potential teratogens
Infectious diseases and vaccinations	Vaccinations up to date; immunity to varicella and rubella; risk for hepatitis B infection
Psychosocial concerns	Depression, interpersonal/family relationships, risk for abuse (physical, sexual, emotional)

Information from Johnson K, Posner SF, Biermann J, et al; CDC/ATSDR Preconception Care Work Group; Select Panel on Preconception Care. Recommendations to improve preconception health and health care—United States. A report of the CDC/ATSDR Preconception Care Work Group and the Select Panel on Preconception Care. MMWR Recomm Rep. 2006;55:1-23. [PMID: 16617292]

TABLE 66. Commonly Used Medications With Potential for Teratogenic Effects

Class/Type	Examples
Antibiotics	Tetracycline, doxycycline, sulfonamides, trimethoprim, para-aminosalicylate
Anticoagulants	Warfarin
Antidepressants	Selective serotonin reuptake inhibitors, lithium
Antihypertensive agents	ACE inhibitors, angiotensin receptor blockers, direct renin inhibitors
Antiepileptic drugs	Valproic acid, phenytoin, carbamazepine
Antithyroid medications	Propylthiouracil, carbimazole, methimazole
Hormones	Androgens, testosterone derivatives
Immunosuppressant/chemotherapeutic agents	Folate antagonists, cyclophosphamide, methotrexate
Others	Vitamin A derivatives, statins, NSAIDs, isotretinoin

TABLE 67. FDA Classification of Drugs in Pregnancy[a]

Class	Fetal Effect of Drug During Pregnancy
A	No disclosed fetal effects
B	Animal studies failed to demonstrate fetal risk
C	Animal studies suggest adverse fetal effects
D	Evidence of human fetal risk
X	Documented fetal abnormalities

[a]In 2015, the FDA published changes in pregnancy and lactation labeling for prescription drugs. A summary of these changes is available at https://www.fda.gov/Drugs/DevelopmentApprovalProcess/DevelopmentResources/Labeling/ucm093307.htm. The pregnancy letter categories will be removed with the new labeling requirements; however, for prescription drugs that were previously approved, these changes will be phased in gradually.

cessation of tobacco, alcohol, or illicit drugs before conception and education on the consequences of not doing so.

Women should be up to date with immunizations. Women who are considering pregnancy should be assessed for immunity to varicella and rubella. For women who are not immune, varicella and rubella vaccination should be administered with the advice that pregnancy be avoided for at least 4 weeks after the vaccine is administered to reduce risk to the fetus. Immunizations to be avoided during pregnancy, in addition to varicella and rubella, include human papillomavirus, measles, mumps, live attenuated influenza, and live attenuated herpes zoster.

Consultation with a genetics counselor may be helpful if there is a personal or family history of genetic disorders.

Patients should also be counseled about new infections, such as Zika virus and its risk for adverse fetal outcomes (for example, microcephaly), and be educated on the risks of travel to endemic areas and modes of transmission, including mosquito bite, sexual intercourse, and blood transfusion. Appropriate preventive measures should be addressed.

Interventions that optimize pregnancy outcomes include daily intake of folic acid (0.4-0.8 mg/d [400-800 µg/d]) to reduce the risk for neural tube defects. Low-dose oral iron supplements can reduce the risk for maternal anemia. Prenatal multivitamins that contain sufficient folic acid are a reasonable option for women contemplating pregnancy.

KEY POINTS

- Contraception counseling involves an understanding of the risk for pregnancy, assessing contraceptive options, identifying the appropriate agent based on benefits and risks, and educating the patient on appropriate use of contraceptives.

- Contraindications to oral combination estrogen-progesterone contraceptive pills include breast cancer, venous thromboembolism, uncontrolled hypertension, liver disease, and migraine with aura; progesterone-only pills can be used for women with a contraindication to estrogen.

(Continued)

- Women who smoke more than 15 cigarettes per day and are older than 35 years should not use estrogen-containing contraceptive preparations.

- Long-acting reversible contraceptives are progestin-only forms of contraception that include depot medroxyprogesterone acetate injections, progestin implants, and intrauterine devices.

- Women considering pregnancy should undergo a comprehensive assessment of risk factors for adverse pregnancy outcomes and begin folic acid supplementation.

Menstrual Disorders

Abnormal Uterine Bleeding

Evaluation

Abnormal uterine bleeding is defined as excessive bleeding in terms of flow volume, frequency, and duration. Among non-pregnant women of reproductive age, abnormal uterine bleeding is classified according to etiology by using the International Federation of Obstetrics and Gynecology system with the acronym PALM-COEIN (polyp, adenomyosis, leiomyoma, malignancy and hyperplasia, coagulopathy, ovulation dysfunction, endometrial, iatrogenic, and not yet classified). Abnormal uterine bleeding in this population can be further classified as ovulatory or anovulatory. Ovulatory bleeding occurs at regular intervals, but the menstrual flow is excessive. This may be related to thyroid disease; bleeding disorders; or structural abnormalities, such as uterine fibroids or polyps. Anovulatory cycles are characteristically irregular in terms of flow and cycle duration, as lack of ovulation and the resultant lack of cyclic progesterone cause endometrial hyperplasia and irregular bleeding. Anovulation occurs with polycystic ovary syndrome, hypothyroidism or hyperthyroidism, hyperprolactinemia, chronic liver or kidney disease, and medications (such as antidepressant and antipsychotic agents, chemotherapy, and tamoxifen). Anovulatory causes of bleeding in the patient of reproductive age increase the risk for endometrial cancer because of the lack of cyclic progesterone-induced withdrawal bleeding and resultant endometrial hyperplasia.

Causes of abnormal uterine bleeding in the postmenopausal patient are similar to those in women of reproductive age, although there is an increased risk for endometrial cancer. Risk factors for endometrial cancer other than age older than 50 years and anovulatory causes of bleeding include such conditions as Lynch or Cowden syndrome; obesity; and reproductive factors, such as nulliparity and late menopause.

Evaluation of abnormal uterine bleeding in the premenopausal woman includes assessment of menstrual cycle length, regularity, intermenstrual bleeding, volume of menstrual flow (including passage of clots), association with pain, presence of an intrauterine device, and postcoital bleeding. Assessment for thyroid disease, liver or kidney disease, and bleeding disorders is also indicated. Pelvic examination is performed to determine whether the source of bleeding is from the vulva, vagina, cervix, or uterus. Pregnancy testing is recommended for all premenopausal women with abnormal uterine bleeding because bleeding may occur with pregnancy-related conditions, such as placenta previa and ectopic gestation. Pelvic ultrasonography is indicated to assess for structural abnormalities in the uterus and to determine endometrial thickness. Endometrial thickness greater than 4 mm in postmenopausal women may indicate endometrial hyperplasia or malignancy. In premenopausal women, endometrial thickness is not a reliable indicator because thickness varies according to the phase of the menstrual cycle.

Evaluation of the postmenopausal patient is similar to that of the premenopausal patient. Because of the increased risk for endometrial cancer, however, any vaginal bleeding occurring in peri- and postmenopausal women warrants evaluation to rule out malignancy, usually with endometrial biopsy.

Management

Management of abnormal uterine bleeding is aimed at the underlying cause. Structural abnormalities, such as endometrial polyps or submucosal fibroids, may be surgically resected. Treatment of underlying endocrine disorders (thyroid disease, polycystic ovary disease) may result in improvement.

For women with anovulatory cycles, treatment is aimed at providing adequate progestin to maintain endometrial stability. The type of therapy depends on the patient's plans for contraception. For women who wish to preserve fertility, medroxyprogesterone acetate used for the second half of the menstrual cycle will restore cyclic withdrawal bleeding. For women interested in contraception, oral contraceptive pills containing estrogen and progesterone or the levonorgestrel intrauterine device may be used. Additionally, NSAIDs may be used because these drugs reduce synthesis of prostaglandins in the endometrium, leading to vasoconstriction and reduced bleeding. Tranexamic acid, an antithrombolytic agent, stabilizes clots and may be used for treatment of heavy vaginal bleeding. For women experiencing acute and severe bleeding, agents such as gonadotropin-releasing hormone or intravenous administration of high-dose estrogens may be used. For women who do not respond to medical therapy, operative procedures such as endometrial ablation or hysterectomy may be performed.

Dysmenorrhea

Dysmenorrhea is characterized by pain during menstruation; it may also be associated with low back pain, headache, nausea, vomiting, and diarrhea. Dysmenorrhea is classified as primary or secondary. Primary dysmenorrhea involves cramping lower abdominal and pelvic pain that occurs during menstrual cycles without an identifiable cause. Secondary dysmenorrhea may result from pelvic conditions, such as endometriosis, inflammatory disease, or uterine fibroids.

A detailed history is necessary to assess the timing of pain and relationship to the menstrual cycle. Sexual history is important to assess for infection and risk for abuse. Primary dysmenorrhea can be treated with NSAIDs and cyclooxygenase-2 inhibitors; persistent symptoms can be treated with oral contraceptive pills. Secondary dysmenorrhea requires treatment of the underlying condition.

KEY POINTS

- Evaluation of all patients with abnormal uterine bleeding includes a detailed history, physical and pelvic examinations, pregnancy testing, and pelvic ultrasonography.
- Risk factors for endometrial cancer include age older than 50 years; anovulatory causes of bleeding; such conditions as Lynch or Cowden syndrome; obesity; and reproductive factors, such as nulliparity and late menopause.
- Any vaginal bleeding occurring in peri- and postmenopausal women warrants evaluation to rule out malignancy, usually with endometrial biopsy.
- Primary dysmenorrhea can be treated with NSAIDs and cyclooxygenase-2 inhibitors, and persistent symptoms can be treated with oral contraceptive pills; secondary dysmenorrhea requires treatment of the underlying condition.

Menopause

Diagnosis

Menopause is the permanent cessation of menses that is diagnosed retrospectively after a woman has not experienced a menstrual period for 12 months. Menopause may be natural, surgical following bilateral oophorectomies, or medical as a result of medications such as chemotherapy. Menopause occurring before age 40 years is considered premature menopause or premature ovarian insufficiency. Perimenopause refers to the phase of menopause transition, extending into early postmenopause; it varies in length and may be associated with irregular menstrual cycles, fluctuating hormone levels, and intermittent hot flushes.

Symptoms of menopause include vasomotor symptoms (hot flushes, night sweats), depression, difficulties with memory and concentration, sleep disturbances, and genitourinary symptoms (vaginal dryness, dyspareunia). Up to 50% of women experience hot flushes during perimenopause, but symptoms generally resolve spontaneously in a few years. Genitourinary syndrome of menopause is the result of estrogen deficiency and is characterized by vaginal symptoms, such as vaginal burning or irritation; sexual symptoms, such as dyspareunia or sexual dysfunction; or urinary symptoms, such as dysuria or recurrent urinary infections. Pelvic examination findings include a pale, dry vaginal lining with reduction in rugae. Increases in LDL cholesterol and bone loss are also associated with menopause.

Routine laboratory testing for the diagnosis of menopause is not recommended. Patients with possible early menopause should have pregnancy excluded and undergo measurement of follicle-stimulating hormone, thyroid-stimulating hormone, and prolactin. Younger patients should undergo evaluation for amenorrhea (see MKSAP 18 Endocrinology and Metabolism).

Management

Management of menopausal symptoms is recommended to improve quality of life. Pregnancy is possible even if menstrual cycles are irregular, and contraception should be discussed if pregnancy is not desired. The U.S. Preventive Services Task Force recommends against the use of combined estrogen and progestin for the primary prevention of chronic conditions (coronary artery disease, dementia, stroke, and fractures) in postmenopausal women and against the use of estrogen alone for the primary prevention of chronic conditions in postmenopausal women who have had a hysterectomy.

Vasomotor Symptoms

The approach to starting menopausal hormone therapy for women aged 50 to 59 years, or within 10 years of menopause onset, who are experiencing menopause symptoms is outlined in **Table 68**. Estrogen is the most effective therapy for vasomotor symptoms; the lowest dose of estrogen to manage symptoms should be used. Contraindications to hormone therapy include pregnancy, unexplained vaginal bleeding, coronary artery disease, stroke, thromboembolic disease, breast cancer, and endometrial cancer.

Transdermal estrogen is preferable to oral estrogen because it may be associated with less thromboembolic risk, but some patients may prefer oral therapy.

For women who experience menopausal symptoms and have an intact uterus, estrogen should be combined with progestin to avoid unopposed estrogen-related endometrial proliferation. Continuous daily estrogen with progestin does not result in cyclic vaginal bleeding and may be a preferred option for many women. Women must be informed that estrogen with cyclic progestin will result in withdrawal bleeding.

Use of hormone therapy in menopause should be reassessed every year to determine benefits and risks and determine the appropriate time to discontinue the medication. Treatment duration is based on continued presence of vasomotor symptoms. Postmenopausal hormone use with combined estrogen-progestin therapy taken for more than 5 years is associated with increased risk for breast cancer and requires that women receive individualized breast cancer risk assessment and counseling.

Nonhormonal drugs can help modulate vasomotor symptoms in women with contraindications to hormone therapy or who wish to avoid the associated risks. Antidepressant agents, including selective serotonin reuptake inhibitors (such as citalopram, escitalopram, and paroxetine) and serotonin-norepinephrine reuptake inhibitors (such as

TABLE 68. Initiating Systemic Hormone Therapy in Women Aged 50 to 59 Years or Within 10 Years of Menopause Onset for Vasomotor Symptoms[a]

Step 1: Confirm that hot flushes/night sweats are moderate to severe in intensity and refractory to lifestyle modifications and/or vaginal symptoms have been refractory to local therapies.

Step 2: Assess for contraindications to systemic hormone therapy.

Step 3: Assess the patient's baseline risk for stroke, cardiovascular disease, and breast cancer (consider using the 10-year ASCVD risk calculator, Framingham stroke risk score, Framingham CHD risk score, and Gail model risk score to quantify this risk). If the Framingham stroke or CHD risk score is >10% or Gail model risk score is elevated, consider alternatives to systemic hormone therapy.[b,c]

Step 4: Use the lowest dose of estrogen that relieves menopausal symptoms.

Step 5: Add systemic progesterone therapy to estrogen therapy in women who have an intact uterus.

Step 6: Assess symptoms and side effects after initiating therapy and adjust the dose of estrogen if symptoms are persistent.

Step 7: Reassess symptoms and risk factors for cardiovascular disease, stroke, and breast cancer annually.

Step 8: Discontinue systemic hormone therapy if the risks of treatment outweigh the benefits.

ASCVD = atherosclerotic cardiovascular disease; CHD = coronary heart disease.

[a]According to the 2017 hormone therapy position statement of The North American Menopause Society, the safety profile of hormone therapy in women who initiate therapy more than 10 or 20 years after menopause onset or at age 60 years or older is not as favorable as for younger women, owing to greater absolute risks for coronary heart disease, stroke, venous thromboembolism, and dementia.

[b]Some experts indicate that systemic hormone therapy is safe in women who have experienced menopause within the last 5 years and have a Framingham CHD risk score of 10% to 20%.

[c]Most participants in the Women's Health Initiative (a set of two hormone therapy trials) had a Gail model risk score of less than 2%.

venlafaxine, desvenlafaxine, and duloxetine), and gabapentin are effective. Research is inconclusive regarding supplements such as soy, black cohosh, and other phytoestrogens for vasomotor symptoms.

Genitourinary Syndrome of Menopause

Management of genitourinary syndrome of menopause (GSM) includes topical nonhormonal and hormonal preparations to relieve symptoms. Nonhormonal approaches include as-needed vaginal lubricants for intercourse and vaginal moisturizers that can alleviate vaginal dryness and irritation when used regularly. The North American Menopause Society recommends nonhormonal vaginal therapies as first-line treatment for GSM.

Hormonal preparations include estradiol or conjugated estrogen in tablet, cream, or ring forms. Low-dose vaginal estrogen is recommended for the management of vaginal atrophy because it builds the vaginal epithelium and restores the acidic pH and microenvironment. Moreover, improving the lining of the lower urethra reduces dysuria and recurrent urinary tract infection. For women with breast cancer, current or

past, low-dose vaginal therapy should be given only with the approval of the treating oncologist. Vaginal dehydroepiandrosterone and the selective estrogen receptor modulator ospemifene are both approved by the FDA for management of dyspareunia associated with GSM; most experts consider these treatment modalities second-line therapies because of their side effects and limited safety experience.

KEY POINTS

- Routine laboratory testing for the diagnosis of menopause is not recommended; patients with possible early menopause should have pregnancy excluded and undergo measurement of follicle-stimulating hormone, thyroid-stimulating hormone, and prolactin levels. **HVC**

- Pregnancy is possible even if menstrual cycles are irregular, and contraception should be discussed if pregnancy is not desired.

- Estrogen is the most effective therapy for vasomotor symptoms of menopause.

- Nonhormonal options for vasomotor symptoms of menopause include antidepressant agents and gabapentin.

- Management of genitourinary syndrome of menopause includes topical nonhormonal and hormonal preparations to achieve symptom relief.

Chronic Pelvic Pain

Chronic pelvic pain (CPP) refers to a syndrome of intermittent or persistent pain below the level of the umbilicus or in the pelvis of at least 6 months' duration that is severe enough to result in functional disability or require medical care. Evaluation and diagnosis of CPP are challenging; CPP may be secondary to a single underlying cause, multiple concurrent disorders, or no clear cause. The identifiable causes can be classified as gynecologic (endometriosis, pelvic inflammatory disease), urologic (recurrent urinary tract infection, interstitial cystitis), gastrointestinal (pelvic adhesions, irritable bowel syndrome), musculoskeletal (myofascial pain, hernia), psychological (depression, sexual abuse), or neurologic (pudendal neuralgia).

Risk factors for CPP include physical, sexual, and/or emotional abuse; pelvic inflammatory disease; history of abdominopelvic surgery; chronic pain syndromes; and psychological conditions, such as anxiety or depression.

Evaluation includes a detailed history to determine characteristics of the pain, including association with menstrual cycle, urination, or bowel movement, as well as assessment for risk factors and known causes of CPP. Physical examination includes detailed abdominal and gynecologic examinations. Laboratory testing is of limited value unless specific disorders are suggested by the history and clinical examination (urinalysis for urinary tract infection, testing for STI). Transvaginal ultrasonography is used to identify anatomic pathology, such as a pelvic mass. In the absence of an abnormality noted on clinical examination or ultrasound, laparoscopy may be helpful for the evaluation of severe symptoms of unclear cause.

Treatment is aimed at the underlying cause and may be challenging if no clear cause is identified. For patients without a clearly identified cause, treatment is aimed at pain management. NSAIDs may be helpful for patients with moderate CPP. Additional therapies include antidepressant agents, physical therapy, cognitive behavioral therapy, biofeedback, acupuncture, hypnosis, and stress reduction therapies.

KEY POINTS

- Risk factors for chronic pelvic pain include physical, sexual, and/or emotional abuse; pelvic inflammatory disease; history of abdominopelvic surgery; chronic pain syndromes; and psychological conditions, such as anxiety or depression.

- NSAIDs may be helpful for patients with moderate chronic pelvic pain without a clearly identified cause.

Female Sexual Dysfunction

Female sexual dysfunction is characterized by persistent or recurrent distressing sexual concerns or difficulties and is likely underappreciated; it affects more than one third of sexually active women. A sexual health history is an important part of the medical evaluation; open-ended questions regarding sexual activity and possible concerns, such as pain with intercourse, are appropriate and may uncover a previously unidentified disorder.

According to the DSM-5, female sexual dysfunction is divided into three categories: female orgasmic disorder, sexual interest/arousal disorder, and genitopelvic pain/penetration disorder. Female orgasmic disorder is the persistent or recurrent delay, infrequency, reduced intensity, or absence of orgasm following a normal excitement phase. Female sexual interest/arousal disorder includes hypoactive sexual desire or arousal dysfunction and is diagnosed if the patient reports at least three of the following symptoms: lack of sexual interest, lack of sexual thoughts or fantasies, decreased initiation of sexual activity or decreased responsiveness to the partner's initiation attempts, reduced excitement or pleasure during sexual activity, reduced response to sexual cues, or decreased genital or nongenital sensations during sexual activity. Genitopelvic pain/penetration disorder is diagnosed when there is persistent or recurrent difficulty in vaginal penetration during intercourse, marked vulvovaginal or pelvic pain during penetration, fear of pain or anxiety about pain in anticipation of or during penetration, or tightening or tensing of pelvic floor muscles during attempted penetration. Diagnosis of a sexual disorder requires that the aforementioned symptoms occur more than 75% of the time for at least 6 months and cause clinically significant distress.

Sexual functioning involves multiple components, including emotions, relationships, past experiences, physiologic responses, overall health, and personal beliefs; therefore, a comprehensive approach is needed to evaluate and treat the condition.

Assessment of female sexual dysfunction includes a detailed sexual history of symptom duration, whether acute or gradual onset, if related to a specific partner or a generalized concern; association with pain; precipitating events; life stressors; medical and surgical history; medications; and history of physical, emotional, and/or sexual abuse. Screening for concurrent depression is indicated. The Female Sexual Function Index questionnaire, a brief validated self-report questionnaire, can be used for clinical assessment of symptoms. Pelvic examination is aimed at assessing for specific sites of pain or tenderness, vaginal dryness, or atrophy suggestive of genitourinary symptoms of menopause. Laboratory testing is of limited value and performed only if an underlying cause is suspected.

Therapy is aimed at treating the underlying cause of female sexual dysfunction, which is often multifactorial. Vaginal dryness and atrophy from genitourinary symptoms of menopause may warrant use of vaginal moisturizers and vaginal estrogen therapy. Lubricants can be used as needed for intercourse, and deep muscle relaxation therapies and objects, such as dilators, to increase the diameter of the vagina may be used for patients with vulvovaginal pain. Systemic hormone therapy in postmenopausal women may help sexual function. Ospemifene is a selective estrogen receptor modulator approved by the FDA for treatment of dyspareunia associated with vulvovaginal atrophy.

Flibanserin is the only drug approved by the FDA for premenopausal women with female sexual interest/arousal disorder. However, caution is warranted when this medication is prescribed because of side effects (dizziness, syncope, hypotension, somnolence) and lack of safety data when flibanserin is combined with alcohol or certain medications (antidepressants). Low-dose testosterone treatment (off-label) increases sexual function scores, but side effects must be discussed. Phosphodiesterase inhibitors, such as sildenafil, have shown inconsistent results in women.

Treatment strategies must also address psychological and behavioral aspects of female sexual dysfunction. Cognitive behavioral therapy can help minimize negative attitudes and help with anxiety. Couples therapy may be beneficial. Sex therapy includes counseling; cognitive behavioral therapy; and treatment of concomitant mental health conditions, such as depression and anxiety.

KEY POINT

- A sexual health history is an important part of the medical evaluation; open-ended questions regarding sexual activity and possible concerns, such as pain with intercourse, are appropriate and may uncover a previously unidentified disorder.

HVC

Vaginitis

Vaginitis describes conditions associated with vulvovaginal symptoms that may include vaginal discharge, burning, itching, or odor. Vaginal discharge can be physiologic, related to ovulation or pregnancy, or infectious, most commonly bacterial vaginosis, candidiasis, or trichomoniasis (**Table 69**). Other causes of vaginal discharge include irritation from use of douches, atrophic vaginitis, malignancy, or a foreign body.

History should include details about the type of vaginal discharge (volume, color, odor), timing related to menstrual cycle, use of douches, at-risk sexual behavior, dysuria, and dyspareunia. Physical examination includes assessment of the

TABLE 69. Clinical Presentation, Evaluation, and Management of Vaginitis

Cause of Vaginitis	Clinical Presentation	Evaluation	Management
Bacterial vaginosis	Malodorous or "fishy" vaginal discharge, often most noticeable after intercourse Increased thin white or gray discharge Symptoms other than malodor may be minimal	pH >4.5 KOH amine whiff test result positive Saline wet mount with >20% epithelial clue cells	Metronidazole: 500 mg orally twice daily for 7 days[a] (avoid alcohol during treatment and for 24 hours after last dose); or vaginal gel (0.75%) 5 g into vagina at bedtime for 5 nights Clindamycin: 300 mg orally twice daily for 7 days; or vaginal cream (2%) 5 g into vagina for 7 nights Note: Use oral regimens in pregnancy.
Vulvovaginal candidiasis	Itching, irritation, dysuria, dyspareunia, vulvodynia, excoriation, erythema, fissures Increased thick white discharge (although may be normal)	pH ≤4.5 KOH amine whiff test result negative KOH wet mount shows hyphae, pseudohyphae, or yeast	**Uncomplicated[b]** Fluconazole: 150 mg orally as a single dose Butoconazole vaginal: (2% cream) 5 g into vagina at bedtime for 3 nights Clotrimazole vaginal: (1% cream) 5 g into vagina at bedtime for 7-14 nights; or 100-mg vaginal tablet into vagina at bedtime for 7 nights; or 200 mg (two vaginal tablets) into vagina once daily at bedtime for 3 nights Miconazole vaginal: (2% cream) 5 g into vagina at bedtime for 7 nights; or 100-mg vaginal suppository into vagina at bedtime for 7 nights; or 200-mg vaginal suppository into vagina at bedtime for 3 nights Note: Single-dose vaginal preparations and non-imidazoles are available but less effective. **Complicated[c]** Longer duration of initial oral or topical treatment, followed by maintenance therapy: Fluconazole: 150 mg orally every 3 days for a total of three doses; or topical imidazole therapy for 7-14 nights Following this, maintenance therapy is based on refractory or recurrent symptoms: Fluconazole: 150 mg orally weekly for 6 months; or 200 mg orally weekly for 8 weeks; or 200 mg orally twice weekly for 4 months; or 200 mg orally once monthly for 6 months
Trichomoniasis	Increased discolored discharge (yellowish, gray, and/or frothy) Dyspareunia, dysuria, itch, erythema, postcoital bleeding, abdominal pain Punctate cervical hemorrhages ("strawberry" cervix)	pH ≥4.5 KOH amine whiff test result negative Saline wet mount with trichomonads, leukocytes NAAT or rapid assay result positive	Metronidazole[a]: 2 g orally as a single dose; treatment failure with 2-g metronidazole is treated with 500 mg orally twice daily for 7 days Note: Avoid alcohol during treatment and for 24 hours after last dose.

KOH = potassium hydroxide; NAAT = nucleic acid amplification test.

[a]Safe in pregnancy.

[b]Uncomplicated vulvovaginal candidiasis: *Candida albicans*, mild to moderate symptom severity, healthy nonpregnant women, four or fewer episodes per year.

[c]Complicated vulvovaginal candidiasis: Severe symptoms, suspected or proven non-albicans *Candida* species, more than four episodes per year, uncontrolled diabetes mellitus, or immunosuppression.

vulva and vagina for erythema, edema, excoriation, papillomas, and the type of discharge. However, clinical findings do not sufficiently distinguish between the common causes of vaginitis, and laboratory testing is necessary to establish a diagnosis. Diagnostic testing includes assessment of vaginal wall secretions for pH, amine (whiff) test, and microscopic evaluation with saline potassium hydroxide (KOH) wet mounts, or specific testing for trichomoniasis.

Bacterial Vaginosis

Bacterial vaginosis is the most common cause of vaginal discharge. It results from the loss of the normal hydrogen peroxide–producing lactobacilli in the vagina with an increase in the vaginal pH that contributes to an overgrowth of *Gardnerella vaginalis* and other anaerobes. Anaerobic overgrowth results in the production of amines, causing the characteristically malodorous discharge. Patients with bacterial vaginosis are at increased risk for STIs, including HIV infection, and for preterm delivery.

More than half of patients with bacterial vaginosis are asymptomatic. Symptomatic patients report a thin, vaginal discharge with a fishy odor. Clinical diagnosis includes the presence of at least three of four features: vaginal pH greater than 4.5, thin and homogeneous vaginal discharge, a positive whiff test result in which application of 10% KOH to vaginal secretions results in a fishy odor, and the finding of at least 20% clue cells on saline wet mount preparation. Clue cells are vaginal epithelial cells that on microscopy have ill-defined cell borders due to adherent coccobacilli (**Figure 16**).

Asymptomatic bacterial vaginosis does not require treatment. See Table 69 for treatment options for symptomatic bacterial vaginosis.

Vulvovaginal Candidiasis

Vulvovaginal candidiasis is the second most common cause of vaginitis; it is usually caused by *Candida albicans* and less commonly by non-albicans *Candida*. Unlike pharyngeal candidiasis, it frequently occurs in immunocompetent women with no risk factors. Factors that may increase the risk for vulvovaginal candidiasis include diabetes mellitus; pregnancy; and use of oral contraceptives, glucocorticoids, or antibiotics. Recurrent vulvovaginal candidiasis, characterized by infections occurring four or more times per year, is also caused by *C. albicans*, but up to 20% may be caused by *Candida glabrata* and other non-albicans *Candida* species.

Vulvovaginal candidiasis is typically characterized by vaginal itching, irritation, and discharge and may be associated with dysuria and dyspareunia. Examination reveals vulvar edema and excoriation, with thick, white, curdy vaginal discharge. Diagnostic testing involves a saline or 10% KOH wet mount of the discharge showing yeast, hyphae, or pseudohyphae (**Figure 17**). Women with negative wet mount results but signs and symptoms of candidiasis should have vaginal cultures for *Candida* performed and should be treated if results are positive. If cultures cannot be performed, empiric treatment is recommended.

Asymptomatic patients should not receive treatment. See Table 69 for treatment options of symptomatic uncomplicated and complicated vulvovaginal candidiasis. Recurrent symptoms after treatment warrant an evaluation for the presence of underlying predisposing factors. No evidence supports treatment of sexual partners of patients with vulvovaginal candidiasis.

Trichomoniasis

Trichomoniasis is a vaginal infection caused by *Trichomonas vaginalis*, a flagellated protozoan. It is a common STI, with a high prevalence among patients in STI clinics and incarcerated individuals. It is associated with increased risk for preterm labor in pregnancy as well as increased risk for HIV transmission.

Women may be asymptomatic or present with copious vaginal discharge that is malodorous, pale yellow or gray, frothy, and associated with vulval itching and burning. Vaginal pH is often elevated but is not helpful diagnostically. Testing may include microscopy, nucleic acid amplification testing (NAAT),

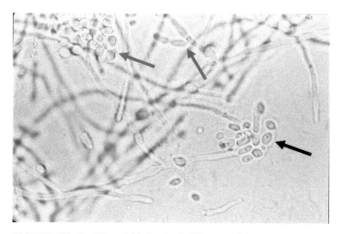

FIGURE 16. Clue cells are vaginal epithelial cells whose surface is studded with adherent coccobacilli bacteria (*arrows*), often obscuring the border of the epithelial cells; they are characteristic of bacterial vaginosis.

FIGURE 17. *Candida* vaginitis showing budding yeast (*blue arrow*), spores (*black arrow*), and elongated spores appearing as pseudohyphae (*red arrow*) with potassium hydroxide.

rapid antigen testing, and culture; choice of diagnostic testing is largely driven by availability. Microscopy with examination of a wet mount of the vaginal fluid showing motile trichomonads can establish the diagnosis when positive, but false-negative test results are common. NAAT or rapid antigen testing may be used as the primary diagnostic test or if the suspicion of trichomoniasis is high but the wet mount result is negative. When *Trichomonas* is identified, testing for other STIs should be considered. See Table 69 for treatment of trichomoniasis. Women should be retested within 3 months of treatment. Treatment of sexual partners is recommended to prevent reinfection.

KEY POINTS

HVC
- Clinical findings do not sufficiently distinguish between the common causes of vaginitis, and laboratory testing is necessary to establish a diagnosis.

HVC
- Clinical diagnosis of bacterial vaginosis includes the presence of at least three of four features: vaginal pH greater than 4.5, thin and homogeneous vaginal discharge, a positive whiff test result, and at least 20% clue cells on saline wet mount preparation.

- Diagnostic testing for vulvovaginal candidiasis involves a saline or 10% potassium hydroxide wet mount of the discharge showing yeast, hyphae, or pseudohyphae.

- Testing for trichomoniasis may include microscopy, nucleic acid amplification testing, rapid antigen testing, and culture; choice of diagnostic testing is largely driven by availability.

Eye Disorders

Eye Emergencies

Acute vision loss requires immediate ophthalmology evaluation. Selected conditions that can cause acute vision loss are listed in **Table 70**.

Trauma or chemical injury to the globe, eyelid, or nasolacrimal system also warrants urgent evaluation by an ophthalmologist. Patients with chemical injury to the eye should immediately receive eye irrigation to neutralize the ocular surface while awaiting ophthalmologic evaluation.

Vision-threatening eye infections requiring immediate intravenous antibiotics and ophthalmology evaluation include endophthalmitis (particularly bacterial infection of the aqueous and vitreous humors) and orbital cellulitis (infection of the fat and muscle cells of the orbit). Periorbital and preseptal cellulitis (infection anterior to the orbital septum) are less of a threat to sight. ☐

KEY POINT

- Eye emergencies requiring immediate ophthalmology evaluation include acute vision loss; trauma or chemical injury to the globe, eyelid, or nasolacrimal system; and vision-threatening eye infections.

TABLE 70. Selected Conditions Requiring Immediate Ophthalmologic Evaluation

Acute angle-closure glaucoma
Central retinal artery occlusion
Central retinal vein occlusion
Chemical injury
Corneal ulcers
Endophthalmitis
Keratitis
Optic neuritis
Orbital cellulitis
Retinal detachment
Scleritis
Trauma
Uveitis

Red Eye

Cardinal features of conditions that cause red eye are listed in **Table 71**.

Conjunctivitis

Conjunctivitis is the most common cause of red eye and is categorized as infectious (viral [**Figure 18**], bacterial [**Figure 19**]) or noninfectious (irritants, allergic). Factors favoring a bacterial cause include glued eyes in the morning, redness completely obscuring the tarsal vessels, purulent discharge, a red eye observed at 20 feet, and occurrence in the winter or spring. Lack of discharge decreases the likelihood of a bacterial cause. Bacterial conjunctivitis is often caused by *Staphylococcus aureus* and usually resolves within a week; however, topical antimicrobial treatment (erythromycin ophthalmic 0.5% ointment, trimethoprim-polymyxin B ophthalmic ointment) shortens the duration of symptoms by up to 1.5 days. Topical fluoroquinolones (such as levofloxacin) are not first-line therapy for routine bacterial conjunctivitis; however, they are indicated for conjunctivitis in contact lens wearers because of the high incidence of *Pseudomonas* infection. The threshold to treat with antibiotics is lowered in health care workers; patients in health care facilities; or patients with immunocompromise, including those with diabetes mellitus. Treatment of viral conjunctivitis is supportive, including cold compresses. Patients with viral conjunctivitis are considered contagious for as long as the eye continues to tear and produce discharge, usually 3 to 7 days. ☐

Keratitis

Keratitis represents infection and inflammation of the cornea. It most commonly results from bacterial infection (especially with *Pseudomonas* species) in contact lens wearers or in those with herpes simplex virus infection. Keratitis is an ocular emergency and requires urgent ophthalmology evaluation.

TABLE 71. Cardinal Features of Conditions That Cause Red Eye

Cause	Pain	Visual Symptoms	Examination Findings	Associated Systemic Conditions	Immediate Ophthalmologic Evaluation?
Conjunctivitis	Irritation only; associated with discharge and crusting	None unless discharge clouds vision	Diffuse erythema of conjunctiva, also involving inner aspect of eyelids	Usually limited to eye	No
Keratitis	Present, often with foreign body sensation	Blurred vision	Corneal stromal infiltrates or, in the case of herpes, corneal dendritic branching; circumferential redness around the border of the sclera and cornea (ciliary flush)	Usually limited to the eye	Yes
Episcleritis	Minimal	None	Superficial redness of episcleral vessels and episclera; may be localized	Minority of patients have underlying disease (rheumatoid arthritis, inflammatory bowel disease)	No
Scleritis	Severe, often worse with eye movement; associated tearing and photophobia	Decreased vision; may be complete loss	Scleral edema with diffuse deep red/violaceous discoloration; globe tenderness	>50% with rheumatologic disease (rheumatoid arthritis, vasculitis)	Yes
Uveitis/iritis	None to moderate	Variable; may include floaters	Ciliary flush; hypopyon (suppurative fluid seen in the dependent portion of the anterior chamber)	Common; infection (HSV, CMV); inflammatory disorders (spondyloarthritis, sarcoidosis)	Yes
Subconjunctival hemorrhage	Mild or none	None	Discrete bright red confluent region without hyperemia	Spontaneous; anticoagulation; trauma; increased pressure (coughing)	No

CMV = cytomegalovirus; HSV = herpes simplex virus.

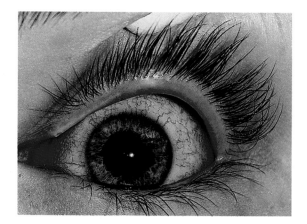

FIGURE 18. Diffuse conjunctival injection and erythema, usually with a watery or mucoserous discharge, are characteristic of viral conjunctivitis.

Reproduced from Joyhill09. Eye with viral conjunctivitis. Digital image. http://commons.wikimedia.org/wiki/File:An_eye_with_viral_conjunctivitis.jpg. February 1, 2010. Accessed July 10, 2018. Licensed under the Creative Commons Attribution-ShareAlike 3.0 Unported (CC BY-SA 3.0) International License (https://creativecommons.org/licenses/by-sa/3.0/deed.en).

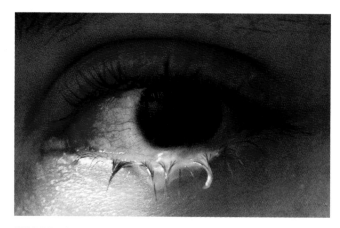

FIGURE 19. In patients with bacterial conjunctivitis, eye discharge is thick and may be yellow or green.

Reproduced from Tanalai. Swollen eye with conjunctivitis. Digital image. http://commons.wikimedia.org/wiki/File:Swollen_eye_with_conjunctivitis.jpg. January 22, 2008. Accessed July 10, 2018. Licensed under the Creative Commons Attribution 3.0 Unported (CC BY 3.0) International License (https://creativecommons.org/licenses/by/3.0/deed.en).

Episcleritis and Scleritis

Episcleritis is a focal, acute area of inflammation involving the superficial layers of the episclera. It is usually self-limited, resolving in a few weeks. Treatment is symptomatic and includes artificial tears; anti-inflammatory agents, such as topical NSAIDs and glucocorticoids, may be needed.

Scleritis is an inflammatory disorder of the sclera, which lies beneath the episcleral and conjunctival layers (**Figure 20**). Scleritis is an acute threat to vision and requires urgent evaluation by an ophthalmologist.

Uveitis

Anterior uveitis (iritis) is characterized by inflammation of the middle eye, including the iris, ciliary body, and choroid. In addition to pain, photophobia, vision impairment, and circumferential redness around the border of the sclera and cornea (ciliary flush), the pupil may have an irregular shape because it has become attached to the anterior surface of the lens or the posterior surface of the cornea. Uveitis requires urgent evaluation by an ophthalmologist.

Subconjunctival Hemorrhage

Subconjunctival hemorrhage is common and not a threat to vision (**Figure 21**). When symptoms are present, warm compresses or ophthalmic lubricants may provide relief. Symptoms should resolve gradually but may recur in patients receiving anticoagulants.

Blepharitis

Blepharitis is a common inflammatory condition of the eyelid margin and may be associated with rosacea. Treatment includes warm compresses, application of diluted shampoo

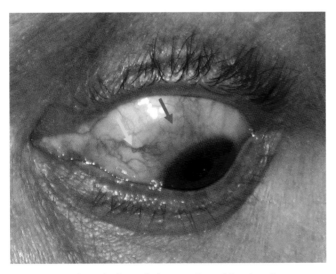

FIGURE 20. The cardinal sign of scleritis is edema of the sclera often associated with a violaceous discoloration of the globe (*red arrow*). Tenderness is invariably present. Typically, there is intense dilation of episcleral blood vessels (*yellow arrow*). Scleral inflammation may be focal or diffuse.

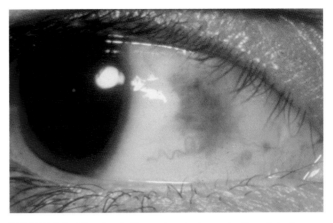

FIGURE 21. Subconjunctival hemorrhage is characterized by unilateral, localized, and sharply circumscribed redness without discharge or pain.

with a cotton-tip applicator, topical antibiotics (for staphylococcal infections), and oral tetracyclines (for infections associated with rosacea).

KEY POINTS

- Conjunctivitis is the most common cause of red eye and is associated with ocular irritation (not pain), discharge, and no impairment of vision.
- Keratitis is an ocular emergency that represents infection and inflammation of the cornea and is characterized by ocular redness, pain, and impaired vision.
- Episcleritis is a focal, acute area of typically asymptomatic inflammation involving the superficial layers of the episclera that is usually self-limited, whereas scleritis is a painful inflammatory disorder of the sclera associated with tearing and photophobia and is an acute threat to vision.

Dry Eye

Dry eye (keratoconjunctivitis sicca) is a multifactorial inflammatory disorder involving the tears and ocular surface. Symptoms may include eye dryness, a sensation of a foreign body in the eye, blurred vision, and light sensitivity. Examination may show decreased tearing, malposition of the lids, conjunctival erythema, blepharitis, or reduced blink rate. Validated symptom questionnaires may be diagnostically helpful. Ophthalmologists can perform more specific lacrimal function testing. Treatment includes artificial tears, environmental strategies (for example, increased humidification), and topical cyclosporine. Oral omega-3 fatty acid supplements may alleviate the symptoms of dry eye syndrome.

KEY POINT

- Treatment of dry eye includes artificial tears, environmental strategies, and topical cyclosporine.

Corneal Abrasion and Ulcer

Corneal abrasions are often caused by trauma from a foreign body. Pain, sensation of a foreign body, watery eyes, red eye, photophobia, and reactive miosis may be present. Corneal examination involves fluorescein dye and a Wood lamp or slit lamp. Management of uncomplicated abrasions includes topical NSAIDs. Current evidence does not support the use of topical antibiotics or eye patching. Topical anesthetics may decrease rate of healing and should be avoided. The presence of a corneal ulcer requires prompt evaluation by an ophthalmologist.

Cataracts

Cataracts are opacifications of the lens and should be suspected in patients presenting with painless gradual worsening of visual acuity. Direct ophthalmoscopy shows lens opacification, a diminished red reflex, and obscured funduscopic examination. Surgery is indicated when vision impairment interferes with the patient's activities of daily living.

Glaucoma

Glaucoma is the leading cause of permanent blindness in the world. It is typically characterized by increased intraocular pressure (IOP) as a result of decreased outflow of aqueous humor from the anterior chamber. However, according to the U.S. Preventive Services Task Force, there is insufficient evidence to recommend screening for glaucoma in adults.

Primary Open-Angle Glaucoma

Primary open-angle glaucoma accounts for more than 80% of glaucoma cases in the United States. Increased resistance to aqueous outflow through the trabecular meshwork leads to increased IOP and vision loss through retinal cell death. Patients may present with bilateral peripheral visual loss that is gradual and painless. Funduscopic examination may demonstrate increased cup-to-disc ratio (CDR) (**Figure 22**), CDR asymmetry, and disc hemorrhage. Treatment is directed by an ophthalmologist and involves medications (topical prostaglandins, β-blockers, and α-adrenergic agonists) to decrease IOP and, when refractory, surgery.

Angle-Closure Glaucoma

Angle-closure glaucoma is caused by mechanical obstruction of the aqueous humor drainage at the angle of the anterior chamber, leading to increased IOP. Blockage is usually secondary to the positioning of the lens on the iris; if blockage is present chronically, patients may be asymptomatic until advanced vision loss has occurred. Acute blockage may occur with exposure to sympathomimetic or anticholinergic medications or with pupillary dilation.

Patients with acute blockage present with severe eye pain, headache, nausea, and blurred vision or halos around lights.

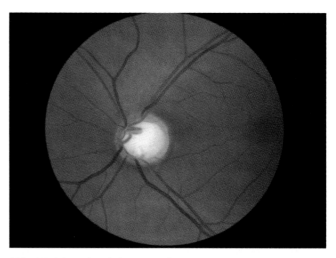

FIGURE 22. A relatively large cup-to-disc ratio and cupping identified by the disappearance of vessels over the edge of the attenuated optic rim are characteristic of glaucoma.

Examination may demonstrate severe conjunctive hyperemia, corneal edema, a mid-dilated (4-6 mm) nonreactive pupil, and severe elevation in IOP. Because of the immediate threat to vision, urgent evaluation by an ophthalmologist is required. **H**

KEY POINTS

- Primary open-angle glaucoma is characterized by increased intraocular pressure, increased cup-to-disc ratio (CDR), CDR asymmetry, and bilateral peripheral visual loss that is gradual and painless.
- Patients with acute angle-closure glaucoma present with severe eye pain, headache, nausea, and blurred vision or halos around lights, and examination may demonstrate severe conjunctive hyperemia, corneal edema, a mid-dilated (4-6 mm) nonreactive pupil, and severe elevation in intraocular pressure; urgent evaluation by an ophthalmologist is required because of the immediate threat to vision.

Age-Related Macular Degeneration

Age-related macular degeneration (AMD) is a progressive chronic disease involving the central retina. Patients with early AMD are often asymptomatic, although yellow drusen may be visible underneath retinal pigment epithelium (**Figure 23**). Patients with atrophic (dry) AMD, which accounts for 80% to 90% of AMD cases, note slowly progressive vision loss over years. About 10% to 20% of patients with atrophic AMD progress to neovascular (wet) AMD, which often presents with more rapid visual loss and may be accompanied by a sudden worsening of central vision associated with straight-line distortion (metamorphopsia), scotoma, or both.

Smoking cessation decreases the risk for developing AMD and should be recommended to all patients who smoke. There

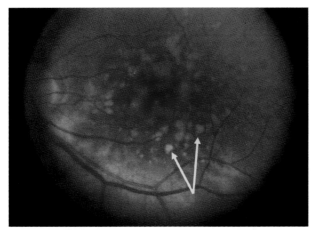

FIGURE 23. Atrophic (dry) age-related macular degeneration showing distinct yellow-white lesions called drusen (*arrows*) surrounding the macular area and areas of pigment mottling.

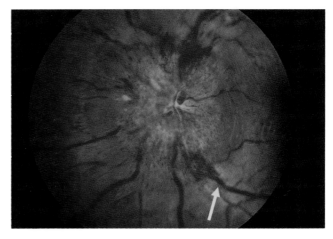

FIGURE 24. Optic nerve papillitis is characterized by hyperemia and swelling of the disc, blurring of disc margins, and distended veins (*arrow*). The normal arteriole-to-venous ratio is approximately 4:5.

is no cure for atrophic AMD; however, dietary supplementation with high-dose antioxidants, vitamins, and zinc can delay the progression of AMD. First-line treatment for neovascular AMD is anti–vascular endothelial growth factor (VEGF) therapies. The treatment burden of the intravitreal injections, however, is high, and the long-term risk for systemic absorption of VEGF inhibitors is unknown.

KEY POINT

HVC
- Smoking cessation decreases the risk for age-related macular degeneration and should be recommended to all patients who smoke.

Optic Neuritis

Optic neuritis is characterized by inflammation and demyelination of the optic nerve. Usually unilateral in onset, it presents with visual loss occurring over hours to days. It is associated with acute pain, particularly with eye movement, as well as loss of color vision. Examination may demonstrate an afferent pupillary defect (paradoxical dilation of the affected pupil when the examining light is rapidly shifted from the unaffected to the affected eye); papillitis (swollen disc with blurred margin) may be seen on funduscopy in one third of patients (**Figure 24**). Two thirds of patients will have retrobulbar neuritis and a normal funduscopic examination. Urgent evaluation by an ophthalmologist is required. Although the diagnosis is clinical, MRI usually reveals demyelination of the optic nerve. Treatment with high-dose intravenous glucocorticoids improves the rate of visual recovery.

Retinal Detachment

Patients with retinal detachment may present with a unilateral increase in floaters followed by a sudden, peripheral visual field defect that resembles a black curtain and may progress across the entire visual field. A retinal tear and elevation of the surrounding retina may be visible on dilated funduscopy. Immediate evaluation by an ophthalmologist is indicated for surgical treatment.

Retinal Vascular Occlusion

Retinal Artery Occlusion

Patients with central retinal artery occlusion present with acute, profound, and painless loss of monocular vision. It is most commonly associated with carotid artery atherosclerosis but may be associated with cardiogenic embolism, thrombophilia, or giant cell arteritis. Examination usually shows an afferent pupillary defect; funduscopic examination may show a "cherry red spot" at the fovea surrounded by retinal pallor. Emergent evaluation by an ophthalmologist is necessary.

Retinal Vein Occlusion

Central retinal vein occlusion (CRVO) is usually associated with thrombus formation in the central retinal vein, whereas branch retinal vein occlusion (BRVO) appears related to compression of the branch vein by nearby crossing arterioles. Both are associated with cardiovascular risk factors, including hypertension, diabetes, and tobacco use. CRVO often presents with acute onset of painless blurred monocular vision. BRVO may be asymptomatic but may present with scotoma or focal field defects of blurriness corresponding to the area of retinal vein occlusion.

Examination may reveal an afferent pupillary defect (particularly in CRVO), retinal vein congestion, retinal hemorrhage, and cotton-wool spots (**Figure 25**). A patient whose presentation suggests CRVO requires immediate evaluation by an ophthalmologist.

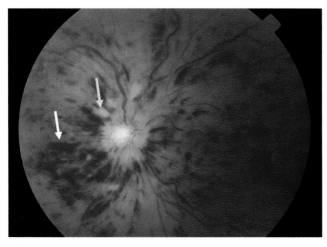

FIGURE 25. Central retinal vein occlusion is characterized by optic disc swelling, dilated and tortuous veins, as well as flame-shaped retinal hemorrhages (*white arrow*) and cotton-wool spots (*yellow arrow*) ("blood and thunder").

KEY POINTS

- Central retinal artery occlusion may present with acute, profound, and painless loss of monocular vision and is most commonly associated with carotid artery atherosclerosis.

(Continued)

KEY POINTS *(continued)*

- Central retinal vein occlusion is usually associated with thrombus formation in the central retinal vein and often presents with acute onset of painless blurred monocular vision; immediate evaluation by an ophthalmologist is required.

Ear, Nose, Mouth, and Throat Disorders

Hearing Loss

Hearing loss is common. It is associated with depression and functional decline but underrecognized by patients and physicians. The U.S. Preventive Services Task Force has concluded that there is insufficient evidence to assess the benefits and harms of screening for hearing loss in asymptomatic older adults.

Hearing loss is categorized according to the anatomic deficit: conductive, sensorineural, or mixed (**Table 72**). Conductive hearing loss is more often associated with pain or ear drainage, whereas sensorineural hearing loss is more often accompanied by tinnitus or vertigo.

TABLE 72.	Causes of Hearing Loss
Cause	**Description**
Conductive Hearing Loss[a]	
Cerumen impaction	May completely obstruct ear canal
Otosclerosis	Associated with overgrowth of bone in the middle ear
Tympanic membrane perforation	Often heals without intervention
Cholesteatoma	Abnormal growth of keratinized squamous epithelium in the middle ear
Sensorineural Hearing Loss[b]	
Presbycusis	Age-related hearing loss; often symmetric, high-frequency loss
Sudden sensorineural hearing loss	Often idiopathic, more often unilateral
Meniere disease	Classically, triad of sensorineural hearing loss, tinnitus, and vertigo; not all are necessarily present at once, may fluctuate
Acoustic neuroma	Benign tumor of Schwann cell sheath surrounding vestibular or cochlear nerve
Noise	May be related to chronic noise exposure or sudden, short noise blast exposure
Ototoxic drugs	Antibiotics (aminoglycosides, erythromycin, vancomycin)
	Chemotherapeutic agents (cisplatin, carboplatin, vincristine)
	Loop diuretics
	Anti-inflammatory agents (aspirin, NSAIDs, quinine)
Mixed or Causing Either Conductive or Sensorineural Hearing Loss	
Infection	Labyrinthitis, otitis media, chronic otitis
Head trauma	May be caused by ossicular disruption leading to conductive hearing loss or by auditory nerve injury causing sensorineural hearing loss

[a]Conductive hearing loss is inadequate mechanical transmission of sound through the tympanic membrane and ossicles of the middle ear.

[b]Sensorineural hearing loss is deficit or injury of the vestibulocochlear nerve.

Assessment of hearing may begin with asking the patient about perceived hearing loss (for example, "Do you have difficulty hearing?"). More formal screening can also be performed (**Table 73**).

In patients with hearing loss, physical examination should include otoscopic examination as well as the Weber and Rinne tests (**Table 74**), which can help differentiate sensorineural from conductive hearing loss. Referral to an audiologist is indicated when hearing loss is identified. Imaging (typically MRI) is rarely required unless the hearing loss is acute, unilateral, progressive, or associated with other neurologic changes. Patients should be evaluated urgently by an otolaryngologist when there is sudden sensorineural hearing loss, hearing loss with vertigo, or hearing loss associated with head trauma. Vertigo is discussed in Common Symptoms.

Treatment options for hearing loss include assistive listening devices, hearing aids, and cochlear implants. Treatment of sudden sensorineural hearing loss involves oral glucocorticoids, although strong evidence of efficacy is lacking.

TABLE 73. Screening Maneuvers to Assess Hearing

Screening Maneuver	Technique
Patient Self-Assessment	
Single-item screening	Patient answers yes or no to the following question: "Do you feel you have hearing loss?"
Hearing Handicap Inventory for the Elderly-Screening Version	Patient answers 10-item question set, with options of yes, no, or sometimes.
Clinician Examination	
Finger rub test	The examiner gently rubs two fingers together at a distance of 15 cm (6 in) from patient's ear. A positive test result is failure to identify rub in more than two of six attempts.
Whispered voice test	The examiner stands an arm's length behind the patient and masks the untested ear by occluding the canal and rubbing the tragus. The examiner whispers six sets of three letter or number combinations. Failure to repeat at least three sets correctly is a positive test result.
Handheld audiometer	The examiner holds the device in the patient's ear while the patient indicates awareness of each tone. A positive test result is a failure to identify the 1000-Hz or 2000-Hz frequency in both ears or the 1000-Hz and 2000-Hz frequency in one ear.

TABLE 74. Distinguishing Between Conductive and Sensorineural Hearing Loss With the Weber and Rinne Tests

Condition	Weber Test[a] Result	Rinne Test[b] Result
Conductive hearing loss	Louder in the affected ear	Decreased in the affected ear (bone conduction > air conduction)
Sensorineural hearing loss	Louder in the unaffected ear	As loud or louder in the affected ear (air conduction > bone conduction)

[a]A 256-Hz vibrating tuning fork (although a 512-Hz tuning fork may be used) is applied to the forehead or scalp at the midline, and the patient is asked if the sound is louder in one ear or the other; a normal test result shows no lateralization.

[b]A 512-Hz vibrating tuning fork is applied to the mastoid process of the affected ear until it is no longer heard. The fork is then repositioned outside of the external auditory canal, and the patient is asked if he or she can again hear the tuning fork; with a normal test result, air conduction is greater than bone conduction, and the tuning fork can be heard.

KEY POINTS

- Assessment of hearing may begin with asking the patient about perceived hearing loss (for example, "Do you have difficulty hearing?"). **HVC**

- Patients should be evaluated urgently by an otolaryngologist when there is sudden sensorineural hearing loss, hearing loss with vertigo, or hearing loss associated with head trauma.

Tinnitus

Tinnitus is the conscious perception of an auditory sensation (for example, buzzing or ringing) without an external stimulus. Evaluation should include assessment for hearing loss and cardiovascular, cerebrovascular, and neurologic disease, including examination of the carotid arteries and temporal bone for bruits. Patients with unilateral tinnitus should undergo prompt audiologic assessment and, if hearing loss is confirmed, MRI to examine for acoustic neuroma. Patients should be evaluated urgently by an otolaryngologist when tinnitus is associated with sudden hearing loss, otorrhea, vestibular dysfunction, focal neurologic deficits, or pulsatile tinnitus (particularly if tinnitus is sudden in onset, which may suggest a vascular cause).

Treatment involves addressing the underlying condition. Medications have not been shown to be of benefit, but antidepressants may reduce associated distress. Cognitive behavioral therapy, relaxation therapy, and tinnitus retraining therapy may also be helpful.

KEY POINT

- Medications have not been shown to be of benefit for tinnitus, but antidepressants may reduce associated distress. **HVC**

Otitis Media and Otitis Externa

Patients with acute otitis media have ear pain along with bulging or intense erythema of the tympanic membrane or new onset of otorrhea not associated with otitis externa. Few published studies guide management in adults. In children, guidelines suggest use of antibiotics when there is otorrhea or severe signs and symptoms (including moderate to severe otalgia lasting for >48 hours or temperature >39 °C [102.2 °F]). In milder cases, management may consist of observation first with antibiotics for worsening or persistent symptoms. An otolaryngologist should evaluate adults with recurrent acute or persistent otitis media with effusion.

Acute otitis externa is cellulitis of the ear canal with associated inflammation and edema. Bacterial infection, usually with *Pseudomonas* or *Staphylococcus aureus*, causes most cases (90%). Topical treatments, including antibiotics, glucocorticoids, antiseptics, and combination therapies, are first-line management for uncomplicated acute otitis externa; aminoglycosides should be avoided if tympanic membrane perforation is present or possible. Pseudomonal infections, especially in patients with diabetes mellitus, may be aggressive and result in spread to contiguous structures, including bone (malignant otitis externa); treatment requires systemic antipseudomonal antibiotics and urgent referral to an otolaryngologist.

KEY POINT

- Malignant otitis externa requires systemic antipseudomonal antibiotics and urgent referral to an otolaryngologist.

Cerumen Impaction

Cerumen has protective, emollient, and bactericidal properties. However, its normal expulsion, assisted by jaw movement, is sometimes hindered, and cerumen accumulation may cause pain, itching, tinnitus, or hearing loss. When symptomatic, cerumen can be removed by irrigation, manual removal, or topical preparations. No topical agent has demonstrated superiority. Irrigation in the presence of a perforated tympanic membrane may cause vertiginous symptoms; mechanical removal is preferred in these instances.

Upper Respiratory Tract Infection

Sinusitis

Acute rhinosinusitis presents with nasal congestion, purulent nasal discharge, facial pain/pressure, fever, or cough. Most cases are caused by viruses, allergies, or irritants. It is usually self-limited; decongestants and mucolytics may alleviate symptoms. Avoidance of unnecessary antibiotics represents high value care. Indications for antibiotic treatment and regimens are described in **Table 75**. Patients who are seriously ill, deteriorate despite appropriate antibiotic therapy, or have recurrent episodes should be evaluated by an otolaryngologist.

Chronic sinusitis manifests with at least 12 weeks of nasal congestion with purulent drainage, diminished sense of smell, or facial pain/pressure. It may be associated with nasal polyposis (with a strong association with asthma). Demonstration

TABLE 75. Acute Sinusitis Treatment[a]

Indications for Antibiotic Treatment	First-Line Therapy[b]	Penicillin Allergy
Persistent symptoms of >10 days' duration Onset of severe symptoms or signs of high fever >39 °C (102.2 °F) with purulent nasal discharge or facial pain lasting for at least 3 consecutive days Onset of worsening symptoms following a typical viral illness that lasted 5 days after initially improving ("double sickening")	Amoxicillin-clavulanate or amoxicillin	Doxycycline (adults only) or Levofloxacin or moxifloxacin or Clindamycin

[a]There is limited evidence to guide therapy, particularly in adults, and guidelines from major professional societies differ.

[b]Adjunctive therapy, such as intranasal saline irrigation or intranasal glucocorticoids, has been shown to alleviate symptoms and potentially decrease antibiotic use.

of mucosal involvement by nasal endoscopy or imaging (typically CT) is necessary for diagnosis. Treatment includes glucocorticoids and antibiotics.

Rhinitis

Allergic rhinitis involves sneezing, congestion, and rhinorrhea often linked to a season or exposure. Nonallergic rhinitis occurs in response to nonallergic stimuli, such as spicy foods and irritants. First-line treatment of allergic and nonallergic rhinitis consists of avoiding precipitating factors and monotherapy with intranasal glucocorticoids (rather than an intranasal glucocorticoid in combination with an oral antihistamine or a leukotriene receptor antagonist). Rhinitis medicamentosa is chronic rhinitis resulting from the inappropriate long-term use of topical nasal decongestants. Treatment consists of cessation of the decongestant and intranasal glucocorticoids when needed.

Pharyngitis

Pharyngitis presents as sore throat that may worsen with swallowing. Symptoms typically last less than 1 week. Features suggesting the more common viral cause include cough, conjunctivitis, coryza, hoarseness, and oral ulcers. Only 5% to 15% of pharyngitis cases are caused by bacteria, most often group A *Streptococcus pyogenes*. In these cases, appropriate antibiotic treatment reduces the risk for rheumatic fever, suppurative complications (such as peritonsillar or retropharyngeal abscess), duration of symptoms, and transmission. Patients with fewer than three of the four Centor criteria (fever by history, tonsillar exudates, tender anterior cervical lymphadenopathy, and absence of cough) do not need to be tested or treated for group A *Streptococcus*. These patients should be treated conservatively with symptom control (such as analgesics [NSAIDs or acetaminophen], lozenges or topical sprays, and increased environmental humidity). Patients with three or more Centor criteria should be tested by using a rapid antigen detection test. Throat culture should be considered in patients who are at high risk for complications (immunocompromised state) in the setting of high clinical suspicion but negative results on rapid antigen detection testing. Antibiotic treatment is reserved for patients with positive test results; penicillin and amoxicillin are first-line therapies.

Fusobacterium necrophorum infection can cause Lemierre syndrome, a rare suppurative complication of pharyngitis caused by local spread of infection with resultant septic thrombosis of the internal jugular vein. Clinicians should suspect Lemierre syndrome in patients with severe pharyngitis and neck pain that do not respond to appropriate antibiotics. Diagnosis is made with contrast CT of the neck. **H**

KEY POINTS

- **HVC** • Acute rhinosinusitis is usually caused by viruses, allergies, or irritants, and avoidance of unnecessary antibiotics represents high value care.

- **HVC** • Patients with pharyngitis who present with fewer than three of the four Centor criteria do not need to be tested or treated for group A *Streptococcus* infection.

Epistaxis

Ninety percent of epistaxis cases occur in the anterior nasal septum. Cases that occur in the posterior nasopharynx are more common in older patients. The history should include local trauma, nose picking, nasal medications, insufficient humidification, infection, drug use, and coagulopathies.

Anterior bleeds can be managed with compression for at least 15 minutes. Concomitant use of topical vasoconstrictors, such as oxymetazoline, may be useful. Refractory bleeding may require cautery or nasal packing and, rarely, embolization or surgical ligation. Posterior bleeds may cause substantial blood loss; most patients will require hospitalization and otolaryngology consultation. Patients with recurrent unilateral epistaxis should undergo CT or MRI imaging and nasal endoscopy.

KEY POINT

- Anterior epistaxis can usually be managed with compression and concomitant administration of topical vasoconstrictors, such as oxymetazoline.

Oral Health

Oral Infection and Ulcers

Oral mucosal findings are discussed in MKSAP 18 Dermatology.

Dental Infections

Dental infections may involve the gingiva, tooth, or supportive bony structures. Infection of the tooth is often asymptomatic until the pulp cavity is involved, which leads to abscess. Abscess often necessitates root canal (removal of the diseased pulp).

Dental caries (**Figure 26**) is caused by bacteria that destroy enamel and dentin, resulting in tooth sensitivity or pain and stained pits and fissures on tooth surfaces. Caries may lead to odontogenic infection and tooth loss.

Periodontal infections are caused by bacteria in subgingival dental plaque, leading to gingivitis (inflamed gums) (**Figure 27**) or periodontitis (loss of supportive bone structure from chronic gingivitis). Chronic periodontal disease is associated with increased risk for cardiovascular disease. Fluoride and good dental hygiene are essential for prevention and treatment.

The presence of dental caries or periodontal disease should prompt dental consultation.

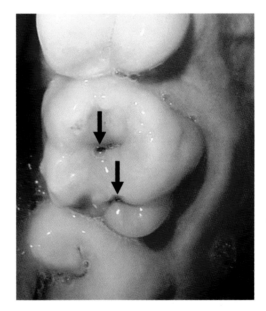

FIGURE 26. Dental caries (cavities or tooth decay) represents localized destruction of dental hard tissues and appears as black or brown spots on the surface of the tooth.

Modified from Nerval. Tooth with extensive evidence of dental carries. Digital image. https://commons.wikimedia.org/wiki/File:Toothdecay_(1).jpg. January 21, 2004. Accessed July 10, 2018. Licensed under the Creative Commons Attribution-ShareAlike 3.0 Unported (CC BY-SA 3.0) International License (https://creativecommons.org/licenses/by-sa/3.0/deed.en).

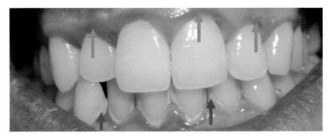

FIGURE 27. Red and swollen gingival tissue (*blue arrows*) that typically bleeds with brushing or flossing is characteristic of gingivitis. Also seen is abundant yellow dental plaque at the gum line and between teeth (*green arrows*).

Reproduced from Wikimedia Commons. Gingivitis before treatment. Digital image. https://commons.wikimedia.org/wiki/Category:Gingivitis#/media/File:Gingivitis-before.JPG. August 8, 2013. Accessed July 10, 2018.

Mental and Behavioral Health

Mood Disorders

Mood disorders are characterized by elevation or depression of mood associated with psychomotor, cognitive, and/or vegetative symptoms that cause significant functional impairment. The two main groups of mood disorders are depressive disorders and bipolar disorder.

Depressive Disorders

The lifetime prevalence of depressive disorders in developed countries is approximately 20%, and women are affected almost twice as often as men. The peak onset is in the fifth decade of life, and incidence decreases in the elderly population. Depression is the leading cause of disability in the United States among individuals aged 15 to 44 years and is a major risk factor for suicide.

Depressive disorders most often initially present in the primary care setting but are underdiagnosed. Depressive symptoms are frequently encountered in patients with chronic medical disease either as a result of the illness itself (such as hypothyroidism) or as a response to the disability caused by the illness. Depression commonly accompanies many medical conditions, including cancer, neurologic diseases (Parkinson disease), heart failure, and HIV infection. Medications, including glucocorticoids and interferon, may also trigger depressive symptoms. Clinicians must exclude these potential causes of depressive symptoms during the evaluation of any patient for depression.

Screening for depression is underperformed, and the U.S. Preventive Services Task Force advises screening all patients for depression during primary care visits, with adequate systems in place to ensure accurate diagnosis, effective treatment, and appropriate follow-up. For such general-population screening, the PHQ-2 is effective and easy to use. If a patient provides a positive response to either of the two questions ("Over the past 2 weeks, have you felt down, depressed, or hopeless?" and "Over the past 2 weeks, have you felt little interest or pleasure in doing things?"), further investigation for depression is warranted.

Diagnosis
Major Depressive Disorder
The DSM-5 criteria for diagnosis of major depressive disorder require at least five of the following symptoms (at least one of which must be depressed mood or anhedonia) during the same 2-week period:

- Depressed mood most of the day, almost every day
- Anhedonia (loss of interest or pleasure in nearly all activities), almost all the time
- Insomnia or hypersomnia almost every day
- Significant change in weight (gain or loss) or appetite (increase or decrease) nearly every day

- Fatigue or decreased energy nearly every day
- Psychomotor agitation or retardation almost every day
- Decreased ability to concentrate almost all the time
- Feelings of worthlessness or of excessive or inappropriate guilt nearly every day
- Recurrent thoughts of death or suicidal ideation (with or without a specific plan), or a suicide attempt

For a diagnosis of major depressive disorder, the symptoms cannot be attributable to a medical condition, medication, or substance use and must cause significant functional impairment. Clinicians must assess patients with depression for any history of elevated mood, which would suggest bipolar disorder; prescribing antidepressant monotherapy to a patient with bipolar disorder may precipitate a manic episode.

Persistent Depressive Disorder
Previously known as dysthymia, persistent depressive disorder is characterized by depressed mood most of the time for at least 2 years with at least two of the following symptoms while depressed: appetite change (increased or decreased), fatigue or low energy, decreased self-esteem, insomnia or hypersomnia, poor concentration, and feelings of hopelessness. These symptoms are milder than in major depressive disorder but still cause impairment of social or occupational functioning. Symptoms can temporarily resolve but do not abate for more than 2 months at a time.

Seasonal Affective Disorder
Seasonal affective disorder (SAD) is defined as major depressive disorder, mania, or hypomania with recurrent seasonal onset and resolution. SAD is not a separate diagnostic entity; rather, it is a subtype of each of these mood disorders (with the specifier "with seasonal pattern"). The most common form of SAD is major depressive disorder in which symptoms arise during autumn or winter and subside the following spring for at least 2 consecutive years (major depressive disorder with seasonal pattern). Seasonal episodes of depression substantially outnumber nonseasonal episodes. The diagnostic criteria are otherwise the same as for major depressive disorder.

Premenstrual Dysphoric Disorder
Premenstrual dysphoric disorder consists of symptoms of mood disturbance that develop the week before menses, remit within a week after menses, and occur with most menstrual cycles during a given year. Diagnosis requires the presence of at least one primary symptom: mood swings, irritability or anger, feelings of hopelessness or depressed mood, and anxiety. Additionally, a patient must have a total of at least five symptoms, which may also include appetite changes, decreased interest in usual activities, fatigue, difficulty concentrating, feelings of loss of control, sleep disturbance, and physical symptoms (breast tenderness, weight gain, bloating, myalgia).

Peripartum Depression

Peripartum depression affects 7% of pregnant or postpartum women and is characterized as a major depressive disorder occurring during pregnancy or within 4 weeks after delivery. It is not considered a separate mood disorder; instead, it is a subtype of major depressive disorder with the specifier "with peripartum onset." Risk factors include previous depression, anxiety, low socioeconomic status, lack of social support, previous physical abuse, and unintended pregnancy. Treatment is similar to that used for other forms of depression but with close attention to drug safety in pregnancy and breastfeeding.

Persistent Complex Bereavement Disorder

Grief is a normal response to interpersonal loss (such as death of a loved one) and may include symptoms of labile emotions, sadness, loneliness, and even fleeting hallucinations of deceased loved ones. The grief process varies, but most patients functionally adapt to loss within 12 months. Pathologic grieving persists longer and is accompanied by intense longing for and preoccupation with the deceased, along with feelings of emptiness and inability to live after the loss. This response to grief is termed "complicated grief," or "persistent complex bereavement disorder" (as proposed in DSM-5 as a future diagnostic classification). Up to 10% of bereaved patients develop persistent complex bereavement disorder, but the incidence is doubled in patients with other mood disorders. Other risk factors include older age, loss of a spouse or child, and sudden death of loved one. A major life loss can induce other mood disorders; therefore, clinicians should maintain a high index of suspicion for these disorders in the bereaved patient.

Management

Most patients with major depressive disorder can be successfully managed in the primary care setting. Referral to a psychiatrist is indicated for patients with severe depression, failure of initial therapy, complex psychiatric comorbidities, and high suicide risk. Before initiating therapy, clinicians must assess medical comorbidities, other medical treatments, and substance use, which may contribute to depression. For initial acute therapy, a 2016 clinical practice guideline from the American College of Physicians recommends either cognitive behavioral therapy (CBT) or second-generation antidepressants (SGAs) after discussing treatment and side effects, cost, accessibility, and patient preferences. It is unclear whether combination therapy with both CBT and medication therapy is more efficacious than either treatment modality alone. Other psychologic therapies are available as second-line options (**Table 76**).

Four classes of SGAs are available: selective serotonin reuptake inhibitors (SSRIs), serotonin-norepinephrine reuptake inhibitors (SNRIs), serotonin modulators, and atypical antidepressants (**Table 77**). Drug selection should be based on side effect profiles and patient-specific characteristics. Side effects are common, and patient education regarding adverse effects can improve adherence. SSRIs are generally well tolerated but can cause reduced sexual desire,

TABLE 76. Common Psychological Interventions to Treat Depression

Intervention	Description
Acceptance and commitment therapy	Uses mindfulness techniques to overcome negative thoughts and accept difficulties
Cognitive therapy	Helps patients correct false self-beliefs and negative thoughts
Cognitive behavioral therapy	Includes a behavioral component in cognitive therapy, such as activity scheduling and homework
Interpersonal therapy	Focuses on relationships and how to address issues related to them
Psychodynamic therapy	Focuses on conscious and unconscious feelings and experiences
Third-wave cognitive behavioral therapy	Targets thought processes to help persons with awareness and acceptance

Reproduced with permission from Qaseem A, Barry MJ, Kansagara D; Clinical Guidelines Committee of the American College of Physicians. Nonpharmacologic versus pharmacologic treatment of adult patients with major depressive disorder: a clinical practice guideline from the American College of Physicians. Ann Intern Med. 2016;164:351. [PMID: 26857948] doi:10.7326/M15-2570. Copyright 2016, American College of Physicians.

anorgasmia, and delayed orgasm. Bupropion causes fewer sexual side effects but is contraindicated in patients with seizure disorders. SSRIs, SNRIs, bupropion, and monoamine oxidase inhibitors all have the potential to cause serotonin syndrome, particularly if used in combination or with other specific medications (including metoclopramide, tramadol, and linezolid).

After starting with a low dosage, the medication should be gradually titrated to achieve a clinical response while monitoring for adverse effects. Therapeutic response can be objectively measured with the PHQ-9 (https://www.integration.samhsa.gov/images/res/PHQ%20-%20Questions.pdf) by comparing scores before and during treatment. A decrease in the score of at least 50% indicates a response to treatment; a decrease to a score of less than 5 indicates remission. If initial monotherapy fails to achieve an adequate response within 6 to 12 weeks, potential next therapeutic steps are guided by the initial choice of therapy and the presence of any response. If a partial response occurs, increasing the dosage of the chosen medication or adding psychotherapy (if not already used) may be appropriate. If no response is seen, switching to another SGA or adding a second agent with or without psychotherapy is indicated. A second-line approach is the addition of an antipsychotic drug. FDA-approved antidepressant-antipsychotic combinations include olanzapine with fluoxetine and aripiprazole or quetiapine with any antidepressant. In cases of resistant depression, electroconvulsive therapy is also safe and effective.

Approximately half of patients who respond to appropriate initial therapy (CBT or SGA monotherapy) develop recurrent depression after 1 year without continued treatment. The American Psychiatric Association recommends continuation

TABLE 77. Dosages and Comparative Adverse Effects of Second-Generation Antidepressants

Drug	Dosage (mg/d)	Comparative or Drug-Specific Adverse Effects[a]
Selective serotonin reuptake inhibitors (SSRIs)		
Citalopram	20-40	Possible increased risk for QT interval prolongation and torsade de pointes (dosages >40 mg/d)
Escitalopram	10-20	N/A
Fluoxetine	10-80	Lowest rates of discontinuation syndrome compared with other SSRIs
Paroxetine	20-60	Highest rates of sexual dysfunction among SSRIs; higher rates of weight gain; highest rates of discontinuation syndrome
Sertraline	50-200	Higher incidence of diarrhea syndrome
Fluvoxamine	40-120	N/A
Serotonin-norepinephrine reuptake inhibitors (SNRIs)		
Venlafaxine	75-375	Higher rates of nausea and vomiting; higher rates of discontinuations due to adverse events than SSRIs as a class; highest rates of discontinuation syndrome; duloxetine has lower rates of adverse events and discontinuation syndrome than other SNRIs
Venlafaxine XR	75-225	
Desvenlafaxine	50-100	Same as venlafaxine
Duloxetine	60-120	Same as venlafaxine
Serotonin modulators		
Nefazodone	200-600	N/A
Atypical antidepressants		
Bupropion	200-450	Lower rate of sexual adverse events than escitalopram, fluoxetine, paroxetine, and sertraline
Bupropion SR	150-400	

N/A = not available; SR = sustained release; XR = extended release.

[a]Common adverse effects associated with second-generation antidepressants include constipation, diarrhea, dizziness, headache, insomnia, nausea, sexual adverse events, and somnolence.

Adapted with permission from Qaseem A, Barry MJ, Kansagara D; Clinical Guidelines Committee of the American College of Physicians. Nonpharmacologic versus pharmacologic treatment of adult patients with major depressive disorder: a clinical practice guideline from the American College of Physicians. Ann Intern Med. 2016;164:350-9. [PMID: 26857948] doi:10.7326/M15-2570. Copyright 2016, American College of Physicians.

therapy (treatment after resolution of a major depressive episode) for 4 to 9 months in patients who responded to acute therapy. The antidepressant dosage that was effective in acute treatment should be maintained in the continuation phase, and if psychotherapy was used, it should also be continued. Patients with three or more previous major depressive episodes, persistent depressive disorder, or residual depressive symptoms should receive long-term maintenance therapy at a similar dosage. When long-term drug therapy is not indicated or must be stopped for other reasons, antidepressant medications should be gradually tapered to avoid discontinuation syndrome. The most common symptoms associated with discontinuation syndrome are dizziness, fatigue, headache, and nausea typically occurring within 1 to 7 days of abruptly stopping or rapidly discontinuing antidepressants.

Special Populations

Persistent complex bereavement disorder may respond to both psychotherapy and pharmacologic therapy, which should be targeted to specific symptoms. SSRIs and SNRIs have demonstrated benefit in patients with depressive symptoms.

Premenstrual and peripartum depression are treated similarly to other forms of depression but with additional attention paid to drug safety during pregnancy. SSRIs and SNRIs are FDA pregnancy category C, except for paroxetine, which is category D. All antidepressant medications are safe with breastfeeding.

Major depressive disorder with seasonal pattern can be effectively treated with CBT and SGAs. However, daily exposure to 10,000 lux of visible light for 30 to 60 minutes is also beneficial.

Patients with concomitant pain syndromes may derive additional analgesic benefit from the use of SNRIs.

Bipolar Disorder

Bipolar disorder is characterized by major depressive episodes and periods of mania or hypomania. The prevalence is 1% to 3%, and women are affected slightly more often than men. Onset typically occurs in early adulthood, and more than half of patients initially present with a major depressive episode. Bipolar disorder is the most expensive mental health problem and carries a high lifetime suicide risk.

Bipolar disorder is divided into two main categories: bipolar 1 and bipolar 2. Diagnosis of bipolar 1 disorder requires at least one episode of mania that is not explained by a medication effect, substance use, or a medical condition. DSM-5 defines mania as an episode of at least 7 consecutive days of irritable, expansive, or elevated mood that interferes with social or occupational functioning and has at least three of the following characteristics (four if the patient reports irritable mood only): inflated self-esteem (grandiosity), increased talkativeness, flight of ideas, distractibility, decreased sleep need, increased goal-directed activity, and excessive risk-taking behaviors (promiscuity, spending sprees). Most patients with bipolar 1 disorder also experience major depressive episodes, and many experience periods of hypomania. Hypomania is defined by the same criteria as mania except the duration is at least 4 consecutive days and symptoms do not cause severe functional impairment.

Patients with bipolar 2 disorder have periods of both hypomania and major depression but never mania. Cyclothymic disorder is a related disorder characterized by multiple episodes of hypomanic and depressive symptoms that do not meet criteria for hypomania or major depression.

Treatment of bipolar disorder should be directed by a psychiatrist. First-line medications include lithium, valproic acid, carbamazepine, and lamotrigine; psychotherapy plays an adjunctive role. Patients with acute mania typically require one of the aforementioned medications plus an atypical antipsychotic agent (aripiprazole, olanzapine, quetiapine). Severe bipolar depression may require a combination of first-line medications or adjunctive antidepressants (fluoxetine plus olanzapine). Quetiapine is also effective as monotherapy for bipolar depression.

KEY POINTS

- **HVC** • The U.S. Preventive Services Task Force advises screening all patients for depression at primary care visits.

- **HVC** • For initial acute treatment of major depressive disorder, options include cognitive behavioral therapy or second-generation antidepressants after consideration and discussion of side effects, cost, accessibility, and patient preferences.

- Peripartum depression may occur during pregnancy or within 4 weeks after delivery; treatment is similar to that for other forms of depression but with close attention paid to drug safety in pregnancy.

- Referral to a psychiatrist is indicated for patients with severe depression, failure of initial therapy, complex psychiatric comorbidities, and high suicide risk.

- Clinicians must assess patients with depression for any history of elevated mood, which would suggest bipolar disorder; prescribing antidepressant monotherapy to a patient with bipolar disorder may precipitate a manic episode.

Anxiety Disorders
Generalized Anxiety Disorder

Generalized anxiety disorder (GAD) is characterized by excessive anxiety about activities or events (occupation, school) that occurs more days than not for at least 6 months and causes significant distress or functional impairment. Patients with GAD typically worry more than expected about minor matters and recognize that this anxiety is difficult to control. DSM-5 diagnostic criteria also require that a patient have at least three of the following symptoms: restlessness, fatigue, irritability, muscle tension, sleep disturbance, or difficulty concentrating. Patients often have comorbid mood and anxiety disorders, including depression, panic disorder, and social anxiety disorder, and clinicians must investigate for other psychiatric illnesses as the source of symptoms. In addition, patients with GAD frequently report various other physical symptoms, including headaches, palpitations, dizziness, and chest and abdominal pain; these may be the presenting symptoms and often prompt evaluation for medical illness. The lifetime prevalence of GAD is 5% to 10%, and women are affected more often than men.

Patients with significant anxiety or multiple unexplained physical symptoms should be screened for GAD using the GAD-7 screening tool (http://www.adaa.org/sites/default/files/GAD-7_Anxiety-updated_0.pdf). The GAD-7 can also be useful for monitoring the severity of the illness during treatment. CBT and pharmacotherapy are equally effective in the treatment of GAD, but patients with comorbid mood disorders are best treated with a medication that targets their concomitant illnesses. SSRIs, SNRIs, buspirone, and tricyclic antidepressants are all effective in the treatment of GAD. SSRIs and SNRIs are preferred first-line drugs because they have fewer side effects than tricyclic antidepressants and effectively treat comorbid behavioral disorders (unlike buspirone). Benzodiazepines are useful for rapidly controlling severe symptoms, especially during initial treatment, while patients await CBT and/or titration of antidepressant dosage. However, benzodiazepines should be used only short term (<4-6 weeks) to avoid dependence and long-term side effects, such as impaired psychomotor performance and amnesia.

Panic Disorder

Panic disorder is commonly encountered in the primary care setting and has a lifetime prevalence of 2%. Panic attacks are a key feature of panic disorder but are not pathognomonic; up to one third of all adults will experience a panic attack during their lifetimes. Depression and other anxiety disorders are frequent comorbidities with panic disorder.

Panic attacks are characterized by sudden onset and rapid escalation (within minutes) of extreme fear or anxiety along with at least four of the following: fear of dying, fear of losing control, palpitations, diaphoresis, tremor, dyspnea, sensation of choking, chest pain, nausea, dizziness, chills or heat sensations, paresthesia, and derealization (the perception that the perceived world is not real). DSM-5 diagnostic criteria for panic disorder include the following: (1) recurrent, unexpected panic attacks and (2) at least one attack followed by 1 or more months of persistent concern about additional panic attacks along with maladaptive behavior changes (for example, avoiding unfamiliar situations). The paroxysmal onset of dyspnea and chest pain may prompt significant medical evaluation. Rarely, panic attacks have a medical cause (hyperthyroidism, pheochromocytoma), and these diagnoses should be considered when other diagnostic findings suggest these conditions.

Treatment of panic disorder involves CBT, pharmacotherapy, or both. SSRIs and SNRIs are first-line medications because of their favorable side effect profile and efficacy. Short courses of benzodiazepines can be used for symptom control, but long-term use is discouraged. Treatment should be continued for at least 1 year after remission is achieved.

Social Anxiety Disorder

Previously known as social phobia, social anxiety disorder is associated with excessive anxiety or fear of criticism or humiliation in social or performance situations. In these situations, patients with social anxiety disorder may experience palpitations, flushing, dyspnea, chest pain, or even panic attacks. To meet DSM-5 diagnostic criteria, these symptoms must be present for at least 6 months and cause significant functional impairment. Patients usually understand that their anxiety is excessive but continue to avoid social situations that trigger anxiety. Both CBT and pharmacotherapy with SSRIs and SNRIs are effective for treatment of social anxiety disorder. For patients with social anxiety disorder restricted to performance situations, CBT is preferred.

Posttraumatic Stress Disorder

Posttraumatic stress disorder (PTSD) is an increasingly recognized anxiety disorder triggered by at least one of the following: direct experience of or witnessing a traumatic situation, learning that a loved one experienced a violent or accidental event, or repeated or excessive exposure to details of a traumatic event (for example, a social worker repeatedly exposed to cases of child abuse). Diagnostic criteria for PTSD also include at least 1 month of intrusive memories of the event (nightmares or flashbacks), avoidance of reminders of the event, adverse changes in cognition or mood related to the event (impaired memory of the event, generalized distrust, anhedonia), and significantly altered arousal and activity (irritability, hypervigilance, sleep disturbance, self-destructive behavior). Risk factors for development of PTSD include greater severity of trauma, poor social support, comorbid psychiatric illness, refugee status, and traumatic brain injury (particularly among military veterans). The symptoms of PTSD typically begin within 4 weeks of the traumatic event. Diagnosis can be challenging because of the patient's desire to avoid discussing the event and the frequency of concomitant psychiatric disorders, including depression, anxiety, substance use disorder, and personality disorders.

Treatment of PTSD generally requires psychotherapy from a specialist with experience in treating the disorder. Antidepressants, including SSRIs and SNRIs, are useful adjunctive therapies. Benzodiazepines are not effective and are not recommended because of the high prevalence of substance use disorders.

Obsessive-Compulsive Disorder

Obsessive-compulsive disorder (OCD) has a lifetime prevalence of approximately 2% and often is accompanied by other mental health disorders. Patients with OCD experience obsessions (recurrent, intrusive thoughts, images, or impulses causing distress) and compulsions (repetitive behaviors [hand washing, counting] done to alleviate obsession-related anxiety). These behaviors cause significant functional impairment through wasted time and disrupted social interactions.

CBT is first-line treatment for OCD. CBT is more effective than pharmacotherapy alone, but SSRIs may be beneficial as adjunct therapy in patients with severe symptoms or inadequate response to CBT. For patients treated with medication, the American Psychiatric Association recommends continued treatment for at least 1 to 2 years.

KEY POINTS

- Cognitive behavioral therapy and pharmacotherapy are equally effective in the treatment of generalized anxiety disorder, but patients with comorbid mood disorders are best treated with a medication that targets their concomitant illnesses. **HVC**

- Cognitive behavioral therapy and pharmacotherapy with selective serotonin reuptake inhibitors and serotonin-norepinephrine reuptake inhibitors are effective for treatment of social anxiety disorder and panic disorder.

- Risk factors for development of posttraumatic stress disorder include greater severity of trauma, poor social support, comorbid psychiatric illness, refugee status, and traumatic brain injury (particularly among military veterans); treatment generally requires psychotherapy from a specialist.

- Cognitive behavioral therapy is first-line treatment for obsessive-compulsive disorder. **HVC**

Substance Use Disorders

Tobacco

Tobacco use remains the most common cause of preventable death in the United States. It is implicated in the development of multiple malignancies, pulmonary diseases, and cardiovascular conditions, and all-cause mortality is three to five times higher in smokers than nonsmokers. Tobacco use has been associated with an increased risk for several cancers, reproductive disorders, peptic ulcer disease, osteoporosis, certain pulmonary infections, diabetes mellitus, and age-related macular degeneration. The benefits of quitting tobacco use begin immediately, and over decades, risks for many of the associated conditions decrease substantially.

The U.S. Preventive Services Task Force recommends that clinicians ask all adults about tobacco use, advise them to stop using tobacco, and provide behavioral interventions and approved pharmacotherapy to adult tobacco users (**Table 78**). Abrupt cessation of tobacco use may result in higher long-term abstinence rates than gradually decreasing use. Combining behavioral counseling with pharmacotherapy is more effective than either modality alone. Effective counseling and behavioral resources include problem-solving guidance (such as developing a quit plan and overcoming barriers), motivational interviewing, social support, and telephone quit lines. There is a dose-response relationship between the intensity and frequency of counseling and quit rates, which seem to plateau after 90 minutes of total counseling.

All smokers without contraindications should additionally receive at least one of seven FDA-approved treatments for smoking cessation (**Table 79**). Varenicline is superior to single forms of nicotine replacement therapy and bupropion; combining more than one type of nicotine replacement therapy (short-acting and long-acting) is more effective than monotherapy.

Although tobacco use has decreased overall in the United States, increasing use of electronic nicotine delivery systems (also known as e-cigarettes and vaping), particularly among young people, is creating new health concerns because their long-term health risks are not yet fully understood. Although e-cigarettes may have a benefit of harm reduction for established smokers, the nicotine-containing aerosol also includes other chemicals (such as formaldehyde, propylene glycol, and heavy metals), which may be harmful. Use of e-cigarettes may also act as a "gateway" for young people, leading toward smoking more traditional tobacco products. The National Academy of Sciences has concluded that e-cigarettes are not without biological effects, including dependence, although not to the extent of combustible tobacco cigarettes. The implications for long-term effects on morbidity and mortality remain unclear.

Alcohol

Unhealthy alcohol use is the third leading cause of preventable death in the United States. Individuals with disordered alcohol use often interact with the health care system but rarely receive appropriate treatment. The U.S. Preventive Services Task Force recommends routine screening for unhealthy alcohol use. Recommended screening tools include the Alcohol Use Disorders Identification Test (AUDIT) (available at https://pubs.niaaa.nih.gov/publications/Audit.pdf), the abbreviated AUDIT-Consumption (AUDIT-C) (available at https://www.integration.samhsa.gov/images/res/tool_auditc.pdf), and the single-question screen "How many times in the past year have you had five [four for women and adults older than age 65 years] or more drinks in 1 day?" (see Routine Care of the Healthy Patient).

Patients with a positive screening result should be assessed for the presence of an alcohol use disorder, the severity of the disorder, and related health consequences, including hepatic, cardiac, and neurologic sequelae. Comorbid psychiatric, chronic pain, and substance use disorders are often present and complicate treatment. Treatment should be tailored to the risk level (**Table 80**).

For patients with at-risk or harmful drinking behavior, brief (6-15 minutes) multicontact behavioral counseling has the best evidence for reducing episodes of heavy drinking and weekly alcohol consumption and improving adherence to recommended drinking levels.

Patients diagnosed with alcohol use disorder often require a multipronged approach with both psychotherapy and medication to ensure safety and minimize relapse. Psychotherapeutic interventions are a key component of effective treatment and may include CBT or 12-step facilitation. Pharmacotherapy for relapse prevention should be considered; naltrexone and acamprosate are the most effective medications (**Table 81**). Naltrexone is preferred because some studies have demonstrated acamprosate to be no more effective than placebo. When at-risk patients do not respond to brief interventions or when patients with alcohol use disorder do not respond to office-based therapies, they should be referred to addiction specialists.

Alcohol withdrawal is a common complication of alcohol use disorder. Alcoholic hallucinosis (hallucinations without clouding of the sensorium) and withdrawal seizures are typically seen within 24 to 48 hours of cessation of alcohol use and are treated expectantly, although a significant percentage of patients will progress to severe withdrawal (delirium tremens). Delirium tremens usually has onset at least 48 hours after the last drink and manifests as autonomic activation (hypertension, tachycardia, fever) and altered mental status. It

TABLE 78. Tobacco Cessation: The 5 As
ASK about tobacco use at every encounter
Identify and document tobacco use
Consider systematic process (such as asking about tobacco use when taking vital signs)
ADVISE patients to quit tobacco use
Strong, clear, personalized message
ASSESS willingness to quit
Not everyone is ready to try to quit
If not ready, offer motivational counseling
ASSIST in quitting
Set a quit date
Behavioral changes: alternatives, skills
Pharmacotherapy
Support: environment, triggers
ARRANGE follow-up
In person, telephone, electronic
Monitor progress, side effects, withdrawal

Reproduced with permission from Patel MS, Steinberg MB. In the clinic. Smoking cessation. Ann Intern Med. 2016;164:ITC36. [PMID: 26926702] doi:10.7326/AITC201603010. Copyright 2016, American College of Physicians.

TABLE 79.	Approved Tobacco Treatment Medications			
Product	**Advantages**	**Disadvantages**	**Precautions**	**Side Effects**
Long-Acting				
Nicotine patch	Place and forget; over the counter; can decrease morning cravings if worn at night	Passive—no action to take when craving occurs	Caution within 2 wk of cardiac event[a]	Skin reaction (50% of patients), vivid dreams or sleep disturbances
Bupropion SR (twice daily) and XL (once daily)	Less weight gain while using; antidepressant benefit	Side effects not uncommon; passive—no action to take with cravings; prescription required	Do not use with seizure disorders, current use of bupropion or MAO inhibitors, electrolyte abnormalities, eating disorders; monitor blood pressure	Insomnia (40%), dry mouth, headache, anxiety, rash
Varenicline	Reduces withdrawal and may prevent relapse	Passive—no action to take with cravings; prescription required	Avoid with severe kidney disease; evaluate for mental illness and monitor mood	Nausea (30%), insomnia, neuropsychiatric effects (e.g., depression, suicidal ideation)[b]
Short-Acting				
Nicotine gum	Use as needed; can self-dose; over the counter	Difficult to chew, poor taste	Caution within 2 wk of cardiac event[a]	Jaw pain; nausea if swallowing saliva
Nicotine inhaler	Use as needed; mimics hand–mouth behavior	Costly, visible; requires prescription	Caution within 2 wk of cardiac event[a]	Cough, throat irritation
Nicotine nasal spray	Use as needed; rapid relief of symptoms	Costly, visible; requires prescription	Caution with asthma, nasal/sinus problems; caution within 2 wk cardiac event[a]	Nasal irritation; possible dependence
Nicotine lozenge	Ease of use; over the counter; flexible dosing	Slightly more costly than gum	Caution within 2 wk of cardiac event[a]	Hiccups, nausea, heartburn

MAO = monoamine oxidase; SR = sustained release; XL = extended release.

[a]Recent myocardial infarction, severe angina, life-threatening arrhythmia.

[b]Postmarketing adverse effect not confirmed in more controlled studies. FDA "black box" warning removed in 2016.

Adapted with permission from Patel MS, Steinberg MB. In the clinic. Smoking cessation. Ann Intern Med. 2016;164:ITC33-ITC48. [PMID: 26926702] doi:10.7326/AITC201603010. Copyright 2016, American College of Physicians.

TABLE 80.	Definitions for Alcohol Use Classifications	
Category	**Definition**	**Health Consequences**
Moderate or lower-risk alcohol use	No more than four drinks on a single day or 14 drinks per week for men; for men older than age 65 years and women, no more than three drinks on a single day or seven drinks in a week	Uncommon
Hazardous or at-risk drinking	When thresholds for lower-risk alcohol use are exceeded	Increased risk for alcohol-related consequences
Harmful alcohol use	Pattern of drinking that causes health consequences	
Alcohol use disorder	When individual meets at least 2 of the 11 DSM-5 criteria	Patients with moderate to severe alcohol use disorder (more than three criteria met) may benefit from more intensive treatment

is often preceded by mild symptoms of withdrawal or withdrawal seizures.

Many patients with alcohol withdrawal require hospitalization, although some low-risk patients can be safely managed in the outpatient setting. Benzodiazepines are the safest and most effective method to manage withdrawal. After initial dosing to acutely control symptoms, a symptom-triggered approach using standardized instruments, such as the Clinical Institute Withdrawal Assessment for Alcohol, Revised (CIWA-Ar), should be used to measure the severity of withdrawal and guide treatment. Phenobarbital, propofol, and dexmedetomidine may be useful in refractory cases. **H**

Drugs

Use of illicit drugs occurs in 9% of the U.S. population. The most commonly used drugs are marijuana, prescription drugs, cocaine, hallucinogens, inhalants, and heroin. Although the evidence base does not currently support screening and brief intervention for drug use, a single-item screening question ("How many times in the past year have you used an illegal drug or used prescription medications for nonmedical reasons?") may be helpful in routine care or when the history, physical

TABLE 81. Pharmacotherapy for Patients With an Alcohol Use Disorder

Medication (Typical Dosage)[a]	Indication	Mechanism	Side Effects	Notes
Benzodiazepines Symptom-triggered: chlordiazepoxide, 50-100 mg; diazepam, 10-20 mg; or lorazepam, 2-4 mg every 1-2 hours until symptoms subside	Treatment or prophylaxis for alcohol withdrawal syndrome	Enhance GABA inhibition of neuronal excitability	Oversedation, paradoxical hyperactivity, depression Addictive potential	Caution in patients with respiratory or hepatic impairment
Naltrexone Oral, 50-100 mg daily Injectable, 380 mg monthly	Relapse prevention	Opioid antagonist that may reduce the subjective reward associated with alcohol use	Nausea, indigestion, headache, fatigue Depressive symptoms Rarely, medication-associated hepatitis Potential for precipitated opioid withdrawal with opioid use	Contraindicated with opioid use Avoid in patients with decompensated cirrhosis; use with caution with hepatitis, compensated cirrhosis
Acamprosate 666 mg three times daily	Relapse prevention	May antagonize glutamate-mediated neuronal hyperexcitability and reduce prolonged (but not acute) withdrawal symptoms	Diarrhea, nausea/vomiting, myalgia, rash, dizziness, palpitations Rarely associated with kidney impairment	Reduce dosage with kidney insufficiency May be used with naltrexone Medication adherence may be challenging
Disulfiram 250-500 mg daily	Prevention of drinking and relapse prevention	Aldehyde dehydrogenase inhibition results in acetaldehyde accumulation with alcohol use, leading to unpleasant symptoms (alcohol-disulfiram reaction)	Drowsiness, rash Rarely, medication-associated severe hepatotoxicity, optic neuritis, peripheral neuropathy	Potential for many drug-drug interactions Patient must be abstinent at least 12 hours before medication administration Avoid in patients with hepatic impairment or cardiovascular disease Most appropriate for patients with strong motivation to be abstinent and with support to promote medication adherence

GABA = γ-aminobutyric acid.

[a]Naltrexone, disulfiram, and acamprosate are all FDA pregnancy category C (animal studies indicate potential fetal risk or have not been conducted, and no or insufficient human studies have been done; drugs in this category should be used in pregnant or lactating women only when potential benefits justify potential risk to the fetus or infant). Benzodiazepines are category X (contraindicated in pregnancy) or D (positive evidence of risk).

Adapted with permission from Edelman EJ, Fiellin DA. In the clinic. Alcohol use. Ann Intern Med. 2016;164:ITC10. [PMID: 26747315] doi:10.7326/AITC201601050. Copyright 2016, American College of Physicians.

examination, or risk profile suggest drug use (see Routine Care of the Healthy Patient for discussion of other screening tools). Internists play a central role in prevention, diagnosis, and management of substance use disorders, including identifying and managing medical comorbidities and reducing harm.

Treatment primarily involves psychotherapeutic support. Internists may also play a role in harm reduction, ensuring that at-risk patients (such as injection drug users) receive appropriate vaccinations and referrals to needle exchange services.

Prescription opioid use has emerged as a major cause of morbidity and mortality, necessitating coordinated medical and policy responses (see Common Symptoms). The risk for overdose is increased with higher doses and with concurrent benzodiazepine prescription. A notable study of trends in benzodiazepine use found that increased prescriptions and the mortality rate associated with overdose increased by a factor of five since 1996. Although nonfatal prescription opioid overdose presents an opportunity for intervention, most of these patients continued to receive opioids, and those receiving the highest dosage had the highest risk for repeated overdose. The nonmedical use of prescription opioids appears to be a strong risk factor for heroin use, although the transition to heroin occurs at a low rate and is influenced by cost and availability of drugs when it occurs.

Internists are increasingly treating opioid use disorder with pharmacotherapy in the office (**Table 82**). Most patients with opioid use disorder will require extended treatment consisting of both psychosocial support and medication-assisted treatment.

Intranasal naloxone is an important adjunct therapy in opioid use disorder, with evidence demonstrating a reduction in overdose death when used. Patients at risk for overdose, including those prescribed high-dose opioids for chronic pain (>50 morphine milligram equivalents per day) and those being

TABLE 82.	Medical Treatment for Opioid Use Disorder			
Medication	**Uses**	**Side Effects and Risks**	**Precautions**	**Notes**
Methadone	Inpatient withdrawal management; maintenance	Sedation, prolongation of the QTc interval, nausea, constipation, weight gain, edema, amenorrhea, decreased bone density, decreased libido Risk for respiratory depression and overdose	Prolonged, variable half-life with incomplete cross-tolerance with other opioids; requires low initiation dose and slow titration Potential for drug interactions with inducers or inhibitors of P-450 system	U.S. schedule II For outpatient addiction treatment, only available through state-licensed programs For pain treatment, available from licensed prescribers
Buprenorphine-naloxone	Inpatient withdrawal management; maintenance	Nausea, constipation, headache, insomnia Rarely associated with overdose, usually in combination with other sedating agents	Risk for precipitated opioid withdrawal if initiated too soon in opioid-tolerant patient after last use of full opioid agonist May be less effective in severe liver disease due to increased bioavailability of naloxone; periodic monitoring of liver enzymes is recommended	U.S. schedule III Requires federal waiver
Buprenorphine	Inpatient withdrawal management; maintenance, particularly for pregnant women	Nausea, constipation, headache, insomnia Rarely associated with overdose, usually in combination with other sedating agents	Risk for precipitated opioid withdrawal if initiated too soon after last use of full opioid agonist Periodic monitoring of liver enzymes is recommended	U.S. schedule III Requires federal waiver Once-monthly injection formulation approved in 2017
Naltrexone				
IM	Maintenance	Nausea, fatigue, dizziness, injection site reaction	Risk for precipitated withdrawal if taken soon after last opioid dose Risk for overdose if dose is missed and patient relapses Periodic monitoring of liver enzymes is recommended; impaired metabolism in liver disease	Some variability in length of time for full opioid blockade
Oral	Bridge before IM naltrexone; maintenance in highly supervised settings	Nausea, headache, dizziness, elevated aminotransferase levels	Periodic monitoring of liver enzymes is recommended; impaired metabolism in liver disease	

IM = intramuscular; QTc = corrected QT interval.

Adapted with permission from Pace CA, Samet JH. In the clinic. Substance use disorders. Ann Intern Med. 2016;164:ITC58-ITC59. [PMID: 27043992] doi:10.7326/AITC201604050. Copyright 2016, American College of Physicians.

treated for or in recovery from opioid use disorders, should be offered naloxone. Friends and family members may also receive prescriptions and training in naloxone use.

KEY POINTS

HVC
- In tobacco cessation, combining behavioral counseling with pharmacotherapy is more effective than either modality alone, and combining more than one type of nicotine replacement therapy (short- and long-acting) is more effective than monotherapy.

- For patients with at-risk or harmful drinking behavior, brief (6-15 minutes) multicontact behavioral counseling has the best evidence for improving adherence to recommended drinking levels.

- Patients diagnosed with alcohol use disorder often require both psychotherapeutic and pharmacologic approaches to ensure safety and minimize relapse.

- Patients at risk for opioid overdose, including those prescribed high-dose opioids for chronic pain and those being treated for or in recovery from opioid use disorders, should be offered naloxone.

- Most patients with opioid use disorder will require extended treatment consisting of both psychosocial support and medication-assisted treatment.

Personality Disorders

Personality disorders involve consistent patterns of interpersonal behavior and perceptions that are inflexible, diverge significantly from the behavioral standards of the person's culture, and cause substantial functional impairment and emotional distress. Development of these disorders usually occurs in adolescence, and the prevalence in the United States is estimated at 10% to 15%. Comorbid psychiatric illness is common. Three clusters of personality disorders are based on symptoms (**Table 83**).

Personality disorders add challenges to patient care and can serve as a substantial barrier to care. Physicians should have open, yet sensitive, discussion of the personality disorder diagnosis with the patient and emphasize the purpose of providing the best possible care. Such discussion may also make the patient more receptive to referral to a mental health professional. Establishing a relationship based on trust and clear boundaries can also help facilitate care. No pharmacotherapy specifically treats personality disorders, but medications may be used for improving specific symptoms (for example, mood stabilizers for impulsivity). Psychotherapy can help patients improve coping mechanisms.

Somatic Symptom and Related Disorders

Previously known as somatoform disorders, somatic symptom and related disorders are characterized by medically

TABLE 83. Personality Disorders
Cluster A: Odd or Eccentric Thinking and Behaviors
Paranoid: pervasive distrust of others; unjustified suspicion of others; unjustified suspicions regarding their partners or spouses; overly hostile reactions to perceived insults
Schizoid: prefer to be alone and lack interest in relationships; seem indifferent, cold, and unresponsive to social cues; take pleasure in few activities
Schizotypal: manifest odd thinking, beliefs (e.g., their thoughts are magical and can influence others, events have hidden meaning), dress, and other behaviors
Cluster B: Dramatic or Unpredictable Thinking and Behaviors, Emotional
Antisocial: engage in behaviors such as lying, stealing, and other aggressive and violent behaviors; disregard others' feelings, rights, and safety; lack remorse for these behaviors; often experience recurrent legal problems
Borderline: have chaotic relationships (idealized and devalued) and a fragile self-image; fear abandonment; experience labile and intense emotions (e.g., anger), sense of emptiness; engage in impulsive and risky behaviors (e.g., gambling, sex); may manifest self-injury and suicidality
Histrionic: excessive emotionality and attention-seeking behavior; dramatic; often seductive or sexually provocative; melodramatic
Narcissistic: grandiose and inflated self-perceptions; desire attention
Cluster C: Anxious and Fearful Thinking and Behaviors
Avoidant: feel inadequate and are sensitive to criticism; extremely shy and socially inhibited and avoid activities that involve interactions with others, especially strangers
Dependent: excessively dependent on others ("clingy") and fear being alone; lack self-confidence and tolerate poor treatment by others
Obsessive-compulsive: perfectionistic and preoccupied with orderliness and rules; controlling of situations and others; rigid regarding values; not the same as obsessive-compulsive disorder, which is an anxiety disorder

Reproduced with permission from Schneider RK, Levenson JL. Psychiatry Essentials for Primary Care. Philadelphia: American College of Physicians, 2008.

unexplained symptoms causing emotional distress and psychosocial impairment. Prevalence is as high as 4%, and primary care is a common setting for presentation. Patients with these disorders have very high use of health care resources yet are dissatisfied with their care. Before diagnosing any of these disorders, clinicians should thoroughly evaluate for and optimize treatment of medical disease and other psychiatric disorders (such as depression and generalized anxiety). Many unexplained medical problems are related to unidentified organic pathology, and patients with known medical disease may have a concurrent somatic symptom or related disorder.

Types

Somatic symptom disorder (previously called somatization disorder) is characterized by one or more somatic symptoms present for at least 6 months causing significant distress or interference with life and associated with excessive thoughts, behaviors, and feelings related to the symptoms. When the main symptom is pain, the specifier "with predominant pain" is applied (previously referred to as pain disorder).

Illness anxiety disorder (formerly known as hypochondriasis) is characterized by excessive concern about health and preoccupation with health-related activities (for example, measuring pulse). In contrast to somatic symptom disorder, no or only mild somatic symptoms are present in illness anxiety disorder.

Conversion disorder involves at least one symptom of neurologic dysfunction (abnormal sensation or motor function) that is unexplained by a medical condition and not consistent with examination findings. Conversion disorder does not represent fabrication of symptoms but rather unexplained symptoms that do not have a pathophysiologic basis. These symptoms, which are functionally limiting, occur during times of substantial physical, emotional, or psychological stress.

Somatic symptom and related disorders must be differentiated from factitious disorder and malingering. Factitious disorder is an intentional fabrication of symptoms or injury to oneself or another without clear external benefit. Malingering occurs when a patient feigns medical problems for gain; thus, malingering is not a psychiatric diagnosis.

Management

Clinicians should acknowledge the patient's symptoms in somatic symptom and related disorders and focus on coping mechanisms and regularly scheduled visits. Diagnostic testing and referral to specialists should not be requested solely to provide reassurance. For somatic symptom disorder, CBT is effective for patients willing to undergo psychotherapy; antidepressant drugs also have demonstrated benefit. Illness anxiety disorder may respond to CBT, whereas disease education is the primary treatment for conversion disorder.

KEY POINT

HVC

- Clinicians should acknowledge the patient's symptoms in somatic symptom and related disorders and focus on coping mechanisms and regularly scheduled visits.

Eating Disorders

Types

Approximately 3% of the U.S. population has an eating disorder. Disorders most likely to be encountered by internists include anorexia nervosa, bulimia nervosa, and binge eating disorder.

Anorexia nervosa is characterized by restriction of caloric intake relative to requirements that leads to below-normal body weight and is also associated with fear of weight gain and a distorted body image. DSM-5 further divides the disorder by subtypes: restricting type (no episodes of food binges or purging) and binge eating/purging type. Women are affected three to four times more often than men, and onset most often occurs in adolescence.

In bulimia nervosa, patients engage in binge eating followed by compensatory behaviors to prevent weight gain, including self-induced vomiting, laxative abuse, fasting, and excessive exercise, at least once weekly for 3 months. Binge eating is defined as eating substantially more food than most people would consume within a period of time. The key difference between the binge eating/purging type of anorexia nervosa and bulimia nervosa is that patients with anorexia have significant weight loss. Similar to anorexia nervosa, patients with bulimia nervosa have a distorted body image. Prevalence is three times greater among women, and the median age at onset is 18 years.

Binge eating disorder is more common than anorexia and bulimia nervosa and is characterized by binge eating and feelings of loss of control that occur an average of at least once weekly for 3 months. Binging episodes include at least three of the following characteristics: abnormally rapid consumption, eating until uncomfortably full, consuming large amounts of food when not hungry, eating alone due to embarrassment, and feelings of guilt related to overconsumption. These characteristics distinguish binge eating disorder from overeating. The lack of compensatory behaviors to avoid weight gain differentiates binge eating disorder from bulimia nervosa. Concurrent psychiatric disease, including personality, mood, and substance use disorders, is common.

Clues to the presence of an eating disorder on physical examination include findings suggesting malnutrition (muscle wasting, xerosis, and lanugo) and/or self-induced vomiting (erosion of dental enamel, parotid gland enlargement, and scarring or calluses on the hand dorsum).

Medical Complications

Multiple medical problems can develop in patients with anorexia nervosa as a result of malnutrition. Patients often exhibit signs of a hypometabolic state, including bradycardia, hypotension, hypothermia, and decreased gastrointestinal mobility. Electrolyte abnormalities (hypokalemia, hypomagnesemia, and hypophosphatemia) can cause dysrhythmia and contribute to increased mortality. Refeeding syndrome can worsen these electrolyte disturbances, and prevention requires gradual, carefully monitored increase of nutritional intake. Osteopenia and osteoporosis are common and may not be fully reversible if anorexia occurred during peak bone development in adolescence. Amenorrhea, anemia, and peripheral edema also occur frequently and usually resolve with recovery from anorexia nervosa.

Purging behaviors may also lead to electrolyte abnormalities. Additionally, upper gastrointestinal problems (esophagitis, esophageal tears) may develop from self-induced vomiting, and laxative abuse may cause colonic dysmotility.

Treatment

The main goal of treatment is reestablishing normal weight and eating behaviors. Psychotherapy and monitored dietary intake are the mainstays of treatment for anorexia nervosa. In some circumstances, this may require hospitalization to ensure adequate emotional support, appropriate intake, and monitoring for refeeding syndrome. Antidepressant therapy has not proved effective in treating anorexia nervosa, although olanzapine may be considered for patients not responding to psychotherapy and nutritional interventions. CBT is the most effective intervention for bulimia nervosa and binge eating disorder; antidepressant therapy may be beneficial. Topiramate has also shown promise as an adjunctive therapy with CBT in patients with binge eating disorder. Bupropion should be avoided because of increased risk for seizures in patients with eating disorders.

KEY POINTS

HVC
- Psychotherapy and monitored dietary intake are the mainstays of treatment for anorexia nervosa; antidepressant therapy has not proved effective.

- Cognitive behavioral therapy is the most effective intervention for bulimia nervosa and binge eating disorder; antidepressant therapy and topiramate may also be beneficial.

Schizophrenia

Schizophrenia is a heterogeneous psychiatric disorder composed of both positive symptoms (hallucinations, disorganized thought, and delusions) and negative symptoms (flattened affect, decreased activity). Worldwide prevalence is approximately 1%, with a slight male predominance. The pathogenesis of schizophrenia is unclear.

DSM-5 diagnostic criteria for schizophrenia require the presence at least two of the following: delusions, hallucinations, disorganized speech, disorganized or catatonic behavior, and negative symptoms. Diagnosis also requires at least one area of functional impairment (occupation, social interactions, or self-care) and duration of at least 6 months (including 1 month of active symptoms).

Schizophrenia is associated with an increased risk for diabetes, cardiovascular disease, and obesity, and these coexisting conditions may be exacerbated by the metabolic complications of antipsychotic therapy. Undertreatment of medical disease is also common in this population. Mortality is significantly increased in patients with schizophrenia due to these conditions along with concurrent behavioral disorders and substance use; approximately 5% of patients with schizophrenia commit suicide.

Schizophrenia is usually co-managed with a psychiatrist. Antipsychotic medications are highly effective at controlling positive symptoms of schizophrenia, but some degree of negative symptoms usually persists. Because the effectiveness of different antipsychotics is relatively similar, choice of therapy is based primarily on patient comorbidities and the adverse effect profile of medications. Typical or first-generation antipsychotic agents have a higher risk for extrapyramidal symptoms (parkinsonism, akathisia), tardive dyskinesia, and hyperprolactinemia than second-generation or atypical antipsychotic agents (**Table 84**). Some newer antipsychotic agents may also cause less sedation and anticholinergic side effects but carry an increased risk for weight gain and metabolic syndrome (particularly olanzapine and quetiapine). Clozapine may be particularly effective for refractory schizophrenia but is associated with significant adverse effects, including agranulocytosis. Close monitoring for common adverse effects is extremely important with use of any antipsychotic agent.

TABLE 84.	Adverse Effects of Common Antipsychotic Medications					
Medication	**EPS**	**Elevated Prolactin**	**Anticholinergic Symptoms**	**Sedation**	**Weight Gain**	**Hyperlipidemia**
First-Generation Antipsychotics						
Fluphenazine	++	++	+/−	+	+	+
Haloperidol	++	++	+/−	++	+	+
Thiothixene	++	++	+	+	++	−
Chlorpromazine	+	++	++	++	++	++
Thioridazine	+	++	++	++	++	−
Second-Generation Antipsychotics						
Clozapine[a]	+/−	+/−	++	++	+++	+++
Risperidone	++	++	++	+	++	+
Olanzapine	+	+	+	++	+++	+++
Quetiapine	+/−	+/−	+/−	++	++	++
Aripiprazole	+	−	−	+	+	−

EPS = extrapyramidal symptoms.

[a]Clozapine can also cause agranulocytosis and requires routine monitoring of blood counts.

KEY POINTS

- Mortality is significantly increased in patients with schizophrenia because of concurrent cardiovascular disease, behavioral disorders, and substance use; approximately 5% of patients with schizophrenia commit suicide.

- Antipsychotic medications are highly effective at controlling positive symptoms of schizophrenia, but some degree of negative symptoms usually persists; the effectiveness of different antipsychotic agents is relatively similar, and choice of therapy is based primarily on patient comorbidities and the adverse effect profile of medications.

Attention-Deficit/Hyperactivity Disorder

Attention-deficit/hyperactivity disorder (ADHD) is characterized by persistent inattention and/or hyperactivity-impulsivity that disrupts functioning or development. Symptoms must interfere with at least two different settings (such as home and work), and some must be present since age 12 years. ADHD is most frequently recognized in childhood, but the diagnosis may be delayed until adulthood. Most patients diagnosed early in life continue to meet diagnostic criteria as adults. Common manifestations in adults include inattention, disorganization, distractibility, emotional dysregulation, and restlessness. The diagnosis is clinical, and rating scales may be useful; anxiety, mood, and substance use disorders should be considered in the differential diagnosis but may also exist concurrently.

Pharmacologic therapy is similar in adults and children, with stimulants (methylphenidate, amphetamine) as first-line therapy. Close monitoring for cardiovascular side effects (hypertension, arrhythmia) is necessary. Given the potential for abuse, these drugs should not be prescribed to patients with a history of substance use; atomoxetine may be preferred in such patients. Bupropion and tricyclic antidepressants are also beneficial in patients with contraindications to stimulants or with concurrent depression. CBT is beneficial alone or in combination with pharmacotherapy for improving executive functioning.

KEY POINTS

- For diagnosis of attention-deficit/hyperactivity disorder, symptoms must interfere with at least two different settings (such as home and work) and be present since age 12 years.

- Stimulants should not be prescribed to patients with a history of substance use; atomoxetine may be preferred in such patients.

Autism Spectrum Disorder

Autism spectrum disorder (ASD) is a heterogeneous group of developmental disorders that feature repetitive behaviors and significant deficiencies in communication and social interaction. The exact prevalence is debated but ranges from 0.5% to 1%. Pathogenesis remains uncertain but is most likely genetic. Diagnosis requires that symptoms be present since early childhood; however, these may be masked until adulthood. Half of patients have intellectual disability, and many have concurrent seizure and sleep disorders. Early intervention with behavioral and educational interventions improves long-term functioning. Complementary therapies, including specialized diets and music therapy, are also commonly used but lack evidence of efficacy. Pharmacotherapy is reserved for targeted symptoms, such as melatonin for sleep disturbance. Even with intervention, most patients require lifelong assistance with functioning.

Clinicians should understand what communication methods a patient uses and incorporate caregivers into health care visits. Consistency in the health care team can prevent confusion and anxiety, and extra time should be allowed for explanation of procedures. Medical causes of acute behavioral changes should always be considered.

Geriatric Medicine

Comprehensive Geriatric Assessment

Comprehensive geriatric assessment is a multidisciplinary diagnostic process to ascertain the physical, cognitive, psychological, environmental, and functional capabilities of older persons in order to develop a plan for preserving function and maximizing independence and quality of life. Common health issues in older adults include impaired mobility and physical functioning, deficits in sensory function (particularly vision and hearing), and cognitive decline. Additionally, polypharmacy and the cumulative effects of chronic diseases may contribute to decreased functional status and loss of independence. Identifying these issues requires a systematic and multidimensional evaluation, which may be performed in the office, in the patient's home, or upon hospital admission or discharge. When completed in the home or in a dedicated inpatient geriatric unit, comprehensive geriatric assessment may reduce mortality and decrease the need for long-term institutional or nursing home placement.

Functional Status

Functional status assessment is evaluation of a patient's ability to perform activities required for basic self-care (activities of daily living [ADLs]) or to live independently (instrumental activities of daily living [IADLs]). ADLs include bathing, grooming, dressing, toileting, feeding, walking, and transferring. IADLs comprise tasks such as managing finances, performing housework, shopping, self-administering medications, using transportation, preparing meals, and communicating by telephone. Standardized screening instruments for assessment of functional status are presented in **Table 85**. Functional assessment may help determine the need for specific services or the appropriate level of care for the patient.

Vision

Older patients are at increased risk for many conditions that cause vision loss, including cataracts, macular degeneration, presbyopia, glaucoma, and disease-related retinopathy (such as diabetic retinopathy). Reduced visual acuity decreases functional status and quality of life and increases risk for falls, depression, and cognitive impairment.

Screening tests and examination techniques to assess vision in the primary care setting include standardized questionnaires, the Snellen eye chart, and direct ophthalmoscopic examination; however, these tests may not detect such disorders as glaucoma and macular degeneration. The U.S. Preventive Services Task Force (USPSTF) concluded that evidence is insufficient to assess the balance of benefits and harms of screening for impaired visual acuity in asymptomatic adults aged 65 years and older. Nonetheless, given the risks associated with decreased vision coupled with the increased risk for common treatable eye conditions in older adults, it is reasonable to ask about changes in vision and refer the patient to an eye specialist when changes are present. In contrast to the USPSTF recommendations, the American Ophthalmologic Association recommends performing a comprehensive eye examination in older adults every 1 to 2 years.

Hearing

Hearing loss is common in older adults, affecting more than 80% of adults by age 80 years. As with vision loss, hearing loss contributes to increased morbidity and decreased quality of life. The inability to hear is also socially isolating, perhaps more so than other sensory losses. Because of the impaired communication abilities inherent to hearing loss, it may be misdiagnosed as cognitive dysfunction.

Diagnostic tests that reliably screen for hearing loss include assessing whether the patient can hear a whispered voice, fingers rubbing together, or a watch ticking. These tests and single-question screening (that is, asking "Do you have difficulty hearing?") perform as well as more complex questionnaires or handheld audiometry in detecting hearing loss, although there is no evidence that identifying hearing loss translates to better hearing-related quality of life. As such, routine screening for hearing loss in asymptomatic patients is not recommended by the USPSTF. Patients with symptoms, however, should be referred to an otologist or audiologist for formal hearing testing and evaluation to determine whether hearing aids would be beneficial.

Depression

The prevalence of depression in adults older than 60 years is as high as 15%. Chronic illness, grief associated with the loss of loved ones, social isolation due to decreased physical and cognitive function, and the need for institutionalization may all contribute to depression. Common symptoms of depression, such as low energy and somatic symptoms, are often mistakenly attributed to aging and chronic illness. Depression in older adults may also be confused with cognitive dysfunction and is itself a risk factor for cognitive dysfunction.

The USPSTF recommends screening for depression in all adults. The PHQ-2 has been validated as a screening instrument in older adults, with similar sensitivity and specificity in this population compared with its performance in younger adults (see Routine Care of the Healthy Patient). In all age

TABLE 85.	Indices to Assess Basic and Instrumental Activities of Daily Living		
Index	**Assessed Functional Activity**	**Scoring**	**Comments**
Katz Index of Independence in Activities of Daily Living	Bathing Dressing Toileting Transferring Continence Feeding	Assign 1 point for each activity if it can be performed independently, which is defined as requiring no supervision, direction, or personal assistance; scores are then added for a range of 0 to 6 (6 = fully functional; 4 = moderately impaired; 2 = severely impaired)	Simple to use/score; brief, takes only a few minutes to complete Less discriminative at low levels of disability
Lawton and Brody Instrumental Activities of Daily Living (IADL) Scale	Ability to use telephone Shopping Food preparation Housekeeping Laundry Transportation Medication management Ability to handle finances	Assign 1 point for each activity if it can be performed at all; scores are then added for a range of 0 to 8, with a score of 8 representing independence and 0 representing total dependence for IADLs	Simple to use; brief, takes only a few minutes to complete

groups, the PHQ-2 has a lower specificity than more comprehensive screening instruments, which may result in overdiagnosis of depression. A positive screening result should therefore prompt further assessment. The PHQ-9 and Geriatric Depression Scale (https://integrationacademy.ahrq.gov/sites/default/files/Update_Geriatric_Depression_Scale-15_0.pdf) have similar sensitivity and specificity in older adults. The Geriatric Depression Scale, with its yes-or-no answer format, may be easier to administer in patients with cognitive impairment.

Older adults with depression are most commonly treated with pharmacotherapy, and antidepressants protect against suicide attempts in this population. Selective serotonin reuptake inhibitors are the most widely studied antidepressants and are considered first-line therapy. Psychotherapy, including cognitive behavioral therapy, may also be considered as primary treatment or as an adjunct to pharmacotherapy.

Cognitive Function

Cognitive impairment is defined as a progressive decline in at least two cognitive domains (memory, attention, language, visual-spatial function, executive function) that negatively affects patient functioning. The strongest risk factor for cognitive impairment is increasing age. In the absence of symptoms, routine screening is not recommended owing to a lack of evidence that screening leads to effective intervention. However, because cognitive impairment is a risk factor for falls, loss of independence, and poor control of chronic diseases, clinicians should have a low threshold for assessing cognitive decline.

The most widely studied instrument for evaluating cognitive function is the Mini–Mental State Examination (MMSE). The proprietary nature of the MMSE and the time required to administer the test (approximately 7 minutes) may preclude its use for routine outpatient screening. The Montreal Cognitive Assessment (MoCA) takes a similar amount of time to complete and is sensitive for detecting cognitive impairment. The Mini-Cog assessment includes a three-item recall test (similar to elements of the MMSE) followed by a clock-drawing test if any one of the three recall items is missed. The Mini-Cog has acceptable sensitivity and specificity in identifying dementia and is available to clinicians without charge, although it is copyright protected.

Evaluation and treatment of mild cognitive impairment (impaired cognition in the absence of impaired function) and dementia are further discussed in MKSAP 18 Neurology.

Fall Prevention

Thirty percent to 40% of adults older than 65 years fall every year, making falls the leading cause of injury in this age group. Modifiable risk factors for falls include chronic musculoskeletal or neurologic conditions, visual impairment, cognitive impairment, frailty, and polypharmacy.

Screening older adults for fall risk is recommended by the USPSTF and is an element of the Medicare annual wellness visit. Patients should be asked about falls and unsteadiness with walking; those who report falls or balance issues should be evaluated with the Timed Up and Go test, in which the patient is asked to rise from a chair with armrests, walk 10 feet (with their usual assistive devices, if applicable), turn, return to the chair, and sit down. A time of more than 12 seconds is considered abnormal. Patients with prolonged times on the Timed Up and Go test may be referred for more comprehensive assessment or formal gait and balance assessment and therapy. An algorithm for fall risk assessment and prevention is presented in **Figure 28**.

The USPSTF recommends exercise to prevent falls in community-dwelling adults aged 65 years or older who are at increased risk for falls. Exercise interventions include supervised individual and group classes as well as physical therapy. The USPSTF also recommends multifactorial interventions to prevent falls. This process typically involves an initial assessment of modifiable risk factors for falls and subsequent customized interventions. The USPSTF acknowledges that the overall benefit of routinely offering multifactorial interventions to prevent falls is small and should take into account the balance of benefits and harms based on the circumstances of previous falls, presence of comorbid medical conditions, and the patient's values and preferences. The USPSTF recommends against vitamin D supplementation to prevent falls in community-dwelling adults aged 65 years or older who are not known to have osteoporosis or vitamin D deficiency.

Assessment of the Older Driver

Driving is one of the most valued IADLs for older adults, and cessation of driving in this population is associated with negative health consequences. However, drivers older than 65 years are responsible for more traffic fatalities than any other group of drivers other than those younger than 25 years. Decreased visual acuity, decreased cognitive abilities, use of centrally acting medications (including alcohol), conditions that increase the risk for loss of consciousness, and mobility issues of the extremities or neck all increase the risk for motor vehicle crashes in older adults. Caregiver or family concern for driving safety, history of traffic citations, self-restricted driving, and impulsive behaviors are also associated with increased risk for crashes. The decision to advise an older driver to "retire from driving," which is the preferred terminology, is qualitative, complex, and largely dependent on clinician judgment. The evaluation should consider the known risk factors and underlying medical conditions.

Physician advice to retire from driving is associated with older drivers appropriately stopping driving; however, given the risk for depression and social isolation associated with driving retirement, this advice should be coupled with support, suggestions for alternate forms of transportation, and follow-up assessment of mood and quality of life. When patients are resistant to retiring from driving or when the appropriate decision is less clear, formal occupational therapy driving assessment may be helpful.

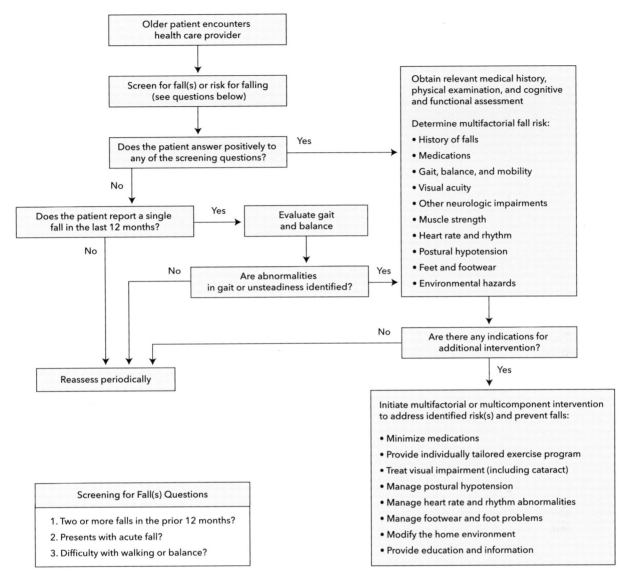

FIGURE 28. Prevention of falls in older persons living in a community.

Adapted with permission from Panel on Prevention of Falls in Older Persons, American Geriatrics Society and British Geriatrics Society. Summary of the updated American Geriatrics Society/British Geriatrics Society clinical practice guideline for prevention of falls in older persons. J Am Geriatr Soc. 2011;59:148-57. [PMID: 21226685] doi:10.1111/j.1532-5415.2010.03234.x. Copyright 2011, John Wiley & Sons, Inc.

Screening for Mistreatment

Older adults are at increased risk for mistreatment, including abuse (infliction of harm), neglect, or financial exploitation, owing to decreased functioning that leads to dependence on others. The prevalence of elder mistreatment is estimated to be roughly 10%. Victims are high utilizers of emergency services, hospital care, and nursing homes and have a higher mortality rate.

There is uncertainty regarding whether screening for elder mistreatment should be routine. The USPSTF concluded that screening cannot be universally recommended for asymptomatic adults; however, screening should be considered in adults with vulnerability for or signs of abuse. Simple screening instruments, such as the Hwalek-Sengstock Elder Abuse Screening Test and the Vulnerability to Abuse Screening Scale, are available but require self-reporting; this complicates assessment in cognitively impaired individuals who cannot independently provide information. Screening may also not occur because of unawareness of these instruments and how to use them, confusion regarding legal and reporting implications (which vary from state to state), and fear of potential harms to the patient and family members that result from false-positive and false-negative screening results.

KEY POINTS

- Comprehensive geriatric assessment is a multidisciplinary diagnostic process to ascertain the physical, cognitive, psychological, environmental, and functional capabilities of older persons in order to develop a plan for preserving function and maximizing independence and quality of life.

(Continued)

KEY POINTS (continued)

- Although routine screening for hearing loss in asymptomatic patients is not recommended, patients with symptoms of hearing loss should be referred to an otologist or audiologist for formal testing and hearing aid placement, if appropriate.
- All older adults should be screened for depression, such as with the PHQ-2.

HVC
- Cognitive impairment is a risk factor for falls, loss of independence, and poor control of chronic diseases; clinicians should inquire about symptoms and perform further evaluation when symptoms are present.

HVC
- The U.S. Preventive Services Task Force recommends exercise to prevent falls in community-dwelling adults aged 65 years or older who are at increased risk for falls.

Frailty Assessment

Frailty is a multifactorial geriatric syndrome characterized by unintentional weight loss, low energy and activity levels, weakness, and slow walking speed. It is important to note that advanced age is not synonymous with frailty. Assessment of frailty may be used to predict response to certain treatments as well as morbidity and mortality in patients with chronic illness. Standardized indices to objectively measure frailty include the Frailty Index, the frailty phenotype, the FRAIL (Fatigue, Resistance, Ambulation, Illness, and Loss of weight) scale, and the Osteoporotic Fractures Frailty Scale. The Frailty Index, a comprehensive assessment of chronic conditions and functioning, has been in use for a longer time than other indices; however, its length and complexity limit its usefulness in routine care. The five-item frailty phenotype was originally validated in the Cardiovascular Health Study of more than 5000 patients aged 65 years and older; it requires measurement of gait speed and grip strength (with a dynamometer), which may not be feasible in primary care. The FRAIL scale consists of five self-reported measures and is easy to administer and score. The Osteoporotic Fractures Frailty Scale, which was developed and validated in an all-female cohort, consists of three elements and is also easy to administer. The rapid screening tools are most easily incorporated into a primary care practice and are useful in the identification of patients who might require more formal comprehensive geriatric assessment (Table 86).

Levels of Care

As the population ages, medical complexity and care needs also increase, necessitating a variety of care delivery models, including home-based and facility-based options.

Several resources are available for older adults who wish to remain in their homes but need medical assistance. Home health agencies offer skilled assistance with medication management, wound care, and physical therapy. These services are provided on an intermittent basis (usually no more than two to three times per week) and are covered by Medicare and Medicaid if the patient is homebound with a documented skilled care need. Patients requiring assistance with ADLs can use custodial care services for help with dressing, bathing, toileting, and cooking; these services are not covered by Medicare but may be paid for by Medicaid. Visiting physicians can also provide outpatient medical care.

For patients who are cared for by family members but require additional resources for gaps in care, adult day care can provide part-time assistance when a patient's primary caregiver is unavailable. If supervision is needed for a longer time, respite care is available at many senior living

TABLE 86.	Examples of Frailty Indices	
Instrument	Description	Scoring
FRAIL (Fatigue, Resistance, Ambulation, Illness, and Loss of weight) scale	Measures presence (1) or absence (0) of: Fatigue: Feeling fatigued most or all of the time over the past 4 weeks. Resistance: Difficulty walking up 10 steps alone without resting or assistance. Ambulation: Difficulty walking several hundred yards without assistance. Illness: Presence of more than five illnesses. Loss of weight: Weight loss >5% in the past year	Each item scored dichotomously as 0 for normal or 1 for abnormal. 1-2 = Prefrail. 3-5 = Frail
Osteoporotic Fractures Frailty Scale	Measures three items: Ability to rise from an armless chair five times (inability = 1). Response to the question "Do you feel full of energy?" (answer of "no" = 1). Weight loss >5% in the past year (presence of weight loss = 1)	Each item scored dichotomously as 0 for normal or 1 for abnormal. 1 = Prefrail. 2-3 = Frail

communities (assisted living facilities and nursing homes). Adult day care and respite care are not typically covered by Medicare or Medicaid.

When long-term daily care needs exceed those that can be provided in a patient's home, three different levels of care are available: independent living, assisted living, and nursing homes. Independent living is suitable only for patients who can independently perform ADLs and simply provides patients with the benefits of living in a community. Assisted living offers a home-like environment but provides varying levels of assistance with medications, ADLs, housekeeping, and meals. For patients requiring additional help with ADLs or medical management, nursing homes provide 24-hour nursing care as well as rehabilitation services. A residential care home (or group home) is a variation of assisted living or the nursing home. Residential care homes use a smaller, home-like environment in the care of patients with similar needs (such as patients with chronic mental illness); however, services provided vary. Independent and assisted living are typically paid for with private funds, or "private pay." Medicare does not usually cover long-term nursing home or residential home care; Medicaid may pay for long-term care depending on patient eligibility and state regulations.

Acute medical care is almost always provided in a hospital setting. Infrequently, serious acute illnesses may be treated in the patient's living environment; however, home hospital care typically occurs only when significant home health resources are available and avoidance of hospitalization has been established as a primary goal in care-planning discussions.

Post-hospitalization care is available in multiple forms. Safe return to a patient's previous living situation can be facilitated with outpatient physical, occupational, and speech therapies in the home or clinic. If a patient requires functional improvement before returning home, rehabilitation can be performed in an acute rehabilitation program or skilled nursing facility (that is, subacute rehabilitation). Acute rehabilitation is provided in a free-standing rehabilitation hospital or a designated hospital unit, and it requires that the patient be able to participate in 3 hours of therapy at least 5 days per week. In patients who cannot tolerate this level of therapy, subacute rehabilitation is appropriate. Medicare covers the costs of both options for up to 100 days, provided that the patient had an inpatient hospitalization of at least 3 days and continues to make progress with goals. Some patients require longer-term, high-intensity medical care, including mechanical ventilation or multiple parenteral therapies, and long-term acute care hospitals are an appropriate option for these patients.

KEY POINT

HVC • Acute rehabilitation requires that the patient be able to participate in 3 hours of therapy at least 5 days per week; in patients who cannot tolerate this level of therapy, subacute rehabilitation is appropriate.

Polypharmacy

The percentage of patients older than 65 years who take five or more prescription medications increased from 24% to 39% between 1999 and 2012. Studies estimate that nursing home patients take eight different medications on average, and medication errors occur in two thirds of such patients. Polypharmacy in older patients is associated with increased health care utilization, costs, medication nonadherence, and functional decline. Patients transitioning between levels of care are particularly vulnerable to inappropriate medication additions, omissions, and dosage changes; the risk for these mistakes increases with the number of medications prescribed. Hazards of polypharmacy include overtreatment or undertreatment of disease, serious drug-drug interactions, and adverse reactions.

Although treatment of comorbid health conditions in older adults often necessitates the use of several medications, clinicians can minimize the potential for adverse effects from polypharmacy. During medication review, clinicians should specifically assess for and reduce medications that should be avoided in older patients, including tricyclic antidepressants, antipsychotics, and benzodiazepines. Drug dosage adjustment is also crucial in older adult patients, given the wide variability in drug metabolism resulting from decreased kidney and liver function as well as the potential for drug interactions. Frequent review of patient medications to confirm their necessity and proper dosing is paramount, especially during care transitions. The 2015 Beers Criteria for Potentially Inappropriate Medication Use in Older Adults from the American Geriatrics Society provides lists of medications that are problematic for elderly patients, as well as recommendations regarding drug interactions to avoid (available at https://geriatricscareonline.org/ProductAbstract/american-geriatrics-society-updated-beers-criteria-for-potentially-inappropriate-medication-use-in-older-adults/CL001).

KEY POINT

• Adverse effects from polypharmacy can be minimized **HVC** with frequent review of the patient's current medications, discontinuation of drugs that are unnecessary or should be avoided, and adjustment of drug dosages as appropriate.

Urinary Incontinence
Epidemiology

Urinary incontinence (UI) is common in older adults, occurring in at least one third of community-dwelling adults older than 65 years and about two thirds of those in nursing homes. Prevalence increases with age in both women and men; however, incidence is higher in women. UI increases risk for falls, depression, and social isolation and reduces health-related quality of life. UI is also a major factor leading to loss of independence and nursing home placement. Risk factors for UI include many common chronic medical conditions (such as diabetes, heart failure, cerebrovascular disease, Parkinson disease, osteoarthritis, and dementia) as well as the medications used in their treatment. Other risk factors are pelvic surgery (including hysterectomy and prostate surgery), pelvic irradiation, pelvic trauma, and obesity.

There are four main classifications of UI: urgency, stress, overflow, and mixed. Functional incontinence, which occurs in patients who cannot reach and use the toilet in a timely manner, may result from cognitive or mobility impairment. Disorders that predispose patients to specific types of incontinence are presented in **Table 87**. Urgency UI and stress UI are the two most common forms, although mixed presentations frequently occur. Urgency UI is associated with intrinsic detrusor muscle instability and is characterized by urine leakage preceded by a sudden urge to void. Urgency UI occurs at increased rates in older patients, with higher rates in women. Stress UI is characterized by urine leakage associated with activities that cause increased intra-abdominal pressure, such as coughing, laughing, or sneezing. Changes in the pelvic floor musculature can contribute to both urgency and stress incontinence. Overflow UI is less common and is associated with comorbidities that alter neurologic control of the bladder and bladder outlet obstruction.

Evaluation

A comprehensive history, including specific questions about the presence and nature of incontinence, should be included in the routine care of the geriatric patient. Because of the social implications of incontinence, patients may be hesitant to volunteer information about symptoms. Validated questionnaires can be used to obtain details on the type of incontinence and the degree of interference with the patient's quality of life, as well as to monitor response to treatment. The 3 Incontinence Questions (3IQ) questionnaire is straightforward and easy to

administer in an office setting; however, several other validated instruments are available.

During the history, female patients should be questioned about pregnancies and gynecologic procedures, and male patients should be asked about symptoms suggestive of prostate enlargement. Additionally, all patients should be screened for chronic conditions associated with increased risk for incontinence (see Table 87). A comprehensive medication history should be obtained, with special attention paid to the use of diuretics and medications with cholinergic or anticholinergic effects, including over-the-counter medications.

The physical examination should incorporate a genitourinary examination, including evaluation of the pelvis in women and the prostate in men. Urinalysis is recommended because transient incontinence may be explained by the presence of urinary tract infection. Additional laboratory investigation or diagnostic testing is usually unnecessary. Postvoid bladder residual volume assessment, which is performed with ultrasonography after spontaneous voiding, may be considered in patients in whom overflow incontinence is suspected. Urodynamic studies are required only for complex cases in which neurologic disease is suspected and surgical intervention is being considered.

Treatment

The American College of Physicians (ACP) recommends nonpharmacologic therapy as the preferred first-line treatment for all types of UI. In cases of urgency UI, pharmacologic therapy may be considered when symptoms are not adequately improved with behavioral therapy. Devices and surgical interventions are third-line therapy. Treatment strategies for UI are listed in **Table 88**.

Behavioral Therapy

Validated behavioral therapy measures include pelvic floor muscle training for stress UI and mixed UI, bladder training with timed voiding for urgency UI, and exercise and weight loss in obese patients with any form of UI.

Pelvic floor muscle training, in which the patient performs sets of contractions of the pelvic floor, is five times more effective than no treatment for stress UI. Patients should be instructed to contract the pelvic floor as if attempting to avoid urination and sustain the contraction for 10 seconds. Contractions should be performed in three or four sets of 10 daily. Patients should be counseled that symptom improvement may not be noticeable until pelvic floor muscle training is consistently performed for several months. Some studies have demonstrated benefits when biofeedback therapy (using a vaginal electromyography probe to provide direct confirmation that the patient is correctly contracting the pelvic floor muscles) is included with these exercises.

Timed voiding or bladder training comprises scheduled voiding attempts at intervals shorter than the usual time between incontinence episodes, regardless of the urge to void,

TABLE 87. Conditions Commonly Associated With Urinary Incontinence

Incontinence Type	Associated Conditions
Stress	Multiparous state, radical prostatectomy
Urgency	Spinal cord injury, stroke, Parkinson disease
	Often idiopathic
Overflow	Diabetes mellitus with neurogenic bladder
	Neurologic disorders (lumbosacral degenerative joint disease, spinal cord injury)
	Prostate hypertrophy with bladder outlet obstruction
Functional	Dementia
	Mobility issues (osteoarthritis, residual deficits from cerebrovascular disease, Parkinson disease)
Mixed	All conditions associated with stress and urgency urinary incontinence

TABLE 88.	Treatment Strategies for Urinary Incontinence		
Incontinence Type	Behavioral Therapy	Pharmacologic Therapy	Other Therapies
Stress	Pelvic floor muscle training +/– biofeedback	No recommended pharmacologic therapies	Pessaries, injectable bulking agents, sling cystourethropexy
Urgency	Bladder training/timed voiding	Antimuscarinics (oxybutynin, darifenacin, solifenacin, tolterodine, fesoterodine, trospium) Mirabegron	Spinal neuromodulators, botulinum toxin injections
Overflow	Double voiding (remaining on the toilet for a few minutes after voiding and then attempting to void again) Triggered voiding (maneuvers to stimulate voiding, including massaging the pubic bone and tugging on pubic hairs)	α-Blocker and 5α-reductase inhibitors for BPH-related symptoms	Transurethral prostatectomy can be considered for BPH-related symptoms Scheduled in-and-out catheterization
Functional	Caregiver-prompted timed voiding	No recommended pharmacologic therapies	None routinely recommended
Mixed	Pelvic floor muscle training +/– biofeedback Bladder training/timed voiding	Consider antimuscarinics or mirabegron	Consider therapies for stress or urgency incontinence depending on predominant symptoms

BPH = benign prostatic hyperplasia.

with a gradual increase in the time between voids. If an episode of urgency occurs before the designated voiding time, patients are encouraged to use pelvic floor muscle contraction until the urge passes and then proceed with voiding directly afterward. In patients with cognitive impairment–related functional UI, timed voiding with prompting by the caregiver may be useful.

Pharmacologic Therapy

No pharmacologic therapies are recommended for the treatment of stress UI. Trials of systemic and vaginal estrogen therapy for stress UI in women generally have been of low quality and yielded mixed results. Vaginal estrogen has been shown to improve symptoms compared with placebo; however, the risks associated with estrogen therapy may outweigh the benefits, especially in patients with breast cancer. Current guidelines do not recommend the use of estrogen therapy for women with continued symptoms of stress UI despite behavioral therapy.

Several classes of pharmacologic agents are available for the treatment of urgency and mixed UI, although medications are recommended only when symptoms persist despite behavioral therapy (see Table 88). No one agent or class of agents has been shown to be superior in head-to-head comparisons. The risk for adverse effects with pharmacologic treatment is low but higher than with behavioral therapies. Anticholinergic and antimuscarinic side effects (dry mouth, constipation, blurred vision) predominate with agents other than mirabegron (a β_3-agonist), whereas mirabegron is associated with gastrointestinal upset and nasopharyngitis. Anticholinergic agents are contraindicated in patients with angle-closure glaucoma and should be used with caution in men with benign prostatic hyperplasia due to the risk for urinary retention.

Pharmacologic treatment of urgency or overflow UI associated with prostatic hyperplasia is discussed in Men's Health. The pharmacologic agents recommended for female patients with urgency UI are also approved for use in men.

Devices, Injectable Agents, and Surgery

Patients with continued symptoms and reduced quality of life despite behavioral and/or pharmacologic therapies should be considered for third-line treatments, including device therapy, injectable agents, and surgery. Ideally, patients should be referred to a urologist or urogynecologist in order to match their clinical symptoms, overall functional status, and personal preferences to an appropriate therapy.

In patients with stress UI, pessary devices are a low-risk treatment option. However, in a systematic review of comparative effectiveness of stress UI treatments, no definitive benefit was demonstrated with pessary devices, vaginal cones, or other intrauterine/intravaginal devices. Limited high-quality evidence supports cystoscopically guided injection of bulking agents into the urethral mucosa at the bladder neck. Injection therapy requires repeat administration in upwards of 70% of patients whose symptoms initially improve. Surgical treatment of stress UI is reserved for patients who do not respond to other therapies and typically consists of sling cystourethropexy. Postoperative adverse effects include increased urinary retention, urgency incontinence, and increased incidence of urinary tract infection.

Resistant urgency UI may be treated with botulinum toxin injections into the detrusor muscle. Repeat dosing is usually performed every 6 to 12 months. Adverse effects include urinary retention requiring self-catheterization. Surgically implanted sacral nerve root neurostimulation

devices may be used in combination with behavioral therapy and pharmacotherapy for resistant urgency UI. Although sacral neuromodulation is associated with symptom improvement, widespread use of these devices is not indicated because of the required surgical intervention, complex programming, high costs, and potential for infection.

Indwelling urinary catheters are not recommended for any type of incontinence, owing to an unacceptably high risk for infection associated with their use.

KEY POINTS

- **HVC** • First-line therapy for urinary incontinence (UI) includes pelvic floor muscle training for stress UI and mixed UI, bladder training with timed voiding for urgency UI, and exercise and weight loss in obese patients with any form of UI.
- **HVC** • No pharmacologic therapies are recommended for the treatment of stress urinary incontinence or functional incontinence.
- Urgency and mixed urinary incontinence may be treated with pharmacologic therapy, including anticholinergic and antimuscarinic agents, when symptoms persist despite behavioral therapy.

Pressure Injuries

Pressure injuries (or pressure ulcers) represent damage to the skin and underlying tissue caused by unrelieved pressure. The most important risk factors for pressure injury are immobility, malnutrition, sensory loss, and reduced skin perfusion, such as occurs with hypovolemia, hypotension, and systemic vasoconstriction. An estimated 2.5 to 3 million pressure injuries are treated each year in acute care facilities in the United States. Among hospitalized patients, prevalence rates range from 3% to 17%; however, rates are much higher in some high-risk groups, approaching 50% in long-term ICU patients. Patients who develop pressure injuries during an acute care stay are much more likely to be discharged to a long-term care facility.

Prevention

Pressure injury prevention is a cost-effective intervention that can positively affect health status. Improved understanding of ulcer pathogenesis and changes in reimbursement have increased the focus on identifying patients at risk and allocating resources to prevention efforts. The Centers for Medicare & Medicaid Services (CMS) has identified pressure ulcer development as a sentinel event (unexpected and preventable occurrence that results in serious patient injury) for health care facilities. As of October 2008, guidelines from CMS dictate that hospitals no longer receive additional payment when a patient has developed a stage III or IV pressure ulcer.

Risk assessment, including a comprehensive history and physical examination, is the first step in pressure injury prevention. In a 2015 clinical practice guideline, the ACP

recommends regular, structured risk assessment to identify at-risk patients. Standardized risk-assessment tools include the Braden, Cubbin and Jackson, Norton, and Waterlow scales. Clinical validation studies have found these instruments to have fairly low positive predictive values (60%-70%); therefore, bedside clinical assessment remains an important part of risk evaluation.

After identification of at-risk patients, pressure redistribution is of paramount importance in the prevention of pressure injuries and may be accomplished with pressure-reducing equipment and proper patient positioning. In patients at increased risk, the ACP recommends using advanced static mattresses or overlays (for example, medical sheepskin overlay) for prevention. Evidence of the efficacy of repositioning, nutritional interventions, and local care (silicone foam dressings or creams) in preventing pressure ulcers is limited. The ACP recommends against the use of alternating air mattresses, primarily based on cost considerations and lack of data demonstrating a clear advantage. There are insufficient data to recommend the routine use of dietary supplements for pressure injury prevention.

Management

Pressure injuries may be classified with the use of a staging system (**Table 89**); advancing stages are characterized by increasing tissue loss, depth, and ulcer size. Successful treatment of established pressure injuries requires interdisciplinary management involving nutrition, pressure-reducing surfaces (including air-fluidized beds), wound care, surgical debridement and repair, and in some cases, vacuum-assisted closure. On the basis of moderate-quality evidence, the ACP

TABLE 89.	Classification of Pressure Injuries
Stage	**Description**
I	Intact skin with nonblanchable redness
II	Partial-thickness loss of dermis. Shallow open ulcer with red-pink wound bed without slough. May also present as intact or ruptured serum-filled blister
III	Full-thickness tissue loss. Visible subcutaneous fat but not bone, tendon, or muscle. May include undermining or tunneling
IV	Full-thickness tissue loss with exposed bone, tendon, or muscle
Unstageable	Full-thickness tissue loss in which the base of the ulcer is covered by slough or eschar
Suspected deep-tissue injury	Purple or maroon localized area of discolored but intact skin or a blood-filled blister due to damage of underlying soft tissue from pressure or shear

Adapted from National Pressure Ulcer Advisory Panel. National Pressure Ulcer Advisory Panel, European Pressure Ulcer Advisory Panel, and Pan Pacific Pressure Injury Alliance. Prevention and Treatment of Pressure Ulcers: Quick Reference Guide. Cambridge Media: Perth, Australia; 2014.

recommends protein-containing supplements to improve wound healing. Moderate-quality evidence has also shown a reduction in pressure injury size with air-fluidized beds compared with other support surfaces. Hydrocolloid and foam dressings are recommended treatments because they have been shown to reduce ulcer size compared with gauze dressings in low-quality studies. Wound electrical stimulation has been demonstrated to be effective as adjunctive therapy to improve healing. Evidence is insufficient to support the use of platelet-derived growth factor dressings, hydrotherapy, hyperbaric oxygen, or maggot therapy. H

KEY POINTS

- Pressure redistribution, such as with advanced static mattresses or overlays, is of paramount importance in the prevention of pressure injuries.
- Protein-containing supplements and hydrocolloid or foam dressings are recommended in the treatment of established pressure injuries.

Perioperative Medicine

General Recommendations

Perioperative medicine comprises preoperative risk assessment, preoperative testing, medical optimization of surgical patients, and postoperative medical care. The role of the internist in the perioperative setting is not to provide surgical clearance but to determine and communicate operative risk to patients and surgical and anesthesia colleagues and to suggest strategies that may mitigate this risk.

Decisions regarding the modality of anesthesia, such as whether to pursue regional or general anesthesia, are best deferred to the anesthesiologist and surgeon, owing to a lack of high-quality evidence that anesthetic choice significantly affects medical outcomes. A recent Cochrane review showed no differences in outcomes, including 30-day mortality, myocardial infarction, pneumonia, and hospital length of stay, with regional anesthesia compared with general anesthesia.

Preoperative Laboratory Testing

Preoperative laboratory testing should be performed on the basis of the patient's medical conditions, physical examination findings, and preoperative symptoms (**Table 90**). Routine laboratory panels expose patients to unnecessary testing and are not recommended.

Perioperative Medication Management

Perioperative medication management begins with eliciting a complete preoperative medication history, including herbal preparations, supplements, and over-the-counter medications. Careful medication reconciliation should be performed to rectify any discrepancies and to prevent medication errors.

TABLE 90. Selected Indications for Preoperative Laboratory Testing

Laboratory Test	Preoperative Indications
Hemoglobin	History of anemia
	Underlying disease that predisposes to anemia (such as kidney disease)
	Suggestive physical examination
	Expected substantial operative blood loss
Platelet count	History of thrombocytopenia or cirrhosis; the presence of signs or symptoms of thrombocytopenia or liver disease
Coagulation studies	Anticoagulant use
	History of abnormal bleeding
	Medical conditions that predispose to coagulopathy (such as liver disease or hemophilia)
Electrolytes	Diseases that predispose to electrolyte derangements (such as kidney disease)
	Use of medications that can cause electrolyte abnormalities (such as diuretics, ACE inhibitors, and angiotensin receptor blockers)
Creatinine	Kidney disease; creatinine is also used in preoperative cardiovascular risk calculators and for calculation of the MELD score
Liver chemistry tests (including bilirubin)	Cirrhosis, history of abnormal liver chemistry test results, or the presence of signs or symptoms of liver disease
	Examination findings suggestive of liver disease
Fasting glucose and hemoglobin A_{1c}	Hyperglycemia suspected based on history and physical examination findings
Urinalysis	Suspected urinary tract infection
	Planned urologic procedures
	Planned implantation of prosthetic devices

MELD = Model for End-stage Liver Disease.

There is a paucity of high-quality evidence to guide perioperative medication management. Most medications are tolerated throughout the perioperative period, with some important exceptions. **Table 91** provides perioperative recommendations for medications with potential surgery-related risk. Patients should be provided with clear instructions on which medications to withhold preoperatively and for what duration.

Postoperative Care

Promotion of patient mobilization, use of lung expansion modalities (see later discussion), improvement in patient nutrition, and enhanced recovery after surgery (ERAS) programs may all decrease the likelihood of postoperative complications. Early mobilization and physical therapy (as necessary) are important components of the postoperative care plan and

TABLE 91. Perioperative Medication Management[a]

Medication	Perioperative Recommendation	Special Considerations
Cardiovascular Agents		
α_1-Blockers	Continue	Risk for intraoperative floppy iris syndrome in cataract surgery; notify surgeon if ocular surgery is planned
α_2-Blockers	Continue	Do not initiate clonidine for preoperative cardiovascular risk reduction (increases risk for perioperative hypotension)
β-Blockers	Continue	Consider initiating preoperatively in patients with ≥3 RCRI risk factors and those with intermediate- or high-risk myocardial ischemia on preoperative stress testing
		Begin β-blocker with enough time to assess tolerability; β-blocker should not be started on the day of surgery (2-7 days before surgery is preferred)
Calcium channel blockers	Continue	Withhold for preoperative hypotension
ACE inhibitors and ARBs	Individualize	Consider withholding if large fluid shifts expected intraoperatively, or if preoperative hypotension, hyperkalemia, or acute kidney injury is present; restart as soon as possible postoperatively
Diuretics	Withhold	Monitor volume status closely if heart failure is present and restart as soon as possible
Nitrates	Continue	Withhold for preoperative hypotension; remove patch and paste formulations
Vasodilators	Continue	Withhold for preoperative hypotension
Statins	Continue	Thought to have beneficial pleiotropic effects in addition to lipid-lowering properties
		Reasonable to start in patients undergoing vascular surgery and those undergoing elevated-risk noncardiac surgery with indication for statin
		Withhold all other lipid-lowering medications
Analgesic Agents		
NSAIDs	Withhold	If possible, withhold 3 days before surgery, especially if increased bleeding risk
Opioids	Individualize	If surgery is elective, may consider preoperative pain rehabilitation and opioid taper
		Continue in most patients receiving long-term opioid therapy
		Risk for poorly controlled postoperative pain and respiratory depression
Acetaminophen	Continue	
Gastrointestinal Agents		
Antacid medications (including H$_2$ blockers and proton pump inhibitors)	Continue	
Hyoscyamine	Withhold	Risk for anticholinergic side effects
Rheumatologic Agents		
Hydroxychloroquine	Continue	
Methotrexate	Individualize	Limited high-quality evidence
		Likely safe to continue in most situations; withhold if significant concern for infection or history of septic complications; dose adjust in cases of kidney injury
TNF-α inhibitors	Withhold	No definitive evidence or guideline recommendations
		Reasonable to withhold one to two half-lives preoperatively
Psychiatric Agents		
Selective serotonin reuptake inhibitors	Usually continue	May increase risk for bleeding, especially in conjunction with antiplatelet agents; risk for withdrawal symptoms with abrupt cessation
Benzodiazepines	Continue	Risk for withdrawal with abrupt cessation; monitor for respiratory depression
Antipsychotics	Continue	Potential for QT prolongation
Supplements		
Herbal preparations	Withhold	Withhold 1 week preoperatively
Vitamins and supplements	Withhold	

ARB = angiotensin receptor blocker; RCRI = Revised Cardiac Risk Index; TNF = tumor necrosis factor.

[a]Perioperative management of antiplatelet agents, anticoagulants, antiepileptic drugs, glucocorticoids, and diabetes medications are discussed later in this chapter.

Information from Fleisher LA, Fleischmann KE, Auerbach AD, Barnason SA, Beckman JA, Bozkurt B, et al; American College of Cardiology. 2014 ACC/AHA guideline on perioperative cardiovascular evaluation and management of patients undergoing noncardiac surgery: a report of the American College of Cardiology/American Heart Association Task Force on practice guidelines. J Am Coll Cardiol. 2014;64:e77-137. [PMID: 25091544] doi:10.1016/j.jacc.2014.07.944 and Devereaux PJ, Sessler DI, Leslie K, Kurz A, Mrkobrada M, Alonso-Coello P, et al; POISE-2 Investigators. Clonidine in patients undergoing noncardiac surgery. N Engl J Med. 2014;370:1504-13. [PMID: 24679061] doi:10.1056/NEJMoa1401106

may decrease the probability of postoperative pneumonia and venous thromboembolism (VTE).

Malnutrition is a risk factor for perioperative morbidity, including infection and poor wound healing, and several nutrition risk stratification tools are available to identify patients at risk for postoperative complications related to malnutrition. The Subjective Global Assessment of Nutritional Status tool incorporates history of calorie intake and physical examination findings, whereas the Nutritional Risk Screening Tool relies on age, BMI and weight loss, and severity of the current medical condition. Serum protein markers, including albumin and prealbumin, are also predictive of postoperative complications. Loss of 15% of body weight over 6 months and a serum albumin level less than 3.0 g/dL (30 g/L) are the most predictive factors of poor surgical outcomes related to malnutrition. Notably, increased enteral calorie intake is effective in reducing postoperative complications.

ERAS programs use evidence-based protocols to standardize care, improve outcomes, and reduce costs in postoperative patients. Best studied in patients undergoing colorectal surgery, ERAS interventions include optimization of nutritional status, physical conditioning, abstinence from alcohol and tobacco, postoperative mobilization, and early removal of urinary catheters. ERAS programs have been demonstrated to decrease length of hospital stay and result in earlier mobilization and return of bowel function in colorectal surgery populations. They are currently being implemented and studied in other surgical populations.

Common complications in the postoperative setting include postoperative urinary retention (POUR), postoperative ileus, and postoperative nausea and vomiting (PONV). POUR is characterized by incomplete bladder emptying after surgery, resulting in increased postvoid residual urine volume. Risk factors include type of surgery (incontinence and anorectal surgery, hernia repair, joint arthroplasty), longer surgery, use of regional anesthesia, administration of more than 750 mL of intraoperative fluids, use of certain postoperative medications (opioids, anticholinergic agents), older age, constipation, pelvic organ prolapse, neurologic disease, history of urinary retention, and history of pelvic surgery. POUR is a urologic emergency. Reversible causes of POUR, such as medication use, should be addressed. In patients with benign prostatic hyperplasia, α_2-blockers should be continued, whereas medications with associated anticholinergic effects, such as oxybutynin, should be withheld. Early removal of indwelling catheters and voiding trials are recommended. For patients in whom a voiding trial is unsuccessful, clean intermittent catheterization is indicated. Urinary tract obstruction should be excluded if POUR is persistent.

Postoperative ileus, or gastrointestinal hypomotility after surgery, is associated with increased length of hospital stay. Ileus is often a physiologic response related to sympathetic nervous system activation, although it can also be caused by activation of inflammatory mediators or the use of medications, such as anesthetics and opioids. Risk factors for the development of postoperative ileus include abdominal and pelvic surgery, open surgical technique, and the presence of other postoperative complications, such as pneumonia. Treatment of ileus includes minimization of postoperative opioids, adequate hydration, bowel rest, electrolyte repletion, postoperative ambulation, and use of chewing gum. Preventive measures for ileus include an appropriate postoperative bowel regimen, which may comprise fiber, stool softeners, osmotic laxatives, and stimulant laxatives. Few data from well-designed clinical trials are available to guide therapy for prolonged postoperative ileus, typically defined as ileus lasting longer than 3 to 5 days. In these patients, it is important to distinguish postoperative ileus from mechanical bowel obstruction.

The prevention and treatment of PONV, a common postoperative event that results in significant patient distress, require a multifaceted approach that involves identifying at-risk patients, reducing baseline risk factors, providing prophylaxis, and treating symptoms. Risk factors for PONV include female sex; young age; nonsmoking status; and use of general anesthesia, postoperative opioids, or volatile anesthetics. Although many risk-mitigation strategies include intraoperative and immediate postoperative care, the internist plays an important role in ensuring adequate postoperative hydration, minimizing the use of opioids, and providing pharmacologic antiemetic therapy. **H**

KEY POINTS

- Preoperative laboratory testing should be performed based on the patient's medical conditions, physical examination findings, and preoperative symptoms; routine laboratory panels expose patients to unnecessary testing and are not recommended. **HVC**

- There is a paucity of high-quality evidence to guide perioperative medication management; in general, most medications are tolerated throughout the perioperative period.

- Optimization of nutritional status, early mobilization, use of lung expansion modalities, and enhanced recovery after surgery programs are important components of the postoperative care plan. **HVC**

- Treatment of postoperative ileus includes minimization of postoperative opioids, adequate hydration, bowel rest, electrolyte repletion, postoperative ambulation, and use of chewing gum.

Cardiovascular Perioperative Management

Cardiovascular Risk Assessment

Preoperative cardiac evaluation entails assessment of patient-specific risk, surgery-specific risk, and urgency of surgery (emergent, urgent, or time sensitive). The approach recommended by the American College of Cardiology (ACC)/American Heart Association (AHA) for perioperative cardiovascular evaluation in patients undergoing noncardiac surgery is presented in **Figure 29**.

Risk calculators, including the Revised Cardiac Risk Index (**Table 92**) and American College of Surgeons National Surgical Quality Improvement Program myocardial infarction and cardiac arrest calculator (https://riskcalculator.facs.org/RiskCalculator), can be used to determine the risk for a perioperative major adverse cardiac event (MACE). Both risk calculators incorporate patient- and surgery-specific risk factors.

Patients with low risk (<1% risk of perioperative MACE) may proceed to surgery without preoperative cardiac stress testing, whereas patients with elevated risk (≥1% risk for perioperative MACE) should undergo assessment of functional capacity. Metabolic equivalents (METs) are used to represent the patient's functional capacity based on the intensity of activity able to be performed. If the patient's functional capacity exceeds 4 METs, the patient may proceed to surgery without further testing. Examples of activities that require 4 METs include walking 4 miles per hour on a flat surface; climbing one to two flights of stairs without stopping; or performing vigorous housework, such as vacuuming. Cardiac stress testing should be considered in patients at elevated risk for MACE with a functional capacity of less than 4 METs or if functional capacity cannot be determined, but only if the results of stress testing will change perioperative management.

Preoperative electrocardiography (ECG) is reasonable in patients with known coronary artery disease, arrhythmia, peripheral artery disease, cerebrovascular disease, or structural heart disease undergoing moderate- to high-risk surgeries. Preoperative ECG may be considered for other asymptomatic patients except those undergoing low-risk procedures. ECG may not alter preoperative decision making, but it provides a useful baseline to guide postoperative management in the event of complications.

Echocardiography to evaluate left ventricular function should not be routinely performed preoperatively. Echocardiography is recommended in certain clinical scenarios, such as in the presence of dyspnea of unknown origin, heart failure with worsening dyspnea or overall change in clinical status, known left ventricular dysfunction without echocardiographic assessment in the last year, and known or suspected moderate to severe valvular stenosis or regurgitation without echocardiographic assessment in the last year or with a change in clinical status.

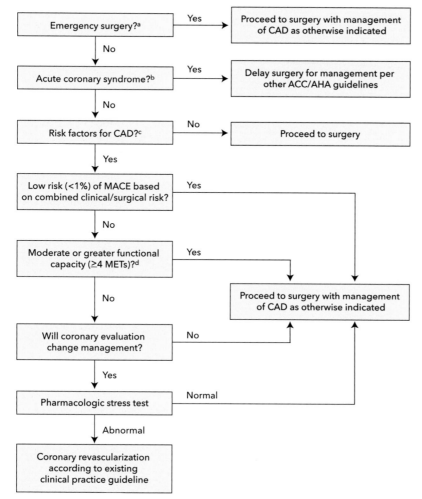

FIGURE 29. Perioperative ischemic cardiac disease evaluation for noncardiac surgery.

ACC = American College of Cardiology; AHA = American Heart Association; CAD = coronary artery disease; MACE = major adverse cardiac event; METs = metabolic equivalents.

[a]Emergency surgery required within 6 hours to avoid loss of life or limb.

[b]Acute coronary syndromes: myocardial infarction <30 days ago, unstable or severe angina.

[c]Risk factors for CAD: not specifically defined in ACC/AHA guidelines; examples include known CAD, cerebrovascular disease (i.e., stroke or transient ischemic attack), chronic kidney disease, diabetes mellitus, and heart failure.

[d]Examples of activities requiring ≥4 METs include climbing a flight of stairs, walking up a hill, walking on level ground at 4 miles per hour, running for a short distance, and playing tennis.

Recommendations from Fleisher LA, Fleischmann KE, Auerbach AD, Barnason SA, Beckman JA, Bozkurt B, et al; American College of Cardiology. 2014 ACC/AHA guideline on perioperative cardiovascular evaluation and management of patients undergoing noncardiac surgery: a report of the American College of Cardiology/American Heart Association Task Force on practice guidelines. J Am Coll Cardiol. 2014;64:e77-137. [PMID: 25091544] doi:10.1016/j.jacc.2014.07.944

TABLE 92. Revised Cardiac Risk Index and Predicted Rate of Major Cardiac Complications Perioperatively

Risk Factor (1 point for each)
High-risk surgery (intrathoracic, intraperitoneal, suprainguinal vascular)
Ischemic heart disease
Heart failure (compensated)
Diabetes mellitus (requiring insulin)
Cerebrovascular disease
Chronic kidney disease (serum creatinine >2.0 mg/dL [176.8 μmol/L])[a]

Number of Points	Risk for Major Cardiac Complications[b]
0	0.4% (95% CI, 0.1-0.8)
1	1.0% (95% CI, 0.5-1.4)
2	2.4% (95% CI, 1.3-3.5)
≥3	5.4% (95% CI, 2.8-7.9)

[a]Estimated glomerular filtration rate <30 mL/min/1.73 m² also shown to predict cardiovascular risk.

[b]Defined as cardiac death, nonfatal myocardial infarction, and nonfatal cardiac arrest.

Data from Lee TH, Marcantonio ER, Mangione CM, et al. Derivation and prospective validation of a simple index for prediction of cardiac risk of major noncardiac surgery. Circulation. 1999;100(10):1043-9. [PMID: 10477528] and Devereaux PJ, Goldman L, Cook DJ, Gilbert K, Leslie K, Guyatt GH. Perioperative cardiac events in patients undergoing noncardiac surgery: a review of the magnitude of the problem, the pathophysiology of the events and methods to estimate and communicate risk. CMAJ. 2005;173:627-34. [PMID: 16157727]

Cardiovascular Risk Management
Coronary Artery Disease
Patients with coronary artery disease (CAD) should not undergo routine coronary angiography or revascularization exclusively to reduce perioperative events. These procedures should be reserved for patients with recognized indications based on existing clinical practice guidelines. In patients who meet the criteria for intervention and in whom noncardiac surgery is time sensitive, balloon angioplasty or bare metal stent implantation should be considered over use of a drug-eluting stent. Elective noncardiac surgery should be delayed 14 days after balloon angioplasty, 30 days after bare metal stent implantation, and optimally 6 to 12 months after drug-eluting stent placement. However, if the risk of surgical delay outweighs the risk for ischemia and stent thrombosis, surgery may be considered 90 days after drug-eluting stent placement.

Patients taking β-blockers, statins, and many antihypertensive medications should continue these medications throughout the perioperative period, unless prohibited by hypotension. In hypotensive patients, dosage reduction is preferred to β-blocker discontinuation. There are also circumstances in which β-blocker or statin therapy should be initiated preoperatively (see Table 91). Postoperative β-blocker administration should be guided by clinical circumstances.

The ACC/AHA perioperative evaluation and management guideline does not recommend routinely obtaining postoperative troponin levels and an ECG in asymptomatic patients. However, these tests are recommended in patients with signs or symptoms of myocardial ischemia, which often presents atypically in the postoperative period (including as delirium in the elderly, hyperglycemia, and blood pressure fluctuations).

Heart Failure
Medical management of decompensated heart failure should be optimized before surgery and may involve diuresis, fluid restriction, and medication adjustments (see MKSAP 18 Cardiovascular Medicine).

Cardiac Arrhythmias
Risk management strategies for patients with a cardiac arrhythmia who are undergoing surgery include continuation of antiarrhythmic medications and, for some patients, continuous cardiac monitoring.

Patients with atrial fibrillation are at risk for rapid ventricular rate due to surgical stress, fluid shifts, and postoperative pain. Maintaining euvolemia, optimizing postoperative pain management, and controlling rates with medications are all appropriate strategies in stable patients. Hemodynamically unstable patients should undergo direct-current cardioversion.

A cardiologist should be consulted in patients with an implantable cardioverter-defibrillator who are undergoing surgery. Patients in whom a device has been deactivated for surgery should undergo continuous cardiac monitoring until the device is reprogrammed.

Valvular Heart Disease
The ACC/AHA guideline states that it is reasonable to perform elevated-risk elective noncardiac surgery in patients with severe asymptomatic aortic stenosis, mitral regurgitation, or aortic regurgitation with preserved left ventricular function. In patients who are candidates for valvular intervention due to symptoms or severity of disease, valvular intervention should be performed before elective noncardiac surgery.

Pulmonary Hypertension
Preoperative evaluation by a pulmonary hypertension specialist is advised for patients with pulmonary hypertension with high-risk features, including group 1 pulmonary hypertension (pulmonary arterial hypertension), pulmonary arterial systolic pressure greater than 70 mm Hg, moderate or severe right ventricular systolic dysfunction, and New York Heart Association functional class III or IV symptoms attributable to pulmonary hypertension. Patients with pulmonary hypertension undergoing noncardiac surgery should be continued on pulmonary vascular targeted therapies, such as phosphodiesterase-5 inhibitors.

Primary Hypertension
In patients with hypertension, urgent blood pressure lowering is not mandatory preoperatively unless there is evidence of

H
CONT. end-organ dysfunction, in which case surgery should be delayed and blood pressure treated. Deferral of surgery may also be considered in patients with a systolic blood pressure of 180 mm Hg or higher or diastolic blood pressure of 110 mm Hg or higher. Moderate preoperative hypertension has not been linked to adverse perioperative outcomes, although evidence is lacking regarding a specific blood pressure threshold. The perioperative use of specific antihypertensive agents is outlined in Table 91. H

KEY POINTS

HVC • Patients with low cardiovascular risk (<1% risk for peri-operative major adverse cardiac event [MACE]) may proceed to surgery without preoperative cardiac stress testing, whereas patients with elevated risk (≥1% risk for perioperative MACE) should undergo assessment of functional capacity to determine necessity for cardiac stress testing.

HVC • Routine electrocardiography is not indicated in asymptomatic patients undergoing low-risk surgical procedures.

HVC • In patients with coronary artery disease, routine coronary angiography or revascularization should be performed for recognized indications based on existing clinical practice guidelines and should not be performed exclusively to reduce perioperative cardiovascular events.

• Patients with hypertension who are undergoing surgery do not require urgent blood pressure lowering preoperatively unless there is evidence of end-organ dysfunction.

Pulmonary Perioperative Management

Perioperative pulmonary complications include pneumonia, respiratory failure, and exacerbation of underlying lung disease. Pulmonary perioperative management involves pulmonary risk assessment, including screening for obstructive sleep apnea (OSA), assessment of any underlying lung disease with optimization of treatment, and optimization of perioperative risk-reduction strategies.

Pulmonary Risk Assessment

Pulmonary risk factors can be categorized as patient-related risk factors or procedure-related risk factors (Table 93). Obesity and well-controlled asthma have not been shown to be independently associated with perioperative pulmonary complications. Risk calculators that include many of the important risk factors as well as other predictors, such as low oxygen saturation and the presence of preoperative sepsis, are available to help determine postoperative risk for respiratory failure, pneumonia, and overall pulmonary complications. The Postoperative Respiratory Failure Risk Calculator is available at www.surgicalriskcalculator.com/prf-risk-calculator, and the Postoperative Pneumonia Risk Calculator is available at www.surgicalriskcalculator.com/postoperative-pneumonia-risk-calculator. These calculators do not consider important

TABLE 93. Pulmonary Risk Factors
Patient-Specific Risk Factors
Age
COPD
Cigarette use
ASA class ≥2[a]
Functional dependence
Obstructive sleep apnea
Heart failure
Poor nutritional status
Procedure-Specific Risk Factors
Surgery in close proximity to the diaphragm (aortic, thoracic, abdominal)
Head and neck surgery
Neurosurgery
Major vascular surgery
Procedure duration >3-4 hours
Emergency surgery

ASA = American Society of Anesthesiologists.

[a]ASA classes are as follows: class 1, normal healthy patient; class 2, patient with mild systemic disease; class 3, patient with severe systemic disease; class 4, patient with systemic disease that is a constant threat to life; and class 5, moribund patient who is not expected to survive for 24 hours with or without operation.

Adapted with permission from Smetana GW, Lawrence VA, Cornell JE; American College of Physicians. Preoperative pulmonary risk stratification for noncardiothoracic surgery: systematic review for the American College of Physicians. Ann Intern Med. 2006;144:584, 587. [PMID: 16618956] Copyright 2006, American College of Physicians.

pulmonary comorbid conditions, such as COPD and OSA, but they are useful in planning for surgery and establishing informed consent.

Spirometry is not useful for predicting risk and should not be routinely ordered for preoperative evaluation, including in patients with COPD. Furthermore, evidence does not support a spirometric threshold below which the risk of surgery is unacceptable. Spirometry is indicated in patients undergoing lung resection, however, to help predict postoperative lung function. Chest radiography is not required in most patients but is indicated in patients with signs or symptoms of pulmonary disease and in patients with underlying cardiac or pulmonary disease and new or unstable symptoms.

All patients should be screened for OSA, which is associated with adverse perioperative outcomes, including cardiac events, pulmonary complications, and ICU admissions. A commonly used screening tool for OSA is the STOP-BANG score (Table 94). In high-risk patients undergoing elective surgery, the American Society of Anesthesiologists recommends further evaluation with polysomnography.

Assessment of Underlying Lung Disease

COPD is the most commonly identified risk factor for postoperative pulmonary complications. Patients should be

TABLE 94. STOP-BANG Obstructive Sleep Apnea Screening Tool	
Survey Items (1 point for each)	
Snoring	
Tiredness or sleepiness during the day	
Observed apnea during sleep	
Pressure, high blood	
BMI >35	
Age >50 years	
Neck circumference >40 cm (15.7 in)	
Gender = male	
STOP-BANG Score	**Risk Correlation**
0-2	Low risk for OSA
≥3	Increased risk for OSA
≥5	Increased risk for moderate-severe OSA

OSA = obstructive sleep apnea.

Adapted with permission from Chung F, Yegneswaran B, Liao P, et al. STOP questionnaire: a tool to screen patients for obstructive sleep apnea. Anesthesiology. 2008 May;108(5):812-21. [PMID: 18431116] *and* Chung F, Subramanyam R, Liao P, Sasaki E, Shapiro C, Sun Y. High STOP-Bang score indicates a high probability of obstructive sleep apnoea. Br J Anaesth. 2012 May;108(5):768-75. [PMID: 22401881]

KEY POINTS

- Preoperative chest radiography is indicated only in patients with signs or symptoms of pulmonary disease and in patients with underlying cardiac or pulmonary disease and new or unstable symptoms. **HVC**

- Spirometry should not be routinely performed preoperatively except in patients undergoing lung resection. **HVC**

- All patients undergoing surgery should be screened for obstructive sleep apnea, which is associated with adverse perioperative outcomes, including cardiac events, pulmonary complications, and ICU admissions.

screened preoperatively for signs and symptoms of COPD exacerbation and instructed to take prescribed inhaled medications on the morning of surgery. In patients with an exacerbation, surgery should be postponed, and treatment should be initiated.

Perioperative Risk-Reduction Strategies

Risk for pulmonary complications should be mitigated with perioperative risk-reduction interventions, including preoperative initiation of lung expansion maneuvers (deep breathing exercises and incentive spirometry), limiting use of nasogastric tubes in abdominal surgery for nausea or abdominal distention, and aspiration precautions. A recent multicenter randomized trial demonstrated that a 30-minute preoperative education and breathing exercise training session can reduce postoperative pulmonary complication rates by 50%. Smoking cessation has been shown to reduce pulmonary risk and should be encouraged as far in advance of surgery as possible. Patients with pulmonary disease should continue outpatient medications.

In patients diagnosed with OSA, continuous positive airway pressure (CPAP) should be initiated preoperatively. Patients at high risk for OSA undergoing nonelective surgery should be placed on continuous pulse oximetry and monitored for oxygen desaturation, apneas, reduced respiration rate, and oversedation in the postanesthesia care unit (PACU); patients with recurrent respiratory events in the PACU benefit from additional monitoring postoperatively. All patients with known OSA should bring their CPAP device to the hospital for use in the perioperative period.

Hematologic Perioperative Management

Venous Thromboembolism Prophylaxis

The American College of Chest Physicians (ACCP) antithrombotic guideline provides recommendations for VTE prophylaxis for both orthopedic and nonorthopedic surgery populations (**Table 95**). In patients undergoing general surgery or abdominal-pelvic surgery, the ACCP recommends using the Caprini score to estimate the patient's risk for postoperative thrombosis (**Table 96**).

Hip fracture surgery, total knee arthroplasty, and total hip arthroplasty pose a high risk for VTE, and both mechanical (nonpharmacologic) and pharmacologic VTE prophylaxis are recommended. Mechanical prophylaxis is provided with an intermittent pneumatic compression device. For pharmacologic prophylaxis, the ACCP recommends low-molecular-weight heparin in preference to other pharmacologic agents. The minimum recommended duration of pharmacologic VTE prophylaxis in patients undergoing orthopedic surgery is 10 to 14 days; however, in patients without increased bleeding risk, extended-duration postoperative prophylaxis (up to 35 days) is preferred over shorter-duration prophylaxis. Intermittent pneumatic compression devices and pharmacologic VTE prophylaxis are recommended during the entire hospital stay. If bleeding risk is especially high, mechanical prophylaxis is recommended over no prophylaxis. In patients who decline or are unable to tolerate low-molecular-weight heparin, the ACCP recommends apixaban, rivaroxaban, dabigatran, or a vitamin K antagonist over alternate forms of prophylaxis.

The ACCP recommends against the routine placement of inferior vena cava filters for VTE prophylaxis. Routine surveillance for VTE with venous compression ultrasonography is also not recommended in patients undergoing orthopedic surgery, general surgery, abdominal-pelvic surgery, and trauma surgery.

Perioperative Management of Anticoagulant Therapy

Anticoagulant therapy increases the risk for perioperative hemorrhage and should be discontinued in most patients before surgery. Minor surgery, including dental extractions

TABLE 95. Postoperative Venous Thromboembolism Prophylaxis Recommendations for Common Noncardiothoracic Surgeries

	Surgery and Risks		Recommended Prophylaxis[a]
General, abdominal-pelvic, urologic, plastic, vascular	Caprini[b] score 0		Early ambulation
	Caprini score 1-2		IPC
	Caprini score 3-4	Average bleeding risk	LMWH, LDUH, IPC
		High bleeding risk[c]	IPC
	Caprini score ≥5	Average bleeding risk	LMWH or LDUH (+ IPC)
		High bleeding risk[c]	IPC
	Cancer surgery		LMWH for 4 wk
Orthopedic	Hip or knee arthroplasty[d]		IPC + LMWH, LDUH, aspirin, NOAC, fondaparinux, warfarin, or IPC alone if high bleeding risk; continue for 10-35 d
	Hip fracture repair[d]		IPC + LMWH, LDUH, warfarin, fondaparinux, or IPC alone if high bleeding risk; continue for 10-35 d
	Isolated lower leg fracture repairs		None
	Knee arthroscopy with no previous VTE		Early ambulation
Spine (elective)	Average VTE risk		IPC
	High VTE risk (e.g., malignancy, anterior-posterior approach)		IPC + LMWH (when bleeding risk sufficiently low)
Major trauma	Average VTE risk		LMWH, LDUH, IPC
	High VTE risk (e.g., spinal cord or brain injury)		LMWH or LDUH (+ IPC)
	High bleeding risk[c]		IPC
Intracranial	Average VTE risk		IPC
	High VTE risk (e.g., malignancy)		LMWH or LDUH (+ IPC)

IPC = intermittent pneumatic compression; LDUH = low-dose unfractionated heparin; LMWH = low-molecular-weight heparin; NOAC = non–vitamin K antagonist oral anticoagulant (dabigatran, rivaroxaban, apixaban); VTE = venous thromboembolism.

[a]Duration is for postoperative hospitalization unless noted otherwise.

[b]See Table 96 for the Caprini Risk Assessment Scoring method.

[c]Risk factors suggesting high bleeding risk: concurrent antithrombotic therapy (e.g., aspirin for cardiac disease), known or suspected bleeding disorder, active bleeding, liver or kidney disease, and sepsis.

[d]LMWH is preferred.

Recommendations from Gould MK, Garcia DA, Wren SM, Karanicolas PJ, Arcelus JI, Heit JA, et al. Prevention of VTE in nonorthopedic surgical patients: antithrombotic therapy and prevention of thrombosis, 9th ed: American College of Chest Physicians evidence-based clinical practice guidelines. Chest. 2012;141:e227S-e277S. [PMID: 22315263] doi:10.1378/chest.11-2297 and Falck-Ytter Y, Francis CW, Johanson NA, Curley C, Dahl OE, Schulman S, et al. Prevention of VTE in orthopedic surgery patients: antithrombotic therapy and prevention of thrombosis, 9th ed: American College of Chest Physicians evidence-based clinical practice guidelines. Chest. 2012;141:e278S-e325S. [PMID: 22315265] doi:10.1378/chest.11-2404

and minor skin surgery, can be completed while a patient is anticoagulated. Vitamin K antagonist (warfarin) therapy may also be continued in some patients undergoing cardiac device implantation, although the best approach to these procedures in patients receiving non–vitamin K antagonist oral anticoagulants (NOACs), including direct thrombin and factor Xa inhibitors, is unclear. In any case, collaboration with the surgeon or proceduralist is crucial to ensure that it is safe for the patient to remain anticoagulated. When it is necessary to discontinue anticoagulation, vitamin K antagonists should be discontinued at least 5 days before surgery; most procedures can be safely performed with an INR of less than 1.5. The duration for which NOACs are discontinued before surgery depends on

the bleeding risk of the procedure, the patient's kidney function, and the medication half-life; generally, NOACs can be stopped 2 to 3 days preoperatively because of their shorter half-lives.

Bridging anticoagulation is the administration of therapeutic doses of short-acting parenteral therapy, usually heparin, when oral anticoagulant therapy is being withheld during the perioperative period in patients with elevated thrombotic risk. Bridging is most commonly indicated in patients taking vitamin K antagonists. It is not indicated in patients taking NOACs because of the rapid onset and short half-life associated with these drugs, but it may be needed when patients are unable to take oral medications for an extended time after surgery, such as with gastrointestinal surgery.

TABLE 96. Caprini Venous Thromboembolism Risk Assessment Scoring Method

Number of Points for Each Risk Factor	Risk Factors
1	Age 41-60 y; minor surgery; BMI >25; leg edema; varicose veins; recent or current pregnancy; estrogen use; recurrent spontaneous abortion; recent sepsis (<1 mo)/pneumonia (<1 mo); severe lung disease; abnormal pulmonary function; inflammatory bowel disease; acute MI; recent HF (<1 mo); medical patient at bed rest
2	Age 61-74 y; arthroscopic surgery; major surgery lasting >45 min; malignancy; bed rest for >72 h; immobilizing cast; central venous access
3	Age ≥75 y; personal history of VTE; family history of VTE; congenital or acquired thrombophilia; HIT
5	Stroke or spinal cord injury within 1 mo; elective arthroplasty; hip, pelvis, or leg fracture

HF = heart failure; HIT = heparin-induced thrombocytopenia; MI = myocardial infarction; VTE = venous thromboembolism.

Adapted from Bahl V, Hu HM, Henke PK, Wakefield TW, Campbell DA Jr, Caprini JA. A validation study of a retrospective venous thromboembolism risk scoring method. Ann Surg. 2010;251:344-50. [PMID: 19779324] doi:10.1097/SLA.0b013e3181b7fca6

TABLE 97. Annual Stroke Risk Based on CHADS$_2$ Score

CHADS$_2$ Score[a]	Unadjusted Annual Stroke Rate in Patients Not Treated With Anticoagulation (per 100 Patient-Years)[b]
0	0.6
1	3.0
2	4.2
3	7.1
4	11.1
5	12.5
6	13.0

[a]One point is given for heart failure, hypertension, age ≥75 years, and diabetes mellitus. Two points are given for previous stroke or transient ischemic attack.

[b]Data from Friberg L, Rosenqvist M, Lip GY. Evaluation of risk stratification schemes for ischaemic stroke and bleeding in 182 678 patients with atrial fibrillation: the Swedish Atrial Fibrillation cohort study. Eur Heart J. 2012;33:1500-10. [PMID: 22246443] doi:10.1093/eurheartj/ehr488

Postprocedural management of anticoagulation is based on thrombotic and bleeding risk, and close collaboration with the surgeon is essential. In patients taking a vitamin K antagonist, bridging anticoagulation may be deferred if thrombotic risk is low; the first dose of a vitamin K antagonist is typically administered 12 to 24 hours after surgery. If bridging is needed and the bleeding risk is low, bridging anticoagulation may be started as soon as 24 hours after the procedure; in the case of high bleeding risk, initiation of bridging anticoagulation is delayed 48 to 72 hours or possibly longer. Postoperative timing of NOAC reinstitution depends on bleeding risk, as NOACs reach therapeutic levels in 1 to 3 hours, at which point the patient is presumed to be fully anticoagulated. NOACs may be resumed once adequate hemostasis is ensured, usually 48 to 72 hours after surgery.

Because of the risk for spinal epidural hematoma, anticoagulant use with concomitant neuraxial (spinal and epidural) anesthesia should be avoided.

Atrial Fibrillation

The decision to initiate bridging anticoagulation in patients with atrial fibrillation is based on bleeding risk and thrombotic risk. Procedures with an intermediate or high risk for bleeding almost always require interruption of anticoagulation, and the CHADS$_2$ score (**Table 97**) and CHA$_2$DS$_2$-VASc score may be used to determine thrombotic risk and the need for bridging anticoagulation in patients with nonvalvular atrial fibrillation. Although use of the CHA$_2$DS$_2$-VASc score for

risk stratification is advocated in several guidelines, it has not been validated in the perioperative setting (see MKSAP 18 Cardiovascular Medicine).

The landmark BRIDGE trial has shifted clinical practice toward a more conservative approach to bridging anticoagulation in patients with nonvalvular atrial fibrillation. This randomized controlled trial determined bleeding and thrombotic outcomes in patients who received bridging anticoagulation compared with those who did not. An increased risk for bleeding was identified in patients who received bridging anticoagulation, and those who received no bridging anticoagulation did not demonstrate an increased risk for thrombosis. Only a small proportion of patients with a higher thrombotic risk (CHADS$_2$ score of 5 and 6) were included in the study, limiting the applicability in this population. Additionally, most patients underwent minor procedures, which likely carry lower thrombotic risk.

Recommendations from the ACCP and ACC on bridging anticoagulation in patients with atrial fibrillation are provided in **Table 98**.

Prosthetic Heart Valves and Venous Thromboembolic Disease

In patients receiving warfarin anticoagulant therapy for a mechanical prosthetic heart valve, continuation of anticoagulation is recommended when the surgical procedure is minor and bleeding can be managed. In patients undergoing surgery with a higher risk for bleeding, the 2017 ACC/AHA guideline on valvular heart disease suggests that bridging should be considered on an individualized basis in patients with a mechanical mitral valve, a mechanical aortic valve with thromboembolic risk factors, or an older-generation mechanical aortic valve. Bridging is not necessary in patients with a bileaflet mechanical aortic valve and no other risk factors for thrombosis. The ACCP provides similar recommendations for bridging anticoagulation in patients with prosthetic heart valves (**Table 99**).

TABLE 98. American College of Chest Physicians and American College of Cardiology Recommendations for Perioperative Bridging in Patients With Atrial Fibrillation

Risk for Thromboembolism	Patient History and Risk Stratification Score	Bridging Anticoagulation Recommendation
High (annual risk >10%)		
ACCP	$CHADS_2$ score of 5 or 6 Recent stroke or TIA Rheumatic valvular heart disease Patient with history of stroke with warfarin interruption	Bridging
ACC	CHA_2DS_2-VASc score of 7-9 Ischemic stroke, TIA, or systemic embolism within the last 3 mo	Bridging
Moderate (annual risk of 5%-10%)		
ACCP	$CHADS_2$ score of 3 or 4	Bridging unless procedure is associated with a high bleeding risk

ACC	CHA_2DS_2-VASc of 5 or 6
	
	History of ischemic stroke, TIA, or systemic embolism ≥3 mo ago
		Increased risk for bleeding: interrupt VKA without bridging
		
		No significant bleeding risk:
		
		    Stroke, TIA, or systemic embolism history: consider bridging[a]
		
		    No stroke, TIA, or systemic embolism history: no bridging[a]

Low (annual risk <5%)		
ACCP	$CHADS_2$ score of 0-2 No stroke or TIA history	No bridging
ACC	CHA_2DS_2-VASc score ≤4 No history of ischemic stroke, TIA, or systemic embolism	No bridging

ACC = American College of Cardiology; ACCP = American College of Chest Physicians; TIA = transient ischemic attack; VKA = vitamin K antagonist.

[a]Clinical judgment is required.

Information from Douketis JD, Spyropoulos AC, Spencer FA, Mayr M, Jaffer AK, Eckman MH, et al. Perioperative management of antithrombotic therapy: antithrombotic therapy and prevention of thrombosis, 9th ed: American College of Chest Physicians evidence-based clinical practice guidelines. Chest. 2012;141:e326S-e350S. [PMID: 22315266] doi:10.1378/chest.11-2298 and Doherty JU, Gluckman TJ, Hucker WJ, Januzzi JL Jr, Ortel TL, Saxonhouse SJ, et al. 2017 ACC expert consensus decision pathway for periprocedural management of anticoagulation in patients with nonvalvular atrial fibrillation: a report of the American College of Cardiology Clinical Expert Consensus Document Task Force. J Am Coll Cardiol. 2017;69:871-898. [PMID: 28081965] doi: 10.1016/j.jacc.2016.11.024

TABLE 99. American College of Chest Physicians Recommendations for Perioperative Bridging in Patients With a Prosthetic Heart Valve

Risk for Thromboembolism	Patient History	Bridging Anticoagulation Recommendation
High (annual risk >10%)	Any mitral valve prosthesis Any caged-ball or tilting disc aortic valve prosthesis Recent (within 6 mo) stroke or TIA	Bridging
Moderate (annual risk of 5%-10%)	Bileaflet aortic valve prosthesis and one or more of the of following risk factors: atrial fibrillation, previous stroke or TIA, hypertension, diabetes mellitus, heart failure, age >75 y	Bridging unless procedure is associated with a high bleeding risk
Low (annual risk <5%)	Bileaflet aortic valve prosthesis without atrial fibrillation and no other risk factors for stroke	No bridging

TIA = transient ischemic attack.

Recommendations from Douketis JD, Spyropoulos AC, Spencer FA, Mayr M, Jaffer AK, Eckman MH, et al. Perioperative management of antithrombotic therapy: antithrombotic therapy and prevention of thrombosis, 9th ed: American College of Chest Physicians evidence-based clinical practice guidelines. Chest. 2012;141:e326S-e350S. [PMID: 22315266] doi:10.1378/chest.11-2298

ACCP recommendations for bridging anticoagulation in those with a history of venous thromboembolism, including patients with thrombophilias, are included in **Table 100**.

Perioperative Management of Antiplatelet Medications

The perioperative management of dual antiplatelet therapy (DAPT), comprising aspirin plus a P2Y$_{12}$ inhibitor (clopidogrel, ticagrelor, or prasugrel), in patients with CAD depends on the presence of a bare metal or drug-eluting coronary stent, time since stent placement, and, to some degree, the indication for DAPT (stable ischemic heart disease [SIHD] or acute coronary syndrome [ACS] within the last year).

In patients who have a stent placed for SIHD, DAPT should be continued uninterrupted for at least 30 days after bare metal stent placement and a minimum of 6 months after drug-eluting stent placement. Elective surgery should be postponed during these time frames. However, if the risk of surgical delay exceeds the risk for stent thrombosis, discontinuation of the P2Y$_{12}$ inhibitor can be considered after a minimum of 3 months in patients with a drug-eluting stent. Aspirin should be continued if at all possible, and DAPT should be restarted as soon as bleeding risk has sufficiency diminished.

In patients with recent ACS, the ACC and AHA recommend continuing DAPT for at least 1 year regardless of whether the ACS was managed with medical therapy or coronary stent placement. If surgery must be performed within this time frame, DAPT should optimally be maintained for a minimum of 6 months. If more than 3 months have passed and the patient cannot be continued on DAPT because of bleeding risk, proceeding with surgery can be considered if the risk of surgical delay is greater than the risk for stent thrombosis.

In patients with recent percutaneous coronary intervention with stent placement for ACS in whom surgery mandates discontinuation of DAPT, aspirin should be continued. In patients with recent ACS treated medically who must undergo surgery for which DAPT must be discontinued, it is similarly reasonable to continue aspirin when the risk for cardiac events outweighs the risk for bleeding.

In most patients receiving long-term aspirin monotherapy for both primary and secondary prevention of cardiovascular events (in the absence of a coronary stent), aspirin should be discontinued at least 5 days before surgery and restarted postoperatively once bleeding risk has decreased. This recommendation is based on the POISE-2 trial, which found that continued perioperative aspirin resulted in increased bleeding without a decrease in cardiac events.

Perioperative Management of Anemia, Coagulopathies, and Thrombocytopenia

In all patients undergoing surgery, a careful preoperative bleeding history, including a family history, should be obtained to evaluate for underlying bleeding disorders and anemia. Laboratory testing should be reserved for patients with a suggestive history. Patients with known factor deficiencies, platelet function defects, and other coagulopathies should be managed by a hematologist.

In orthopedic and cardiac surgery patients and those with a history of stable CAD, the American Association of Blood Banks recommends a restrictive transfusion threshold (hemoglobin level of 8 g/dL [80 g/L]), as studies indicate that a restrictive threshold results in equivalent or improved patient outcomes. Similarly, in hospitalized hemodynamically stable patients, a transfusion threshold of 7 g/dL (70 g/L) is recommended.

The American Association of Blood Banks recommends a platelet transfusion threshold of 50,000/μL (50×10^9/L) for patients undergoing major non-neurologic surgery or lumbar puncture. Patients with mild thrombocytopenia due to

---

TABLE 100. American College of Chest Physicians Recommendations for Perioperative Bridging in Patients With Venous Thromboembolism

Risk for Thromboembolism	Patient History	Bridging Anticoagulation Recommendation
High (annual risk >10%)	Recent (within 3 mo) VTE	Bridging
	Severe thrombophilia (e.g., deficiency of protein C, protein S, or antithrombin; antiphospholipid antibodies; multiple abnormalities)	
Moderate (annual risk of 5%-10%)	VTE within the past 3-12 mo	Bridging unless procedure is associated with a high bleeding risk
	Nonsevere thrombophilia (e.g., heterozygous factor V Leiden or prothrombin gene mutation)	
	Recurrent VTE	
	Active cancer (treated within 6 mo or palliative)	
Low (annual risk <5%)	VTE >12 mo ago and no other risk factors	No bridging

VTE = venous thromboembolism.

Recommendations from Douketis JD, Spyropoulos AC, Spencer FA, Mayr M, Jaffer AK, Eckman MH, et al. Perioperative management of antithrombotic therapy: antithrombotic therapy and prevention of thrombosis, 9th ed: American College of Chest Physicians evidence-based clinical practice guidelines. Chest. 2012;141:e326S-e350S. [PMID: 22315266] doi:10.1378/chest.11-2298

immune thrombocytopenia are typically able to proceed to surgery at the recommended threshold. Postoperative thrombocytopenia warrants further evaluation, especially in patients with heparin exposure owing to the risk for heparin-induced thrombocytopenia. See MKSAP 18 Hematology and Oncology for a discussion of heparin-induced thrombocytopenia. 🄷

KEY POINTS

- Patients undergoing general surgery or abdominal-pelvic surgery who are at high risk for venous thromboembolism should receive pharmacologic prophylaxis (with low-molecular-weight heparin or low-dose unfractionated heparin) in combination with mechanical prophylaxis.
- The minimum recommended duration of pharmacologic venous thromboembolism prophylaxis in patients undergoing orthopedic surgery is 10 to 14 days; however, in patients without increased bleeding risk, extended-duration postoperative prophylaxis (up to 35 days) is preferred.
- In patients with atrial fibrillation undergoing a procedure with an intermediate or high risk for bleeding, interruption of anticoagulation is almost always required, and the $CHADS_2$ and CHA_2DS_2-VASc scores may be used to determine thrombotic risk and the need for bridging anticoagulation.
- In patients treated with percutaneous coronary intervention who are undergoing elective noncardiac surgery, dual antiplatelet therapy should be continued uninterrupted for at least 30 days after bare metal stent placement and a minimum of 6 months after drug-eluting stent placement.
- HVC • In orthopedic and cardiac surgery patients and those with a history of CAD, the American Association of Blood Banks recommends a restrictive transfusion threshold (hemoglobin level of 8 g/dL [80 g/L]).

Perioperative Management of Endocrine Diseases

Diabetes Mellitus

Evidence demonstrates that patients with uncontrolled diabetes are at increased risk for perioperative complications, including surgical and nonsurgical infections, and postoperative mortality. Patients at high risk for diabetes, such as those with a history of impaired fasting glucose, should be evaluated for diabetes before elective surgery. In patients with established diabetes, it is reasonable to measure hemoglobin A_{1c} within 3 months of surgery. There is not high-quality evidence on whether delaying surgery to improve glycemic control improves outcomes, although efforts should be made to optimize glycemic control before major elective surgery.

Oral and injectable noninsulin medications should be withheld 12 to 72 hours before surgery, replaced with supplemental insulin, and resumed at hospital discharge or when the patient has resumed a full diet. In patients taking insulin therapy, basal insulin should be continued perioperatively. The basal insulin dosage should not be reduced in patients with type 1 diabetes. Preoperative dosage reduction (often 25%-50%) may be considered in patients with type 2 diabetes who have a history of hypoglycemia with skipped or delayed meals.

Postoperatively, if the patient is eating, the ideal insulin regimen is a basal-bolus regimen, with prandial coverage and correction boluses for premeal hyperglycemia. For a discussion of the management of hyperglycemia in the hospital setting, see MKSAP 18 Endocrinology and Metabolism.

Thyroid Disease

Preoperative screening for thyroid disease is not recommended in the absence of symptoms. In patients with symptoms suggestive of thyroid disease or patients with hypothyroidism and a recent change in levothyroxine dosage, it is reasonable to obtain a preoperative thyroid-stimulating hormone level, although there are no guidelines to support such an approach.

In patients with hypothyroidism treated with levothyroxine, therapy should continue uninterrupted. Patients with untreated, asymptomatic mild hypothyroidism may proceed to surgery. A recent retrospective cohort study demonstrated that mild hypothyroidism (median thyroid-stimulating hormone level of 8.6 µU/mL [8.6 mU/L]) was not associated with an increase in perioperative mortality, cardiovascular morbidity, or infectious morbidity. In the presence of severe hypothyroidism, elective surgery should be postponed to prevent myxedema coma, arrhythmias, perioperative hypotension, and other complications.

Patients with well-controlled hyperthyroidism should be continued on therapy, including β-blockers and thionamides. Patients with uncontrolled hyperthyroidism are at risk for thyroid storm in the perioperative period, and surgery should be deferred until thyroid disease can be controlled.

Consultation with an endocrinologist is advised if emergent surgery is required in patients with severe thyroid disease.

Adrenal Insufficiency

Patients with adrenal insufficiency should be evaluated for the need for perioperative supplemental glucocorticoid dosing, known as stress dosing. The decision to initiate perioperative stress dosing is guided by limited evidence, although one strategy uses patient characteristics and the degree of surgical stress to determine management (**Table 101**). Perioperative supplemental glucocorticoid dosing recommendations are provided in **Table 102**.

TABLE 101. Stress Dosing Strategies in Patients at Risk for Adrenal Insufficiency

Patient Risk	Patient Characteristics	Management
High risk	Primary adrenal insufficiency	Stress dosing
	Hypothalamic-pituitary-adrenal axis disease	
	Cushingoid features	
	Equivalent of >5 mg/d of prednisone for >3 wk during the previous 3 mo	
	High-dose inhaled glucocorticoid therapy	
Moderate risk	Equivalent of >5 mg/d of prednisone for <3 wk during the previous 3 mo	Stress dosing may be indicated[a]
	High-dose topical glucocorticoid therapy	Perform preoperative adrenal axis testing
	Injectable glucocorticoid therapy in the last 3 mo	
Low risk	Equivalent of <5 mg/d of prednisone for any duration	No stress dosing
	Low-dose inhaled or topical glucocorticoid therapy	

[a]In patients at moderate risk who require emergent or urgent surgery, no further testing is recommended, and stress-dose glucocorticoids should be administered. In other patients, it is reasonable to measure morning serum cortisol preoperatively to test the hypothalamic-pituitary-adrenal axis.

TABLE 102. Perioperative Supplemental Glucocorticoid Dosing

Surgical Stress Anticipated	Daily Intravenous Hydrocortisone Dose	Duration of Stress Dosing (in Days)
Minor (e.g., ambulatory procedures)	25 mg	1
Moderate (e.g., orthopedic surgery)	50-75 mg	1-2
High (e.g., cardiac bypass graft surgery)	100 mg, followed by 50 mg every 6 hours	2-3

KEY POINTS

- In patients with diabetes mellitus who are undergoing surgery, oral and injectable noninsulin medications should be withheld, replaced with supplemental insulin, and resumed at hospital discharge or when the patient has resumed a full diet.

HVC
- Patients with untreated, asymptomatic mild hypothyroidism may proceed to surgery without further testing or treatment.

- Surgery should be deferred in patients with severe uncontrolled hypo- or hyperthyroidism.

Perioperative Management of Kidney Disease

Patients with chronic kidney disease (CKD) are at increased perioperative risk for fluid and electrolyte imbalance, metabolic acidosis, anemia, bleeding diathesis, and cardiac events, depending on the severity of the underlying disease. For patients undergoing hemodialysis, it is advisable to consult a nephrologist for review of the dialysate prescription, adjustment of fluid removal, and management of peridialysis heparin. Patients with less advanced CKD require correction of electrolyte abnormalities and optimization of volume status preoperatively. In all patients with kidney disease undergoing surgery, it is important to avoid iodinated contrast dye and other nephrotoxic agents and minimize perioperative hypotension.

Perioperative acute kidney injury portends an increased risk for postoperative CKD and, in those with underlying CKD, end-stage kidney disease. The two most important means of mitigating the risk for acute kidney injury are maintenance of renal blood flow and avoidance of further insults to the kidneys. Renal blood flow is maintained by avoiding renal hypoperfusion; effectively managing diuresis and antihypertensive medications; and treating anemia, which may impair peripheral vasodilation. Careful medication review is also warranted to ensure appropriate dosing based on renal clearance. ▪

KEY POINT

- The two most important means of mitigating the risk for acute kidney injury in the perioperative period are maintenance of renal blood flow and avoidance of further insults to the kidneys.

Perioperative Management of Liver Disease

Liver disease increases risk for perioperative infection, encephalopathy, bleeding, fluid retention, and acute kidney and liver decompensation. Patients with chronic liver disease require careful preoperative evaluation and risk stratification using the Model for End-stage Liver Disease (MELD) score and Child-Turcotte-Pugh classification. Patients with compensated liver disease, including those with a MELD score of less than 8 to 10, are often able to proceed with surgery with optimal medical management. In patients with intermediate risk, referral to a hepatologist is reasonable before proceeding with surgery. Those with severe liver disease are at increased and often prohibitive risk for perioperative complications and death; patients with Child-Turcotte-Pugh class C disease and a MELD score greater than 15 are generally advised to avoid elective surgery and should be referred for transplant evaluation if appropriate.

Complications of liver disease should be optimally managed in all patients; however, the American Association for the Study of Liver Diseases recommends against perioperative transjugular intrahepatic portosystemic shunt placement because of a lack of evidence that the procedure improves outcomes.

In general, patients with liver disease should be advised to abstain from alcohol consumption for at least 12 weeks before elective surgery.

Perioperative Management of Neurologic Disease

Patients with neurologic disease are at increased perioperative risk for loss of disease control, among other complications. In patients with epilepsy, perioperative seizure risk is thought to be driven by the severity of the underlying disease and seizure frequency, rather than by anesthesia or surgery type; an important exception is intracranial surgery, which may provoke seizures depending on the location of the surgery, underlying pathologic conditions, and required degree of brain manipulation. Antiepileptic medications should be continued uninterrupted. In patients who are unable to tolerate oral intake, alternate formulations should be used.

Patients with Parkinson disease are predisposed to perioperative delirium, hallucinations, orthostatic hypotension, and complications related to dysphagia. It is essential that patients maintain their normal treatment regimen. Surgery should be scheduled for as early in the day as possible to minimize missed doses, and antidopaminergic antiemetics should be avoided. Parkinson-hyperpyrexia syndrome is a potentially life-threatening complication resulting from withdrawal of or reduction in the dosage of dopamine agonists; it is characterized by rigidity, fever, altered mental status, and autonomic instability.

Asymptomatic carotid bruit is a common finding in older adults but is not predictive of perioperative stroke and therefore requires no preoperative evaluation. Perioperative stroke is discussed in MKSAP 18 Neurology.

Delirium commonly occurs in the postoperative setting, especially in the elderly. Risk factors and treatment are similar to those for delirium in the general hospital setting (see MKSAP 18 Neurology).

KEY POINTS

- Patients with Parkinson disease should continue antiparkinson agents through surgery, and surgery should be scheduled for as early in the day as possible to minimize missed doses.

- **HVC** Asymptomatic carotid bruit is a common finding in older adults but is not predictive of perioperative stroke and therefore requires no preoperative evaluation.

Perioperative Management of the Pregnant Patient

In women of child-bearing age, an accurate menstrual history should be obtained, and pregnancy testing should be performed if pregnancy is suspected. Many institutions require preoperative pregnancy testing in this population.

Elective surgery should be delayed until after pregnancy. Pregnant patients who require surgery should undergo the same preoperative medical evaluation as nonpregnant patients; additional diagnostic testing is unnecessary unless directed by the obstetrician. Modifications to surgical and anesthetic techniques may be required because of the anatomic and physiologic changes of pregnancy. Close collaboration among the obstetrician, surgeon, anesthesiologist, and internist is essential. Notably, pregnancy is considered a hypercoagulable state, and the ACCP recommends perioperative mechanical or pharmacologic VTE prophylaxis for pregnant patients. Although high-quality evidence is lacking, the current body of evidence suggests that surgery does not negatively affect obstetric or maternal outcomes.

KEY POINT

- **HVC** Pregnant patients who require surgery should undergo the same preoperative medical evaluation as nonpregnant patients; additional diagnostic testing is unnecessary, but close collaboration with the patient's obstetrician is advised.

Bibliography

High Value Care in Internal Medicine

The Commonwealth Fund. U.S. spends more on health care than other high-income nations but has lower life expectancy, worse health [Press release]. October 8, 2015. Retrieved from http://www.commonwealthfund.org/~/media/files/news/news-releases/2015/oct/oecd_spending_release_10_6_15_links-ds.pdf.

Qaseem A, Alguire P, Dallas P, Feinberg LE, Fitzgerald FT, Horwitch C, et al. Appropriate use of screening and diagnostic tests to foster high-value, cost-conscious care. Ann Intern Med. 2012;156:147-9. [PMID: 22250146] doi:10.7326/0003-4819-156-2-201201170-00011

Interpretation of the Medical Literature

Barratt A, Wyer PC, Hatala R, McGinn T, Dans AL, Keitz S, et al; Evidence-Based Medicine Teaching Tips Working Group. Tips for learners of evidence-based medicine: 1. Relative risk reduction, absolute risk reduction and number needed to treat. CMAJ. 2004;171:353-8. [PMID: 15313996]

Centre for Evidence Based Medicine. Study designs. http://www.cebm.net/study-designs/. Accessed January 23, 2018.

Citrome L, Ketter TA. When does a difference make a difference? Interpretation of number needed to treat, number needed to harm, and likelihood to be helped or harmed. Int J Clin Pract. 2013;67:407-11. [PMID: 23574101] doi:10.1111/ijcp.12142

Howick J, Chalmers I, Glasziou P, Greenhalgh G, Heneghan C, Liberati A, et al. Explanation of the 2011 Oxford Centre for Evidence-Based Medicine (OCEBM) levels of evidence (background document). Oxford Centre for Evidence-Based Medicine. https://www.cebm.net/wp-content/uploads/2014/06/CEBM-Levels-of-Evidence-Background-Document-2.1.pdf. Accessed January 23, 2018.

Richardson WS, Wilson MC, Keitz SA, Wyer PC; EBM Teaching Scripts Working Group. Tips for teachers of evidence-based medicine: making sense of diagnostic test results using likelihood ratios. J Gen Intern Med. 2008;23:87-92. [PMID: 18064524]

Uman LS. Systematic reviews and meta-analyses. J Can Acad Child Adolesc Psychiatry. 2011;20:57-9. [PMID: 21286370]

Routine Care of the Healthy Patient

Bibbins-Domingo K, Grossman DC, Curry SJ, Davidson KW, Epling JW Jr, García FAR, et al; US Preventive Services Task Force. Screening for colorectal cancer: US Preventive Services Task Force recommendation statement. JAMA. 2016;315:2564-2575. [PMID: 27304597] doi:10.1001/jama.2016.5989

Bibbins-Domingo K, Grossman DC, Curry SJ, Davidson KW, Epling JW Jr, García FA, et al; US Preventive Services Task Force. Screening for obstructive sleep apnea in adults: US Preventive Services Task Force recommendation statement. JAMA. 2017;317:407-414. [PMID: 28118461] doi:10.1001/jama.2016.20325

Bibbins-Domingo K; U.S. Preventive Services Task Force. Aspirin use for the primary prevention of cardiovascular disease and colorectal cancer: U.S. Preventive Services Task Force recommendation statement. Ann Intern Med. 2016;164:836-45. [PMID: 27064677] doi:10.7326/M16-0577

Crowley RA; Health and Public Policy Committee of the American College of Physicians. Climate change and health: a position paper of the American College of Physicians. Ann Intern Med. 2016;164:608-10. [PMID: 27089232] doi:10.7326/M15-2766

Curry SJ, Krist AH, Owens DK, Barry MJ, Caughey AB, Davidson KW, et al; US Preventive Services Task Force. Screening for cervical cancer: US Preventive Services Task Force recommendation statement. JAMA. 2018;320:674-686. [PMID: 30140884] doi:10.1001/jama.2018.10897

Curry SJ, Krist AH, Owens DK, Barry MJ, Caughey AB, Davidson KW, et al; US Preventive Services Task Force. Screening for osteoporosis to prevent fractures: US Preventive Services Task Force recommendation statement. JAMA. 2018;319:2521-2531. [PMID: 29946735] doi:10.1001/jama.2018.7498

DiazGranados CA, Dunning AJ, Kimmel M, Kirby D, Treanor J, Collins A, et al. Efficacy of high-dose versus standard-dose influenza vaccine in older adults. N Engl J Med. 2014;371:635-45. [PMID: 25119609] doi:10.1056/NEJMoa1315727

Grossman DC, Curry SJ, Owens DK, Bibbins-Domingo K, Caughey AB, Davidson KW, et al; US Preventive Services Task Force. Screening for prostate cancer: US Preventive Services Task Force recommendation statement. JAMA. 2018;319:1901-1913. [PMID: 29801017] doi:10.1001/jama.2018.3710

Ikeda Y, Shimada K, Teramoto T, Uchiyama S, Yamazaki T, Oikawa S, et al. Low-dose aspirin for primary prevention of cardiovascular events in Japanese patients 60 years or older with atherosclerotic risk factors: a randomized clinical trial. JAMA. 2014;312:2510-20. [PMID: 25401325] doi:10.1001/jama.2014.15690

Jørgensen T, Jacobsen RK, Toft U, Aadahl M, Glümer C, Pisinger C. Effect of screening and lifestyle counselling on incidence of ischaemic heart disease in general population: Inter99 randomised trial. BMJ. 2014;348:g3617. [PMID: 24912589] doi:10.1136/bmj.g3617

Kim DK, Riley LE, Hunter P. Advisory Committee on Immunization Practices recommended immunization schedule for adults aged 19 years or older - United States, 2018. MMWR Morb Mortal Wkly Rep. 2018;67:158-160. [PMID: 29420462] doi:10.15585/mmwr.mm6705e3

Krogsbøll LT, Jørgensen KJ, Grønhøj Larsen C, Gøtzsche PC. General health checks in adults for reducing morbidity and mortality from disease: Cochrane systematic review and meta-analysis. BMJ. 2012;345:e7191. [PMID: 23169868] doi:10.1136/bmj.e7191

LeFevre ML; U.S. Preventive Services Task Force. Screening for abdominal aortic aneurysm: U.S. Preventive Services Task Force recommendation statement. Ann Intern Med. 2014;161:281-90. [PMID: 24957320] doi:10.7326/M14-1204

Moyer VA; U.S. Preventive Services Task Force. Risk assessment, genetic counseling, and genetic testing for BRCA-related cancer in women: U.S. Preventive Services Task Force recommendation statement. Ann Intern Med. 2014;160:271-81. [PMID: 24366376]

Oeffinger KC, Fontham ET, Etzioni R, Herzig A, Michaelson JS, Shih YC, et al; American Cancer Society. Breast cancer screening for women at average risk: 2015 guideline update from the American Cancer Society. JAMA. 2015;314:1599-614. [PMID: 26501536] doi:10.1001/jama.2015.12783

Saito Y, Okada S, Ogawa H, Soejima H, Sakuma M, Nakayama M, et al; JPAD Trial Investigators. Low-dose aspirin for primary prevention of cardiovascular events in patients with type 2 diabetes mellitus: 10-year follow-up of a randomized controlled trial. Circulation. 2017;135:659-670. [PMID: 27881565] doi:10.1161/CIRCULATIONAHA.116.025760

Siu AL, Bibbins-Domingo K, Grossman DC, Baumann LC, Davidson KW, Ebell M, et al; US Preventive Services Task Force (USPSTF). Screening for depression in adults: US Preventive Services Task Force recommendation statement. JAMA. 2016;315:380-7. [PMID: 26813211] doi:10.1001/jama.2015.18392

Siu AL; U.S. Preventive Services Task Force. Screening for abnormal blood glucose and type 2 diabetes mellitus: U.S. Preventive Services Task Force recommendation statement. Ann Intern Med. 2015;163:861-8. [PMID: 26501513] doi:10.7326/M15-2345

Siu AL; U.S. Preventive Services Task Force. Screening for breast cancer: U.S. Preventive Services Task Force recommendation statement. Ann Intern Med. 2016;164:279-96. [PMID: 26757170] doi:10.7326/M15-2886

Siu AL; U.S. Preventive Services Task Force. Screening for high blood pressure in adults: U.S. Preventive Services Task Force recommendation statement. Ann Intern Med. 2015;163:778-86. [PMID: 26458123] doi:10.7326/M15-2223

Teng K, Acheson LS. Genomics in primary care practice. Prim Care. 2014;41:421-35. [PMID: 24830615] doi:10.1016/j.pop.2014.02.012

van der Wouden CH, Carere DA, Maitland-van der Zee AH, Ruffin MT 4th, Roberts JS, Green RC; Impact of Personal Genomics Study Group. Consumer perceptions of interactions with primary care providers after direct-to-consumer personal genomic testing. Ann Intern Med. 2016;164:513-22. [PMID: 26928821] doi:10.7326/M15-0995

Patient Safety and Quality Improvement

The Joint Commission. Patient safety systems. Comprehensive Accreditation Manual for Hospitals. Update 2, January 2016; PS 1-53. www.jointcommission.org/assets/1/18/PSC_for_Web.pdf. Accessed May 23, 2018.

National Academies of Sciences, Engineering, and Medicine. Improving Diagnosis in Health Care. Washington, DC: The National Academies Press; 2015.

U.S. Department of Health and Human Services, Health Resources and Services Administration. Quality improvement. www.hrsa.gov/quality/toolbox/508pdfs/qualityimprovement.pdf. Published April 2011. Accessed May 23, 2018.

U.S. Department of Health and Human Services, Office of Disease Prevention and Health Promotion. National action plan to improve health literacy. https://health.gov/communication/hlactionplan/pdf/Health_Literacy_Action_Plan.pdf. Published May 2010. Accessed May 23, 2018.

Professionalism and Ethics

ABIM Foundation. American Board of Internal Medicine. Medical professionalism in the new millennium: a physician charter. Ann Intern Med. 2002;136:243-6. [PMID: 11827500]

Appelbaum PS. Clinical practice. Assessment of patients' competence to consent to treatment. N Engl J Med. 2007;357:1834-40. [PMID: 17978292]

Daniel H, Sulmasy LS; Health and Public Policy Committee of the American College of Physicians. Policy recommendations to guide the use of telemedicine in primary care settings: an American College of Physicians position paper. Ann Intern Med. 2015;163:787-9. [PMID: 26344925] doi:10.7326/M15-0498

DeMartino ES, Dudzinski DM, Doyle CK, Sperry BP, Gregory SE, Siegler M, et al. Who Decides When a Patient Can't? Statutes on Alternate Decision Makers. N Engl J Med. 2017;376:1478-1482. [PMID: 28402767] doi:10.1056/NEJMms1611497

Farnan JM, Snyder Sulmasy L, Worster BK, Chaudhry HJ, Rhyne JA, Arora VM; American College of Physicians Ethics, Professionalism and Human Rights Committee. Online medical professionalism: patient and public relationships: policy statement from the American College of Physicians and the Federation of State Medical Boards. Ann Intern Med. 2013;158:620-7. [PMID: 23579867] doi:10.7326/0003-4819-158-8-201304160-00100

Halpern SD, Emanuel EJ. Can the United States buy better advance care planning? Ann Intern Med. 2015;162:224-5. [PMID: 25486099] doi:10.7326/M14-2476

Owens DK, Qaseem A, Chou R, Shekelle P; Clinical Guidelines Committee of the American College of Physicians. High-value, cost-conscious health care: concepts for clinicians to evaluate the benefits, harms, and costs of medical interventions. Ann Intern Med. 2011;154:174-80. [PMID: 21282697] doi:10.7326/0003-4819-154-3-201102010-00007

Snyder Sulmasy L, Mueller PS; Ethics, Professionalism and Human Rights Committee of the American College of Physicians. Ethics and the legalization of physician-assisted suicide: an American College of Physicians position paper. Ann Intern Med. 2017;167(8):576-578. [PMID: 28975242] doi: 10.7326/M17-0938

Palliative Medicine

Bernacki RE, Block SD; American College of Physicians High Value Care Task Force. Communication about serious illness care goals: a review and synthesis of best practices. JAMA Intern Med. 2014;174:1994-2003. [PMID: 25330167] doi:10.1001/jamainternmed.2014.5271

Kavalieratos D, Corbelli J, Zhang D, Dionne-Odom JN, Ernecoff NC, Hanmer J, et al. Association between palliative care and patient and caregiver outcomes: a systematic review and meta-analysis. JAMA. 2016;316:2104-2114. [PMID: 27893131] doi:10.1001/jama.2016.16840

Quill TE, Abernethy AP. Generalist plus specialist palliative care—creating a more sustainable model. N Engl J Med. 2013;368:1173-5. [PMID: 23465068] doi:10.1056/NEJMp1215620

Strand JJ, Kamdar MM, Carey EC. Top 10 things palliative care clinicians wished everyone knew about palliative care. Mayo Clin Proc. 2013;88:859-65. [PMID: 23910412] doi:10.1016/j.mayocp.2013.05.020

Swetz KM, Kamal AH. Palliative care. Ann Intern Med. 2018;168:ITC33-ITC48. [PMID: 29507970] doi:10.7326/AITC201803060

Temel JS, Greer JA, Muzikansky A, Gallagher ER, Admane S, Jackson VA, et al. Early palliative care for patients with metastatic non-small-cell lung cancer. N Engl J Med. 2010;363:733-42. [PMID: 20818875] doi:10.1056/NEJMoa1000678

Common Symptoms

Abernethy AP, McDonald CF, Frith PA, Clark K, Herndon JE 2nd, Marcello J, et al. Effect of palliative oxygen versus room air in relief of breathlessness in patients with refractory dyspnoea: a double-blind, randomised controlled trial. Lancet. 2010;376:784-93. [PMID: 20816546] doi:10.1016/S0140-6736(10)61115-4

Chow AW, Benninger MS, Brook I, Brozek JL, Goldstein EJ, Hicks LA, et al; Infectious Diseases Society of America. IDSA clinical practice guideline for acute bacterial rhinosinusitis in children and adults. Clin Infect Dis. 2012;54:e72-e112. [PMID: 22438350] doi:10.1093/cid/cir1043

Committee on the Diagnostic Criteria for Myalgic Encephalomyelitis/Chronic Fatigue Syndrome, Board on the Health of Select Populations, Institute of Medicine. Beyond Myalgic Encephalomyelitis/Chronic Fatigue Syndrome: Redefining an Illness. Washington (DC): National Academies Press (US); 2015 Feb 10. [PMID: 25695122]

Costantino G, Sun BC, Barbic F, Bossi I, Casazza G, Dipaola F, et al. Syncope clinical management in the emergency department: a consensus from the first international workshop on syncope risk stratification in the emergency department. Eur Heart J. 2016;37:1493-8. [PMID: 26242712] doi:10.1093/eurheartj/ehv378

Dowell D, Haegerich TM, Chou R. CDC guideline for prescribing opioids for chronic pain-United States, 2016. JAMA. 2016;315:1624-45. [PMID: 26977696] doi:10.1001/jama.2016.1464

Evens A, Vendetta L, Krebs K, Herath P. Medically unexplained neurologic symptoms: a primer for physicians who make the initial encounter. Am J Med. 2015;128:1059-64. [PMID: 25910791] doi:10.1016/j.amjmed.2015.03.030

Gibson P, Wang G, McGarvey L, Vertigan AE, Altman KW, Birring SS; CHEST Expert Cough Panel. Treatment of unexplained chronic cough: CHEST guideline and expert panel report. Chest. 2016;149:27-44. [PMID: 26426314] doi:10.1378/chest.15-1496

Hallenbeck J. Pathophysiologies of dyspnea explained: why might opioids relieve dyspnea and not hasten death? J Palliat Med. 2012;15:848-53. [PMID: 22594628] doi:10.1089/jpm.2011.0167

Haller H, Cramer H, Lauche R, Dobos G. Somatoform disorders and medically unexplained symptoms in primary care. Dtsch Arztebl Int. 2015;112:279-87. [PMID: 25939319] doi:10.3238/arztebl.2015.0279

Hooten M, Thorson D, Bianco J, Bonte B, Clavel Jr A, Hora J, et al. Pain: assessment, non-opioid treatment approaches and opioid management. Bloomington (MN): Institute for Clinical Systems Improvement (ICSI); 2016 Sep. 160 p. Available at https://www.icsi.org/guidelines_more/catalog_guidelines_and_more/catalog_guidelines/catalog_neurological_guidelines/pain/.

Kim JS, Zee DS. Clinical practice. Benign paroxysmal positional vertigo. N Engl J Med. 2014;370:1138-47. [PMID: 24645946] doi:10.1056/NEJMcp1309481

Lipsitt DR, Joseph R, Meyer D, Notman MT. Medically unexplained symptoms: barriers to effective treatment when nothing is the matter. Harv Rev Psychiatry. 2015;23:438-48. [PMID: 26378814] doi:10.1097/HRP.0000000000000055

Masters PA. In the clinic. Insomnia. Ann Intern Med. 2014;161:ITC1-15; quiz ITC16. [PMID: 25285559] doi:10.7326/0003-4819-161-7-201410070-01004

Nable JV, Tupe CL, Gehle BD, Brady WJ. In-flight medical emergencies during commercial travel. N Engl J Med. 2015;373:939-45. [PMID: 26332548] doi:10.1056/NEJMra1409213

Parshall MB, Schwartzstein RM, Adams L, Banzett RB, Manning HL, Bourbeau J, et al; American Thoracic Society Committee on Dyspnea. An official American Thoracic Society statement: update on the mechanisms, assessment, and management of dyspnea. Am J Respir Crit Care Med. 2012;185:435-52. [PMID: 22336677] doi:10.1164/rccm.201111-2042ST

Prandoni P, Lensing AW, Prins MH, Ciammaichella M, Perlati M, Mumoli N, et al; PESIT Investigators. Prevalence of pulmonary embolism among patients hospitalized for syncope. N Engl J Med. 2016;375:1524-1531. [PMID: 27797317]

Qaseem A, Kansagara D, Forciea MA, Cooke M, Denberg TD; Clinical Guidelines Committee of the American College of Physicians. Management of chronic insomnia disorder in adults: a clinical practice guideline from the American College of Physicians. Ann Intern Med. 2016;165:125-33. [PMID: 27136449] doi:10.7326/M15-2175

Sharon JD, Trevino C, Schubert MC, Carey JP. Treatment of Ménière's disease. Curr Treat Options Neurol. 2015;17:341. [PMID: 25749846] doi:10.1007/s11940-015-0341-x

Shen WK, Sheldon RS, Benditt DG, Cohen MI, Forman DE, Goldberger ZD, et al. 2017 ACC/AHA/HRS guideline for the evaluation and management of patients with syncope: executive summary: a report of the American College of Cardiology/American Heart Association Task Force on Clinical Practice Guidelines and the Heart Rhythm Society. Circulation. 2017;136:e25-e59. [PMID: 28280232] doi:10.1161/CIR.0000000000000498

Sun BC. Quality-of-life, health service use, and costs associated with syncope. Prog Cardiovasc Dis. 2013;55:370-5. [PMID: 23472773] doi:10.1016/j.pcad.2012.10.009

Trauer JM, Qian MY, Doyle JS, Rajaratnam SM, Cunnington D. Cognitive behavioral therapy for chronic insomnia: a systematic review and meta-analysis. Ann Intern Med. 2015;163:191-204. [PMID: 26054060] doi:10.7326/M14-2841

Venhovens J, Meulstee J, Verhagen WI. Acute vestibular syndrome: a critical review and diagnostic algorithm concerning the clinical differentiation of peripheral versus central aetiologies in the emergency department. J Neurol. 2016;263:2151-2157. [PMID: 26984607]

Whiting PF, Wolff RF, Deshpande S, Di Nisio M, Duffy S, Hernandez AV, et al. Cannabinoids for medical use: a systematic review and meta-analysis. JAMA. 2015;313:2456-73. [PMID: 26103030] doi:10.1001/jama.2015.6358

Musculoskeletal Pain

Abdel Shaheed C, Maher CG, Williams KA, Day R, McLachlan AJ. Efficacy, tolerability, and dose-dependent effects of opioid analgesics for low back pain: a systematic review and meta-analysis. JAMA Intern Med. 2016;176:958-68. [PMID: 27213267] doi:10.1001/jamainternmed.2016.1251

Buller LT, Jose J, Baraga M, Lesniak B. Thoracic outlet syndrome: current concepts, imaging features, and therapeutic strategies. Am J Orthop (Belle Mead NJ). 2015;44:376-82. [PMID: 26251937]

Chou R. In the clinic. Low back pain. Ann Intern Med. 2014;160:ITC6-1. [PMID: 25009837]

Cohen SP. Epidemiology, diagnosis, and treatment of neck pain. Mayo Clin Proc. 2015;90:284-99. [PMID: 25659245] doi:10.1016/j.mayocp.2014.09.008

Deyo RA, Mirza SK. Clinical practice. Herniated lumbar intervertebral disk. N Engl J Med. 2016;374:1763-72. [PMID: 27144851] doi:10.1056/NEJMcp1512658

Goossens P, Keijsers E, van Geenen RJ, Zijta A, van den Broek M, Verhagen AP, et al. Validity of the Thessaly test in evaluating meniscal tears compared with arthroscopy: a diagnostic accuracy study. J Orthop Sports Phys Ther. 2015;45:18-24, B1. [PMID: 25420009] doi:10.2519/jospt.2015.5215

Gross AR, Paquin JP, Dupont G, Blanchette S, Lalonde P, Cristie T, et al; Cervical Overview Group. Exercises for mechanical neck disorders: A Cochrane review update. Man Ther. 2016;24:25-45. [PMID: 27317503] doi:10.1016/j.math.2016.04.005

Hong E, Kraft MC. Evaluating anterior knee pain. Med Clin North Am. 2014;98:697-717, xi. [PMID: 24994047] doi:10.1016/j.mcna.2014.03.001

Iyer S, Kim HJ. Cervical radiculopathy. Curr Rev Musculoskelet Med. 2016;9:272-80. [PMID: 27250042] doi:10.1007/s12178-016-9349-4

Krebs EE, Gravely A, Nugent S, Jensen AC, DeRonne B, Goldsmith ES, et al. Effect of opioid vs nonopioid medications on pain-related function in patients with chronic back pain or hip or knee osteoarthritis pain: the SPACE randomized clinical trial. JAMA. 2018;319:872-882. [PMID: 29509867] doi:10.1001/jama.2018.0899

Li HY, Hua YH. Achilles tendinopathy: current concepts about the basic science and clinical treatments. Biomed Res Int. 2016;2016:6492597. [PMID: 27885357]

Maher C, Underwood M, Buchbinder R. Non-specific low back pain. Lancet. 2017;389:736-747. [PMID: 27745712] doi:10.1016/S0140-6736(16)30970-9

Olaussen M, Holmedal O, Lindbaek M, Brage S, Solvang H. Treating lateral epicondylitis with corticosteroid injections or non-electrotherapeutical physiotherapy: a systematic review. BMJ Open. 2013;3:e003564. [PMID: 24171937] doi:10.1136/bmjopen-2013-003564

Page MJ, Green S, Kramer S, Johnston RV, McBain B, Chau M, et al. Manual therapy and exercise for adhesive capsulitis (frozen shoulder). Cochrane Database Syst Rev. 2014:CD011275. [PMID: 25157702] doi:10.1002/14651858.CD011275

Qaseem A, Wilt TJ, McLean RM, Forciea MA; Clinical Guidelines Committee of the American College of Physicians. Noninvasive treatments for acute, subacute, and chronic low back pain: a clinical practice guideline from the American College of Physicians. Ann Intern Med. 2017;166:514-530. [PMID: 28192789] doi:10.7326/M16-2367

Tenforde AS, Yin A, Hunt KJ. Foot and ankle injuries in runners. Phys Med Rehabil Clin N Am. 2016;27:121-37. [PMID: 26616180] doi:10.1016/j.pmr.2015.08.007

Verdugo RJ, Salinas RA, Castillo JL, Cea JG. Surgical versus non-surgical treatment for carpal tunnel syndrome. Cochrane Database Syst Rev. 2008:CD001552. [PMID: 18843618] doi:10.1002/14651858.CD001552.pub2

Wilson JJ, Furukawa M. Evaluation of the patient with hip pain. Am Fam Physician. 2014;89:27-34. [PMID: 24444505]

Dyslipidemia

Bibbins-Domingo K, Grossman DC, Curry SJ, Davidson KW, Epling JW Jr, García FA, et al; US Preventive Services Task Force. Statin use for the primary prevention of cardiovascular disease in adults: US Preventive Services Task Force recommendation statement. JAMA. 2016;316:1997-2007. [PMID: 27838723] doi:10.1001/jama.2016.15450

Eckel RH, Jakicic JM, Ard JD, de Jesus JM, Houston Miller N, Hubbard VS, et al; American College of Cardiology/American Heart Association Task Force on Practice Guidelines. 2013 AHA/ACC guideline on lifestyle management to reduce cardiovascular risk: a report of the American College of Cardiology/ American Heart Association Task Force on Practice Guidelines. Circulation. 2014;129:S76-99. [PMID: 24222015] doi:10.1161/01.cir.0000437740.48606.d1

Jellinger PS, Handelsman Y, Rosenblit PD, Bloomgarden ZT, Fonseca VA, Garber AJ, et al. American Association of Clinical Endocrinologists and American College of Endocrinology guidelines for management of dyslipidemia and prevention of cardiovascular disease. Endocr Pract. 2017;23:1-87. [PMID: 28437620] doi:10.4158/EP171764.APPGL

Lloyd-Jones DM, Morris PB, Ballantyne CM, Birtcher KK, Daly DD Jr, DePalma SM, et al. 2017 Focused update of the 2016 ACC expert consensus decision pathway on the role of non-statin therapies for LDL-cholesterol lowering in the management of atherosclerotic cardiovascular disease risk: a report of the American College of Cardiology Task Force on Expert Consensus Decision Pathways. J Am Coll Cardiol. 2017;70:1785-1822. [PMID: 28886926] doi:10.1016/j.jacc.2017.07.745

Stone NJ, Robinson JG, Lichtenstein AH, Bairey Merz CN, Blum CB, Eckel RH, et al; American College of Cardiology/American Heart Association Task Force on Practice Guidelines. 2013 ACC/AHA guideline on the treatment of blood cholesterol to reduce atherosclerotic cardiovascular risk in adults: a report of the American College of Cardiology/American Heart Association Task Force on Practice Guidelines. Circulation. 2014;129:S1-45. [PMID: 24222016] doi:10.1161/01.cir.0000437738.63853.7a

Van Horn L, Carson JA, Appel LJ, Burke LE, Economos C, Karmally W, et al; American Heart Association Nutrition Committee of the Council on Lifestyle and Cardiometabolic Health; Council on Cardiovascular Disease in the Young; Council on Cardiovascular and Stroke Nursing; Council on Clinical Cardiology; and Stroke Council. Recommended dietary pattern to achieve adherence to the American Heart Association/American College of Cardiology (AHA/ACC) guidelines: a scientific statement from the American Heart Association. Circulation. 2016;134:e505-e529. [PMID: 27789558]

Obesity

Behary J, Kumbhari V. Advances in the endoscopic management of obesity. Gastroenterol Res Pract. 2015;2015:757821. [PMID: 26106413] doi:10.1155/2015/757821

Chang SH, Stoll CR, Song J, Varela JE, Eagon CJ, Colditz GA. The effectiveness and risks of bariatric surgery: an updated systematic review and meta-analysis, 2003-2012. JAMA Surg. 2014;149:275-87. [PMID: 24352617] doi:10.1001/jamasurg.2013.3654

Flegal KM, Kruszon-Moran D, Carroll MD, Fryar CD, Ogden CL. Trends in obesity among adults in the United States, 2005 to 2014. JAMA. 2016;315:2284-91. [PMID: 27272580] doi:10.1001/jama.2016.6458

Jacob JA. Obesity-related medical care costs Medicaid $8 billion a year. Health agencies update. JAMA 2015;314(24):2607. doi:10.1001/jama.2015.16829

Jensen MD, Ryan DH, Apovian CM, Ard JD, Comuzzie AG, Donato KA, et al; American College of Cardiology/American Heart Association Task Force on Practice Guidelines. 2013 AHA/ACC/TOS guideline for the management of overweight and obesity in adults: a report of the American College of Cardiology/American Heart Association Task Force on Practice Guidelines and The Obesity Society. Circulation. 2014;129:S102-38. [PMID: 24222017] doi:10.1161/01.cir.0000437739.71477.ee

Johnston BC, Kanters S, Bandayrel K, Wu P, Naji F, Siemieniuk RA, et al. Comparison of weight loss among named diet programs in overweight and obese adults: a meta-analysis. JAMA. 2014;312:923-33. [PMID: 25182101] doi:10.1001/jama.2014.10397

Khera R, Murad MH, Chandar AK, Dulai PS, Wang Z, Prokop LJ, et al. Association of pharmacological treatments for obesity with weight loss and adverse events: a systematic review and meta-analysis. JAMA. 2016;315:2424-34. [PMID: 27299618] doi:10.1001/jama.2016.7602

Marcotte E, Chand B. Management and prevention of surgical and nutritional complications after bariatric surgery. Surg Clin North Am. 2016;96:843-56. [PMID: 27473805] doi:10.1016/j.suc.2016.03.006

Moyer VA; U.S. Preventive Services Task Force. Screening for and management of obesity in adults: U.S. Preventive Services Task Force recommendation statement. Ann Intern Med. 2012;157:373-8. [PMID: 22733087]

Men's Health

Crawford P, Crop JA. Evaluation of scrotal masses. Am Fam Physician. 2014;89:723-7. [PMID: 24784335]

McVary KT, Roehrborn CG, Avins AL, et al. American Urological Association guideline: management of benign prostatic hyperplasia (BPH). Linthicum, MD: American Urological Association; 2010. https://www.auanet.org/education/guidelines/benign-prostatic-hyperplasia.cfm. Accessed January 20, 2017.

Nehra A, Jackson G, Miner M, Billups KL, Burnett AL, Buvat J, et al. The Princeton III Consensus recommendations for the management of erectile dysfunction and cardiovascular disease. Mayo Clin Proc. 2012;87:766-78. [PMID: 22862865] doi:10.1016/j.mayocp.2012.06.015

Pearson R, Williams PM. Common questions about the diagnosis and management of benign prostatic hyperplasia. Am Fam Physician. 2014;90:769-74. [PMID: 25611711]

Sharp VJ, Takacs EB, Powell CR. Prostatitis: diagnosis and treatment. Am Fam Physician. 2010;82:397-406. [PMID: 20704171]

Snyder PJ, Bhasin S, Cunningham GR, Matsumoto AM, Stephens-Shields AJ, Cauley JA, et al; Testosterone Trials Investigators. Effects of testosterone treatment in older men. N Engl J Med. 2016;374:611-24. [PMID: 26886521] doi:10.1056/NEJMoa1506119

Women's Health

American College of Radiology. ACR Appropriateness Criteria. Palpable breast masses. Available at https://acsearch.acr.org/docs/69495/Narrative/. Accessed March 15, 2018.

Goyal A. Breast pain. Am Fam Physician. 2016;93:872-3. [PMID: 27175723]

Grossman DC, Curry SJ, Owens DK, Barry MJ, Davidson KW, Doubeni CA, et al; US Preventive Services Task Force. Hormone therapy for the primary prevention of chronic conditions in postmenopausal women: US Preventive Services Task Force recommendation statement. JAMA. 2017;318:2224-2233. [PMID: 29234814]

Joffe HV, Chang C, Sewell C, Easley O, Nguyen C, Dunn S, et al. FDA approval of flibanserin--treating hypoactive sexual desire disorder. N Engl J Med. 2016;374:101-4. [PMID: 26649985]

Mitchell CM, Reed SD, Diem S, Larson JC, Newton KM, Ensrud KE, et al. Efficacy of vaginal estradiol or vaginal moisturizer vs placebo for treating postmenopausal vulvovaginal symptoms: a randomized clinical trial. JAMA Intern Med. 2018;178:681-690. [PMID: 29554173] doi:10.1001/jamainternmed.2018.0116

Munro MG, Critchley HO, Broder MS, Fraser IS; FIGO Working Group on Menstrual Disorders. FIGO classification system (PALM-COEIN) for causes of abnormal uterine bleeding in nongravid women of reproductive age. Int J Gynaecol Obstet. 2011;113:3-13. [PMID: 21345435]

The NAMS 2017 Hormone Therapy Position Statement Advisory Panel. The 2017 hormone therapy position statement of The North American Menopause Society. Menopause. 2017;24:728-753. [PMID: 28650869]

Neal L, Sandhu NP, Hieken TJ, Glazebrook KN, Mac Bride MB, Dilaveri CA, et al. Diagnosis and management of benign, atypical, and indeterminate breast lesions detected on core needle biopsy. Mayo Clin Proc. 2014;89:536-47. [PMID: 24684875]

Portman DJ, Gass ML; Vulvovaginal Atrophy Terminology Consensus Conference Panel. Genitourinary syndrome of menopause: new terminology for vulvovaginal atrophy from the International Society for the Study of Women's Sexual Health and the North American Menopause Society. Menopause. 2014;21:1063-8. [PMID: 25160739]

Steege JF, Siedhoff MT. Chronic pelvic pain. Obstet Gynecol. 2014;124:616-29. [PMID: 25162265]

Workowski KA, Bolan GA; Centers for Disease Control and Prevention. Sexually transmitted diseases treatment guidelines, 2015. MMWR Recomm Rep. 2015;64:1-137. [PMID: 26042815]

Eye Disorders

Azari AA, Barney NP. Conjunctivitis: a systematic review of diagnosis and treatment. JAMA. 2013;310:1721-9. [PMID: 24150468] doi:10.1001/jama.2013.280318

Gelston CD. Common eye emergencies. Am Fam Physician. 2013;88:515-9. [PMID: 24364572]

Lim LS, Mitchell P, Seddon JM, Holz FG, Wong TY. Age-related macular degeneration. Lancet. 2012;379:1728-38. [PMID: 22559899] doi:10.1016/S0140-6736(12)60282-7

Moyer VA; U.S. Preventive Services Task Force. Screening for glaucoma: U.S. Preventive Services Task Force recommendation statement. Ann Intern Med. 2013;159:484-9. [PMID: 24325017]

Narayana S, McGee S. Bedside diagnosis of the 'red eye': a systematic review. Am J Med. 2015;128:1220-1224.e1. [PMID: 26169885] doi:10.1016/j.amjmed.2015.06.026

Bibliography

Weinreb RN, Aung T, Medeiros FA. The pathophysiology and treatment of glaucoma: a review. JAMA. 2014;311:1901-11. [PMID: 24825645] doi:10.1001/jama.2014.3192

Ear, Nose, Mouth, and Throat Disorders

Baguley D, McFerran D, Hall D. Tinnitus. Lancet. 2013;382:1600-7. [PMID: 23827090] doi:10.1016/S0140-6736(13)60142-7

Gauer RL, Semidey MJ. Diagnosis and treatment of temporomandibular disorders. Am Fam Physician. 2015;91:378-86. [PMID: 25822556]

Harris AM, Hicks LA, Qaseem A; High Value Care Task Force of the American College of Physicians and for the Centers for Disease Control and Prevention. Appropriate antibiotic use for acute respiratory tract infection in adults: advice for high-value care from the American College of Physicians and the Centers for Disease Control and Prevention. Ann Intern Med. 2016;164:425-34. [PMID: 26785402] doi:10.7326/M15-1840

Kociolek LK, Shulman ST. In the clinic. Pharyngitis. Ann Intern Med. 2012;157:ITC3-1 - ITC3-16. [PMID: 22944886] doi:10.7326/0003-4819-157-5-20120904-01003

Moyer VA; U.S. Preventive Services Task Force. Screening for hearing loss in older adults: U.S. Preventive Services Task Force recommendation statement. Ann Intern Med. 2012;157:655-61. [PMID: 22893115]

Uy J, Forciea MA. In the clinic. Hearing loss. Ann Intern Med. 2013;158:ITC4-1; quiz ITC4-16. [PMID: 23546583] doi:10.7326/0003-4819-158-7-201304020-01004

Wilson JF. In the clinic. Acute sinusitis. Ann Intern Med. 2010;153:ITC31-15; quiz ITC316. [PMID: 20820036] doi:10.7326/0003-4819-153-5-201009070-01003

Mental and Behavioral Health

Bachhuber MA, Hennessy S, Cunningham CO, Starrels JL. Increasing benzodiazepine prescriptions and overdose mortality in the United States, 1996-2013. Am J Public Health. 2016;106:686-8. [PMID: 26890165] doi:10.2105/AJPH.2016.303061

Dickstein LP, Franco KN, Rome ES, Auron M. Recognizing, managing medical consequences of eating disorders in primary care. Cleve Clin J Med. 2014;81:255-63. [PMID: 24692444] doi:10.3949/ccjm.81a.12132

Edelman EJ, Fiellin DA. In the clinic. Alcohol use. Ann Intern Med. 2016;164:ITC1-16. [PMID: 26747315] doi:10.7326/AITC201601050

Larochelle MR, Liebschutz JM, Zhang F, Ross-Degnan D, Wharam JF. Opioid prescribing after nonfatal overdose and association with repeated overdose: a cohort study. Ann Intern Med. 2016;164:1-9. [PMID: 26720742] doi:10.7326/M15-0038

Lindson-Hawley N, Banting M, West R, Michie S, Shinkins B, Aveyard P. Gradual versus abrupt smoking cessation: a randomized, controlled noninferiority trial. Ann Intern Med. 2016;164:585-92. [PMID: 26975007] doi:10.7326/M14-2805

Moyer VA; Preventive Services Task Force. Screening and behavioral counseling interventions in primary care to reduce alcohol misuse: U.S. Preventive Services Task Force recommendation statement. Ann Intern Med. 2013;159:210-8. [PMID: 23698791] doi:10.7326/0003-4819-159-3-201308060-00652

Pace CA, Samet JH. In the clinic. Substance use disorders. Ann Intern Med. 2016;164:ITC49-ITC64. [PMID: 27043992] doi:10.7326/AITC201604050

Patel MS, Steinberg MB. In the clinic. Smoking cessation. Ann Intern Med. 2016;164:ITC33-ITC48. [PMID: 26926702] doi:10.7326/AITC201603010

Qaseem A, Barry MJ, Kansagara D; Clinical Guidelines Committee of the American College of Physicians. Nonpharmacologic versus pharmacologic treatment of adult patients with major depressive disorder: a clinical practice guideline from the American College of Physicians. Ann Intern Med. 2016;164:350-9. [PMID: 26857948] doi:10.7326/M15-2570

Schuckit MA. Treatment of opioid-use disorders. N Engl J Med. 2016;375:357-68. [PMID: 27464203] doi:10.1056/NEJMra1604339

Siu AL; U.S. Preventive Services Task Force. Behavioral and pharmacotherapy interventions for tobacco smoking cessation in adults, including pregnant women: U.S. Preventive Services Task Force recommendation statement. Ann Intern Med. 2015;163:622-34. [PMID: 26389730] doi:10.7326/M15-2023

Geriatric Medicine

Buta BJ, Walston JD, Godino JG, Park M, Kalyani RR, Xue QL, et al. Frailty assessment instruments: systematic characterization of the uses and contexts of highly-cited instruments. Ageing Res Rev. 2016;26:53-61. [PMID: 26674984] doi:10.1016/j.arr.2015.12.003

Carlson C, Merel SE, Yukawa M. Geriatric syndromes and geriatric assessment for the generalist. Med Clin North Am. 2015;99:263-79. [PMID: 25700583] doi:10.1016/j.mcna.2014.11.003

Chou R, Dana T, Bougatsos C, Grusing S, Blazina I. Screening for impaired visual acuity in older adults: updated evidence report and systematic review for the US Preventive Services Task Force. JAMA. 2016;315:915-33. [PMID: 26934261] doi:10.1001/jama.2016.0783

Dong X. Screening for elder abuse in healthcare settings: why should we care, and is it a missed quality indicator? J Am Geriatr Soc. 2015;63:1686-8. [PMID: 26277299] doi:10.1111/jgs.13538

Gormley EA, Lightner DJ, Faraday M, Vasavada SP; American Urological Association. Diagnosis and treatment of overactive bladder (non-neurogenic) in adults: AUA/SUFU guideline amendment. J Urol. 2015;193:1572-80. [PMID: 25623739] doi:10.1016/j.juro.2015.01.087

Lin JS, O'Connor E, Rossom RC, Perdue LA, Eckstrom E. Screening for cognitive impairment in older adults: a systematic review for the U.S. Preventive Services Task Force. Ann Intern Med. 2013;159:601-12. [PMID: 24145578]

Martin AJ, Marottoli R, O'Neill D. Driving assessment for maintaining mobility and safety in drivers with dementia. Cochrane Database Syst Rev. 2013:CD006222. [PMID: 23990315] doi:10.1002/14651858.CD006222.pub4

Moyer VA; U.S. Preventive Services Task Force. Screening for hearing loss in older adults: U.S. Preventive Services Task Force recommendation statement. Ann Intern Med. 2012;157:655-61. [PMID: 22893115]

Moyer VA; U.S. Preventive Services Task Force. Screening for intimate partner violence and abuse of elderly and vulnerable adults: U.S. Preventive Services Task Force recommendation statement. Ann Intern Med. 2013;158:478-86. [PMID: 23338828] doi:10.7326/0003-4819-158-6-201303190-00588

Qaseem A, Dallas P, Forciea MA, Starkey M, Denberg TD, Shekelle P; Clinical Guidelines Committee of the American College of Physicians. Nonsurgical management of urinary incontinence in women: a clinical practice guideline from the American College of Physicians. Ann Intern Med. 2014;161:429-40. [PMID: 25222388] doi:10.7326/M13-2410

Qaseem A, Humphrey LL, Forciea MA, Starkey M, Denberg TD; Clinical Guidelines Committee of the American College of Physicians. Treatment of pressure ulcers: a clinical practice guideline from the American College of Physicians. Ann Intern Med. 2015;162:370-9. [PMID: 25732279] doi:10.7326/M14-1568

Qaseem A, Mir TP, Starkey M, Denberg TD; Clinical Guidelines Committee of the American College of Physicians. Risk assessment and prevention of pressure ulcers: a clinical practice guideline from the American College of Physicians. Ann Intern Med. 2015;162:359-69. [PMID: 25732278] doi:10.7326/M14-1567

Siu AL, Bibbins-Domingo K, Grossman DC, Baumann LC, Davidson KW, Ebell M, et al; US Preventive Services Task Force (USPSTF). Screening for depression in adults: US Preventive Services Task Force recommendation statement. JAMA. 2016;315:380-7. [PMID: 26813211] doi:10.1001/jama.2015.18392

Perioperative Medicine

Apfelbaum JL, Connis RT, Nickinovich DG, Pasternak LR, Arens JF, Caplan RA, et al; Committee on Standards and Practice Parameters. Practice advisory for preanesthesia evaluation: an updated report by the American Society of Anesthesiologists Task Force on Preanesthesia Evaluation. Anesthesiology. 2012;116:522-38. [PMID: 22273990] doi:10.1097/ALN.0b013e31823c1067

Botto F, Alonso-Coello P, Chan MT, Villar JC, Xavier D, Srinathan S, et al; Vascular events In noncardiac Surgery patients cOhort evaluatioN (VISION) Writing Group, on behalf of The Vascular events In noncardiac Surgery patients cOhort evaluatioN (VISION) Investigators. Myocardial injury after noncardiac surgery: a large, international, prospective cohort study establishing diagnostic criteria, characteristics, predictors, and 30-day outcomes. Anesthesiology. 2014;120:564-78. [PMID: 24534856] doi:10.1097/ALN.0000000000000113

Daniels PR. Peri-procedural management of patients taking oral anticoagulants. BMJ. 2015;351:h2391. [PMID: 26174061] doi:10.1136/bmj.h2391

Devereaux PJ, Mrkobrada M, Sessler DI, Leslie K, Alonso-Coello P, Kurz A, et al; POISE-2 Investigators. Aspirin in patients undergoing noncardiac surgery. N Engl J Med. 2014;370:1494-503. [PMID: 24679062] doi:10.1056/NEJMoa1401105

Doherty JU, Gluckman TJ, Hucker WJ, Januzzi JL Jr, Ortel TL, Saxonhouse SJ, et al. 2017 ACC expert consensus decision pathway for periprocedural management of anticoagulation in patients with nonvalvular atrial fibrillation: a report of the American College of Cardiology Clinical Expert Consensus Document Task Force. J Am Coll Cardiol. 2017;69:871-898. [PMID: 28081965] doi:10.1016/j.jacc.2016.11.024

Douketis JD, Spyropoulos AC, Kaatz S, Becker RC, Caprini JA, Dunn AS, et al; BRIDGE Investigators. Perioperative bridging anticoagulation in patients with atrial fibrillation. N Engl J Med. 2015;373:823-33. [PMID: 26095867] doi:10.1056/NEJMoa1501035

Douketis JD, Spyropoulos AC, Spencer FA, Mayr M, Jaffer AK, Eckman MH, et al. Perioperative management of antithrombotic therapy: antithrombotic therapy and prevention of thrombosis, 9th ed: American College of Chest Physicians evidence-based clinical practice guidelines. Chest. 2012;141:e326S-e350S. [PMID: 22315266] doi:10.1378/chest.11-2298

Falck-Ytter Y, Francis CW, Johanson NA, Curley C, Dahl OE, Schulman S, et al. Prevention of VTE in orthopedic surgery patients: antithrombotic therapy and prevention of thrombosis, 9th ed: American College of Chest Physicians evidence-based clinical practice guidelines. Chest. 2012;141:e278S-e325S. [PMID: 22315265] doi:10.1378/chest.11-2404

Fleisher LA, Fleischmann KE, Auerbach AD, Barnason SA, Beckman JA, Bozkurt B, et al; American College of Cardiology. 2014 ACC/AHA guideline on perioperative cardiovascular evaluation and management of patients undergoing noncardiac surgery: a report of the American College of Cardiology/American Heart Association Task Force on practice guidelines. J Am Coll Cardiol. 2014;64:e77-137. [PMID: 25091544] doi:10.1016/j.jacc.2014.07.944

Gould MK, Garcia DA, Wren SM, Karanicolas PJ, Arcelus JI, Heit JA, et al. Prevention of VTE in nonorthopedic surgical patients: antithrombotic therapy and prevention of thrombosis, 9th ed: American College of Chest Physicians evidence-based clinical practice guidelines. Chest. 2012;141:e227S-e277S. [PMID: 22315263] doi:10.1378/chest.11-2297

Kaufman RM, Djulbegovic B, Gernsheimer T, Kleinman S, Tinmouth AT, Capocelli KE, et al; AABB. Platelet transfusion: a clinical practice guideline from the AABB. Ann Intern Med. 2015;162:205-13. [PMID: 25383671] doi:10.7326/M14-1589

Kaw R, Chung F, Pasupuleti V, Mehta J, Gay PC, Hernandez AV. Meta-analysis of the association between obstructive sleep apnoea and postoperative outcome. Br J Anaesth. 2012;109:897-906. [PMID: 22956642] doi:10.1093/bja/aes308

Levine GN, Bates ER, Bittl JA, Brindis RG, Fihn SD, Fleisher LA, et al. 2016 ACC/AHA guideline focused update on duration of dual antiplatelet therapy in patients with coronary artery disease: a report of the American College of Cardiology/American Heart Association Task Force on Clinical Practice Guidelines. J Am Coll Cardiol. 2016;68:1082-115. [PMID: 27036918] doi:10.1016/j.jacc.2016.03.513

Whelton PK, Carey RM, Aronow WS, Casey DE Jr, Collins KJ, Dennison Himmelfarb C, et al. 2017 ACC/AHA/AAPA/ABC/ACPM/AGS/APhA/ASH/ASPC/NMA/PCNA guideline for the prevention, detection, evaluation, and management of high blood pressure in adults: a report of the American College of Cardiology/American Heart Association Task Force on Clinical Practice Guidelines. J Am Coll Cardiol. 2017. [PMID: 29146535] doi:10.1016/j.jacc.2017.11.006

Zielsdorf SM, Kubasiak JC, Janssen I, Myers JA, Luu MB. A NSQIP analysis of MELD and perioperative outcomes in general surgery. Am Surg. 2015;81:755-9. [PMID: 26215235]

General Internal Medicine Self-Assessment Test

This self-assessment test contains one-best-answer multiple-choice questions. Please read these directions carefully before answering the questions. Answers, critiques, and bibliographies immediately follow these multiple-choice questions. The American College of Physicians (ACP) is accredited by the Accreditation Council for Continuing Medical Education (ACCME) to provide continuing medical education for physicians.

The American College of Physicians designates MKSAP 18 General Internal Medicine for a maximum of 36 *AMA PRA Category 1 Credits*™. Physicians should claim only the credit commensurate with the extent of their participation in the activity.

Successful completion of the CME activity, which includes participation in the evaluation component, enables the participant to earn up to 36 medical knowledge MOC points in the American Board of Internal Medicine's Maintenance of Certification (MOC) program. It is the CME activity provider's responsibility to submit participant completion information to ACCME for the purpose of granting MOC credit.

Earn Instantaneous CME Credits or MOC Points Online

Print subscribers can enter their answers online to earn instantaneous CME credits or MOC points. You can submit your answers using online answer sheets that are provided at mksap.acponline.org, where a record of your MKSAP 18 credits will be available. To earn CME credits or to apply for MOC points, you need to answer all of the questions in a test and earn a score of at least 50% correct (number of correct answers divided by the total number of questions). Please note that if you are applying for MOC points, you must also enter your birth date and ABIM candidate number.

Take either of the following approaches:

- Use the printed answer sheet at the back of this book to record your answers. Go to mksap.acponline.org, access the appropriate online answer sheet, transcribe your answers, and submit your test for instantaneous CME credits or MOC points. There is no additional fee for this service.

- Go to mksap.acponline.org, access the appropriate online answer sheet, directly enter your answers, and submit your test for instantaneous CME credits or MOC points. There is no additional fee for this service.

Earn CME Credits or MOC Points by Mail or Fax

Pay a $20 processing fee per answer sheet and submit the printed answer sheet at the back of this book by mail or fax, as instructed on the answer sheet. Make sure you calculate your score and enter your birth date and ABIM candidate number, and fax the answer sheet to 215-351-2799 or mail the answer sheet to Member and Customer Service, American College of Physicians, 190 N. Independence Mall West, Philadelphia, PA 19106-1572, using the courtesy envelope provided in your MKSAP 18 slipcase. You will need your 10-digit order number and 8-digit ACP ID number, which are printed on your packing slip. Please allow 4 to 6 weeks for your score report to be emailed back to you. Be sure to include your email address for a response.

If you do not have a 10-digit order number and 8-digit ACP ID number, or if you need help creating a username and password to access the MKSAP 18 online answer sheets, go to mksap.acponline.org or email custserv@acponline.org.

CME credits and MOC points are available from the publication date of December 31, 2018, until December 31, 2021. You may submit your answer sheet or enter your answers online at any time during this period.

Directions

Each of the numbered items is followed by lettered answers. Select the **ONE** *lettered answer that is* **BEST** *in each case.*

Self-Assessment Test

Item 1

A 35-year-old woman is evaluated after laboratory test results showed an elevated LDL cholesterol level during routine screening. Family history is remarkable for myocardial infarction in her father at age 45 years. She takes no medications.

On physical examination, vital signs are normal. BMI is 30. The remainder of the examination is unremarkable.

Laboratory studies:

Alanine aminotransferase	30 U/L
Thyroid-stimulating hormone	Normal
Total cholesterol	294 mg/dL (7.61 mmol/L)
LDL cholesterol	195 mg/dL (5.05 mmol/L)
HDL cholesterol	55 mg/dL (1.42 mmol/L)
Triglycerides	220 mg/dL (2.49 mmol/L)

The patient is instructed in therapeutic lifestyle changes to lower her risk for atherosclerotic cardiovascular disease (ASCVD).

According to the American College of Cardiology/American Heart Association cholesterol treatment guideline, which of the following is the most appropriate additional treatment for primary prevention of ASCVD in this patient?

(A) Evolocumab
(B) High-intensity rosuvastatin
(C) Moderate-intensity atorvastatin
(D) No additional treatment is necessary

Item 2

A 40-year-old woman seeks advice on whether she should undergo breast cancer screening with mammography. Her family history is negative for breast and ovarian cancers, and she has no other risk factors for breast cancer.

On physical examination, vital signs and the remainder of the examination are normal.

The patient is engaged in a discussion of the potential benefits and harms of initiating mammography now, including the potential for false-positive results and overdiagnosis. After the discussion, she states that she is not overly concerned about her risk for breast cancer but is anxious about the potential harms associated with screening.

Which of the following is the most appropriate screening test for this patient?

(A) Breast self-examination
(B) Breast tomosynthesis
(C) Screening mammography
(D) No testing

Item 3

A 49-year-old man is scheduled for total right knee arthroplasty. Medical history is otherwise unremarkable. He takes no medications.

On physical examination, vital signs are normal. The right knee demonstrates bony hypertrophy and crepitus with passive movement.

Low-molecular-weight heparin and intermittent pneumatic compression will be initiated and continued during the hospital stay.

Which of the following is the recommended duration of low-molecular-weight heparin prophylaxis for this patient?

(A) Total of 10 days
(B) Total of 14 days
(C) Total of 35 days
(D) Until fully ambulatory
(E) Until hospital discharge

Item 4

A 67-year-old man is evaluated for a 2-year history of worsening pain in his feet. He describes the pain as long-standing aching and burning. The pain is persistent, sometimes waking him from sleep. Medical history is otherwise significant for type 2 diabetes mellitus, hypertension, and hyperlipidemia. Medications are insulin glargine, insulin aspart, valsartan, aspirin, and simvastatin.

On physical examination, vital signs are normal. The feet are insensate to monofilament testing, and vibratory sensation is absent in the feet and ankles. No evidence of skin breakdown is noted.

Which of the following is the most appropriate treatment?

(A) Oral duloxetine
(B) Oral hydromorphone
(C) Oral lamotrigine
(D) Oral tramadol
(E) Topical diclofenac

Item 5

A 23-year-old woman is evaluated for depression as she prepares for discharge from the hospital to home hospice care. She was diagnosed with metastatic ovarian cancer 2 years ago, and she progressed through four lines of chemotherapy, a trial of immunotherapy, and a failed attempt at a phase 1 clinical trial. Her life expectancy is measured in weeks. She is currently hospitalized with volume depletion, and after consultation with her oncologist and palliative care team, she has decided to be discharged home with hospice care.

On physical examination, the patient exhibits substantial fatigue and poor concentration. She has a flat affect except when intermittently tearful. Previously upbeat despite all of the setbacks, she is now withdrawn and describes feeling hopeless. She has pervasive guilt over the burden she believes she has caused her family. Medications are a fentanyl patch, oxycodone, ondansetron, polyethylene glycol, senna, and zolpidem.

Self-Assessment Test

Which of the following is the most appropriate treatment?

(A) Citalopram
(B) Cognitive behavioral therapy
(C) Methylphenidate
(D) Sertraline

Item 6

A 52-year-old man is evaluated for a 2-day history of painless red eye, which began on the right side and quickly spread to the left. He reports that his eyes have a thin mucopurulent discharge and that his eyelids are matted shut in the morning upon waking. He has had no photophobia, change in visual acuity, or itching in the eyes, but he has experienced some mild rhinorrhea. He does not use contact lenses. He is sexually monogamous. Medical history is significant for type 2 diabetes mellitus treated with metformin.

On physical examination, vital signs are normal. There is redness of the sclerae bilaterally, with a white crust-like residue along the edges of the eyelids. The tarsal vessels are obscured by the conjunctival erythema. Visual acuity is intact, and there is no tenderness around the globes.

Which of the following is the most appropriate treatment?

(A) Ceftriaxone
(B) Levofloxacin ophthalmic drops
(C) Olopatadine ophthalmic drops
(D) Trimethoprim–polymyxin B ophthalmic drops

Item 7

Two new treatments for patients with heart failure with preserved ejection fraction were compared in a randomized controlled trial. The primary outcome was reduction in heart failure–related hospitalizations.

Compared with treatment B, treatment A was associated with a statistically significant absolute risk reduction of 6%, and the number needed to treat to prevent one hospitalization was 17.

Which of the following is needed to conclude that treatment A is superior to treatment B?

(A) Confidence interval
(B) Harms and cost of treatment
(C) *P* value
(D) Relative risk reduction

Item 8

A 68-year-old man is evaluated for fever, perineal pain, dysuria, frequency, and intermittent straining that began yesterday. Symptoms began 48 hours after a prostate biopsy due to an elevated prostate-specific antigen level detected during routine screening.

On physical examination, temperature is 38.7 °C (101.7 °F), blood pressure is 145/82 mm Hg, pulse rate is 105/min, and respiration rate is normal. The prostate is enlarged and boggy, and it is tender to gentle palpation. There is no penile discharge, and no scrotal pain occurs with palpation.

Dipstick urinalysis is positive for leukocyte esterase and nitrates. Urine Gram stain reveals gram-negative rods. Urine culture is pending.

Which of the following is the most appropriate treatment?

(A) Amoxicillin
(B) Ceftriaxone and doxycycline
(C) Cephalexin
(D) Trimethoprim-sulfamethoxazole

Item 9

A 22-year-old man is evaluated during a pre-employment examination. The patient is starting a new job as a registered nurse. He is asymptomatic. He received the tetanus toxoid, reduced diphtheria toxoid, and acellular pertussis (Tdap) vaccine 7 years ago and the influenza vaccine during the last influenza season. Approximately 6 months ago, he received one dose of the measles, mumps, and rubella (MMR) vaccine because of lack of documented immunity on serologic testing. Medical history is negative for chronic medical conditions. He is a nonsmoker, and he does not plan to travel outside of the United States in the near future. He takes no medications.

Physical examination is normal.

Laboratory studies are significant for a positive result on a hepatitis B surface antibody test. Hepatitis B surface antigen, hepatitis B core antibody, and hepatitis A IgG antibody levels are undetectable.

Which of the following is the most appropriate vaccination strategy for this health care worker?

(A) Administer a second dose of MMR vaccine
(B) Administer the hepatitis A vaccine
(C) Administer the hepatitis B vaccine
(D) Administer the 23-valent pneumococcal polysaccharide vaccine
(E) No vaccination at this time

Item 10

A 32-year-old woman is evaluated during a domestic airline flight for an episode of weakness and lightheadedness. She is pregnant at 35 weeks' gestation. She has had several contractions since take-off but without regularity. She reports no abdominal pain. She has no medical problems, and her only medication is a prenatal vitamin.

On physical examination, the patient appears weak. Temperature is normal, blood pressure is 105/60 mm Hg, pulse rate is 99/min, and respiration rate is 14/min. Her skin is clammy. Cardiovascular examination is unremarkable. Lungs are clear to auscultation. On abdominal examination, she has a gravid uterus.

Oxygen, 2 L/min by nasal cannula, is started. An intravenous line is placed, and fluids are initiated.

Which of the following is the most appropriate next step in management?

(A) Ask the pilot to descend to a lower altitude
(B) Connect with the ground-based physician
(C) Recommend flight diversion
(D) No further management

Item 11

An 82-year-old man is evaluated during a routine evaluation. He is accompanied to the visit by his son. The patient lives alone, and his son expresses reservations about his father continuing to drive. The patient no longer drives after dark or on the interstate highway. He limits his driving to within a 10-mile radius of his home and mainly drives for local errands and to church on Sundays. He has had no traffic accidents, but he had two recent incidents in which he misjudged the angle of his car in the grocery store parking lot and ran into the shopping cart stand. Medical history is significant for coronary artery disease, hypertension, and mild cognitive impairment. Medications are atorvastatin, aspirin, hydrochlorothiazide, lisinopril, and metoprolol.

On physical examination, blood pressure is 132/82 mm Hg, and pulse rate is 64/min; other vital signs are normal. The patient appears frail with a pleasant demeanor. He wears eyeglasses and hearing aids, and he has impaired hearing as measured by the whispered voice test. On musculoskeletal examination, limited mobility of the cervical spine is noted. He scores 26/30 on the Mini–Mental State Examination. The remainder of the examination is unremarkable.

Which of the following is the most appropriate management regarding this patient's driving?

(A) Advise the patient to retire from driving
(B) Obtain neuropsychological testing
(C) Obtain occupational therapy driving evaluation
(D) Reassure the patient he is competent to drive with self-imposed limitations

Item 12

A 36-year-old woman is evaluated for a 3-year history of fatigue that worsens after activity and does not improve with rest. She also notes intermittent diffuse myalgia and arthralgia, constipation, dizziness, headaches, urinary urgency, memory problems, and paresthesias. Her musculoskeletal symptoms, dizziness, and headache worsen in the upright position and improve when she lies back down. She has almost entirely eliminated social activities. Medical history is significant for episodic migraine and irritable bowel syndrome. Medications are sumatriptan, polyethylene glycol, and hyoscyamine.

On physical examination, vital signs are normal. BMI is 24. Neck circumference is 36 cm (14 in). The remainder of the examination is normal.

Laboratory studies obtained 6 months ago showed a normal complete blood count, electrolyte levels, kidney function test results, liver chemistry test results, fasting glucose level, serum creatine kinase level, and serum thyroid-stimulating hormone level.

Which of the following is the most appropriate diagnostic test to perform next?

(A) Antinuclear antibody assay
(B) Polysomnography
(C) Serum cortisol level measurement
(D) No further testing is recommended

Item 13

A 62-year-old man is evaluated for severe low back pain that began 2 days ago and is progressively worsening. The pain began when he was lifting concrete blocks at his job. The pain is located in his lower back and radiates into the lateral aspects of his legs bilaterally. He also has numbness and tingling in the groin. His last bowel movement was 2 days ago, and he has not urinated for the last 24 hours. Prior to the onset of the pain, the patient felt well.

On physical examination, vital signs are normal. There is decreased pinprick sensation surrounding the anus, decreased anal sphincter tone, and decreased ankle reflexes bilaterally; knee reflexes are normal. Bilateral dorsiflexion and plantar flexion weakness are present. Straight leg raise test reproduces pain bilaterally. There is no spinal tenderness.

Which of the following is the most appropriate diagnostic test to perform next?

(A) CT of the lumbosacral spine
(B) MRI of the lumbosacral spine
(C) Plain radiography of the lumbosacral spine
(D) No imaging studies are indicated

Item 14

A 24-year-old woman is evaluated for a breast lump. She has had no breast trauma or discharge from the nipples. She is nulliparous and has regular menstrual cycles. Medical history is otherwise unremarkable. The patient's mother was recently diagnosed with breast cancer at age 58 years; no other family members have breast or ovarian cancer. Her only medication is an oral contraceptive pill.

On physical examination, vital signs are normal. BMI is 25. A breast examination reveals no skin changes, with dense breast tissue bilaterally. She has a firm, 2-cm, non-tender, mobile mass with well-defined margins in the upper outer quadrant of the left breast. There is no evidence of axillary, cervical, or supraclavicular lymphadenopathy.

Which of the following is the most appropriate test to perform in this patient?

(A) Biopsy
(B) Mammography
(C) Mammography and ultrasonography
(D) Ultrasonography

Item 15

A 24-year-old man is evaluated for a 6-week history of severely depressed mood and loss of interest in work, family, and friends. During this time period, he has been sleeping more than usual (up to 11 hours per day) but still feels like he has no energy. He feels that he is a burden to his family and coworkers and admits to sometimes thinking about suicide. He had similar symptoms 2 years ago, for which he was treated with escitalopram. He remained on this therapy for only 2 weeks because his symptoms rapidly abated, and he had a "surge of energy." One year ago, he had a 4-week period during which he had a similar increase in energy level. During that time, he slept only 4 hours per night and decided that he would become a competitive triathlete. He used most of his money to start a boot camp fitness business, which closed within 2 months. He has never had hallucinations. He takes no medications and does not use alcohol or recreational drugs.

Which of the following is the most likely diagnosis?

(A) Bipolar disorder
(B) Generalized anxiety disorder
(C) Major depressive disorder
(D) Schizophrenia

Item 16

A 27-year-old man is evaluated during a routine follow-up visit for obesity. On his previous two visits, he had a BMI of 38. Despite enrollment in a 6-month comprehensive supervised weight loss program that included nutritional counseling, he has gained 2.3 kg (5.0 lb). He briefly tried orlistat but discontinued this medication because of gastrointestinal side effects. Medical history is significant for type 2 diabetes mellitus and hypertension. Medications are liraglutide, lisinopril, and metformin.

On physical examination, blood pressure is 146/91 mm Hg; other vital signs are normal. BMI is 39. The remainder of the physical examination is unremarkable.

Laboratory studies reveal a hemoglobin A_{1c} value of 8.2%.

Which of the following is the most appropriate management?

(A) Bariatric surgery
(B) Lorcaserin
(C) Referral to a dietician
(D) Very-low-calorie diet

Item 17

A 39-year-old man is evaluated for a 3-month history of dry, intermittent cough. He reports no other associated symptoms and has had no unusual environmental exposures. He is a lifelong nonsmoker. Medical history is significant for hypertension, for which he was started on lisinopril and hydrochlorothiazide 4 months ago. He has no known allergies.

On physical examination, vital signs are normal. There is no pharyngeal erythema or exudate. Lungs are clear to auscultation.

A chest radiograph is normal.

Which of the following is the most appropriate management?

(A) Discontinue lisinopril
(B) Initiate intranasal glucocorticoid therapy
(C) Obtain spirometry
(D) Start proton pump inhibitor therapy

Item 18

A 46-year-old man seeks advice on whether he should undergo prostate cancer screening. He recently underwent direct-to-consumer genetic testing, which revealed that his risk for prostate cancer is 33% higher than that of the average person. He is asymptomatic. Medical history is unremarkable. Family history is significant for prostate cancer diagnosed in his paternal grandfather at age 72 years. He takes no medications.

On physical examination, vital signs and the remainder of the examination are normal.

Which of the following is the most appropriate management?

(A) Digital rectal examination (DRE)
(B) Serum prostate-specific antigen level measurement
(C) Serum prostate-specific antigen level measurement and DRE
(D) Patient education and no further testing

Item 19

A 55-year-old woman is evaluated for left-sided tinnitus that has gradually emerged over the last 6 months. She describes the tinnitus as a high-pitched continuous (nonpulsatile) buzzing. The patient reports no hearing loss, balance difficulties, dizziness, or headaches. Her medical history is otherwise unremarkable.

On physical examination, vital signs are normal. Direct visualization of the external ear canals and tympanic membranes is unremarkable. Findings on Weber and Rinne testing suggest left sensorineural hearing loss. The whispered voice test suggests hearing loss on the left side. Results of the Romberg, cerebellar, and cranial nerve tests are all normal. Audiologic tests confirm mild to moderate left sensorineural hearing loss.

Which of the following is the most appropriate management?

(A) CT angiography of the posterior fossa
(B) MRI of the internal auditory canal
(C) Referral for hearing aid placement
(D) Urgent referral to an otolaryngologist

Item 20

An 82-year-old woman is evaluated for severe and progressive shortness of breath on ambulation. She has COPD and has been hospitalized only once in the past 18 months for an acute exacerbation. She has not experienced an acute worsening of her symptoms, and she has minimal nonproductive cough. She stopped smoking 15 years ago. She notes that her dyspnea is a substantial impediment to her quality of life. Medical history is otherwise significant for heart failure with preserved ejection fraction. Medications are umeclidinium/vilanterol and albuterol inhalers, lisinopril, and chlorthalidone.

On physical examination, temperature is 37.0 °C (98.6 °F), blood pressure is 128/78 mm Hg, pulse rate is 74/min, and respiration rate is 20/min. Oxygen saturation is 96% breathing 1 L/min of oxygen by nasal cannula and is maintained at 96% during a 6-minute walk test. Pulmonary examination reveals a prolonged expiratory phase and intermittent scattered rhonchi throughout her lung fields, with hyperresonance to percussion. Cardiac examination reveals an S_4 but no murmur or jugular venous distention.

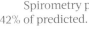

Spirometry performed 2 months ago showed an FEV_1 of 42% of predicted.

Which of the following is the most appropriate treatment?

(A) Furosemide
(B) Oxygen at 2 L/min by nasal cannula
(C) Prednisone
(D) Pulmonary rehabilitation

Item 21

A 50-year-old man is seen for preoperative medical evaluation before left shoulder arthroplasty. History is significant for alcohol-related cirrhosis and osteoarthritis. Medications are lactulose, furosemide, and spironolactone. The patient stopped drinking alcohol 5 months ago but has difficulty with medication adherence. He reports increasing ascites and lower extremity edema.

On physical examination, vital signs are normal. There is no jaundice or scleral icterus. Spider telangiectasias are noted on the face and chest. The abdomen is distended with flank dullness. There is 1+ pitting edema to the knees bilaterally. Mental status examination is normal.

The calculated Model for End-stage Liver Disease (MELD) score is 22.

The patient is instructed to increase his furosemide.

Which of the following is the most appropriate preoperative management?

(A) Cancel surgery and refer for liver transplant evaluation
(B) Delay surgery until after patient achieves 1 year of sobriety
(C) Delay surgery until after placement of a transjugular intrahepatic portosystemic shunt
(D) Proceed to surgery

Item 22

A 24-year-old person is evaluated as an add-on patient for a 1-week history of nasal congestion, watery eyes, and cough productive of yellow sputum. The patient is new to the practice and has indicated on the intake form that his gender is transmale. He responds to questioning that he would prefer to be addressed as "he" or "him," but he seems nervous. He reports no fevers, chills, shortness of breath, or rash. He takes no medications.

On physical examination, vital signs are normal. There is oropharyngeal erythema, and nasal turbinates are boggy. No tonsillar exudate or cervical lymphadenopathy is noted. Lungs are clear to auscultation bilaterally.

Which of the following is the most appropriate next step in management at this visit?

(A) Obtain a hormonal and surgical history
(B) Obtain a social and sexual history
(C) Perform a genital examination
(D) Screen for sexually transmitted infections
(E) Symptomatic treatment

Item 23

A 75-year-old man is being discharged following treatment for acute decompensated heart failure. The patient and his wife are alerted to symptoms that indicate acute worsening of his heart failure and are informed of when he should seek immediate medical assistance. The discharge medication list and the side effects of these medications are reviewed, and the patient and his wife acknowledge an understanding. A nursing education visit regarding the hospital stay and evaluations is completed. A copy of the discharge summary is given to the patient, and a follow-up appointment is scheduled with his internist in 7 days.

Which of the following is also recommended to improve patient safety and reduce rehospitalization in this patient?

(A) Follow-up telephone call and one home nursing visitation
(B) Home telemonitoring
(C) Postdischarge patient education
(D) Timely discharge summary for the primary care physician

Item 24

A 54-year-old man is evaluated for a 6-month history of right shoulder pain. He describes the pain as moderately severe aching that is diffusely localized over the shoulder without radiation to the arm. The pain is constant, although it is worse at night and with any shoulder movement. The pain was insidious in onset and has been progressively worsening. He has had no neurologic or constitutional symptoms. Ibuprofen provides some pain relief.

On physical examination, vital signs are normal. Pain and limited range of motion are noted with both active and passive movement in all planes of motion, as is diffuse tenderness over the anterior and posterior areas of the right shoulder. There is no tenderness to palpation of the bony or soft tissue structures, nor is there cervical spine tenderness. There are no neck symptoms or findings.

Which of the following is the most likely diagnosis?

(A) Acromioclavicular joint degeneration
(B) Adhesive capsulitis
(C) Bicipital tendinitis
(D) Rotator cuff disease

Item 25

A 32-year-old man is evaluated for ongoing intermittent premature ejaculation of 3 years' duration, which he describes as distressing to him and his spouse. He reports no other symptoms. The patient also has depression, which is currently well controlled with amitriptyline. A previous trial of sertraline caused mood instability, prompting its discontinuation. He takes no other medications.

On physical examination, vital signs are normal. Growth and pattern of body hair and testicular size are normal. No gynecomastia is noted.

Laboratory studies show a normal 8:00 AM serum total testosterone level.

163

Which of the following is the most appropriate additional treatment?

(A) Paroxetine

(B) Testosterone gel

(C) Topical lidocaine

(D) No additional treatment is indicated

Item 26

A 67-year-old woman is evaluated for urinary incontinence that has progressively worsened over the past 2 years. She experiences incontinence when she laughs or sneezes but reports no dysuria, hematuria, or loss of continence at night. She has been postmenopausal for 12 years. She had four spontaneous term vaginal deliveries between age 24 and 32 years. She has no other problems and takes no medications.

On physical examination, all vital signs are normal. BMI is 20. Pelvic examination reveals vaginal atrophy. The remainder of the examination is normal.

Which of the following is the most appropriate treatment?

(A) Bladder training

(B) Oral estradiol

(C) Oxybutynin

(D) Pelvic floor muscle training (Kegel exercises)

(E) Weight loss

Item 27

An 81-year-old woman was admitted to the ICU 8 days ago for multisystem organ failure associated with a severe episode of multilobar pneumonia. She has required mechanical ventilation since admission. Efforts to wean the patient from mechanical ventilation have not succeeded, and the patient remains somnolent and unresponsive to verbal stimuli. Medical history is significant for dementia, diabetes mellitus, COPD, chronic kidney disease, and heart failure.

The care team concludes and shares with the patient's family that she will not have a meaningful recovery; however, the patient's children request continued ICU-level care. The patient does not have an advance directive, and her wishes are unknown. After a family meeting with the care team to discuss the patient's prognosis, the children continue to request all treatment.

Which of the following is the most appropriate management?

(A) Consult with the hospital ethics committee

(B) Discontinue ICU care in 48 hours if there is no improvement

(C) Transfer the patient to another institution

(D) Continue current level of care

Item 28

A 54-year-old woman is evaluated for a 9-month history of vaginal irritation and itching. She also has pain during intercourse and uses vaginal lubricants without much relief. At age 50 years, she developed severe menopause-related vasomotor symptoms that responded to a 2-year course of estrogen replacement therapy; she currently has no vasomotor symptoms. Family history is significant for breast cancer. She takes no medications.

On physical examination, vital signs are normal. Pelvic examination shows diminished elasticity of the vulvar skin; thinning of the labia minora; introital narrowing; and dry, pale-colored vaginal lining with decreased rugae.

Which of the following is the most appropriate treatment?

(A) Clobetasol

(B) Ospemifene

(C) Systemic estrogen therapy

(D) Vaginal estrogen therapy

Item 29

A 30-year-old woman is evaluated for a 1-year history of severe anxiety about multiple aspects of her life, including her marriage, work, and health. She also reports irritability, poor sleep, and difficulty concentrating, and she finds it difficult to complete her daily home and occupational tasks. She has had multiple visits with her internist for various symptoms, including atypical chest pain, shortness of breath, palpitations, and intermittent diarrhea. She does not use alcohol, tobacco, or recreational drugs. She drinks one cup of coffee every morning. Her Generalized Anxiety Disorder 7-item scale score is 15, corresponding to severe anxiety.

Laboratory studies reveal a normal serum thyroid-stimulating hormone level.

Which of the following is the most appropriate long-term pharmacologic treatment?

(A) Amitriptyline

(B) Clonazepam

(C) Lithium

(D) Sertraline

Item 30

A 66-year-old woman is evaluated during a follow-up visit for a 5-year history of chronic autoimmune pancreatitis. She has constant, severe, aching midabdominal pain that radiates to the back. Her only surgical option is a pancreaticojejunostomy, a procedure that she is not ready to accept. She has previously tried several tricyclic antidepressants, venlafaxine, gabapentin, oral morphine, and tramadol. A fentanyl patch was substituted for oral morphine during a recent hospitalization, and over the past 6 weeks, she has noted reduced pain and improved function with its use. She lives with her husband and oldest daughter at her home. She does not smoke, drink alcohol, or use illicit drugs. Her only medications are a fentanyl patch, 25 μg/h changed every 72 hours (approximately 75 morphine milligram equivalents/day); prednisone; and pancreatic enzyme replacement.

On physical examination, the patient is frail appearing. Vital signs are normal. BMI is 21. The abdomen is scaphoid; bowel sounds are present. Midepigastric palpation reveals tenderness.

Which of the following is the most appropriate next step in management?

(A) Add lorazepam

(B) Prescribe naloxone and provide caregiver education on its use

(C) Recommend weekly nursing visits before each opioid prescription

(D) Switch the fentanyl patch to short-acting hydromorphone

Item 31

A 60-year-old man is evaluated for abdominal cramping and diarrhea that began after starting ezetimibe. The patient has had persistently elevated LDL cholesterol levels while taking maximally tolerated statin therapy. One year ago, he began receiving atorvastatin, 80 mg/d, with an initial LDL cholesterol level of 180 mg/dL (4.66 mmol/L). However, he developed severe muscle pain, and the dosage was decreased to 40 mg/d and ultimately 20 mg/d. Three months ago, his LDL cholesterol was 140 mg/dL (3.63 mmol/L), at which time ezetimibe was added. Medical history is otherwise significant for myocardial infarction treated with drug-eluting stent placement 1 year ago. Medications are aspirin, clopidogrel, atorvastatin, ezetimibe, metoprolol, and lisinopril.

On physical examination, vital signs are normal. BMI is 27. There is mild, diffuse abdominal tenderness to palpation without rebound or guarding. The remainder of the examination is unremarkable.

In addition to discontinuing ezetimibe, which of the following is the most appropriate management?

(A) Add alirocumab

(B) Add cholestyramine

(C) Add niacin

(D) No further intervention

Item 32

A 65-year-old man is evaluated during a visit to establish care. He is interested in colorectal cancer screening; however, he adamantly refuses to undergo colon preparation, and he does not want to modify his diet for screening. He has never undergone colorectal cancer screening. Medical and family histories are unremarkable. He takes no medications.

Physical examination, including vital signs, is normal.

After discussing the colon preparation process and dietary restrictions with the patient and exploring his concerns, he is steadfast in his refusal.

Which of the following is the most appropriate screening test for this patient?

(A) Circulating methylated *SEPT9* DNA test

(B) CT colonography

(C) Fecal immunochemical test

(D) Sensitive guaiac-based fecal occult blood test

Item 33

A 35-year-old woman is evaluated during a follow-up visit for anxiety. Her symptoms have been well controlled with cognitive behavioral therapy, and she has been drinking kava tea every morning and practicing mindfulness daily. Medical history is significant for nonalcoholic steatohepatitis. Other supplements are folic acid and echinacea.

On physical examination, vital signs are normal. BMI is 36. The remainder of the examination is unremarkable.

Which of the following is the most appropriate recommendation for this patient?

(A) Discontinue echinacea

(B) Discontinue folic acid

(C) Discontinue kava tea

(D) No changes to current therapy

Item 34

A 70-year-old man is seen for a preoperative medical evaluation before laminectomy for spinal stenosis. History is also significant for coronary artery disease and a non–ST-elevation myocardial infarction that occurred 5 years ago. He swims for 30 minutes every other day. He reports no chest pain with activity. Medications are aspirin, simvastatin, metoprolol, and lisinopril.

Physical examination, including vital signs, is normal.

Electrocardiogram performed 2 years ago demonstrated a left anterior fascicular block, several premature atrial contractions, and sinus rhythm.

Which of the following is the most appropriate preoperative cardiac testing for this patient?

(A) Dobutamine stress echocardiography

(B) Electrocardiography

(C) Exercise stress testing

(D) No further testing

Item 35

A 44-year-old man is evaluated for right medial elbow pain that began 2 months ago with a dull ache and has gradually worsened. The pain is worse with elbow flexion, and his right fourth and fifth fingers are numb.

On physical examination, vital signs are normal. Decreased sensation over the volar aspect of the right fourth and fifth fingers is noted, with adduction and abduction weakness of the fingers. The right elbow has full range of motion and no notable erythema, swelling, or tenderness.

Which of the following is the most likely diagnosis?

(A) Carpal tunnel syndrome

(B) Medial epicondylitis

(C) Olecranon bursitis

(D) Ulnar nerve entrapment

Item 36

A 63-year-old woman is evaluated in the emergency department after an unwitnessed syncopal event. She recalls feeling a sensation of warmth and generalized weakness prior to the event but had no chest pain, dyspnea, or palpitations. Medical history is significant for hypertension, hyperlipidemia, and carotid artery stenosis treated with endarterectomy. Medications are lisinopril, hydrochlorothiazide, atorvastatin, and aspirin.

Vital signs and screening cardiovascular and neurologic examinations are normal.

Which of the following tests should be included in the initial evaluation of this patient?

(A) Ambulatory electrocardiographic monitoring and echocardiography

(B) B-type natriuretic peptide and cardiac enzyme measurement

(C) Magnetic resonance carotid angiography and MRI of the brain

(D) Orthostatic blood pressure measurement and electrocardiography

Item 37

A 37-year-old woman is evaluated for contraceptive advice. She is married and has a 1-year-old child. The patient describes the conception of this child as an "accident" because she often missed taking her previous oral contraceptive. Her menstrual periods have resumed and are regular but heavy and, in that regard, bothersome to her. Medical history is unremarkable. She drinks a glass of wine every night and smokes a pack of cigarettes daily. She has no other health issues and takes no medications.

The result of a pregnancy test performed today is negative.

The patient is provided with a brief smoking cessation intervention. She is not ready to stop smoking but will consider it again at a later time.

Which of the following is the most appropriate female contraceptive option for this patient?

(A) Estrogen–progestin oral contraceptive

(B) Estrogen–progestin vaginal ring

(C) Progesterone-containing intrauterine device

(D) Progesterone-only "mini pill"

Item 38

A 43-year-old woman is evaluated during a follow-up appointment for obesity. She has been following a reduced-calorie, low-fat diet and participating in a 45-minute aerobic exercise class three times weekly for the past 6 months. After her last follow-up appointment 1 month ago, she added 30 minutes of brisk walking on the weekend to her exercise regimen. She brings a food diary and weekly weight records to her appointment. She lost an average of 0.2 kg (0.5 lb) per week over the first 3 to 4 weeks, but her weight loss tapered thereafter and her weight has increased by 0.5 kg (1 lb) since her last visit. The total amount of weight lost over the past 8 months is 2.7 kg (6 lb), or 3% of her original weight. The patient reports that she is unable to achieve the calorie reduction recommended, stating that she

is "hungry all the time." Medical history is also significant for type 2 diabetes mellitus and hypertension. Medications are amlodipine, lisinopril, and metformin.

On physical examination, blood pressure is 141/92 mm Hg, and other vital signs are normal. BMI is 31. The remainder of the examination is unremarkable.

Which of the following is the most appropriate next step in treatment?

(A) Bariatric surgery

(B) Liraglutide

(C) Switch to a low-carbohydrate diet

(D) Switch to a very-low-calorie diet

Item 39

A 37-year-old man inquires about palliative medicine referral during a follow-up visit after hospital discharge. He was recently diagnosed with metastatic non–small cell lung cancer, and 1.5 L of fluid was removed with therapeutic thoracentesis, with substantial relief of dyspnea. He has met with his medical oncologist, with plans to initiate disease-directed treatment soon. Medications are dexamethasone, hydromorphone, and senna.

When is the most appropriate time for palliative medicine referral?

(A) Now

(B) At initiation of chemotherapy

(C) At onset of symptoms

(D) Palliative medicine is not indicated for patients undergoing active cancer treatment

Item 40

A 51-year-old woman is evaluated during a routine follow-up visit for diabetes mellitus. She also has hypertension and hyperlipidemia. Medications are metformin, enalapril, chlorthalidone, and high-intensity rosuvastatin. She has no drug allergies.

On physical examination, blood pressure is 126/74 mm Hg. The remainder of the examination is unremarkable.

Her 10-year risk for atherosclerotic cardiovascular disease is 11% according to the Pooled Cohort Equations. She has been instructed in intensive lifestyle modifications.

Which of the following is the most appropriate preventive measure to reduce this patient's cardiovascular risk?

(A) Clopidogrel

(B) Low-dose aspirin

(C) Low-dose aspirin and clopidogrel

(D) Regular-dose aspirin

(E) No additional therapy

Item 41

A 37-year-old woman is evaluated for a 6-year history of difficulty initiating sleep and significant daytime sleepiness. She works as a registered nurse, and she notes that her daytime sleepiness is exacerbated when she works several night shifts in a row at the hospital. She does not drink alcohol, use tobacco, or consume caffeinated products. She recently initiated a new exercise program and exercises three to four mornings each week. She has no other symptoms and takes no medications.

On physical examination, vital signs are normal. BMI is 30. Oxygen saturation breathing ambient air is 97%. The remainder of the physical examination is normal.

Which of the following is the most appropriate next step in management?

(A) Multiple sleep latency testing
(B) Overnight oximetry
(C) Polysomnography
(D) Serum ferritin level measurement
(E) Two-week sleep diary

Item 42

A 32-year-old man emails to request an opinion on his medical conditions. He is not an established patient but decided to contact the physician after viewing an online profile. His message indicates that he has a several-year history of abdominal pain with intermittent diarrhea and constipation, for which he takes polyethylene glycol, fiber, and dicyclomine. He notes that he has seen a primary care physician and gastroenterologist and undergone extensive testing, including an endoscopy and colonoscopy. He requests a recommendation for a new test or treatment.

Which of the following is the most appropriate management?

(A) Advise the patient to obtain celiac disease assessment
(B) Ask the patient to email his medical records before providing advice
(C) Request that the patient call the office to establish care
(D) Do not respond to the patient's email

Item 43

A 38-year-old woman is evaluated for a 2-day history of worsening eye pain and decreasing visual acuity in her left eye. The pain is worse with eye movement. She reports no fever or trauma. Vision loss is mostly central, and her ability to distinguish colors has diminished. She does not feel the sensation of a foreign body in the eyes. She wears contact lenses. Her medical history is otherwise unremarkable.

On physical examination, vital signs are normal. Eye movement is intact but painful, with visual acuity of 20/20 in the right eye and 20/60 in the left. Afferent pupillary defect is noted in the left eye. There is no corneal injection or discharge, and the optic discs appear normal.

Which of the following is the most likely diagnosis?

(A) Corneal abrasion
(B) Herpes simplex keratitis
(C) Optic neuritis
(D) Orbital cellulitis

Item 44

During a routine health examination, a patient asks about an article that recommended avoiding statin therapy because of the risk for memory loss. The findings were based on cross-sectional data analysis of a well-validated national health survey, which was conducted by random sampling of patients according to zip code of residence. The analysis showed that patients who self-reported memory loss were more likely to also report having taken statin drugs (odds ratio, 1.8; 95% CI, 1.2-2.7; $P = 0.046$).

Which of the following is the most likely threat to the validity of this study?

(A) Confounding
(B) Selection bias
(C) Self-reported data
(D) Statistical significance

Item 45

A 75-year-old woman underwent total hip arthroplasty 4 hours ago and is now evaluated because she has been unable to void since the operation. Bladder ultrasound reveals 900 mL of urine. Other than manageable postoperative pain, she has no symptoms. Current medications are acetaminophen, oxycodone, and enoxaparin.

Which of the following is the most appropriate management?

(A) Suprapubic catheter placement
(B) Suprapubic warm wet gauze application
(C) Tamsulosin administration
(D) Urethral bladder catheterization

Item 46

A 66-year-old woman is transitioning care after her previous physician retired and undergoes a new patient evaluation. She is asymptomatic. She is unclear when her last Pap smear was performed or the result. Medical history is unremarkable, and she takes no medications.

The physical examination, including vital signs, is normal.

Which of the following is the most appropriate cervical cancer screening strategy for this patient?

(A) Obtain high-risk human papillomavirus (hrHPV) testing now
(B) Obtain Pap smear and hrHPV testing now
(C) Obtain Pap smear now
(D) Obtain results of last cervical cancer screening examination
(E) No further screening

Item 47

A 51-year-old woman is referred for evaluation. She has a 10-year history of chronic pain that she describes as head-to-toe aching, twisting, and sometimes burning that involves several large muscle groups. The pain is constant, and she rates the severity as a 6 on a 10-point scale. She is able to work despite the pain but is constantly fatigued. Her current regimen of oxycodone provides minimal relief. She has tried three other opioid medications as well as gabapentin and milnacipran, all of which provided only minimal improvement in her pain. Medical history is also significant for generalized anxiety disorder treated with sertraline.

On physical examination, vital signs are normal. There is tenderness in multiple large muscle groups. The remainder of the physical examination is normal.

In addition to slow tapering of oxycodone, which of the following is the most appropriate next step in treatment?

(A) Lorazepam
(B) Physical therapy
(C) Transcutaneous electrical nerve stimulation
(D) Transdermal fentanyl

Item 48

A 79-year-old woman is accompanied to the office by her son for an evaluation of her memory. The patient forgot to attend her last two scheduled appointments. The patient lives alone; her son visits her daily and sets up a weekly pill box with her medications. The son reports that on several occasions lately, pills that his mother should have taken have been left in the compartments. The patient admits that she sometimes gets confused as to which section of the pill box is the correct one for that day. Medical history is significant for hypothyroidism, hypertension, gastroesophageal reflux disease, and osteoarthritis. Medications are levothyroxine, amlodipine, omeprazole, vitamin D, and acetaminophen.

On physical examination, vital signs are normal. The patient is pleasant and interactive. The physical examination is normal, including neurologic and gait assessment. Depression screening with PHQ-2 is negative.

Which of the following is the most appropriate test to perform next?

(A) Apolipoprotein E (*APOE*-ε4) genotyping
(B) Fluorodeoxyglucose-PET brain imaging
(C) Formal neurocognitive testing
(D) Mini-Cog testing

Item 49

A 36-year-old woman is evaluated for posterior neck pain and stiffness that began 1 week ago while she was doing sit-ups. The pain is worse with movement of the head. She has limited range of motion of the neck in all directions. The pain does not radiate down her arms, and she has not had arm weakness, parethesias, or other neurologic symptoms. She reports no systemic symptoms. The pain is lessened with ibuprofen.

On physical examination, vital signs are normal. On palpation, tenderness of the cervical paraspinal muscles is noted. There is no cervical spine tenderness. Symptoms are not reproduced when the examiner bends the patient's head to either side while also extending the neck and applying a downward axial load (Spurling test). Neurologic examination is normal.

Which of the following is the most likely diagnosis?

(A) Cervical myelopathy
(B) Cervical radiculopathy
(C) Cervical sprain
(D) Whiplash-associated neck pain

Item 50

A 32-year-old woman is evaluated for bothersome vaginal discharge of 2 weeks' duration. Her last Pap smear was obtained 15 months ago and was normal. Nucleic acid amplification test results confirm *Trichomonas vaginalis* infection. Treatment of the patient is initiated.

Which of the following is the most appropriate additional management?

(A) Pap testing
(B) Test sexual partner for trichomoniasis
(C) Treat sexual partner for trichomoniasis
(D) No further testing or intervention is necessary

Item 51

A 46-year-old woman is evaluated for a 3-day history of paresthesia of the right lateral nipple. She has experienced this symptom approximately three times per year for the past 7 years. The paresthesia generally lasts 7 to 10 days. She has no other right breast concerns and reports no milky or bloody discharge, fever, chills, or antecedent trauma. She has undergone extensive evaluation, including laboratory testing, mammography, breast ultrasonography, and dermatologic and neurologic examinations; all results have been normal. She has no other medical problems and takes no medications. She works full time, and her symptom has not limited her functioning.

On physical examination, vital signs are normal. Breast examination is normal bilaterally.

Which of the following is the most likely diagnosis?

(A) Conversion disorder
(B) Illness anxiety disorder
(C) Medically unexplained symptom
(D) Somatic symptom disorder

Item 52

A 45-year-old woman is evaluated for a 2-month history of bothersome lower extremity edema. The edema does not vary with time of day or activity level. Medical history is notable for fibromyalgia treated with pregabalin. She otherwise feels well and is active in a physical therapy program.

On physical examination, vital signs are normal. Pitting edema is present to just above the ankles bilaterally without evidence of calf swelling, varicosities, or hyperpigmentation. There is no tenderness to palpation of the lower extremities. No jugular venous distention, extracardiac sounds, or pulmonary crackles are noted.

Which of the following is the most appropriate next step in management?

(A) Begin hydrochlorothiazide

(B) Perform lower extremity duplex Doppler ultrasonography

(C) Prescribe compression stockings

(D) Switch pregabalin to duloxetine

Item 53

A 40-year-old woman is evaluated for a 6-month history of poor sleep, lack of energy, constant feelings of sadness, and difficulty concentrating at work. These symptoms began shortly after she was passed over for a promotion at work. She has lost interest in her usual hobbies of running and gardening and has withdrawn from her family and friends. She reports feeling like she is "not worth anything" and sometimes thinks about "ending it all." She says she has never felt like this before; she was previously a positive and optimistic person. She reports never having periods of increased energy, decreased need for sleep, or drastically elevated mood. She has had no hallucinations. She does not use alcohol, tobacco, or recreational drugs.

Laboratory studies reveal a normal serum thyroid-stimulating hormone level.

Which of the following is the most likely diagnosis?

(A) Bipolar disorder

(B) Generalized anxiety disorder

(C) Major depressive disorder

(D) Persistent depressive disorder

Item 54

A 24-year-old woman is evaluated for an 8-month history of chronic fatigue, unrefreshing sleep, short-term memory loss, and postexertional malaise. She also has symptoms of lightheadedness and dizziness that worsen with upright posture and improve after lying down. Her symptoms do not improve with rest and began suddenly 1 month after being diagnosed with early localized Lyme disease, for which she received a 14-day course of doxycycline. As a result of her symptoms, she has had to curtail many of her social activities and has taken numerous days off work. She takes no medications and has no known allergies.

On physical examination, vital signs are normal. The remainder of the examination is unremarkable.

Laboratory studies reveal a normal complete blood count, electrolyte levels, kidney function test results, liver chemistry test results, and serum thyroid-stimulating hormone level. A pregnancy test result is negative.

Her PHQ-9 score and her Generalized Anxiety Disorder 7-item scale score are both normal.

Which of the following is the most likely diagnosis?

(A) Chronic multifactorial fatigue

(B) Mood disorder

(C) Post–Lyme disease syndrome

(D) Systemic exertion intolerance disease

Item 55

A 29-year-old man is evaluated in an urgent care center for a 2-day history of pain and swelling of the right hemiscrotum. The pain is stable in intensity, neither worsening nor improving. Other symptoms include low-grade fever and dysuria. He reports no abdominal pain, nausea, or vomiting.

On physical examination, temperature is 38.3 °C (100.9 °F), and pulse rate is 103/min. Blood pressure and respiration rate are normal. There are erythema and swelling of the right hemiscrotum and moderate tenderness to palpation of the superolateral aspect of the right hemiscrotum. The hemiscrotum is not elevated, and there is no scrotal mass, rash, or penile discharge.

Which of the following tests is most likely to have a positive finding?

(A) Cremasteric reflex test

(B) Pain relief with testicular elevation

(C) Scrotal examination in standing and supine positions

(D) Transillumination study

Item 56

A 44-year-old man is evaluated during a follow-up visit for a 6-month history of low back pain. The pain worsens with standing and is relieved by lying down. He describes the pain as moderate aching. The pain does not radiate down the legs, and he has not had bowel or bladder dysfunction, fevers, leg weakness, night sweats, saddle anesthesia, or weight loss. The pain has been interfering with his ability to work. He participated in acupuncture, mindfulness-based stress reduction, and spinal manipulation, all of which provided only minimal relief.

On physical examination, vital signs are normal. On palpation, bilateral paraspinal muscle tenderness is noted. The musculoskeletal and neurologic examinations are otherwise normal.

Which of the following is the most appropriate pharmacologic option for this patient?

(A) Acetaminophen

(B) Duloxetine

(C) Hydrocodone

(D) Ibuprofen

(E) Tramadol

Item 57

A 59-year-old man is evaluated for recurring epistaxis over the last several months, usually on the right side. He has been able to stop the bleeding by applying pressure to the nares, but on one occasion, he required treatment in the emergency department. Typically, blood loss has been minimal. He does not use intranasal medications and reports no substance use. He has otherwise been well. There is no family history of epistaxis or rheumatologic or bleeding disorders. His only medication is low-dose aspirin.

On physical examination, vital signs are normal. On nasal examination, there are no clear lesions, erythema, petechiae, scabs, telangiectasias, ulcers, or visible bleeding.

Which of the following is the most appropriate management?

(A) Discontinue aspirin
(B) Obtain coagulation studies
(C) Obtain complete blood count
(D) Perform nasal endoscopy

Item 58

A hospital system is attempting to reduce the number of hospital-acquired infections, including catheter-related urinary tract infections, bloodstream infections, *Clostridium difficile* infections, and ventilator-associated pneumonia. A common possible factor appears to be the low rate of hand hygiene (78%) documented among hospital staff.

Which of the following measures is most likely to improve hand hygiene rates at this hospital?

(A) Create a spaghetti diagram
(B) Implement the Lean model and create a value stream map
(C) Reiterate the importance of hand hygiene in an email to the hospital staff
(D) Use a Plan-Do-Study-Act cycle

Item 59

A 91-year-old woman is evaluated to establish care following discharge from a hospital to a skilled nursing facility. She had been living in her own home until 2 weeks ago when she fell and sustained a left intertrochanteric femur fracture. Her fracture was surgically stabilized, and her postoperative course was complicated by delirium and urinary tract infection. Since discharge, she has had no major medical problems. Left hip pain is controlled with acetaminophen as needed. Medical history is otherwise significant for hypertension and type 2 diabetes mellitus. Medications before hospital admission were amlodipine, lisinopril, and metformin. In the hospital, acetaminophen was added for pain and quetiapine for agitated postoperative delirium.

On physical examination, blood pressure is 148/78 mm Hg without orthostatic changes; other vital signs are normal. She has mildly antalgic gait. Cardiac, neurologic, and pulmonary examinations are normal.

Which of the patient's prescribed medications should be discontinued to prevent adverse effects?

(A) Acetaminophen
(B) Amlodipine
(C) Lisinopril
(D) Quetiapine

Item 60

A 59-year-old woman is evaluated during a follow-up visit for mouth pain of 2 years' duration. Her mouth pain was previously localized to the tongue and floor of the mouth; however, it is now diffuse, burning, and constant. The pain has also worsened over the past year despite continued dosage escalation of a transdermal fentanyl patch and oral hydromorphone. She has no pain with swallowing. Medical history is significant for squamous cell carcinoma of the tongue treated with chemotherapy and radiation therapy; her treatment course was complicated by severe mucositis. She has been without evidence of disease for the past 2 years.

On physical examination, vital signs are normal. The patient is alert and oriented but inattentive and slow to answer questions. Reflexes are exaggerated in the upper and lower extremities, and myoclonic jerking of the legs and clonus at the ankles are noted. Strength is normal. Mouth examination reveals erythematous oral mucosa with no focal areas of erosion or masses.

A CT scan of the head and neck shows no evidence of recurrent disease.

Which of the following is the most likely diagnosis?

(A) Malingering
(B) Opioid-induced hyperalgesia
(C) Opioid withdrawal
(D) Pseudoaddiction

Item 61

A 61-year-old man is seen for medical evaluation before a pancreaticoduodenectomy for suspected pancreatic cancer scheduled in 7 days. He reports no recent chest pain or bleeding complications after undergoing drug-eluting stent placement to the left anterior descending artery for an ST-elevation myocardial infarction 5 months ago. He has been riding his bike 10 miles daily since recovering from the myocardial infarction. Medications are aspirin, clopidogrel, losartan, atorvastatin, and atenolol.

On physical examination, vital signs are normal. Scleral icterus and jaundice are noted. Cardiac examination is normal, the lungs are clear, and the abdomen is nontender. There is no lower extremity edema.

Which of the following is the most appropriate perioperative management of this patient's antiplatelet therapy?

(A) Continue clopidogrel and aspirin
(B) Withhold aspirin and clopidogrel now
(C) Withhold aspirin now; continue clopidogrel
(D) Withhold clopidogrel now; continue aspirin

Item 62

A 55-year-old man is seen for a general wellness visit. He is asymptomatic. Family history is significant for prostate cancer diagnosed in his father at age 85 years.

The physical examination is normal.

Which of the following is the most appropriate action regarding prostate cancer screening?

(A) Discuss the benefits and harms of screening
(B) Obtain a serum prostate-specific antigen level
(C) Perform a digital rectal examination
(D) Recommend against screening

Item 63

An 84-year-old woman in hospice care is evaluated for "death rattle" that is disturbing to family members. She is in the active phases of dying, and her family is distressed by her noisy respiratory secretions; they are worried that she is choking. Medications are haloperidol, hydromorphone, lactulose, and acetaminophen.

On physical examination, respiration rate is 12/min. She is not responsive but does not appear uncomfortable. Extremities are cool. There are oropharyngeal secretions that produce a rattling and gurgling sound with inspiration.

Which of the following is the most appropriate initial management?

(A) Atropine ophthalmic drops given sublingually
(B) Glycopyrronium
(C) Scopolamine patch
(D) Suctioning by catheter
(E) Symptom explanation and reassurance

Item 64

A 48-year-old man is evaluated during a follow-up visit for hypertension. He has no symptoms. He received the tetanus toxoid, reduced diphtheria toxoid, and acellular pertussis vaccine 9 years ago and the influenza vaccine during the most recent influenza season. He is a current smoker with a 25-pack-year history. His only medication is chlorthalidone.

On physical examination, vital signs are normal, and the remainder of the examination is unremarkable.

Which of the following is the most appropriate vaccine to administer to this patient?

(A) Recombinant zoster vaccine
(B) Tetanus and diphtheria toxoids booster
(C) 13-Valent pneumococcal conjugate vaccine
(D) 23-Valent pneumococcal polysaccharide vaccine
(E) No vaccines are indicated

Item 65

A 17-year-old girl is seen for a health maintenance evaluation. She reports no health issues. In discussing dietary habits, she states that she frequently eats very large amounts of food until she is uncomfortably full. These episodes have occurred at least twice per week for the past year; during them, she feels a loss of control over her eating and guilt about her overconsumption. She often eats large amounts of food despite not being hungry, and she prefers eating alone because she is embarrassed of her eating. She does not take laxatives or induce vomiting after such episodes. She rarely exercises. BMI is 30.

Which of the following is the most likely diagnosis?

(A) Anorexia nervosa, binging subtype
(B) Binge eating disorder
(C) Bulimia nervosa
(D) Overeating

Item 66

A 33-year-old woman is evaluated for a 10-month history of bilateral diffuse breast pain. The pain is severe in intensity, occurring about a week before her menstrual cycle and resolving afterward. She has generally lumpy breasts without a dominant mass and no nipple discharge. Her menstrual cycles are regular. She drinks a cup of coffee in the morning and another at noon. Medical history is otherwise unremarkable. She has no family history of breast cancer.

On physical examination, vital signs are normal. BMI is 29. Examination of the breasts shows dense nodularity in the upper outer quadrant of both breasts and no skin changes. Tenderness is elicited on examination of the upper outer quadrants of the breasts. There is no evidence of cervical, supraclavicular, or axillary lymphadenopathy.

Which of the following is the most appropriate next step in management?

(A) Advise avoidance of caffeine
(B) Advise use of a well-fitting bra
(C) Breast ultrasonography
(D) Diagnostic mammography
(E) Initiate danazol

Item 67

A 67-year-old man is evaluated for a 3-hour history of episodic dizziness. He notes a room-spinning sensation started suddenly without antecedent trauma and has been accompanied by nausea. Medical history is significant for hypertension, hyperlipidemia, and type 2 diabetes mellitus. Medications are lisinopril, atorvastatin, and metformin.

On physical examination, temperature is normal, blood pressure is 174/88 mm Hg, pulse rate is 101/min, and respiration rate is normal. The Dix-Hallpike maneuver evokes immediate nystagmus with no fatigability. The nystagmus is vertical without a torsional component, but the direction varies depending on the direction of the patient's gaze. The neurologic examination is limited but grossly nonfocal.

Which of the following is the most likely diagnosis?

(A) Acoustic neuroma
(B) Acute labyrinthitis
(C) Benign paroxysmal positional vertigo
(D) Vertebrobasilar ischemia
(E) Vestibular neuronitis

Item 68

A 46-year-old man is evaluated for a 2-month history of right anterior knee swelling. The swelling began insidiously and has gradually worsened. It is now the size of a golf ball and interferes with his ability to kneel, which is vital to his job as a carpet layer. The knee is painful only when he kneels; he has no problems with knee motion or stability. He feels well otherwise.

On physical examination, vital signs are normal. He has a 4-cm swelling on the anterior aspect of the right knee. The overlying skin is erythematous and warm. The knee exhibits full range of motion. There is no medial or lateral joint tenderness; knee joint effusion; or laxity with anterior, posterior, valgus, or varus forces.

Which of the following is the most appropriate initial management?

- (A) Activity modification
- (B) Fluid aspiration
- (C) Ibuprofen
- (D) Plain radiography
- (E) Serum uric acid measurement

Item 69

A 49-year-old man was admitted to the ICU 3 days ago with sepsis secondary to health care–associated pneumonia. He is now being transferred to the general medical floor. Medical history is significant for spinal cord injury with associated lower extremity paralysis and neurogenic bladder. He is able to perform intermittent bladder catheterization. Medications are baclofen, enoxaparin, and levofloxacin.

On physical examination, vital signs are normal. BMI is 19. Left lower lobe crackles are present on lung auscultation. There is flaccid paralysis of the lower extremities. Skin is intact without erythema over pressure points.

Which of the following is the most appropriate intervention to prevent the development of a pressure injury?

- (A) Advanced static mattress
- (B) Alternating air mattress
- (C) Frequent repositioning
- (D) Zinc supplementation

Item 70

A 24-year-old man is evaluated during a routine examination. He is asymptomatic. He is sexually active with men and has had multiple partners in the past year. He reports using condoms half of the time. Medical history is unremarkable. He takes no medications.

On physical examination, vital signs and the remainder of the examination are normal.

Results of combination HIV antibody immunoassay/ p24 antigen testing are negative.

Which of the following is the most appropriate interval for HIV screening in this patient?

- (A) At least annually
- (B) Every 2 years
- (C) Every 3 years
- (D) Every 5 years
- (E) No further screening

Item 71

A 65-year-old woman is evaluated during a wellness visit. She has no symptoms. Medical history is significant for hypertension and impaired fasting glucose. She has never smoked cigarettes. Medications are hydrochlorothiazide and metformin.

On physical examination, blood pressure is 130/80 mm Hg; other vital signs are normal. BMI is 26. The remainder of the physical examination is normal.

Laboratory studies:

Total cholesterol	271 mg/dL (7.02 mmol/L)
LDL cholesterol	155 mg/dL (4.01 mmol/L)
HDL cholesterol	50 mg/dL (1.29 mmol/L)
Triglycerides	330 mg/dL (3.73 mmol/L)

Her estimated 10-year risk for atherosclerotic cardiovascular disease (ASCVD) using the Pooled Cohort Equations is 11.1%.

In addition to therapeutic lifestyle changes, which of the following is the most appropriate therapy for primary prevention of ASCVD in this patient?

- (A) Alirocumab
- (B) Ezetimibe
- (C) Gemfibrozil
- (D) Simvastatin

Item 72

A 72-year-old woman is evaluated for a 2-week history of intermittent dizziness. She has had no falls. Medical history is notable for hypertension and diabetes mellitus, for which she takes amlodipine, lisinopril, and metformin. A review of the patient's medical record reveals that the dosage of amlodipine was increased 3 weeks ago by a colleague's order. The patient's documented blood pressure was normal 3 weeks ago, and the care plan notes that the dosage of the antihypertensive agents should remain the same.

On physical examination, blood pressure is 115/70 mm Hg supine and 90/55 mm Hg standing, and pulse rate is 85/min supine and 105/min standing.

Which of the following is the most appropriate management?

- (A) Explain that a colleague committed an error and steps will be taken to reduce the chance of recurrence
- (B) Explain that the pharmacy committed an error by providing the incorrect dosage
- (C) Report the error to the National Practitioner Data Bank without further patient disclosure
- (D) Restore the previous dose of amlodipine without further patient disclosure

Item 73

A 68-year-old woman is evaluated for a 6-month history of incontinence typified by continuous leakage and dribbling. She reports no back pain, dysuria, or fever. Medical history is significant for a 30-year history of type 2 diabetes mellitus and a 10-year history of hypertension and hyperlipidemia. Medications include benazepril, metformin, and rosuvastatin.

On physical examination, blood pressure is 147/76 mm Hg, and pulse rate is 92/min. On abdominal examination, the bladder is palpable just above the pubic symphysis. Foot examination demonstrates dry feet, loss of sensation to monofilament testing, and vibration up to the ankles. Lower extremity tendon reflexes are absent.

Urinalysis results are normal.

Which of the following is the most appropriate management?

(A) Botulinum toxin injection
(B) Oxybutynin
(C) Postvoid residual urine volume measurement
(D) Urodynamic testing

Item 74

A 44-year-old man is evaluated for a 6-year history of constant low-grade perineal pain with intermittent exacerbations and intermittent urinary symptoms of dysuria, frequency, and urgency. He had a documented case of acute bacterial prostatitis 6 years ago; since then, he has undergone extensive urologic evaluation during many of his exacerbations, all with negative findings. He has been treated numerous times with antibiotics, anti-inflammatory agents, and α-blockers without symptomatic benefit. He has no other medical problems and currently takes no medications.

On physical examination, vital signs are normal. Prostate examination yields mild and poorly localized tenderness without masses or nodules. There is no penile discharge or scrotal pain on palpation.

Results of previous laboratory studies reveal a normal erythrocyte sedimentation rate, C-reactive protein level, leukocyte count, serum creatinine level, electrolyte levels, and serum prostate-specific antigen level. A postvoid residual ultrasound was normal.

Which of the following is the most appropriate pharmacologic treatment?

(A) Lidocaine-hydrocortisone suppository
(B) Pregabalin
(C) Tamsulosin
(D) Trimethoprim-sulfamethoxazole

Item 75

A 51-year-old woman is evaluated for a 2-year history of intermittent chest pain that lasts up to 6 hours. The chest pain is not triggered by exertion, stress, or other inciting factors and is not accompanied by other symptoms. The patient also reports cramping lower abdominal and pelvic pain of 4 years' duration without nausea or bowel habit changes. She has undergone evaluation by four different physicians for these symptoms. Over the past year, she has undergone electrocardiography, chest radiography, mammography, exercise stress testing, echocardiography, CT of the abdomen and chest, upper endoscopy, and colonoscopy; all findings were normal. Recent complete blood count, comprehensive metabolic panel, and C-reactive protein level were also normal. She is unhappy with the medical care she has received and spends much of her free time reading articles related to her symptoms. She is afraid that she has a life-threatening illness that no one has been able to diagnose. Medications are acetaminophen, a multivitamin, and probiotics.

On physical examination, vital signs and all other findings are normal.

Which of the following is the most appropriate next step in management?

(A) Cognitive behavioral therapy
(B) *MEFV* gene analysis
(C) Pregabalin
(D) Whole-body PET

Item 76

A 64-year-old man is evaluated in the emergency department for acute onset of vision loss in the right eye, which began 1 hour ago. He can barely see his own hands in front of his eye. He has no eye pain. One week ago, he had an episode of monocular vision loss in the right eye that resolved after 5 minutes. He has had no other recent medical concerns. He has no history of floaters, headaches, jaw claudication, muscular weakness, or weight loss. Medical history is significant for hyperlipidemia and hypertension. Medications are atorvastatin and lisinopril.

On physical examination, vital signs are normal. There is loss of visual acuity in the right eye, and pupillary examination reveals an afferent pupillary defect. The optic disc is shown. There is no conjunctival erythema or scalp tenderness.

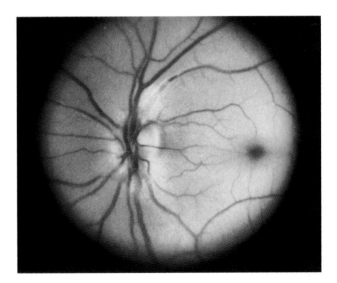

Laboratory studies reveal an erythrocyte sedimentation rate of 22 mm/h.

Which of the following is the most likely diagnosis?

(A) Acute angle-closure glaucoma
(B) Central retinal artery occlusion
(C) Idiopathic intracranial hypertension
(D) Retinal detachment

Item 77

A 74-year-old man is evaluated for severe chronic shortness of breath. Medical history is significant for New York Heart Association functional class III heart failure and severe COPD. He was hospitalized 3 weeks ago for an exacerbation of his COPD. He has returned to his baseline oxygen requirements, but his continued shortness of breath is a significant impediment to his quality of life. The patient's goal is comfort. He does not desire any additional interventions for his heart failure or COPD. Medications are tiotropium, fluticasone propionate/salmeterol, albuterol, amlodipine, lisinopril, hydrochlorothiazide, and oxygen by nasal cannula.

On physical examination, the patient is comfortable at rest but develops dyspnea while ambulating, with associated anxiety. Temperature is 36.9 °C (98.4 °F), blood pressure is 124/68 mm Hg, pulse rate is 98/min, and respiration rate is 32/min. Oxygen saturation is 93% breathing 4 L/min of oxygen by nasal cannula. Pulmonary examination reveals distant breath sounds and a prolonged expiratory phase; the lungs are otherwise clear to auscultation. The estimated central venous pressure is 6 cm H_2O. Cardiac examination reveals an S_4 but is otherwise normal. There is no peripheral edema.

Chest radiograph shows evidence of hyperinflation but no signs of heart failure, pneumonia, or pneumothorax.

Which of the following is the most appropriate treatment of this patient's dyspnea?

(A) Oral furosemide
(B) Oral hydromorphone
(C) Oral lorazepam
(D) Nebulized morphine

Item 78

A 69-year-old man is evaluated during a routine visit. He is asymptomatic. Medical history is remarkable for hypertension, atrial fibrillation, and type 2 diabetes mellitus. He has a 25-pack-year smoking history but quit smoking 3 years ago. Medications are amlodipine, metoprolol, rivaroxaban, and atorvastatin.

Physical examination, including vital signs, is normal.

His estimated 10-year risk for atherosclerotic cardiovascular disease (ASCVD) according to the Pooled Cohort Equations is 14.6%.

Which of the following is most appropriate for primary prevention of ASCVD in this patient?

(A) Add aspirin
(B) Add fish oil
(C) Switch rivaroxaban to aspirin
(D) No further intervention

Item 79

A 28-year-old man is evaluated in the emergency department for a right ankle sprain that occurred earlier in the day while he was refereeing a soccer game. When running down the field, his right cleat stuck in the turf, and his foot rotated laterally. He was able to bear weight immediately after the injury, but he had to leave the game. The ankle has begun to swell, making it difficult for the patient to ambulate.

On physical examination, vital signs are normal. The patient walks with antalgic gait, although he is able to bear weight. Swelling is present over the anterior and lateral distal leg above the right ankle. Pain is reproduced both by squeezing the leg at mid-calf level and by having the patient cross his right leg with the lateral malleolus resting on the left knee. There is no tenderness to palpation over the malleoli, the navicular bone, or the fifth metatarsal base.

Which of the following is the most likely diagnosis?

(A) Achilles tendon rupture
(B) Ankle fracture
(C) High ankle sprain
(D) Lateral ankle sprain

Item 80

A 23-year-old woman is evaluated for a 2-week history of persistent thick, white vaginal discharge; burning in the vulvar and vaginal regions; and vaginal itching. She has never had these symptoms before. She is in a monogamous sexual relationship. Medical history is otherwise unremarkable, and she takes no medications.

On physical examination, vital signs are normal. Pelvic examination reveals vulvar edema with a few excoriations. Speculum examination demonstrates thick, white, curdy vaginal discharge. The remainder of the examination is unremarkable.

Laboratory studies reveal a vaginal pH of 4.4; whiff test result is negative. Potassium hydroxide microscopy shows hyphae. Results of tests for *Chlamydia trachomatis* and *Neisseria gonorrhoeae* are negative.

Which of the following is the most appropriate treatment?

(A) Intravaginal clotrimazole
(B) Intravaginal nystatin
(C) Oral metronidazole
(D) Oral voriconazole

Item 81

A 53-year-old man is evaluated for possible opioid therapy initiation for a several-year history of chest and back pain. Both types of pain significantly impair his ability to sleep, and he has not been able to work for the last 6 months. Over the past few years, he has undergone extensive evaluation, and no modifiable cause of the pain has been discovered. The patient has tried various nonpharmacologic interventions (acupuncture, cognitive behavioral therapy, exercise) and nonopioid pharmacologic therapies (duloxetine, gabapentin, ibuprofen), but he continues to have poor quality of life. These interventions are ongoing. He has no history of anxiety, depression, or substance use disorder. Results of screening tests for depression and anxiety disorders performed today are negative. His only medications are duloxetine, gabapentin, and ibuprofen.

The risks and known benefits of long-term opioid therapy are reviewed with the patient. Treatment goals are discussed, and there is an understanding that opioid therapy will be stopped if the goals are not achieved or the risks exceed the benefit. A check with the state's prescription drug monitoring program confirms that the patient is not receiving opioids or benzodiazepine therapy.

Which of the following is recommended before starting opioid therapy in this patient?

(A) Baseline urine drug screening
(B) Discontinuation of all other pain medications
(C) Discontinuation of all nonpharmacologic therapies
(D) Psychiatric evaluation

Item 82

A 60-year-old woman is seen for a preoperative medical evaluation before elective total left knee arthroplasty. She experiences occasional dizziness after swimming for 30 minutes. History is also significant for benign paroxysmal positional vertigo. She has no other medical problems or symptoms and takes no medications.

On physical examination, temperature is normal, blood pressure is 130/75 mm Hg, pulse rate is 75/min, and respiration rate is 16/min. Cardiac examination reveals a grade 3/6 late-peaking harsh systolic murmur heard throughout the precordium, with radiation to the bilateral carotid arteries. The lungs are clear. There is no lower extremity edema.

Transthoracic echocardiogram obtained 2 years ago demonstrated moderate aortic stenosis with a valve area of 1.3 cm^2 and gradient of 25 mm Hg.

In addition to electrocardiography, which of the following is the most appropriate preoperative testing for this patient?

(A) B-type natriuretic peptide level measurement
(B) Dobutamine stress echocardiography
(C) Transthoracic echocardiography
(D) No further testing

Item 83

A 29-year-old man is evaluated during a new patient visit. He is concerned about gradual weight gain over the last several years. He does not pay much attention to his diet and describes his lifestyle as generally sedentary. He does not use tobacco products and does not drink more than one to two alcoholic drinks per week. He reports no problems with nonrestorative sleep or daytime hypersomnolence. He takes no medications.

On physical examination, blood pressure is 149/90 mm Hg, and pulse rate is 87/min. BMI is 35. His waist circumference is 107 cm (42 in). The remainder of the physical examination is normal.

Which of the following is the most appropriate test to perform next?

(A) Exercise stress test
(B) Hepatic ultrasonography
(C) Overnight polysomnography
(D) Serum lipid panel
(E) Thyroid function studies

Item 84

A 59-year-old woman is evaluated for an 8-month history of minimally productive cough. Her cough has persisted despite empiric treatment with intranasal and inhaled glucocorticoids, inhaled bronchodilators, a proton pump inhibitor, antihistamines, and decongestants. She reports no wheezing, heartburn, or nasal discharge. She is a lifelong nonsmoker and has no history of unusual environmental exposures. She has no known allergies and currently takes no medications.

On physical examination, vital signs are normal. Tympanic membranes are clear. The remainder of the examination is unremarkable.

Chest radiograph, spirometry, bronchial hyperresponsiveness testing, sinus CT scan, and esophageal pH monitoring are normal. Sputum analysis is negative for eosinophils.

Which of the following is the most appropriate treatment?

(A) Azithromycin
(B) Inhaled ipratropium
(C) Morphine
(D) Multimodal speech therapy

Item 85

A 47-year-old woman is evaluated during a follow-up visit for major depressive disorder that was diagnosed 2 months ago. At that time, she reported a 4-month history of anhedonia, depressed mood, decreased energy, insomnia, and weight loss. Her PHQ-9 score was 14, indicating moderate depression. She was prescribed sertraline, and her symptoms improved; her PHQ-9 score is now 9 (mild depression). However, she is distressed because she has had anorgasmia since starting sertraline.

Which of the following is the most appropriate next step in management?

(A) Continue sertraline and initiate cognitive behavioral therapy
(B) Discontinue sertraline and initiate bupropion
(C) Discontinue sertraline and initiate paroxetine
(D) Discontinue sertraline and refer for electroconvulsive therapy

Item 86

A 53-year-old woman is evaluated during follow-up for several chronic medical problems without a medical explanation despite extensive evaluation. Symptoms include nonpositional lightheadedness, difficulty concentrating, and total body numbness. Her symptoms have been stable for the past 2 years. She has a history of anxiety and depression, and her mood is well controlled with medical therapy. Medications are sertraline and acetaminophen as needed.

The physical examination, including vital signs, is normal. Findings on brain MRI obtained 2 years ago were normal.

Which of the following is the most appropriate management?

(A) Anti-Hu antibody assay
(B) Anti–N-methyl-D-aspartate receptor antibody assay
(C) Cognitive behavioral therapy
(D) No further management

Item 87

A 42-year-old man is evaluated for low back pain that began 4 days ago after he shoveled snow. The pain is mild to moderate in severity and does not radiate. He has not had any fevers, leg weakness, night sweats, or bowel or bladder dysfunction. Ibuprofen lessens the pain, as does a heating pad. He has no history of illicit substance use, and his medical history is unremarkable. He takes no additional medications.

On physical examination, vital signs are normal. Bilateral lumbar paraspinal muscle tenderness is noted; the musculoskeletal and neurologic examinations are otherwise normal.

Which of the following is the most appropriate test to perform next?

(A) CT of the lumbar spine
(B) Erythrocyte sedimentation rate measurement
(C) MRI of the lumbar spine
(D) Plain radiography of the lumbar spine
(E) No additional testing

Item 88

A 26-year-old man requests genetic testing for familial adenomatous polyposis. He is asymptomatic. Medical history is unremarkable. His 34-year-old brother recently underwent genetic testing, which revealed a mutation of the adenomatous polyposis coli (*APC*) gene. His father died of colon cancer at age 45 years, and two paternal uncles died of colon cancer at age 46 years and age 47 years. There is no family history of colon cancer in his maternal family members. He takes no medications.

Which of the following is the most appropriate management?

(A) Begin sulindac
(B) Obtain colonoscopy at age 40 years
(C) Obtain genetic testing
(D) Refer for genetic counseling

Item 89

A 70-year-old man is evaluated before discharge from the hospital after treatment for community-acquired pneumonia. Medical history is significant for mild dementia. The patient lives alone and has a daughter who lives nearby. Remaining in his home is very important to him.

The care team recommends that the patient be discharged to a short-term rehabilitation facility to gain strength and prepare him to safely return to his home. The patient refuses. Decision-making capacity is assessed; he is able to articulate the risks, benefits, and alternatives to short-term rehabilitation as well as an understanding of his current medical condition.

Which of the following is the most appropriate management?

(A) Administer the Mini–Mental State Examination
(B) Ask the patient's daughter to make a decision on his behalf

(C) Discharge the patient home with home care services
(D) Obtain a court order for the patient to be discharged to a rehabilitation facility
(E) Refer the patient to a psychiatrist for a capacity assessment

Item 90

A 55-year-old woman is evaluated during a routine examination. Medical history is significant for hypertension, hyperlipidemia, diabetes mellitus, and a non–ST-elevation myocardial infarction 2 weeks ago. She is a current smoker with a 35-pack-year smoking history. She is ready to stop smoking. Medications are metformin, rosuvastatin, aspirin, clopidogrel, metoprolol, and lisinopril.

On physical examination, vital signs and other findings are normal.

Which of the following is the most effective smoking cessation therapy for this patient?

(A) Bupropion
(B) Electronic cigarettes
(C) Nicotine replacement therapy
(D) Varenicline

Item 91

A 69-year-old man is evaluated during a routine examination. The patient reports being healthy and has no symptoms. He has a 10-pack-year smoking history but quit smoking at age 42 years. Medical history is otherwise unremarkable. He takes no medications.

On physical examination, vital signs are normal. BMI is 22. The remainder of the examination is normal.

Which of the following is the most appropriate screening test for this patient?

(A) Abdominal duplex ultrasonography
(B) Chest radiography
(C) Dual-energy x-ray absorptiometry
(D) Low-dose lung CT
(E) No screening is recommended

Item 92

A 62-year-old woman is admitted to the hospital for pneumonia. Her medical history is significant for stage I estrogen receptor–positive invasive breast cancer, for which she was treated with breast-conserving surgery and radiation therapy and then started on tamoxifen. During her hospital stay, antibiotic therapy is initiated, and tamoxifen is withheld. Following discharge, the patient is evaluated in the office, and it is noted that she is no longer taking tamoxifen.

Which of the following measures would have most likely prevented this medication error?

(A) Computerized physician order entry
(B) Electronic medication administration record use
(C) Improved medication labeling
(D) Medication reconciliation

Item 93

An 87-year-old woman is evaluated during a follow-up visit after a recent diagnosis of breast cancer. In the 18 months before her diagnosis, she noted a generalized decline in her energy level and appetite. She no longer is able keep up with others when walking any distance, and she now requires some assistance with dressing because of generalized weakness. She has unintentionally lost 3.6 kg (8 lb) in the last 6 months. Medical history is significant for breast cancer, coronary artery bypass graft surgery at age 74 years, COPD, and hypertension. Medications are albuterol, tiotropium, salmeterol, atorvastatin, aspirin, lisinopril, and metoprolol.

On physical examination, vital signs are normal. BMI is 19. The remainder of the examination is unremarkable.

Which of the following is most likely to predict the patient's overall morbidity, mortality, and response to breast cancer treatment?

(A) FRAIL scale score
(B) Pharmacologic cardiac stress test
(C) Six-minute walk test
(D) Timed Up and Go test

Item 94

A 30-year-old man is evaluated for feeling "moody" and having persistent difficulty staying focused and keeping track of tasks. He reports often feeling restless and catching himself jumping between tasks before completing them. He describes himself as "hopelessly disorganized." As a result, he has lost or not paid home utility bills and has not always completed work tasks to the satisfaction of his supervisor. He recalls having these problems since childhood. He is otherwise well. He does not use coffee, alcohol, tobacco, or recreational drugs and does not take any medications.

In addition to cognitive behavioral therapy, which of the following is the most appropriate treatment?

(A) Clonazepam
(B) Escitalopram
(C) Methylphenidate
(D) Ropinirole

Item 95

A 26-year-old woman is evaluated for left lateral knee and distal thigh pain that began 6 weeks ago. She is a long-distance runner who trains 6 days per week. The pain began insidiously and has slowly worsened over time. The pain is worst when she is running downhill. She experiences no pain while resting. She has not had any knee trauma and reports no catching, grinding, or locking.

On physical examination, vital signs are normal. On palpation, tenderness is noted 2 cm proximal to the lateral femoral condyle. With the patient supine, pain is reproduced with repeated flexion and extension of the knee as thumb pressure is applied to the lateral femoral epicondyle. There is weakness with left hip abduction. There is no joint line tenderness, joint effusion, or ligament laxity with applied stress.

Which of the following is the most likely diagnosis?

(A) Iliotibial band syndrome
(B) Lateral collateral ligament tear
(C) Lateral meniscal tear
(D) Meralgia paresthetica

Item 96

A 28-year-old woman is evaluated for persistent pain in the left upper outer breast of 9 weeks' duration. The pain is nonradiating and is not associated with aggravating factors or trauma. She has not noted breast lumps, fever, nipple discharge, or skin changes. Medical history is unremarkable, and she has no family history of breast or ovarian cancer. She takes no medications.

On physical examination, vital signs are normal. BMI is 24. The breast tissue is dense, with no overlying skin changes or underlying masses. Focal tenderness is elicited on palpation of the upper quadrant of the left breast, but no mass or chest wall tenderness is present. There is no evidence of axillary, cervical, or supraclavicular lymphadenopathy. The remainder of the examination is unremarkable.

Which of the following is the most appropriate management?

(A) Advise elimination of caffeine
(B) Breast ultrasonography
(C) Initiate danazol
(D) Mammography and breast ultrasonography
(E) Reassurance

Item 97

A 52-year-old man is evaluated for substernal chest pain. The pain is not consistently associated with exertion, nor is it always relieved by rest; it sometimes occurs when he is eating or when he is anxious. He has a 30-pack-year smoking history, but he quit smoking 2 years ago. Medical history is significant for hypertension and hyperlipidemia, for which he takes lisinopril and rosuvastatin, respectively.

On physical examination, vital signs and cardiovascular examination are normal.

An electrocardiogram reveals left ventricular hypertrophy with associated ST-T-wave changes, findings that are unchanged from an electrocardiogram obtained 2 years ago.

The patient's pretest probability of ischemic coronary artery disease is estimated to be 50%. Treadmill stress echocardiography is performed. This test has a positive likelihood ratio of 10.0 and a negative likelihood ratio of 0.1. The patient's stress test result is positive.

Which of the following best approximates the patient's posttest probability of ischemic coronary artery disease?

(A) 65%
(B) 75%
(C) 85%
(D) 95%

Item 98

A 34-year-old woman is hospitalized for a small bowel resection due to multiple strictures. She has a 10-year history of Crohn disease. History is also significant for a provoked pulmonary embolism that occurred 5 years ago. Medications are azathioprine and certolizumab.

On physical examination, vital signs are normal. The abdomen is soft. Mild diffuse pain without rebound or guarding is noted.

The patient's Caprini risk score for venous thromboembolism is 6 (high risk).

Which of the following is the most appropriate postoperative venous thromboembolism prophylaxis for this patient?

(A) Graduated compression stockings
(B) Graduated compression stockings and low-molecular-weight heparin
(C) Intermittent pneumatic compression
(D) Low-molecular-weight heparin
(E) Low-molecular-weight heparin and intermittent pneumatic compression

Item 99

A 49-year-old man is hospitalized for a 4-day history of poorly controlled nausea, vomiting, fatigue, and volume depletion. He has locally advanced esophageal adenocarcinoma and is undergoing neoadjuvant chemoradiation therapy. Radiation therapy is administered daily, and chemotherapy with low-dose carboplatin plus paclitaxel is administered weekly. His nausea and vomiting are temporally related to the radiation therapy. Medical history is otherwise significant for previous tobacco use. Other medications are acetaminophen, docusate sodium, bisacodyl, oxycodone, and prochlorperazine.

On physical examination, the patient appears fatigued. Blood pressure is 110/68 mm Hg, and pulse rate is 96/min; the remaining vital signs are normal. Pain is elicited with deep palpation of the epigastrium.

Which of the following is the most appropriate initial treatment of this patient's nausea?

(A) Haloperidol
(B) Olanzapine
(C) Ondansetron
(D) Synthetic oral cannabinoids

Item 100

A 30-year-old woman is evaluated for a 2-day history of sore throat and fatigue. She reports anorexia, chills, fever, rhinorrhea, and a dry persistent cough that keeps her awake at night. She works as a school bus driver. She has tried over-the-counter cough and cold products without benefit. Medical history is unremarkable, and she takes no medications.

On physical examination, temperature is 37.2 °C (99.0 °F); all other vital signs are normal. She has nasal and pharyngeal erythema with sparse whitish exudate. There is no lymphadenopathy or rash. The remainder of the examination is normal.

Which of the following is the most appropriate management?

(A) Amoxicillin
(B) Streptococcal rapid antigen detection test
(C) Symptom control
(D) Throat culture

Item 101

A 22-year-old woman is evaluated in the emergency department after an episode of syncope. She experienced a prodrome of nausea, diaphoresis, and warmth while waiting in line to attend a concert in a crowded, warm corridor. Her boyfriend reports that she recovered quickly and was not confused after the event. Before the episode, she had skipped dinner to arrive at the concert early. She experienced a similar episode of syncope at age 14 years when she had venipuncture for routine laboratory testing. She describes no other symptoms at the time of the episode, and her only reported symptom at this time is fatigue. She takes no medications.

On physical examination, blood pressure is 118/65 mm Hg sitting and 108/60 mm Hg after standing for 3 minutes, and pulse rate is 78/min sitting and 82/min after standing for 3 minutes. Other vital signs and the remainder of the examination are normal.

An electrocardiogram is normal.

Which of the following is the most likely diagnosis?

(A) Hypoglycemia-induced syncope
(B) Neurally mediated syncope
(C) Orthostatic syncope
(D) Postural orthostatic tachycardia syndrome

Item 102

A 67-year-old man is evaluated in follow-up for urinary incontinence. Six months ago, he began tamsulosin for occasional nocturia, frequency, and urgency related to benign prostatic hyperplasia. Tamsulosin decreased the frequency of nocturia, but he continued to have daytime urinary urgency with a few occasions of urine leakage. He attempted to control his symptoms with behavioral modification, including bladder training and scheduled voiding, but he still has episodes of urgency and leakage. He prefers not to undergo any surgical intervention. Medical history is otherwise significant for heart failure with preserved ejection fraction. Medications include benazepril, carvedilol, furosemide, spironolactone, tamsulosin, and aspirin.

On physical examination, blood pressure is 102/60 mm Hg, and pulse rate is 72/min. Other vital signs and the remainder of the physical examination are normal.

Bladder ultrasonography shows a postvoid residual urine volume of 30 mL.

Which of the following is the most appropriate treatment?

(A) Dutasteride
(B) Intermittent bladder catheterization
(C) Mirabegron
(D) Sacral nerve root neurostimulation

Item 103

A 29-year-old woman is evaluated during a routine examination. She is asymptomatic. Her last Pap smear was obtained 3 years ago and was normal. She completed the human papillomavirus (HPV) vaccine series at age 26 years. Medical and family histories are unremarkable. She takes no medications.

Which of the following is the most appropriate cervical cancer screening strategy at this time?

(A) Cervical cytology
(B) Cervical cytology and HPV testing
(C) High-risk HPV testing
(D) No further testing

Item 104

A 31-year-old man is evaluated for dull, aching, left-sided scrotal discomfort and fullness with intermittent swelling. His symptoms began 6 months ago. He is sexually inactive.

On physical examination, vital signs are normal. Testicular size is normal bilaterally. On his left hemiscrotum, there are tenderness to palpation in the superolateral region and soft, compressible swelling along the spermatic cord, which increases with standing and the Valsalva maneuver. Transillumination and the Prehn sign (diminished scrotal discomfort with elevation) are negative.

Which of the following is the most appropriate treatment?

(A) Ceftriaxone plus doxycycline
(B) Ibuprofen and scrotal support
(C) Ligation of the left gonadal vein
(D) Topical lidocaine

Item 105

A 60-year-old woman is evaluated for left wrist pain that began 3 months ago. She describes the pain as aching, with an intermittent tingling sensation over her left thumb, index, and middle fingers. Symptoms are worse at night and with repetitive motion of the wrist. She types frequently during her work as an administrative assistant.

On physical examination, vital signs are normal. The left wrist exhibits full range of motion, with no visible swelling. There is no evidence of sensory loss, muscle atrophy, or weakness.

Which of the following is the most appropriate initial management?

(A) Electromyography
(B) Glucocorticoid injection
(C) Splinting of the wrist
(D) Surgical decompression of the median nerve

Item 106

A 45-year-old woman is evaluated for a 2-day history of deep boring pain in the right eye. She also describes eye redness and photophobia but no recent trauma to the eye. She has a 10-year history of rheumatoid arthritis, treated with etanercept.

On physical examination, vital signs are normal. Diffuse right eye redness is noted, and there is pain on extraocular movement testing. Gentle pressure over the eye with the lid closed results in pain. There is no scleromalacia in either eye. There is diminished visual acuity of the right eye.

Which of the following is the most likely diagnosis?

(A) Episcleritis
(B) Scleritis
(C) Subconjunctival hemorrhage
(D) Viral conjunctivitis

Item 107

A 57-year-old man is evaluated prior to a right partial nephrectomy for renal cell carcinoma. He is asymptomatic. Medical history is significant for stage 3 chronic kidney disease, hypertension, hyperlipidemia, and degenerative joint disease. He has no history of abnormal bleeding and tolerated left knee arthroplasty 3 years ago without complications. Family history is negative for bleeding diatheses. Medications are lisinopril, hydrochlorothiazide, and simvastatin.

On physical examination, temperature is normal, blood pressure is 125/75 mm Hg, pulse rate is 63/min, and respiration rate is 18/min. BMI is 29. Cardiac examination reveals a regular rate and rhythm with no murmurs. Lungs are clear to auscultation. There is no lower extremity edema, conjunctival pallor, abdominal mass or tenderness, or hepatomegaly.

Which of the following is the most appropriate preoperative testing for this patient?

(A) Alanine aminotransferase and aspartate aminotransferase levels
(B) Prothrombin time and activated partial thromboplastin time
(C) Serum creatinine and electrolyte levels
(D) No preoperative testing

Item 108

A 46-year-old woman is evaluated for knee pain. Seven months ago, she underwent sleeve gastrectomy for obesity. Before the procedure, her BMI was 36. She recently initiated a running program to enhance her weight loss and is now experiencing knee pain, which she treats with ibuprofen as needed. Medical history is significant for hypertension, obesity, and type 2 diabetes mellitus. Medications are atorvastatin, ibuprofen, lisinopril, and metformin.

On physical examination, blood pressure is 118/64 mm Hg; other vital signs are normal. Knee examination is remarkable for tenderness with compression of the patella. There is no joint instability or tenderness along the medial or lateral joint lines.

Which of the following medications should be discontinued in this patient?

(A) Atorvastatin
(B) Ibuprofen
(C) Lisinopril
(D) Metformin

Item 109

A 38-year-old man is evaluated for an 8-week history of insomnia and irritability. He previously saw another physician in the practice, whom he describes as a "terrible doctor." He was treated for depression for several years and has a history of several low-lethality suicide attempts, usually related to interpersonal conflicts. He also reports having turbulent relationships with his parents and siblings.

During the appointment, he makes several compliments about your bedside manner and calls you the best doctor he has ever had. In discussing his symptoms, he attributes many of them to the break-up with his previous girlfriend. After the break-up, he engaged in a 3-day drinking and gambling binge. The patient says he is doing great now because he is in a new relationship with "the perfect woman."

Which of the following is the most likely diagnosis?

(A) Bipolar disorder
(B) Borderline personality disorder
(C) Generalized anxiety disorder
(D) Histrionic personality disorder

Item 110

A 33-year-old woman is evaluated for a 16-month history of chronic fatigue, unrefreshing sleep, difficulty concentrating, and postexertional malaise. As a result of her symptoms, she has become isolated, restricting her social and personal activities. She has also taken sick days from work with increasing frequency in recent months. Medical and family histories are unremarkable. She takes no medications.

On physical examination, the patient has depressed mood. Vital signs are normal. Neurologic examination and the remainder of the examination are normal.

Her PHQ-9 score is 6, consistent with mild depression.

After a careful evaluation, the patient is diagnosed with systemic exertion intolerance disease.

In addition to a graded exercise program, which of the following is the most appropriate treatment?

(A) Cognitive behavioral therapy
(B) Methylphenidate
(C) Mirtazapine
(D) Prednisone
(E) Sertraline

Item 111

A 35-year-old woman is evaluated during a routine follow-up examination for hypothyroidism and requests a prescription for birth control pills. She is in a new sexual relationship. She has regular menstrual cycles, and her last menstrual period was 4 weeks ago. Her most recent Pap smear was obtained 2 years ago and was normal. Her only medical problem is hypothyroidism treated with levothyroxine. Her mother had breast cancer at age 67 years.

On physical examination, vital signs are normal. BMI is 25. The remainder of the examination is unremarkable.

Which of the following is the most appropriate next step in her management?

(A) Advise against hormonal contraception
(B) Mammography
(C) Pelvic examination and Pap test
(D) Pregnancy test

Item 112

A 38-year-old woman is evaluated for low back pain that began 7 days ago when she bent over to pick up a piece of paper. She describes the pain as moderate aching that is localized to the right lower back. A sharp pain intermittently radiates down the lateral aspect of the right leg. She has not had bowel or bladder dysfunction, fevers, leg weakness, night sweats, saddle anesthesia, or weight loss. She has no history of trauma, and she does not use intravenous drugs.

On physical examination, vital signs are normal. BMI is 21. Musculoskeletal and neurologic examinations are normal.

Which of the following is the most appropriate initial treatment?

(A) Acetaminophen
(B) Duloxetine
(C) Nonpharmacologic modalities
(D) Oxycodone

Item 113

A 59-year-old man is evaluated following recent diagnoses of type 2 diabetes mellitus and hypertension. He is asymptomatic. He has never smoked cigarettes. Medications are metformin, chlorthalidone, and low-dose aspirin.

On physical examination, blood pressure is 130/80 mm Hg; other vital signs are normal. BMI is 36. The remainder of the physical examination is unremarkable.

Laboratory studies:

Total cholesterol	243 mg/dL (6.29 mmol/L)
LDL cholesterol	140 mg/dL (3.63 mmol/L)
HDL cholesterol	45 mg/dL (1.17 mmol/L)
Triglycerides	290 mg/dL (3.28 mmol/L)

His 10-year risk for atherosclerotic cardiovascular disease (ASCVD) based on the Pooled Cohort Equations is 22.4%.

The patient is instructed in therapeutic lifestyle changes to lower his risk for ASCVD.

Which of the following is the most appropriate additional treatment for primary prevention of ASCVD in this patient?

(A) Fenofibrate
(B) Fish oil supplementation
(C) Moderate- or high-intensity atorvastatin
(D) No additional treatment is required

Item 114

A 49-year-old man is evaluated for a 2-year history of poor sleep with associated daytime fatigue and sleepiness that often interfere with his performance at work. He recorded a sleep diary, which reveals difficulty with sleep initiation and multiple awakenings throughout the night. He has no other physical symptoms that affect his sleep, and his partner does not notice him snoring or gasping.

Physical examination, including vital signs, is normal.

Which of the following is the most appropriate next step in management?

(A) Cognitive behavioral therapy
(B) Diphenhydramine
(C) Melatonin
(D) Mirtazapine
(E) Zolpidem

Item 115

A 52-year-old man fails to attend a scheduled appointment. He was initially evaluated for bilateral knee osteoarthritis 1 year ago, and treatment with weight loss, NSAIDs, and physical therapy was recommended. Over the past year, the patient missed three scheduled appointments, did not attend physical therapy, arrived for urgent care assessment twice with requests for stronger pain medications, and did not complete sufficient trials of oral nonopioid pharmacologic agents. Attempts to reach the patient by phone to discuss adherence to his care plan have not been successful. The visit today was scheduled to discuss the difficulties in his treatment and assess his barriers to care. Medical history is significant for bipolar disorder. In past visits, he has not appeared manic or suicidal.

Which of the following is the most appropriate management?

(A) Refer the patient to a psychiatrist
(B) Report the patient to the local mental health crisis team
(C) Send the patient a letter warning that the relationship may be terminated
(D) Terminate the patient relationship immediately

Item 116

A 35-year-old woman is evaluated for numbness, tingling, and weakness in her left arm that radiates from the shoulder to the fingers. Her symptoms began 3 months ago and appear to be worsening. They occur with repetitive use of the arm, especially with overhead activities. She has been painting a ceiling mural for the past 6 months. She has no history of arm or shoulder trauma. She takes no medications.

On physical examination, vital signs are normal. When the patient holds her arms above her head for several minutes during the examination, the symptoms are reproduced. The neck demonstrates full range of motion, and muscle bulk and tone in the upper extremities are normal bilaterally. Neurologic examination is normal, and all upper extremity pulses are full and equal.

Results of electrodiagnostic studies are normal.

Which is the most appropriate therapy for this patient?

(A) Gabapentin
(B) Interscalene injection of botulinum toxin type A

(C) Physical therapy
(D) Surgical decompression

Item 117

A 52-year-old woman is evaluated for acute onset of right-sided hearing loss that began yesterday. Soon afterward, she also noted a sensation of ear fullness and ringing in the same ear. She has no other focal neurologic symptoms. She reports no rhinorrhea, fever, pharyngitis, or ear pain. Medical history is significant for hypertension. She takes chlorthalidone. She has had no other exposures to medications or supplements.

On physical examination, vital signs are normal. There is decreased hearing in the right ear; the Weber test lateralizes to the left ear, and air conduction is louder than bone conduction bilaterally. The ear canals are unobstructed, and the tympanic membranes are normal appearing. The neurologic examination is unremarkable.

Which of the following is the most likely diagnosis?

(A) Meniere disease
(B) Otosclerosis
(C) Ototoxicity
(D) Sudden sensorineural hearing loss

Item 118

A 60-year-old man is evaluated in the hospital for a pressure injury. The pressure injury developed during a prolonged hospitalization after a motor vehicle accident that resulted in a closed head injury and pelvic and spinal fractures. Medications are heparin, oxycodone, and ibuprofen or acetaminophen as needed.

On physical examination, vital signs are normal. A painful 4-cm sacral ulcer with full-thickness loss of skin and adipose tissue is present (stage III). The ulcer has no purulence or surrounding induration.

Which of the following is the most appropriate treatment?

(A) Hydrocolloid dressing
(B) Platelet-derived growth factor dressing
(C) Standard gauze dressing
(D) Zinc-infused dressing

Item 119

A 25-year-old man is evaluated during a new patient visit. He is experiencing severe anxiety about the start of a new job next month. Specifically, he is concerned about his ability to arrive on time because every morning before leaving his apartment, he feels compelled to perform multiple checks to ensure that all electronic devices are turned off and all windows and doors are locked. These activities consume approximately 1 hour of time. He performs these same activities each night before going to bed and often repeats them several times because of overwhelming feelings that he has forgotten something and his apartment will catch fire or be robbed. As a result of his anxieties, the patient rarely socializes outside of his home. When he is away from home, he uses a surveillance application to monitor his apartment 11 minutes after every hour.

Which of the following is the most appropriate management?

(A) Buspirone
(B) Clonazepam
(C) Cognitive behavioral therapy
(D) Risperidone

Item 120

A 58-year-old man is evaluated in an urgent care center for a 3-day history of right-sided scrotal swelling, pain, and dysuria. He reports no antecedent trauma, nausea, or vomiting. He is sexually active with both men and women and uses condoms intermittently. He does not take any medications.

On physical examination, temperature is 38.5 °C (101.3 °F), pulse rate is 101/min, and other vital signs are normal. The right hemiscrotum is edematous, with tenderness to palpation of the superolateral aspect. The scrotal pain lessens with elevation of the scrotum. There is no penile discharge.

Results of nucleic acid amplification testing for chlamydia and gonorrhea are pending.

Which of the following is the most appropriate treatment?

(A) Ceftriaxone
(B) Ceftriaxone and doxycycline
(C) Ceftriaxone and levofloxacin
(D) Ibuprofen and scrotal support

Item 121

A 44-year-old woman is evaluated for a breast lump she noticed 1 week ago. There is no nipple discharge. She birthed two children, the first at age 25 years, and her menstrual cycles are regular. She has no family members with breast or ovarian cancer. She has no other medical problems and takes no medications.

On physical examination, vital signs are normal. BMI is 28. Examination of the breasts reveals dense tissue bilaterally and no skin changes. A mass is noted in the upper inner area of the right breast, measuring 1.8 cm; it is firm, mobile, and nontender, with ill-defined margins. There is no evidence of axillary, cervical, or supraclavicular lymphadenopathy. The remainder of the examination is unremarkable.

Which of the following is the most appropriate diagnostic test to perform next?

(A) Breast MRI
(B) Core-needle biopsy
(C) Diagnostic mammography and ultrasonography
(D) Ultrasonography

Item 122

A 34-year-old woman is evaluated during a follow-up visit for blood pressure control. She states that she hopes to become pregnant and would like to stop her oral contraceptive. She

does not smoke, drink alcohol, or use illicit drugs. She is in a monogamous sexual relationship and has had no sexually transmitted infections. Medical history is significant for hypertension, type 2 diabetes mellitus, and depression since childhood. Medications are an oral contraceptive, lisinopril, metformin, citalopram, and acetaminophen as needed.

On physical examination, vital signs are normal. The remainder of the examination is unremarkable.

In addition to starting folic acid, which of the following medications should be stopped at this time?

(A) Acetaminophen
(B) Citalopram
(C) Lisinopril
(D) Metformin

Item 123

A 77-year-old woman is seen for a preoperative medical evaluation before resection of the sigmoid colon for recurrent diverticulitis scheduled 5 days from now. She has nonvalvular atrial fibrillation and is receiving long-term warfarin, without a history of bleeding complications. She has no history of stroke, transient ischemic attack, or intracardiac thrombus. History is also significant for hypertension. Medications are warfarin, chlorthalidone, and metoprolol.

The physical examination, including vital signs, is normal.

The INR measurement is 2.3. Calculated $CHADS_2$ score is 2, and CHA_2DS_2-VASc score is 4.

In addition to withholding warfarin before surgery, which of the following is the most appropriate management of this patient's perioperative anticoagulation?

(A) Begin aspirin, 81 mg/d
(B) Begin enoxaparin when the INR drops below 2.0
(C) Begin unfractionated heparin when the INR drops below 2.0
(D) No additional interventions

Item 124

A 26-year-old man is evaluated during a routine examination. He is asymptomatic. The patient is sexually active with men and has had multiple partners in the past year. He engages in both oral and anal sex, and he reports using condoms most of the time. He does not use illicit drugs. He is unsure about his vaccination status and has never been tested for HIV infection, syphilis, or infectious hepatitis. Medical history is unremarkable. He takes no medications.

The physical examination, including vital signs, is normal.

Screening is arranged for HIV infection, syphilis, and hepatitis A and B.

Which of the following additional screening tests is most appropriate, as recommended by the Centers for Disease Control and Prevention?

(A) Anal cytology
(B) Hepatitis C antibody assay

(C) Nucleic acid amplification test for chlamydia and gonorrhea

(D) No additional tests are indicated

Item 125

A 31-year-old man is evaluated during a follow-up visit for depression. He previously experienced two episodes of major depressive disorder that were effectively treated with fluoxetine. Three months ago, he presented with recurrent symptoms of depression. His PHQ-9 score was 14, indicating moderate depression. Fluoxetine was initiated and uptitrated to an effective dosage. The patient now reports significant improvement in his symptoms. His PHQ-9 score is 6, indicating mild depression; he reports no adverse effects from the medication.

Which of the following is the most appropriate next step in management?

(A) Complete 8 months of fluoxetine therapy

(B) Complete 8 months of fluoxetine, then switch to bupropion for long-term maintenance therapy

(C) Continue fluoxetine as long-term maintenance therapy

(D) Discontinue fluoxetine

Item 126

A 38-year-old man is evaluated during a new-patient visit for a 5-year history of fatigue, dizziness, nonexertional chest pain, intermittent and transient abdominal swelling, insomnia, and fleeting numbness of the extremities. He has been evaluated by two different internal medicine physicians, a gastroenterologist, a rheumatologist, and a pulmonologist. Despite extensive blood testing and imaging, a unifying diagnosis has never been established. Medical history is significant for depression, migraine, and cholecystectomy. He does not use tobacco, alcohol, or illicit drugs. Current medications are ibuprofen and sumatriptan as needed, acetaminophen, and citalopram.

Physical examination, including vital signs, is normal.

In addition to eliciting the patient's concerns, which of the following is the most appropriate initial management?

(A) Comprehensive metabolic profile and C-reactive protein level

(B) *MEFV1* genetic testing

(C) Obtain all previous medical records

(D) Psychiatry consultation

(E) Rheumatoid factor and antinuclear antibody titer

Item 127

A 49-year-old man is evaluated for a 2-day history of posterior neck stiffness and pain that radiates down his left arm and into the fourth and fifth fingers of his left hand. He is left-handed and works as a roofer. The pain worsens when he turns his head to the left and improves when he lies down, although he sometimes has pain when rising from a prone position. He has not had any arm or hand weakness or problems writing. He has no systemic symptoms.

On physical examination, vital signs are normal. On palpation, the pain is reproduced when the examiner applies downward pressure with the patient's head bent to the left and extended (Spurling test). Pain is relieved when the patient holds his left arm above the plane of his shoulder. Neck range of motion is limited with both left and right lateral rotation. There is no cervical spine tenderness to palpation. The neurologic examination is normal.

Which of the following is the most appropriate management?

(A) Cervical collar

(B) Cervical MRI

(C) Electrodiagnostic testing

(D) Gabapentin

(E) Neck exercises

Item 128

A 25-year-old woman is evaluated during a routine wellness visit. She received the tetanus toxoid, reduced diphtheria toxoid, and acellular pertussis (Tdap) vaccine at age 18 years; the meningococcal conjugate vaccine at age 11 years with a booster dose at age 16 years; and an influenza vaccine during the most recent influenza season. She is single, lives in an apartment with a roommate, and is a nonsmoker. She has no upcoming travel plans. She has no medical problems and takes no medications.

Physical examination, including vital signs, is normal.

Which of the following vaccinations should be offered to this patient?

(A) Human papillomavirus vaccine

(B) Quadrivalent meningococcal conjugate vaccine

(C) Tdap vaccine

(D) 23-Valent pneumococcal polysaccharide vaccine

Item 129

A 49-year-old woman is seeking therapy for a 6-month history of increasing hot flushes, now occurring six to eight times per day. She also has night sweats that occur three to five times per night and result in disrupted sleep and daytime fatigue. Her last menstrual period was 14 months ago. She has no personal or family history of breast or ovarian malignancies. She takes no medications.

On physical examination, vital signs are normal, as are pelvic and breast examinations.

Which of the following is the most appropriate management?

(A) Hormone therapy with estrogen alone

(B) Hormone therapy with estrogen and progesterone

(C) Ospemifene

(D) Vaginal estrogen therapy

Item 130

A 55-year-old man is evaluated in the emergency department for a 2-day history of dizziness accompanied by nausea and vomiting. He works as an electrician, and his symptoms started suddenly while installing an overhead light fixture with his head tilted back for a prolonged period. He describes the dizziness as a constant whirling sensation that is unaffected by changes in position. He also reports symptoms of a recent upper respiratory tract infection but no fever. He has no other medical problems and takes no medications.

On physical examination, temperature is normal, blood pressure is 155/84 mm Hg, pulse rate is 99/min, and respiration rate is normal. Hearing is diminished on the left side. Spontaneous combined horizontal and torsional nystagmus is noted but lessens with a fixed gaze. The patient declines further examination because of severe nausea.

Which of the following is the most likely diagnosis?

(A) Benign paroxysmal positional vertigo
(B) Labyrinthitis
(C) Meniere disease
(D) Posterior circulation stroke
(E) Vestibular neuronitis

Item 131

A 47-year-old man is evaluated for a 2-day history of cough productive of small amounts of yellow sputum, as well as sinus congestion, frontal headache, rhinorrhea, and malaise. He has had no fevers, chest pain, or shortness of breath. Medical history is otherwise unremarkable.

On physical examination, vital signs are normal. There is tenderness over the maxillary sinuses bilaterally. The nasal mucosa is diffusely edematous with moderate amounts of clear discharge. Pharyngeal examination reveals erythema without tonsillar exudate. The tympanic membranes appear normal. No cervical lymphadenopathy is noted. The remainder of the examination is normal.

Which of the following is the most appropriate treatment?

(A) Amoxicillin
(B) Codeine
(C) Inhaled albuterol
(D) Intranasal fluticasone

Item 132

A 67-year-old woman with multiple myeloma is evaluated for back pain. The pain began several months ago but has dramatically worsened in the past 2 weeks. It is located in the lumbar and thoracic spine with associated paraspinal muscle spasms. The pain does not radiate into the buttocks or legs, and there has been no change in gait or bowel or bladder function. She rates the pain as an 8 on a 10-point scale at its worst. Medical history is significant for multiple myeloma and end-stage kidney disease on hemodialysis. Medications are acetaminophen, amlodipine, aspirin, metoprolol, sertraline, bortezomib, dexamethasone, and lenalidomide.

On physical examination, vital signs are normal. Palpation elicits tenderness over the thoracic and lumbar spine. The abdomen is not distended, and there are no palpable masses. Neurologic examination is normal.

Restaging CT scans from 2 months ago reveal lytic lesions in the lumbar spine and left iliac crest.

Spine MRI is scheduled.

Which of the following is the most appropriate treatment of this patient's pain?

(A) Fentanyl patch
(B) Gabapentin
(C) Hydromorphone
(D) Morphine
(E) Tramadol

Item 133

A 68-year-old man is evaluated before elective left total hip arthroplasty. He reports left groin pain and new fatigue and dyspnea that limit ambulation to one flight of stairs and one block. Medical history is significant for type 2 diabetes mellitus, ischemic stroke, hypertension, hyperlipidemia, peripheral artery disease, degenerative joint disease, and chronic kidney disease. Medications are insulin glargine, insulin lispro, aspirin, lisinopril, simvastatin, and tramadol.

On physical examination, temperature is normal, blood pressure is 145/85 mm Hg, pulse rate is 89/min, and respiration rate is 18/min. BMI is 35. Cardiopulmonary examination is normal. There is no lower extremity edema.

Laboratory studies are notable for a serum creatinine level of 2.1 mg/dL (185.6 µmol/L).

An electrocardiogram demonstrates Q waves in leads II and III.

Which of the following is the most appropriate diagnostic test to perform next?

(A) Dobutamine stress echocardiography
(B) Exercise electrocardiography
(C) Transthoracic echocardiography
(D) No further testing

Item 134

A physician has noticed that a 67-year-old colleague in the medical practice has been increasingly forgetful in recent months. The colleague has had more difficulty remembering the names of her new patients and the medical students who are doing rotations in the practice, and she has also frequently missed meetings because of scheduling mix-ups. She admits that she cannot keep track of all of the new medications for diabetes mellitus without using a reference. The physician is unaware of the colleague's personal medical history but is concerned about her memory and cognitive status.

Which of the following is the most appropriate management?

(A) Continue to monitor the colleague
(B) Directly approach the colleague and help her plan for confidential evaluation
(C) Offer to confidentially evaluate the colleague
(D) Report the colleague to the state medical board

Item 135

A 64-year-old man is evaluated for a 5-year history of intermittent erectile dysfunction. He experiences nocturnal and early-morning penile tumescence, and he is able to achieve and maintain an erection sufficient for sexual activity approximately 50% of the time. Medical history is significant for coronary artery disease, depression, hyperlipidemia, hypertension, obstructive sleep apnea, peripheral vascular disease, and type 2 diabetes mellitus. Medications are aspirin, atorvastatin, isosorbide mononitrate, lisinopril, metformin, metoprolol, and sertraline. He does not use continuous positive airway pressure.

On physical examination, all vital signs are normal. BMI is 26. He has normal body hair growth and pattern, normal testicular size, and no gynecomastia.

Laboratory studies reveal an 8:00 AM serum fasting total testosterone level of 380 ng/dL (13.2 nmol/L).

Which of the following is the most appropriate treatment?

(A) Alprostadil
(B) Psychotherapy
(C) Sildenafil
(D) Testosterone gel

Item 136

A 42-year-old woman is evaluated for a 2-month history of left foot pain between the third and fourth toes, accompanied by a burning sensation and the sensation of walking on a pebble. She has not experienced any trauma in the area, and she does not have edema or erythema. Symptom onset was insidious, and the pain only occurs when she is standing or walking. She works as a restaurant hostess and wears high-heeled shoes for her job.

On physical examination, vital signs are normal. The left foot appears normal, with no palpable abnormalities or tenderness between the third and fourth toes. Sensation is intact throughout the foot, and posterior tibial and dorsalis pedis pulses are palpable.

Which of the following is the most likely diagnosis?

(A) Bunion deformity
(B) Hammertoe deformity
(C) Morton neuroma
(D) Plantar fasciitis

Item 137

A hospital system's initial analysis of costs related to prolonged hospital stays revealed that surgical wound infections account for a large proportion of costs. Assessment of the surgical data for the hospital showed that the postoperative wound infection rate is 19%.

Which of the following is the most appropriate tool to assist in reducing postoperative wound sepsis at this institution?

(A) Clinical audit
(B) Control chart
(C) Lean model
(D) Model for Improvement

Item 138

A 92-year-old woman is evaluated for urinary incontinence. Six months ago, the patient occasionally lost control of small amounts of urine, which was managed with an adult diaper. At present, the patient seems to have lost the ability to recognize that she needs to urinate until it is too late to reach the bathroom. There have been no recent noticeable changes in cognition. Medical history is significant for dementia treated with donepezil.

On physical examination, vital signs are normal. The patient appears frail. She is not oriented to place or time. Gait is stable and narrow based. She is slow to rise from a chair, and she requires the arm rests to get up.

Which of the following is the most appropriate treatment?

(A) Oxybutynin
(B) Pelvic floor muscle training (Kegel exercises)
(C) Prompted voiding
(D) Sling cystourethropexy

Item 139

A 23-year-old man is evaluated during a new patient visit. He was honorably discharged from the Army 2 months ago after serving two tours of duty in Afghanistan. Four months ago, his platoon's vehicle was struck by an improvised explosive device. He sustained a severe concussion and multiple lacerations, and three members of his platoon were killed. For the last 3 months, the patient has had daily nightmares in which he relives the event and can see his comrades being killed. He has also experienced flashbacks of the event when he hears loud noises, such as fireworks and thunder. He has had great difficulty sleeping and is increasingly irritable.

The patient has been unable to find employment because he avoids social situations. He has also withdrawn from family and friends because he is afraid they will ask about his military service, and he does not wish to discuss the events he experienced. He has been drinking alcohol more frequently, having up to four beers before bedtime to induce sleep. He does not use tobacco or recreational drugs.

Medical history is otherwise unremarkable, and physical examination is normal.

Which of the following is the most appropriate treatment?

(A) Clonazepam
(B) Propranolol
(C) Psychotherapy
(D) Topiramate

Item 140

A 61-year-old man is evaluated in an urgent care center for acute frontal headache and pain in the right eye that began a few hours earlier while he was watching his grandson's basketball game. The pain extends through the anterior scalp and downward across the nose. The patient is also nauseated and vomiting acutely. He has photophobia and notes that lights appear "fuzzy." Medical history is significant for hypertension and anxiety. Medications are hydrochlorothiazide and citalopram.

On physical examination, blood pressure is 150/90 mm Hg; other vital signs are normal. Severe conjunctival erythema; photophobia; a mid-dilated, nonreactive pupil on the right side; and corneal cloudiness are noted. Upon gentle palpation of the eyes, tenderness and increased firmness are noted over the right globe compared with the left. Right eye visual acuity is grossly decreased. No discharge is noted.

Which of the following is the most likely diagnosis?

(A) Acute angle-closure glaucoma
(B) Bacterial endophthalmitis
(C) Central retinal vein occlusion
(D) Scleritis

Item 141

A 31-year-old woman requests genetic testing for Huntington disease. She has a close friend who recently had a positive genetic test result for the *huntingtin* gene mutation, and she would like to undergo testing for assurance that she is without the disease. She is asymptomatic. Medical history is unremarkable. She takes no medications.

On physical examination, vital signs are normal. Neurologic examination and the remainder of the examination are normal.

Which of the following is the most appropriate management?

(A) Obtain a brain MRI
(B) Obtain a three-generation family history
(C) Obtain genetic testing
(D) Refer for genetic counseling

Item 142

A 45-year-old woman is evaluated for heavy menstrual bleeding. She reports having heavy unpredictable bleeding of variable flow and duration for the past year. Her last period was 12 days ago. She has a history of provoked deep venous thrombosis 3 years ago following an intercontinental flight. She is a current smoker with a 10-pack-year history and does not wish to quit smoking at this time. She has never been pregnant and does not wish to become pregnant in the future.

On physical examination, vital signs are normal. BMI is 24. Breast and pelvic examinations are normal.

Laboratory studies reveal a hemoglobin level of 10.2 g/dL (102 g/L) and mean corpuscular volume of 68 fL. Pregnancy test result is negative.

A subsequent evaluation for secondary causes of abnormal uterine bleeding, including endometrial cancer, was negative.

In addition to oral iron supplements, which of the following is the most appropriate management?

(A) Combination oral contraceptive pill
(B) Endometrial ablation
(C) Levonorgestrel-containing intrauterine device
(D) Medroxyprogesterone acetate for the second half of the menstrual cycle

Item 143

A 28-year-old man is evaluated for a 10-month history of dizziness. He describes the dizziness as a sense of nonvertiginous imbalance and notes that it worsens with personal motion, movement of objects around him, and sitting or standing upright. The dizziness has persisted since he experienced a concussion without loss of consciousness while playing soccer 10 months ago. He reports no focal neurologic symptoms. He takes no medications.

On physical examination, vital signs are normal. On neurologic examination, cranial nerve examination findings are normal, motor strength is intact, and deep tendon reflexes are normal. Romberg test result is negative. Gait is normal.

Findings on a brain MRI are normal.

In addition to vestibular and balance rehabilitation therapy, which of the following is the most appropriate treatment?

(A) Amitriptyline
(B) Canalith repositioning maneuver (Epley maneuver)
(C) Lorazepam
(D) Sertraline

Item 144

H

An 82-year-old man is evaluated for discharge planning. He was hospitalized with community-acquired pneumonia complicated by respiratory failure and sepsis, which required prolonged mechanical ventilation. He eventually required a tracheostomy and remains on mechanical ventilation, but his respiratory status is otherwise stable. He is severely deconditioned and has been unable to participate even minimally in physical therapy. Although he is expected to require mechanical ventilation for at least several more weeks, he is medically stable for discharge. Medical history is significant for chronic kidney disease, heart failure, hypertension, and type 2 diabetes mellitus. Medications are insulin aspart, insulin glargine, carvedilol, furosemide, and lisinopril.

On physical examination, the patient is alert and cooperative but appears frail on mechanical ventilation. Vital signs and the remainder of the examination are normal.

Which of the following is the most appropriate discharge disposition for this patient?

(A) Acute rehabilitation facility
(B) In-home rehabilitation services
(C) Rehabilitation at a long-term acute care hospital
(D) Skilled nursing facility

Item 145

A proposed new screening protocol for ovarian cancer involves universal pelvic ultrasonography for asymptomatic women starting at age 30 years. The protocol is based on a national study of randomly selected 30-year-old women. The authors of the study note that unilateral oophorectomy performed for suspicious lesions resulted in longer survival than oophorectomy performed for patients with symptoms, based on historical data. The study authors conclude that the screening protocol will reduce ovarian cancer–related deaths.

Which of the following is most likely to threaten the validity of the authors' conclusions?

(A) Lead-time bias
(B) Length-time bias
(C) Recall bias
(D) Selection bias

Item 146

A 42-year-old woman is approaching discharge from the hospital for alcohol withdrawal. She has had severe alcohol use disorder for several years but says she is willing to do whatever it takes to quit. Medical history is also significant for hypertension and chronic kidney disease. Medications are amlodipine and chlorthalidone.

Physical examination, including vital signs, is normal.

A complete blood count and comprehensive metabolic profile are normal. The estimated glomerular filtration rate is 50 mL/min/1.73 m^2.

Which of the following is the most appropriate pharmacologic treatment?

(A) Acamprosate
(B) Chlordiazepoxide
(C) Disulfiram
(D) Naltrexone

Item 147

A 72-year-old man is hospitalized for the third time in 3 months for shortness of breath. He has stage 3 chronic kidney disease, end-stage COPD, and New York Heart Association functional class III heart failure. The patient does not have an advance directive, and the resuscitation preference most recently noted from a visit 6 months ago is "full code." Medications are acetaminophen, aspirin, lisinopril, metoprolol, and torsemide.

Which of the following is the most appropriate initial strategy to develop goals of care?

(A) Ask about hospice referral timing
(B) Ask about resuscitation preferences
(C) Ask what he understands about his illnesses
(D) Provide information about prognosis

Item 148

A 50-year-old woman is evaluated in the hospital following a non–ST-elevation myocardial infarction treated with drug-eluting stent placement. She is currently asymptomatic. Medical history is significant only for hypertension. Medications are clopidogrel, aspirin, lisinopril, and metoprolol.

Physical examination, including vital signs, is normal. BMI is 29.

Laboratory studies:

Total cholesterol	239 mg/dL (6.19 mmol/L)
LDL cholesterol	155 mg/dL (4.01 mmol/L)
HDL cholesterol	45 mg/dL (1.17 mmol/L)
Triglycerides	195 mg/dL (2.20 mmol/L)

Which of the following is the most appropriate additional diagnostic testing to perform before initiating high-intensity statin therapy in this patient?

(A) Alanine aminotransferase level measurement
(B) Alanine aminotransferase and creatine kinase level measurement
(C) Creatine kinase level measurement
(D) No further laboratory studies are indicated

Item 149

A 40-year-old man is evaluated during a routine examination. He is healthy and asymptomatic, although he leads a sedentary lifestyle. Family history is noncontributory. He takes no medications.

On physical examination, temperature is normal, blood pressure is 120/74 mm Hg, pulse rate is 68/min, and respiration rate is normal. BMI is 32. The remainder of the physical examination is unremarkable.

When should this patient be screened for diabetes mellitus?

(A) At age 45 years
(B) At this visit
(C) If he develops an additional risk factor for diabetes
(D) No screening is indicated

Item 150

A 19-year-old man is evaluated in the emergency department after his roommate became concerned about his behavior. The patient began college 7 months ago, and since then, his roommate has watched the patient become increasingly isolated from others and lacking in emotion. The patient has frequently expressed concerns that the government is tracking his movements and even his thoughts. In the past 2 months, he has stopped attending classes and spends long periods in bed. The roommate called the patient's parents after the patient sealed up the ventilation in their room because he believed government agents were injecting gas into the building. The patient says he does not feel depressed. He had no behavioral problems before starting college, and he does not use alcohol, recreational drugs, or over-the-counter medications.

Which of the following is the most likely diagnosis?

(A) Bipolar disorder
(B) Major depressive disorder
(C) Paranoid personality disorder
(D) Schizophrenia

Item 151

A 39-year-old woman is evaluated for a 3-week history of malodorous vaginal discharge. She was treated with antibiotics for a urinary tract infection 3 weeks before the onset of symptoms. She is in a monogamous sexual relationship. Medical history is unremarkable. Her only medication is an oral contraceptive.

On physical examination, vital signs are normal. Pelvic examination reveals thin, homogenous, grayish vaginal discharge. There is no adnexal or cervical motion tenderness. The rest of the examination is unremarkable.

Laboratory testing reveals a vaginal pH of 5.6; whiff test result is negative.

Which of the following is the most appropriate test to confirm the diagnosis?

(A) Culture for *Gardnerella vaginalis*
(B) Nucleic acid amplification test for trichomoniasis
(C) Potassium hydroxide wet mount study for yeast
(D) Saline microscopy for clue cells

Item 152

A 60-year-old man is evaluated for a 6-month history of worsening urinary frequency, urgency, hesitancy, incomplete emptying, nocturia, and weakened stream. He reports no dysuria, incontinence, or acute urinary retention. Medical history is also significant for erectile dysfunction. He takes no medications.

On physical examination, vital signs are normal. Rectal examination reveals a diffusely enlarged prostate that is nontender to palpation, with no masses or nodules noted. Testicular size is normal. A comprehensive metabolic profile and urinalysis are normal; an 8:00 AM total testosterone level is also normal.

Which of the following is the most appropriate treatment?

(A) Finasteride
(B) Oxybutynin
(C) Tadalafil
(D) Tamsulosin

Item 153

A 55-year-old man is hospitalized after he was injured at a construction site structure collapse. He has a fractured pelvis, a shoulder dislocation, a mild concussion, and multiple abrasions. He is scheduled to undergo surgery for the fractured pelvis tomorrow morning. History is significant for hyperlipidemia, hypertension, coronary artery disease, and a non–ST-elevation myocardial infarction 2 years ago treated with drug-eluting stent placement. Current medications are atorvastatin, metoprolol, amlodipine, and aspirin.

On physical examination, temperature is normal, blood pressure is 170/90 mm Hg, pulse rate is 102/min, and respiration rate is 20/min. Oxygen saturation is 96% breathing ambient air. Multiple abrasions and ecchymosis are noted. Cardiac examination reveals tachycardia but is otherwise normal.

Which of the following is the most appropriate management of this patient's medications before surgery?

(A) Continue amlodipine, aspirin, and metoprolol; withhold atorvastatin
(B) Continue amlodipine, atorvastatin, and metoprolol; withhold aspirin
(C) Continue atorvastatin, metoprolol, and aspirin; withhold amlodipine
(D) Continue all medications

Item 154

A 50-year-old woman is seen following screening digital mammography. She is asymptomatic and has no medical problems. Other than her age and sex, she has no additional risk factors for breast cancer and no family history of breast cancer. The mammogram report notes no suspicious lesions but indicates that the breasts are heterogeneously dense (density category C).

On previous physical examination, vital signs and breast examination were normal.

In addition to education on breast density, which of the following is the most appropriate adjunctive breast cancer screening?

(A) Breast MRI
(B) Digital breast tomosynthesis
(C) Repeat digital mammography in 6 months
(D) No further testing

Item 155

A 49-year-old woman is evaluated for a 3-year history of pelvic pain. An extensive evaluation has not found a clearly defined pathophysiologic or anatomic cause, and therapy has been targeted to general pain management lately. She has been a willing and cooperative participant in biofeedback, cognitive behavioral therapy, physical therapy, hypnosis, acupuncture, meditation, and stress-reduction techniques, without significant pain relief. Her pain has been unresponsive to multiple trials of nonopioid analgesics and antidepressants, and she has tried oral tapentadol and tramadol, which were also ineffective. She currently takes acetaminophen and gabapentin. Medical history is significant for end-stage kidney disease, for which she receives hemodialysis, and hypertension. Other medications are metoprolol succinate, amlodipine, intravenous iron, and an erythropoiesis-stimulating agent.

Which of the following is the most reasonable treatment option for this patient's chronic pain?

(A) Oral immediate-release morphine sulfate
(B) Oral medical cannabis oil
(C) Oral methadone
(D) Topical lidocaine

Item 156

A 66-year-old man is evaluated for right posterior knee swelling that began 3 days ago. The knee is not painful, unstable, warm, or red. He has no systemic symptoms. History is significant for bilateral knee osteoarthritis. His only medication is aspirin, which adequately controls his osteoarthritis pain.

On physical examination, vital signs are normal. A large bulge is visible on the posterior aspect of the right knee, without erythema, tenderness, or warmth. Crepitus of the knees is noted bilaterally. There is no joint instability or increased laxity with stress forces.

Which of the following is the most appropriate management?

(A) Aspiration of fluid
(B) Glucocorticoid injection
(C) Ibuprofen
(D) Plain radiography of the knee
(E) No treatment

Item 157

A 56-year-old woman is evaluated during a wellness examination. She reports no vaginal bleeding, discharge, or other symptoms since reaching menopause at age 52 years. Over the past 3 months, she has noted a lack of interest in sexual activity that has been occasionally distressing for her. She uses vaginal lubricant for intercourse, which reduces the mild discomfort with sexual activity. She has no history of pelvic surgery, sexually transmitted infections, or sexual trauma. Results of screening tests for anxiety and depression are negative. Medical history is otherwise unremarkable, and she takes no medications.

On physical examination, the external genitalia are normal. Pelvic examination reveals pale vaginal walls and a decrease in vaginal lubrication. The remainder of the examination is unremarkable.

Which of the following is the most likely female sexual disorder diagnosis?

(A) Female orgasmic disorder
(B) Genitopelvic pain/penetration disorder
(C) Sexual interest/arousal disorder
(D) No female sexual disorder

Item 158

A 78-year-old man is evaluated in the emergency department for a 1-day history of worsening dizziness. The patient describes the dizziness as a room-spinning sensation and notes that he has some accompanying nausea and imbalance. He reports no other symptoms. Medical history is notable for hypertension, hyperlipidemia, and type 2 diabetes mellitus. Medications are aspirin, lisinopril, atorvastatin, and metformin.

On physical examination, blood pressure is 172/88 mm Hg; other vital signs are normal. The patient has difficulty with tandem walking. With extraocular movement testing, the patient has vertical nystagmus. The neurologic examination is otherwise nonfocal and without mental status changes.

Which of the following is the most appropriate diagnostic test to perform next?

(A) CT of the head
(B) MRI of the brain

(C) Vestibular laboratory testing
(D) No further testing

Item 159

A 27-year-old woman is evaluated for help with weight loss. After a visit 3 months ago, she enrolled in an online weight loss program and began a walking program. She currently walks 30 minutes per session 5 days per week. She admits that she has difficulty adhering to the diet restrictions. She avoids weighing herself because she finds it discouraging. She has lost 0.2 kg (0.5 lb) since her visit 3 months ago. Medical history is unremarkable, and she takes no medications.

On physical examination, vital signs are normal. BMI is 32. The remainder of the examination is unremarkable.

Which of the following is the most appropriate management?

(A) Bariatric surgery
(B) Behavioral therapy
(C) Exercise for 45 minutes/day
(D) Low-carbohydrate diet
(E) Phentermine-topiramate

Item 160

A 45-year-old man was hospitalized following a head-on motor vehicle crash. On day 4, he survived cardiac arrest but experienced anoxic brain injury. The care team concludes that he has a poor neurologic prognosis and is unlikely to regain consciousness or interact with his environment.

A family meeting is planned to discuss the decision to perform a tracheostomy and percutaneous endoscopic gastrostomy for enteral feeding. His wife reports that the patient has previously stated that he would not want to be kept alive if he could not interact with her or their children. The patient does not have an advance directive.

Which of the following should be the basis for the decision regarding this patient's management?

(A) Patient's best interests
(B) Patient's medical condition
(C) Patient's previously expressed wishes
(D) Risk management

Item 161

A 58-year-old man is admitted to the hospital for a 2-week history of worsening constipation. He has end-stage heart failure (New York Heart Association functional class IV) and stage 3 chronic kidney disease. Medications include bisoprolol, furosemide, losartan, spironolactone, hydromorphone (for dyspnea palliation), bisacodyl, lactulose, senna, docusate, and tap water enema.

On physical examination, respiration rate is 20/min; other vital signs are normal. Oxygen saturation is 92% breathing ambient air. Cardiac examination reveals an S_3, jugular venous distention, and peripheral edema. Crackles are auscultated at the lung bases. Moderate abdominal distention is noted, with tenderness to palpation.

H CONT.

Which of the following is the most appropriate treatment of this patient's constipation?

(A) Lubiprostone
(B) Methylnaltrexone
(C) Polyethylene glycol
(D) Sodium phosphate enema

Item 162

An 18-year-old man is brought to the office by his mother, who is concerned about his behavior in school. Since age 6 years, the patient has had difficulty interacting with people and exhibits several unusual, repetitive behaviors, including tapping his fork three times with each bite of food. He has scored well on aptitude tests but has struggled in classroom activities that require working with other students. He has no friends, and his parents find it difficult to engage in conversation with him.

On physical examination, the patient exhibits paucity of speech; he answers yes-or-no questions appropriately. There is no evidence of disordered thinking.

Which of the following is the most likely diagnosis?

(A) Antisocial personality disorder
(B) Autism spectrum disorder
(C) Obsessive-compulsive disorder
(D) Social anxiety disorder

Item 163

A 42-year-old man is seen to discuss recent test results. He is asymptomatic. He has no known medical problems and takes no medications. He does not use tobacco products.

On physical examination, blood pressure is 128/74 mm Hg; other vital signs are also normal. BMI is 24. The remainder of the examination is unremarkable.

Laboratory studies:

Total cholesterol	270 mg/dL (6.99 mmol/L)
LDL cholesterol	170 mg/dL (4.40 mmol/L)
HDL cholesterol	40 mg/dL (1.04 mmol/L)
Triglycerides	300 mg/dL (3.39 mmol/L)

His 10-year risk for atherosclerotic cardiovascular disease based on the Pooled Cohort Equations is 3.4%.

Which of the following is the most appropriate treatment of this patient's hyperlipidemia?

(A) Low-intensity statin therapy
(B) Moderate-intensity statin therapy
(C) High-intensity statin therapy
(D) Therapeutic lifestyle changes

Item 164

A 58-year-old woman is evaluated for a 4-week history of left lateral hip pain. She describes the pain as a moderate ache that intermittently radiates down the lateral aspect of the left leg. It began insidiously and has gradually worsened. The pain worsens when she is climbing stairs or lying on the affected

side. She reports no previous trauma to the area. She has not had any leg weakness or swelling or any constitutional symptoms. She has not taken any analgesics for the pain.

On physical examination, vital signs are normal. On palpation, there is tenderness over the left greater trochanter. There is painless full range of motion with abduction, flexion, and external rotation of the left hip. The remainder of the examination is normal.

In addition to activity modification, which of the following is the most appropriate management?

(A) Ibuprofen
(B) Glucocorticoid injection
(C) Hydrocodone/acetaminophen
(D) Plain radiography of the left hip

Item 165

A 56-year-old woman is evaluated for severe vaginal itching and discomfort. Her symptoms have progressively worsened over the last 4 months. There is no associated vaginal discharge or vaginal odor. She is experiencing significant vaginal dryness, and intercourse has become painful despite the use of lubricants. She has been menopausal since age 53 years. She takes no medications.

On physical examination, vital signs are normal. Physical examination reveals dry vaginal epithelium that is smooth and shiny. Blood vessels are visible beneath the pale vaginal mucosa, and increased friability is evident.

Vaginal pH is 6.0. Wet mount shows occasional leukocytes. Whiff test result is negative. There are no clue cells and no hyphae on potassium hydroxide preparation.

Which of the following is the most likely diagnosis?

(A) Acute allergic contact dermatitis
(B) Genitourinary syndrome of menopause
(C) Vulvar lichen planus
(D) Vulvar lichen sclerosus

Item 166

A 64-year-old man is evaluated to establish care. Medical history is significant for long-standing low back pain secondary to traumatic vertebral compression fractures. He has chronic pain that partially responds to heat and relaxation, but he also has several acute exacerbations of pain daily that "immobilize" him and prevent him from working. These episodes do not respond to nonpharmacologic therapy. He has tried multiple nonopioid analgesic agents but discontinued these drugs because of lack of efficacy or side effects. He works from his home as an editor for a sports magazine.

Long-term opioid therapy is considered. Treatment goals, as well as the possibility of discontinuing therapy in the absence of meaningful improvements or if the risks exceed the benefits, are discussed with the patient.

Which of the following is also recommended before prescribing opioid therapy to this patient?

(A) Current Opioid Misuse Measure survey
(B) Naloxone prescription and education

(C) Opioid risk assessment

(D) Psychiatry referral

(C) 5 Days

(D) 7 Days

Item 167

A 55-year-old woman is evaluated before partial colectomy for recurrent episodes of diverticulitis. Medical history is otherwise significant for atrial fibrillation and hypertension. Medications are apixaban, hydrochlorothiazide, and metoprolol.

On physical examination, vital signs are normal. BMI is 25. Cardiac examination reveals an irregularly irregular rhythm. Pulmonary examination is normal.

Laboratory studies demonstrate a serum creatinine level of 1.0 mg/dL (88.4 µmol/L), an estimated glomerular filtration rate greater than 60 mL/min/1.73 m², and a hemoglobin level of 13.0 g/dL (130 g/L).

When should this patient's anticoagulant therapy be discontinued before surgery?

(A) 1 Day

(B) 3 Days

Item 168

A 36-year-old man is evaluated for a 3-month history of severely depressed mood; hypersomnia; poor appetite; 6.8-kg (15-lb) weight loss; and loss of interest in family, hobbies, and work. He has not had thoughts of suicide. He has never had similar problems and does not use alcohol, tobacco, or recreational drugs. He wants help but is concerned about the side effects of psychotropic medications. His PHQ-9 score is 13, indicating moderate depression.

Laboratory studies reveal a normal serum thyroid-stimulating hormone level.

Which of the following is the most appropriate treatment?

(A) Amitriptyline

(B) Cognitive behavioral therapy

(C) Paroxetine

(D) Quetiapine

Answers and Critiques

Item 1   Answer: B

Educational Objective: Treat a patient with an LDL cholesterol level higher than 190 mg/dL (4.92 mmol/L).

The most appropriate treatment for primary prevention of atherosclerotic cardiovascular disease (ASCVD) in this patient is high-intensity statin therapy with rosuvastatin or atorvastatin. According to the American College of Cardiology (ACC)/American Heart Association (AHA) cholesterol treatment guideline, patients aged 21 years or older with severe LDL cholesterol elevation (≥190 mg/dL [4.92 mmol/L]) should receive the maximum tolerated statin therapy for primary prevention of ASCVD, regardless of 10-year risk for ASCVD. High-intensity statin therapy is recommended unless there are contraindications to its use. It is reasonable to intensify statin therapy as tolerated to achieve an LDL cholesterol reduction of at least 50%. In contrast to the ACC/AHA recommendation, the U.S. Preventive Services Task Force recommends initiating low- to moderate-intensity statin therapy in adults aged 40 to 75 years without a history of ASCVD who have one or more ASCVD risk factors (dyslipidemia, diabetes mellitus, hypertension, or smoking) and a calculated 10-year ASCVD event risk of 10% or higher.

In the absence of familial hypercholesterolemia, proprotein convertase subtilisin/kexin type 9 (PCSK9) inhibitors, such as alirocumab and evolocumab, are not indicated in primary prevention of ASCVD. Cost, treatment burden (injections), and absence of long-term safety data argue against their use in primary prevention. Such treatment might be considered if the patient cannot tolerate statin therapy or if LDL cholesterol cannot be sufficiently reduced in the highest-risk patients.

In patients with an LDL cholesterol level of 190 mg/dL (4.92 mmol/L) or higher, initial treatment with a moderate-intensity statin is less preferred; however, if the patient is unable to tolerate high-intensity therapy, down-titration to moderate-intensity therapy could be considered, especially if adequate LDL cholesterol reduction can be achieved.

An evaluation for secondary causes of hyperlipidemia is also indicated in patients with an LDL cholesterol level of 190 mg/dL (4.92 mmol/L) or higher. The most common secondary causes are obesity, hypothyroidism, biliary obstruction, and nephrotic syndrome. Medications can also increase LDL cholesterol level, and some of the most commonly implicated drugs include cyclosporine, HIV medications (such as protease inhibitors), glucocorticoids, and amiodarone. If a secondary cause is not identified, LDL cholesterol level elevation is considered primary, and family members should undergo screening because severe hypercholesterolemia is often genetically determined, as may be the case with this patient who has a first-degree relative with premature ASCVD.

KEY POINT

- The American College of Cardiology and American Heart Association recommend that patients aged 21 years or older with an LDL cholesterol level of 190 mg/dL (4.92 mmol/L) or higher should receive high-intensity statin therapy for primary prevention of atherosclerotic cardiovascular disease.

Bibliography

Stone NJ, Robinson JG, Lichtenstein AH, Bairey Merz CN, Blum CB, Eckel RH, et al; American College of Cardiology/American Heart Association Task Force on Practice Guidelines. 2013 ACC/AHA guideline on the treatment of blood cholesterol to reduce atherosclerotic cardiovascular risk in adults: a report of the American College of Cardiology/American Heart Association Task Force on Practice Guidelines. Circulation. 2014;129:S1-45. [PMID: 24222016] doi:10.1161/01.cir.0000437738.63853.7a

Item 2   Answer: D

Educational Objective: Use a shared decision-making approach to guide the initiation of breast cancer screening in a younger woman.

This patient should not be screened for breast cancer at this time. In women aged 50 to 74 years, there is a clear benefit to screening mammography, and all breast cancer guidelines recommend screening mammography in this age group. Biennial screening mammography imparts most of the benefit of annual screening mammography with fewer harms, although the recommended screening frequency differs between guidelines. In women younger than 50 years or aged 75 years or older, the balance of benefits and harms is less clear, and screening recommendations vary widely. Most guidelines, including the recommendation statement of the U.S. Preventive Services Task Force (USPSTF), recommend individualized screening decisions for women aged 40 to 49 years based on patient context and values regarding specific benefits and harms. Compared with screening mammography in older women, the USPSTF concludes that, for women in their 40s, the number of women who benefit from screening mammography is smaller, and the harm is higher; however, the benefit still outweighs the harm. Therefore, the value the patient places on averting death from breast cancer compared with the importance she places on avoiding potential harms (false-positive results, anxiety, and overdiagnosis) can help guide her decision. This patient places more importance on avoiding potential harms and therefore should not pursue screening mammography or breast tomosynthesis at this time; no further testing is the best option.

The USPSTF recommends against teaching breast self-examination (BSE), as BSE does not reduce breast cancer mortality and is associated with increased rates of breast biopsy.

The USPSTF found insufficient evidence to assess the balance of benefits and harms of using breast tomosynthesis, or three-dimensional mammography, as a primary screening method for breast cancer; however, National Comprehensive Cancer Network guidelines indicate that breast tomosynthesis can be considered as an initial screening strategy for average-risk women. In studies, breast tomosynthesis is often associated with double the rate of radiation but lower recall rates.

As women progress through their 40s, the number of women who benefit from screening mammography increases, while the chance for harms slightly decreases. A woman's values and preferences may also shift over time; therefore, breast cancer screening should be periodically discussed.

KEY POINT

- The decision to initiate breast cancer screening in women aged 40 to 49 years should be an individualized one based on patient context and values regarding specific benefits and harms.

Bibliography

Nelson HD, Pappas M, Cantor A, Griffin J, Daeges M, Humphrey L. Harms of breast cancer screening: systematic review to update the 2009 U.S. Preventive Services Task Force recommendation. Ann Intern Med. 2016;164:256-67. [PMID: 26756737] doi:10.7326/M15-0970

Item 3   Answer: C

Educational Objective: Provide extended-duration postoperative pharmacologic venous thromboembolism prophylaxis in a patient undergoing major orthopedic surgery.

The recommended postoperative duration of venous thromboembolism (VTE) prophylaxis with low-molecular-weight heparin (LMWH) following major orthopedic surgery is 35 days in patients who are not at increased bleeding risk and have not experienced perioperative bleeding complications. The American College of Chest Physicians (ACCP) antithrombotic guideline provides recommendations for VTE prophylaxis for both orthopedic and nonorthopedic surgery populations. The ACCP guideline identifies hip arthroplasty, knee arthroplasty, and hip fracture surgery as major orthopedic surgeries. These surgeries pose a high VTE risk, and both pharmacologic and mechanical VTE prophylaxis are recommended during hospitalization. The ACCP recommends LMWH over other pharmacologic agents, although there are other acceptable agents, including aspirin for those unable or unwilling to take heparin. For patients without increased bleeding risk, extended duration of postoperative prophylaxis for up to 35 days is recommended over shorter-duration prophylaxis of 10 to 14 days, which is the minimum recommended duration of pharmacologic VTE prophylaxis in orthopedic surgery. Randomized trials, systematic reviews, and meta-analyses have shown that compared with placebo, aspirin, and warfarin, extended prophylaxis up to 35 days

with LMWH reduces the rate of VTE disease without excess bleeding in patients who undergo major orthopedic surgery. If bleeding risk is especially high, mechanical prophylaxis is recommended over no prophylaxis. In patients who decline LMWH injections or who are unable to tolerate LMWH, the oral direct thrombin inhibitor dabigatran, a factor Xa inhibitor (apixaban, rivaroxaban, edoxaban), or a vitamin K antagonist (warfarin) is recommended over alternate forms of prophylaxis. For this patient undergoing major orthopedic surgery, dual perioperative VTE prophylaxis with LMWH and intermittent pneumatic compression is recommended during hospitalization, with LMWH continued for up to 35 days.

Because of the elevated risk for VTE in many patients undergoing orthopedic surgery, a short course of VTE prophylaxis, such as 10 or 14 days, is insufficient because thrombotic risk remains elevated beyond this time frame.

KEY POINT

- For patients undergoing orthopedic surgery without increased bleeding risk, postoperative dual venous thromboembolism prophylaxis with intermittent pneumatic compression and low-molecular-weight heparin is recommended during hospitalization; low-molecular-weight heparin should be continued for up to 35 days.

Bibliography

Falck-Ytter Y, Francis CW, Johanson NA, Curley C, Dahl OE, Schulman S, et al. Prevention of VTE in orthopedic surgery patients: antithrombotic therapy and prevention of thrombosis, 9th ed: American College of Chest Physicians evidence-based clinical practice guidelines. Chest. 2012;141: e278S-e325S. [PMID: 22315265]

Item 4   Answer: A

Educational Objective: Treat a patient with neuropathic pain with duloxetine.

The most appropriate treatment for this patient with evidence of painful diabetic peripheral neuropathy and substantial neuropathic pain is initiation of oral duloxetine. Diabetes mellitus can cause various types of neuropathy. The most common pattern is symmetric distal sensory or sensorimotor. It is characterized by a stocking-glove distribution that ascends proximally. Diabetic sensorimotor neuropathy frequently presents as a sensation of numbness, tingling, burning, heaviness, pain, or sensitivity to light touch. The pain may worsen at night and with walking. Glycemic control and minimizing cardiovascular risk factors can slow the progression and improve the symptoms of diabetic neuropathy. Treatment of painful neuropathies is symptomatic. Tricyclic antidepressants (amitriptyline, nortriptyline), serotonin-norepinephrine reuptake inhibitors (venlafaxine, duloxetine), antiepileptic drugs (pregabalin, gabapentin, valproic acid), opioids (tapentadol), and topical capsaicin are commonly used. However, only pregabalin, duloxetine, and tapentadol (extended release) have FDA approval for painful diabetic neuropathy. Although duloxetine and gabapentinoids are considered first-line therapy, they are costly. The dosage of duloxetine is started at 20 mg/d or 30 mg/d and increased to a goal dosage of 60 mg/d. Dosages higher than 60 mg/d have not been shown to be more effective for analgesia.

Hydromorphone is a potent opioid agonist that is typically used in the treatment of cancer-associated pain, whereas tramadol is a weak opioid agonist with analgesic activity that is influenced by inhibition of serotonin and norepinephrine reuptake. Although potentially effective in the treatment of neuropathic pain syndromes, opioids are considered third-line therapy after maximization and combination of neuropathic agents. Studies have shown that most patients with peripheral neuropathies are not treated with appropriate neuropathic agents or adequate dosages of these drugs, and dosages should be maximized before initiating opioids.

The effectiveness of lamotrigine for chronic neuropathic pain was evaluated in a systematic review. The studies included patients with central poststroke pain, diabetic neuropathy, HIV-related neuropathy, intractable neuropathic pain, spinal cord injury–related pain, and trigeminal neuralgia. Only one study of patients with HIV-related neuropathy had a statistically significant result, which was restricted to patients receiving antiretroviral therapy. The authors concluded that there is no role for lamotrigine in the treatment of chronic neuropathic pain.

Topical NSAIDs such as diclofenac (available as a solution, spray, gel, or patch) provide similar pain relief for inflammatory conditions as oral medications with fewer gastrointestinal effects. However, they are significantly more expensive than oral NSAIDs. More importantly, anti-inflammatory agents have not been shown to be effective in the treatment of peripheral neuropathies and would not be indicated in this patient with a neuropathic pain syndrome.

KEY POINT

- Gabapentinoids and serotonin-norepinephrine reuptake inhibitors are first-line therapy for neuropathic pain syndromes.

Bibliography
Watson JC, Dyck PJ. Peripheral neuropathy: a practical approach to diagnosis and symptom management. Mayo Clin Proc. 2015;90:940-51. [PMID: 26141332]

Item 5   Answer: C

Educational Objective: Treat depression at the end of life with methylphenidate.

The most appropriate treatment for this patient's depression is methylphenidate. Patients with a serious, life-threatening illness and untreated depression have poorer quality of life, which can lead to increased caregiver stress and burden. Diagnosing depression in terminally ill patients, however, is challenging. Although anticipatory grief is common in patients at the end of life and is considered a normal part of most end-of-life experiences, it can be distinguished from clinical depression by the patient's ability to find enjoyment and a fluctuating mood. Patients with depression at the end of life have symptoms that include hopelessness, pervasive guilt, and worthlessness. Depression in terminally ill patients responds well to both pharmacologic and nonpharmacologic treatments. Tricyclic antidepressants, selective serotonin reuptake inhibitors, serotonin-norepinephrine reuptake inhibitors, and mirtazapine are all effective agents. Prognosis should be taken into account because these medications take weeks to reach peak effect. This patient has symptoms consistent with clinical depression as well as a limited life expectancy. Methylphenidate is a rapid-acting psychostimulant that is well tolerated and effective in the treatment of depression; once initiated, results can be seen within 24 to 48 hours. Methylphenidate may also have the benefit of improving cancer-associated fatigue.

Selective serotonin reuptake inhibitors, such as citalopram and sertraline, are effective in the treatment of depression; however, they can take many weeks and dose titration to reach effectiveness. Given this patient's limited life expectancy, a more rapid-acting agent is needed.

Cognitive behavioral therapy, when available, is an effective therapy for patients with depression and a serious medical illness. However, most trials showing benefit are centered on multiweek, if not several-months-long, interventions and are of limited availability for patients on home hospice.

KEY POINT

- Methylphenidate is a rapid-acting psychostimulant that is well tolerated and effective in the treatment of depression at the end of life; results can be seen as quickly as 24 to 48 hours after initiation.

Bibliography
Swetz KM, Kamal AH. Palliative care. Ann Intern Med. 2018;168:ITC33-ITC48. [PMID: 29507970] doi:10.7326/AITC201803060

Item 6   Answer: D

Educational Objective: Treat bacterial conjunctivitis.

The most appropriate treatment is trimethoprim-polymyxin B ophthalmic drops. This patient has acute, painless eye redness and several other signs of bacterial conjunctivitis. Studies have identified features that increase the probability of a bacterial cause of conjunctivitis, including redness of the conjunctival membrane obscuring the tarsal vessels, matting of both eyes in the morning, and purulent discharge. Inability to see redness of the eyes at 20 feet decreases the likelihood of a bacterial cause. Antibiotic treatment of bacterial conjunctivitis with topical trimethoprim-polymyxin B or erythromycin can shorten the duration of symptoms, but overall, bacterial conjunctivitis is a self-limited condition from which most patients recover within 2 weeks. Antibiotics should be enlisted when there

Answers and Critiques

is a higher risk for complications, such as in patients who wear contact lenses; immunocompromised patients, such as those with diabetes mellitus; and patients with copious, hyperpurulent discharge of the eye.

Ceftriaxone is used to treat gonococcal infection. Typical patients with gonococcal conjunctivitis are young men with copious purulent discharge and marked conjunctival inflammation. Periocular edema and tenderness, gaze restriction, and preauricular lymphadenopathy are common with gonococcal conjunctivitis.

Because of concerns about antimicrobial resistance and cost, topical fluoroquinolones (such as levofloxacin) are not first-line therapy for routine cases of bacterial conjunctivitis. Topical fluoroquinolones are indicated for conjunctivitis in contact lens wearers as a result of the high incidence of *Pseudomonas* infection.

Olopatadine ophthalmic drops are used for seasonal allergies; the mucopurulent discharge, morning matting of the eyes, and lack of itching make allergic conjunctivitis a less likely cause of this patient's symptoms.

KEY POINT

- Bacterial conjunctivitis is characterized by redness of the conjunctival membrane obscuring the tarsal vessels, matting of both eyes in the morning, and thin mucopurulent discharge; treatment may include topical antibiotics, such as trimethoprim–polymyxin B or erythromycin.

Bibliography

Narayana S, McGee S. Bedside diagnosis of the 'red eye': a systematic review. Am J Med. 2015;128:1220-1224.e1. [PMID: 26169885] doi:10.1016/j.amjmed.2015.06.026

Item 7   Answer: B

Educational Objective: Understand the limitations of the number needed to treat to inform clinical decision making.

The harms and cost of treatment are needed to conclude that treatment A is superior to treatment B. When assessing the clinical impact of an intervention, the number needed to treat (NNT) provides a quantifiable measure of the treatment effect that is easily understood by physicians and patients; it represents the number of patients who must receive a treatment to cause one additional patient to benefit. The acceptability of the NNT as a means of comparing one treatment with another depends on the risks associated with the condition, the cost and side effects of the treatment, and other treatments available. When comparing one treatment with another, head-to-head comparisons provide the best evidence of superiority. In this head-to-head comparison of two treatments, the absolute risk reduction for heart failure–related hospitalizations is 6% with treatment A compared with treatment B. This translates to 17 patients (NNT = 1/absolute risk reduction) who need to receive treatment A to result in 1 less heart failure–related hospitalization compared

with treatment B. Although this information is informative, other data, such as cost and harms, must be evaluated before a conclusion that treatment A is superior to treatment B can be reached. If harms are more frequent or more severe with treatment A, the reduction in hospitalization for heart failure may become clinically meaningless.

Confidence intervals (CIs) are a method for indicating the range in which a value derived from a study is likely to lie; narrower ranges imply greater confidence, or certainty, that the reported value is closer to the true value. The *P* value expresses the probability that the findings in a study can be explained by chance alone and represents the level of statistical significance. *P* values offer less information than do CIs because CIs can demonstrate the plausible range of values for an event or outcome, whereas *P* values indicate only statistical significance. Although CIs provide more precise information about the range of expected benefit, the *P* value and CI are of less importance than understanding the harms, costs, and alternative therapies that might be available.

A disadvantage of relative comparisons, including relative risk, is the potential for exaggerated outcomes. For instance, interventions that reduce the rate of an outcome from 40% to 20% or from 4% to 2% have a relative risk reduction of 50%. However, the absolute risk reduction for the first case is 20%, whereas the absolute risk reduction for the second case is 2%.

KEY POINT

- The acceptability of the number needed to treat as a means of comparing one treatment with another depends on the risks associated with the condition, the cost and side effects of the treatment, and other treatments available.

Bibliography

Citrome L, Ketter TA. When does a difference make a difference? Interpretation of number needed to treat, number needed to harm, and likelihood to be helped or harmed. Int J Clin Pract. 2013;67:407-11. [PMID: 23574101] doi: 10.1111/ijcp.12142

Item 8   Answer: D

Educational Objective: Treat acute bacterial prostatitis after a urologic procedure.

This patient's history and physical examination findings indicate acute bacterial prostatitis, and the most appropriate treatment regimen is trimethoprim-sulfamethoxazole. Patient groups at high risk for acute bacterial prostatitis include those with diabetes mellitus, immunosuppression, or cirrhosis. Risk factors include unprotected sexual intercourse, urogenital instrumentation (chronic indwelling bladder catheterization, intermittent bladder catheterization, prostate biopsy), urinary tract manipulation (prostate resection), urinary stasis (obstruction), and benign prostatic hyperplasia. The most common infectious cause for acute bacterial prostatitis is *Escherichia coli* or other gram-negative bacilli. Diagnosis is typically established with urine Gram stain and culture in patients with a compatible history. The treatment of choice for acute bacterial prostatitis is a prolonged course of trimethoprim-sulfamethoxazole or ciprofloxacin. Data on treatment duration are sparse, but 6 weeks is reasonable and recommended by experts. Given the prolonged duration of antimicrobial therapy required in cases of acute bacterial prostatitis, it is most prudent to select an antibiotic with appropriate coverage, while also attempting to minimize the potential for serious adverse effects. Prolonged ciprofloxacin use has been associated with QT prolongation as well as tendinopathy/tendon rupture, especially in older adults. As such, given the treatment duration needed for acute bacterial prostatitis, trimethoprim-sulfamethoxazole would be the most appropriate choice.

Amoxicillin would be an appropriate choice for patients with acute prostatitis and gram-positive cocci in chains. This finding would suggest an enterococcal infection, and treatment with amoxicillin or ampicillin would be appropriate. Neither of these antibiotics would be effective for acute bacterial prostatitis caused by *E. coli* or other gram-negative bacilli.

Men younger than 35 years who are sexually active and men older than 35 years who engage in high-risk sexual behavior should be treated with regimens that cover *Neisseria gonorrhoeae* and *Chlamydia trachomatis*. Ceftriaxone and doxycycline, or ceftriaxone and azithromycin, would be appropriate treatment choices in cases of acute epididymitis, specifically targeting *C. trachomatis* or *N. gonorrhoeae*. Neither regimen would be appropriate in this case.

Cephalexin would be an appropriate choice for patients with acute prostatitis and gram-positive cocci in clusters suggesting infection with *Staphylococcus aureus* or coagulase-negative staphylococci (*Staphylococcus epidermidis* or *Staphylococcus saprophyticus*).

KEY POINT

- The most common infectious cause of acute bacterial prostatitis is *Escherichia coli* or other gram-negative bacilli; the treatment of choice is a prolonged course of trimethoprim-sulfamethoxazole or ciprofloxacin.

Bibliography
Gill BC, Shoskes DA. Bacterial prostatitis. Curr Opin Infect Dis. 2016;29:86-91. [PMID: 26555038] doi:10.1097/QCO.0000000000000222

Item 9   Answer: A

Educational Objective: Manage vaccination of a health care worker.

This patient should receive a second dose of the measles, mumps, and rubella (MMR) vaccine. In all immunocompetent adults who lack documented immunity against measles, mumps, and rubella, at least one dose of the MMR vaccine should be administered. Health care workers are at increased risk for acquiring and transmitting measles, mumps, and rubella and should receive a second dose of the MMR vaccine at least 28 days after the first dose. A second dose should also be administered to postsecondary students and international travelers. For persons who have been previously vaccinated with two doses of a mumps virus–containing vaccine but are at increased risk because of an outbreak, the Advisory Committee on Immunization Practices recommends administering a third dose of mumps virus–containing vaccine to improve protection.

This patient's status as a health care worker does not necessitate administration of the hepatitis A vaccine, despite serologic tests indicating that he lacks immunity. The hepatitis A vaccine should be administered to patients who are at increased risk for infection or complications of infection, such as those who work or travel to endemic areas, men who have sex with men, individuals with chronic liver disease, illicit drug users, persons with clotting disorders, persons who conduct hepatitis A–related research, and household or close contacts of adopted children from endemic areas. Hepatitis A vaccination is also indicated in persons who desire vaccination and could be administered to this patient if he wishes.

Hepatitis B vaccination is indicated in all health care workers who lack immunity. This patient has a positive hepatitis B surface antibody test result, whereas his surface antigen and core antibody levels are undetectable. This pattern is consistent with prior vaccination with an appropriate immune response. As such, hepatitis B vaccination is unnecessary in this patient.

Pneumococcal vaccination is recommended in all adults aged 65 years and older and adults aged 19 to 64 years with certain high-risk conditions. This patient does not have any chronic medical conditions and is also a nonsmoker; therefore, vaccination with the 23-valent pneumococcal polysaccharide vaccine is not indicated.

KEY POINT

- Health care workers are at increased risk for acquiring and transmitting measles, mumps, and rubella and should receive a second dose of the MMR (measles, mumps, and rubella) vaccine.

Bibliography
Kim DK, Riley LE, Hunter P; Advisory Committee on Immunization Practices. Recommended immunization schedule for adults aged 19 years or older, United States, 2018. Ann Intern Med. 2018;168:210-220. [PMID: 29404596] doi:10.7326/M17-3439

Item 10   Answer: B

Educational Objective: Manage an in-flight medical emergency by connecting to the ground-based physician.

The most appropriate next step in management is to connect with the ground-based physician. In-flight medical emergencies are relatively common during air travel, occurring in an estimated 1 of 600 flights. Airlines based in the United States are mandated by the Federal Aviation Administration to carry at least one automated external defibrillator; supplemental oxygen; and a medical kit that contains a stethoscope, sphygmomanometer, gloves, airway supplies, intravenous access supplies, and some basic medications. In the case of an in-flight emergency, the physician's role generally involves assessing the patient, establishing a diagnosis when possible, administering basic medical treatments, providing reassurance as appropriate, and recommending flight diversion if necessary. Physicians should practice within their scope of training, be mindful of patient privacy, and document the patient encounter. Although not a Federal Aviation Administration requirement, most airlines have contracts with 24-hour call centers with a ground-based physician to aid in the event of an in-flight emergency. Often, ground-based physicians trained in emergency or aerospace medicine can assist the on-board physician remotely and help direct care, which can be particularly helpful when the medical problem is outside the scope of the physician's practice.

The principles of hypobaric hypoxia apply to commercial airplanes, in which cabins are pressurized to the equivalent of 1500 to 2500 meters (approximately 5000 to 8200 feet) in altitude, resulting in an inspired oxygen tension between 110 and 120 mm Hg (about 70% of the levels encountered at sea level). Although this correlates with an arterial P_{O_2} of approximately 60 mm Hg (8.0 kPa) in healthy individuals, those with underlying pulmonary disease are at risk for significant hypoxemia during a flight. This patient will have no difficulty maintaining her oxyhemoglobin saturation above 90%, and asking the pilot to descend to a lower altitude will serve no useful purpose. A better strategy is to contact the ground-based physician.

Although this patient is dizzy and weak, her clinical status and vital signs appear stable. She needs further medical evaluation and management; however, flight diversion is probably not indicated at this time. Furthermore, the ground-based medical team can also help determine whether flight diversion is needed.

KEY POINT

- In most in-flight medical emergencies, the physician's role involves assessing the patient, establishing a diagnosis when possible, administering basic medical treatments, providing reassurance as appropriate, and recommending flight diversion if necessary.

Bibliography
Nable JV, Tupe CL, Gehle BD, Brady WJ. In-flight medical emergencies during commercial travel. N Engl J Med. 2015;373:939-45. [PMID: 26332548] doi: 10.1056/NEJMra1409213

Item 11   Answer: A

Educational Objective: Counsel an older patient with risk factors for a motor vehicle accident.

This patient should be advised to retire from driving. Driving assessments are qualitative and rely heavily on clinical judgment. The more risk factors for a motor vehicle accident that an older driver has, the higher the risk for an adverse event while driving. Drivers at highest risk should be counseled to retire from driving. This patient has multiple risk factors for unsafe driving, including cognitive impairment,

self-restrictions in driving (does not drive after dark or on the interstate highway, drives within a 10-mile radius of home), minor accidents, and concerns from family members about driving safety. His other risk factors include impaired mobility, hearing decline, and medical conditions with increased risk for loss of consciousness. Physician advice to retire from driving is associated with older drivers appropriately discontinuing driving. Given the risk for depression and social isolation associated with driving retirement, however, this advice should be coupled with suggestions for alternate forms of transportation and follow-up assessment of his mood and quality of life.

Detailed neuropsychological testing is especially useful for the following patients: (1) those with milder cognitive symptoms to determine whether cognitive difficulties are within the realm of normal age-associated cognitive decline versus mild cognitive impairment; (2) those with definite dementia, diagnosed on the basis of clinical impression and results of screening cognitive tests, who have clinical features overlapping two or more underlying pathologic processes; and (3) those with cognitive symptoms whose clinical picture is confounded by significant depression. The results of neuropsychological testing are unlikely to change the recommendation to retire from driving considering this patient's multiple risk factors.

If a patient is resistant to advice to retire from driving, a formal occupational therapy driving evaluation may be helpful.

Given his numerous observable risk factors, this patient should not be reassured that he is competent to drive.

KEY POINT

- The more risk factors for a motor vehicle accident that an older driver has, the higher the risk for an adverse event while driving.

Bibliography
Martin AJ, Marottoli R, O'Neill D. Driving assessment for maintaining mobility and safety in drivers with dementia. Cochrane Database Syst Rev. 2013:CD006222. [PMID: 23990315] doi:10.1002/14651858.CD006222.pub4

Item 12   Answer: D

Educational Objective: Evaluate a patient with symptoms of systemic exertion intolerance disease.

No further diagnostic testing is required in this patient. She meets the diagnostic criteria for systemic exertion intolerance disease (SEID), with fatigue of at least 6 months' duration accompanied by substantial reduction in preillness activities, postexertional malaise, unrefreshing sleep, and either cognitive impairment or orthostatic intolerance. Although the pathophysiology of SEID remains unclear, the phenomenon of central sensitization (the pathophysiologic dysregulation of the thalamus, hypothalamus, and amygdala) is gaining acceptance as a potential cause of SEID as well as of other highly prevalent comorbid conditions, including fibromyalgia, mood disturbances, irritable bowel syndrome, and interstitial cystitis. This patient's history, examination, and previous diagnostic test results point to central sensitization, as demonstrated by the constellation of such symptoms as diffuse arthralgia and myalgia, chronic fatigue, bowel and bladder irritability, chronic headaches, brain fog, paresthesias, and unrefreshing sleep. In patients with SEID, the history and physical examination should guide the choice of diagnostic tests. It is reasonable to obtain a complete blood count, creatine kinase (for myalgia), electrolyte panel, thyroid-stimulating hormone level, fasting glucose level, and kidney and liver chemistry tests; however, unnecessary laboratory, imaging, and invasive studies should be avoided because most patients will have unrevealing findings, which provide no lasting reassurance to patients. In this case, the diagnostic evaluation should be limited unless there is compelling new information to warrant further testing.

Antinuclear antibody testing is an effective screening tool for systemic lupus erythematosus; however, myalgia, arthralgia, and fatigue are insufficient reasons to test for antinuclear antibodies unless accompanied by objective findings of systemic lupus erythematosus.

Patients at moderate to high risk for obstructive sleep apnea should undergo further testing, including a home sleep study or polysomnography. On the basis of this patient's presentation (female, young, normal BMI and neck circumference, lack of daytime sleepiness), she is considered to be at low risk for obstructive sleep apnea, and further sleep testing is not warranted.

Serum cortisol testing is unnecessary in this patient who is not manifesting findings that are suggestive of adrenal failure or insufficiency, such as hypotension, tachycardia, hyponatremia, and hyperkalemia.

KEY POINT

- In patients with fatigue without a clear cause, it is reasonable to obtain a complete blood count, electrolyte panel, thyroid-stimulating hormone level, fasting glucose level, and kidney and liver chemistry tests; unnecessary laboratory, imaging, and invasive studies should be avoided.

Bibliography

Committee on the Diagnostic Criteria for Myalgic Encephalomyelitis/Chronic Fatigue Syndrome, Board on the Health of Select Populations, Institute of Medicine. Beyond Myalgic Encephalomyelitis/Chronic Fatigue Syndrome: Redefining an Illness. Washington, DC: National Academies Press; 2015. [PMID: 25695122]

Item 13   Answer: B

Educational Objective: Evaluate a patient suspected of having cauda equina syndrome.

This patient should undergo emergent MRI of the lumbosacral spine. His history and physical examination findings are concerning for cauda equina syndrome, which is a surgical emergency. Cauda equina syndrome is most commonly caused by a large disk herniation, but it can also result from direct trauma, infection, or malignancy. Symptoms include low back pain with radiation to the legs, saddle anesthesia, bowel and/or bladder dysfunction, erectile dysfunction, and leg weakness. On physical examination, absent or decreased perianal sensation, diminished anal sphincter tone, hypoactive or absent ankle reflexes, and focal sensory and muscle weakness are commonly present. MRI is considered the gold standard for diagnosing cauda equina syndrome.

CT can be obtained in patients suspected of having cauda equina syndrome who are unable to undergo MRI. However, MRI is considered to be better at visualizing the soft tissue structures of the cauda equina than CT and is therefore the preferred imaging modality in patients who can undergo either procedure, such as this one.

Although plain radiography can be performed when there is concern for metastatic cancer to the vertebral bodies, it has no value in visualizing the soft tissue structures of the cauda equina and therefore is not the preferred imaging modality in cases of suspected cauda equina syndrome.

Signs that urgent surgical intervention may be necessary include bowel- or bladder-sphincter dysfunction, particularly urine retention or urinary incontinence; diminished perineal sensation, sciatica, or sensory motor deficits; and bilateral or unilateral motor deficits that are severe and progressive. Forgoing imaging in this patient and failing to provide definitive surgical intervention could result in permanent neurologic deficits.

KEY POINT

- Nerve root involvement of the cauda equina requires immediate imaging, preferably with MRI, and surgical intervention to prevent permanent neurologic damage.

Bibliography

Chou R. In the clinic. Low back pain. Ann Intern Med. 2014;160:ITC6-1. [PMID: 25009837]

Item 14   Answer: D

Educational Objective: Evaluate a breast mass in a woman younger than 30 years.

The most appropriate diagnostic test for this young woman with a breast mass is ultrasonography. A breast mass is characterized by a lesion that persists throughout the menstrual cycle and differs from the surrounding breast tissue and the corresponding area in the contralateral breast. The differential diagnosis of a palpable breast mass includes abscess, cyst, fat necrosis, fibroadenoma, and neoplasm. Evaluation of a palpable breast mass varies based on the patient's age and risk factors and the degree of clinical suspicion. Mammography and ultrasonography are the initial imaging modalities. Ultrasonography is often preferred in women younger than 30 years because increased breast tissue density in younger women limits the usefulness of mammography. Ultrasonography may also be a better choice for young women and

Answers and Critiques

pregnant patients in order to avoid radiation exposure. The main utility of ultrasonography is its ability to differentiate cystic from solid lesions. A cyst is likely to be benign if it has symmetric, round borders with no internal echoes. A solid lesion with uniform borders and uniformly sized internal echoes is consistent with a benign fibroadenoma. In this patient with relatively low-risk clinical symptoms, ultrasonography is preferred. The description of the mass (firm, nontender, mobile mass with well-defined margins and no lymphadenopathy) suggests a benign finding, such as a fibroadenoma or cyst. If the ultrasound shows a simple cyst, no further evaluation is necessary, unless the patient is symptomatic. If the ultrasound reveals a solid lesion, it must be evaluated completely with biopsy.

An image-directed core-needle biopsy of a breast mass would be recommended if an ultrasound shows a solid-appearing, suspicious (Breast Imaging Reporting and Data System [BI-RADS] category 4) or highly suspicious (BI-RADS category 5) mass. This patient must undergo ultrasonography to determine the BI-RADS category of the mass before a decision on whether to perform a biopsy can be made.

The dense breast tissue often found in young women limits the sensitivity, and hence the effectiveness, of mammography. Therefore, mammography is generally not needed for young women with a low-risk breast mass.

For women aged 30 years or older with a palpable breast abnormality, both diagnostic mammography and ultrasonography would be recommended. Because this patient is younger than 30 years, only ultrasonography is warranted at this time.

KEY POINT

- For women younger than 30 years with a low-risk breast mass, ultrasonography is usually the only imaging required.

Bibliography
Lehman CD, Lee AY, Lee CI. Imaging management of palpable breast abnormalities. AJR Am J Roentgenol. 2014;203:1142-53. [PMID: 25341156] doi:10.2214/AJR.14.12725

Item 15   Answer: A
Educational Objective: Diagnose bipolar disorder.

The most likely diagnosis is bipolar disorder. This patient exhibits multiple symptoms of depression (anhedonia, sleep disturbance, feelings of worthlessness, suicidal ideation), but he also has a history of at least one previous manic episode, manifested by increased energy, decreased need for sleep, grandiose thinking, and risky behavior. This patient's clinical picture of depression and one or more episodes of mania is most consistent with a diagnosis of bipolar disorder. In patients with bipolar disorder, dysfunction is often extreme, and the associated lifetime risk for suicide is high (6%-15%). Referral to a psychiatrist should be strongly considered when resources are available.

Generalized anxiety disorder is characterized by excessive anxiety about activities or events occurring more days than not for at least 6 months and causing significant distress or functional impairment. Patients with this disorder often experience fatigue and sleep disturbance but do not have a history of mania or meet diagnostic criteria for a major depressive disorder.

More than half of patients with bipolar disorder initially present with a depressive episode. However, presence of manic episodes in this patient excludes major depressive disorder as the diagnosis. Recognition of previous manic or hypomanic episodes is crucial because the treatment of depression in bipolar disorder requires mood stabilizers (such as carbamazepine, lithium, or valproic acid), either alone or in combination with antidepressants. Treatment with antidepressants alone may increase the risk for mania and hypomania.

Patients with schizophrenia have negative symptoms, such as flattened affect and decreased activity, in combination with positive symptoms, including hallucinations and disorganized thought. This patient has no positive symptoms.

KEY POINT

- More than half of patients with bipolar disorder initially present with a depressive episode; however, recognition of previous manic or hypomanic episodes is crucial because the treatment of bipolar disorder requires mood stabilizers, either alone or in combination with antidepressants.

Bibliography
Frye MA. Clinical practice. Bipolar disorder—a focus on depression. N Engl J Med. 2011;364:51-9. [PMID: 21208108] doi:10.1056/NEJMcp1000402

Item 16   Answer: A
Educational Objective: Treat an obese patient with bariatric surgery.

This patient with obesity-related comorbid conditions and no weight loss success after a trial of comprehensive lifestyle modifications meets the criteria for referral for bariatric surgery. Bariatric surgery should be considered for patients who do not lose weight with lifestyle modifications, with or without pharmacologic therapy, and have a BMI of 40 or greater or a BMI of 35 or greater with obesity-related comorbid conditions, such as type 2 diabetes mellitus, coronary artery disease, obstructive sleep apnea, or osteoarthritis. Studies comparing bariatric surgery with nonsurgical treatment (diet, exercise, behavioral modification, and medications) have shown that participants randomly assigned to bariatric surgery lost more weight and were more likely to experience remission of type 2 diabetes and metabolic syndrome, improved quality of life, and reduced medication use. Evidence suggests that bariatric surgery is also associated with reduced mortality and improvement of obstructive sleep apnea, osteoarthritis, and other conditions.

Lorcaserin is approved as adjunctive therapy to comprehensive lifestyle modification in the treatment of overweight and obesity. This patient is already taking liraglutide, another approved pharmacologic agent for obesity, and has tried but not responded to a third approved agent, orlistat. He is unlikely to benefit from the addition of lorcaserin to his medication regimen.

Behavioral therapy for obesity may include the use of a trained interventionist, such as a nutritionist or dietician. This patient is already participating in a comprehensive behavioral therapy plan that includes nutritional counseling; a separate referral to a dietician is unnecessary. Behavioral therapy is also less likely than bariatric surgery to be successful in this patient.

Very-low-calorie diets are recommended when rapid weight loss is medically indicated. Their use requires close medical supervision with frequent office visits and laboratory monitoring. In this patient, there is no indication for rapid weight loss that would warrant the use of a very-low-calorie diet.

KEY POINT

- Bariatric surgery should be considered in patients who do not lose weight with lifestyle modifications and have a BMI of 40 or greater, or a BMI of 35 or greater with obesity-related comorbid conditions, such as type 2 diabetes mellitus, coronary artery disease, obstructive sleep apnea, or osteoarthritis.

Bibliography

Jensen MD, Ryan DH, Apovian CM, Ard JD, Comuzzie AG, Donato KA, et al; American College of Cardiology/American Heart Association Task Force on Practice Guidelines. 2013 AHA/ACC/TOS guideline for the management of overweight and obesity in adults: a report of the American College of Cardiology/American Heart Association Task Force on Practice Guidelines and The Obesity Society. Circulation. 2014;129:S102-38. [PMID: 24222017] doi:10.1161/01.cir.0000437739.71477.ee

Item 17   Answer: A

Educational Objective: Treat ACE inhibitor–induced chronic cough.

The most appropriate management is discontinuation of lisinopril. This patient has chronic cough, defined as cough lasting more than 8 weeks. When smoking and use of an ACE inhibitor are eliminated, the most common causes of chronic cough are upper airway cough syndrome (UACS), gastroesophageal reflux disease, and asthma. Evaluation of chronic cough begins with a thorough history, physical examination, and chest radiography. If the initial evaluation is unrevealing and the patient is taking ACE inhibitor therapy, discontinuation of the ACE inhibitor is the most appropriate first step in management. Up to 20% of patients taking an ACE inhibitor develop a dry cough, usually within 1 to 2 weeks of therapy initiation. Onset of cough, however, may be delayed by months in a small percentage of patients. Cessation of ACE inhibitor therapy usually results in resolution of the cough within 2 weeks. Rechallenge with an ACE inhibitor will result in return of the cough in two thirds of patients and is not recommended. In patients whose blood

pressure responded to ACE inhibitor therapy or who require renin-angiotensin system inhibition, an angiotensin receptor blocker can be tried because this class of drugs is associated with a lower incidence of cough.

If a cause of chronic cough is not determined after initial evaluation, and smoking and ACE inhibitor therapy have been discontinued, a stepwise approach is pursued, beginning with a 2-week trial of empiric treatment for UACS. UACS related to allergic rhinitis is best treated with intranasal glucocorticoids, whereas UACS due to nonallergic rhinitis should be treated with first-generation antihistamines and decongestants. This patient has no findings suggestive of allergic rhinitis and has not yet discontinued ACE inhibitor therapy; therefore, an intranasal glucocorticoid should not be initiated.

If chronic cough does not respond to empiric treatment for UACS, evaluation of asthma with spirometry (or empiric treatment) is warranted. If results of spirometry are negative for asthma, bronchial hyperresponsiveness testing should be pursued.

Proton pump inhibitor therapy is indicated in patients with chronic cough when symptoms of gastroesophageal reflux are present or when chronic cough persists despite empiric therapy for UACS or empiric treatment for asthma and nonasthmatic eosinophilic bronchitis with inhaled glucocorticoids.

KEY POINT

- In patients with chronic cough who have a normal chest radiograph and are taking an ACE inhibitor, the first intervention is discontinuation of the ACE inhibitor.

Bibliography

Irwin RS, Baumann MH, Bolser DC, Boulet LP, Braman SS, Brightling CE, et al. Diagnosis and management of cough executive summary: ACCP evidence-based clinical practice guidelines. Chest. 2006;129:1S-23S. [PMID: 16428686] doi:10.1378/chest.129.1_suppl.1S

Item 18   Answer: D

Educational Objective: Manage a patient who has undergone direct-to-consumer genetic testing.

This patient should be advised that no further testing is necessary and should be educated on the limitations of direct-to-consumer (DTC) genetic testing. DTC genetic testing is a commercial service that allows patients to obtain genetic information for a low cost and without referral from a physician. These tests estimate the risk for many common medical conditions by genotyping polymorphic nucleotides. Single-nucleotide polymorphisms (SNPs) that are disproportionately found in affected individuals are identified, and odds ratios for each SNP are determined. The SNPs are usually common but have low penetrance (that is, most people with an SNP do not develop disease). Individually, SNPs contribute very little to overall disease risk; most SNPs have an odds ratio of less than 1.5. Because

Answers and Critiques

counseling or education is not typically provided before or after the DTC genetic test is obtained, patients are generally unable to accurately interpret the results and may request guidance or additional testing from their physicians. This patient's absolute risk for developing prostate cancer based on the test results is extremely small; therefore, no further testing is required.

Screening for prostate cancer in asymptomatic, average-risk men is controversial, and recommendations vary among professional organizations and frequently change. However, no guidelines support performing a digital rectal examination (DRE) to screen for prostate cancer. The overall sensitivity of DRE does not exceed 60%, whereas the specificity is greater than 90%; the positive predictive value of an abnormal DRE is 28%. As such, there is no indication for this test either alone or in combination with serum prostate-specific antigen (PSA) level measurement.

The U.S. Preventive Services Task Force recommends that clinicians discuss potential benefits and harms of PSA-based screening for prostate cancer in men aged 55 to 69 years. The decision to proceed with PSA level measurement should be individualized based on the patient's beliefs and values. In this 46-year-old patient, obtaining a serum PSA level is not indicated. The patient's family history of prostate cancer at an advanced age does not significantly increase his risk for cancer. He has a low pretest probability of prostate cancer, and a positive test result will likely be false positive. Nevertheless, patients with positive test results often undergo biopsy with the attendant risks of infection, bleeding, pain, and anxiety.

KEY POINT

- Patients who undergo direct-to-consumer genetic testing should be advised of the risks and limitations of these tests, including the possibility for misinterpretation.

Bibliography
Burke W, Trinidad SB. The deceptive appeal of direct-to-consumer genetics. Ann Intern Med. 2016;164:564-5. [PMID: 26925528] doi: 10.7326/M16-0257

Item 19   Answer: B

Educational Objective: Evaluate unilateral tinnitus and hearing loss.

The most appropriate management is MRI of the internal auditory canal. The assessment of tinnitus must differentiate more dangerous causes (such as neoplasms or cerebrovascular conditions) from more benign causes (such as infections or drugs). Most commonly, tinnitus is bilateral; unilateral tinnitus may indicate more serious pathology. Patients with unilateral tinnitus should undergo prompt hearing testing; if hearing loss is documented, as in this case, the patient should undergo MRI of the internal auditory canal to rule out an acoustic neuroma. It is important to note that patients who present with tinnitus may not report hearing loss that is subsequently revealed on audiologic testing.

The type of tinnitus is an important factor in the evaluation. Pulsatile tinnitus, when synchronous with the heartbeat, may suggest a vascular anomaly, including atherosclerotic disease, arteriovenous fistulas, or paragangliomas, most commonly in the jugular bulb or tympanic arteries of the middle ear. A patient with pulsatile tinnitus should be examined for bruits over the neck, periauricular area, temple, orbit, and mastoid areas. If the physical examination findings do not explain the pulsatile tinnitus, noninvasive intracranial imaging, including CT angiography or MR angiography, should be performed. This patient does not have pulsatile tinnitus but does have unilateral hearing loss. Therefore, imaging of the internal auditory canal for acoustic neuroma will be of higher diagnostic yield than vascular imaging.

This patient's primary symptom is tinnitus, with accompanying asymptomatic hearing loss. A hearing aid is more likely to be of use in a patient with symptomatic hearing loss. More importantly, the priority in this patient is excluding an acoustic neuroma, not hearing aid placement.

This patient's tinnitus is gradual in onset and requires further evaluation. However, the patient does not need urgent referral to an otolaryngologist. Patients should be urgently referred when tinnitus is associated with symptoms suggesting serious, reversible underlying pathology, including sudden sensorineural hearing loss, pulsatile tinnitus, vestibular symptoms, ear pain, or drainage or malodor that fails to resolve.

KEY POINT

- Tinnitus associated with unilateral sensorineural hearing loss suggests acoustic neuroma and requires advanced imaging with MRI.

Bibliography
Baguley D, McFerran D, Hall D. Tinnitus. Lancet. 2013;382:1600-7. [PMID: 23827090] doi:10.1016/S0140-6736(13)60142-7

Item 20   Answer: D

Educational Objective: Treat severe dyspnea.

The most appropriate treatment for this patient is pulmonary rehabilitation. Pulmonary rehabilitation is recommended for all symptomatic patients with an FEV_1 less than 50% of predicted and specifically for those hospitalized with an acute exacerbation of COPD. These programs include education, functional assessment, nutrition counseling, and follow-up to reinforce behavioral techniques for change. They also include an exercise training component that has been shown to improve endurance, flexibility, and upper and lower body strength. Exercise training can provide sustained benefit for postexacerbation symptoms (such as breathlessness) following the completion of even a single rehabilitation program. When combined with other forms of therapy (medical therapy, smoking cessation, nutrition counseling, and education), pulmonary rehabilitation decreases patients' perceived intensity of breathlessness, reduces dyspnea and fatigue, facilitates increased participation in daily activities, and enhances health-related quality of life, including improvements in anxiety and depression.

This patient has heart failure with preserved ejection fraction but no physical examination findings that suggest volume overload. Thus, initiation of furosemide is not indicated at this time.

. Although this patient has severe dyspnea in the setting of advanced COPD, her oxygen saturation is preserved with 1 L/min oxygen by nasal cannula at rest and during a 6-minute walk test. Additional oxygen therapy will not relieve dyspnea or improve clinical outcomes.

Glucocorticoids, such as prednisone, can be an effective treatment in the setting of a COPD exacerbation, which is defined as a sustained worsening of a patient's COPD. Exacerbations are marked by increased breathlessness and are usually accompanied by increased cough and sputum production. This patient has stable chronic dyspnea on exertion and no other findings that would suggest an exacerbation.

KEY POINT

- Pulmonary rehabilitation can provide significant benefits for patients with chronic lung disease and has been shown to improve subjective dyspnea in patients with severe COPD and following an acute exacerbation of COPD.

Bibliography

Cortopassi F, Gurung P, Pinto-Plata V. Chronic obstructive pulmonary disease in elderly patients. Clin Geriatr Med. 2017;33:539-552. [PMID: 28991649]

Item 21   Answer: A

Educational Objective: Evaluate a patient with decompensated liver disease who is scheduled for elective surgery.

The most appropriate preoperative management is to cancel surgery and refer the patient for liver transplant evaluation. Patients with cirrhosis but no complications are referred to as having compensated cirrhosis; they may be asymptomatic or may have nonspecific symptoms, such as fatigue, poor sleep, muscle cramps, feeling cold, or itching. Patients with complications of cirrhosis (hepatic encephalopathy, variceal hemorrhage, ascites, spontaneous bacterial peritonitis, hepatorenal syndrome, jaundice, or hepatocellular carcinoma) are referred to as having decompensated cirrhosis. Referral to a transplant center is indicated for patients with decompensation or a Model for End-stage Liver Disease (MELD) score of greater than 15. The MELD score is an equation that incorporates bilirubin, INR, and serum creatinine levels, and it accurately predicts 3-month survival. This patient, who has decompensated liver disease with a MELD score of 22, which confers a 30-day surgical mortality risk of more than 50%, should avoid elective surgery. Patients with decompensated liver disease have not only a higher perioperative mortality rate but also a significantly increased risk

for other complications, including encephalopathy, electrolyte derangements, fluid imbalance, coagulopathy, infection, acute kidney injury, and hepatorenal syndrome. It is reasonable to refer patients at intermediate risk to a hepatologist before proceeding with surgery. Patients with compensated liver disease are often able to proceed with surgery with optimal medical management.

The deciding factor in this case is not the patient's duration of sobriety but the presence of decompensated liver disease and an unacceptably high MELD score. Elective surgery should be avoided until these risks are mitigated with liver transplantation.

The American Association for the Study of Liver Diseases recommends against perioperative transjugular intrahepatic portosystemic shunts, stating that there is no reliable perioperative evidence of improved clinical outcomes.

KEY POINT

- Patients with decompensated liver disease should avoid elective surgery and be referred for liver transplant evaluation.

Bibliography

Rai R, Nagral S, Nagral A. Surgery in a patient with liver disease. J Clin Exp Hepatol. 2012;2:238-46. [PMID: 25755440]

Item 22   Answer: E

Educational Objective: Provide culturally sensitive care to a transgender patient.

This patient requires symptomatic treatment of his viral upper respiratory tract symptoms. In general, examination of an organ system should be related to the patient's symptoms. This patient's gender identity is not relevant to the reason for the visit; therefore, obtaining a detailed gender-related history (hormonal, surgical, social, and sexual) and performing a genital examination are unnecessary. Additionally, these interventions may make this nervous patient feel more uncomfortable and potentially dissuade him from returning for important ongoing health care.

A comprehensive history of a transgender person is usually not possible to obtain in one visit; it is best obtained over time in order to build rapport with the patient. In general, history taking is similar in transgender and nontransgender patients and should include family, reproductive, sexual, psychiatric, and social histories. Elements of the history that are unique to the transgender population are hormonal and surgical therapies related to gender transition.

Recommendations for sexually transmitted infection (STI) screening are the same for transgender patients as for nontransgender patients. Screening should take into account the patient's anatomy and sexual history. As it would be inappropriate to perform STI screening in a nontransgender patient during a first-time visit for unrelated episodic care, it would also be inappropriate to screen this patient today. STI screening is important and should be performed; however, it can wait until patient rapport has been established and a more detailed history has been obtained to guide screening.

Many online resources are available for learning about transgender persons and providing culturally sensitive medical care. The University of California, San Francisco, has published guidelines for primary and gender-affirming care of transgender and gender nonbinary persons at http://transhealth.ucsf.edu/protocols. Additionally, the National Lesbian, Gay, Bisexual, and Transgender (LGBT) Health Education Center, a program of the Fenway Institute, provides learning modules at www.lgbthealtheducation.org/lgbt-education/learning-modules/.

> **KEY POINT**
>
> • Irrespective of gender presentation, physicians should provide care for all patients in a sensitive, respectful, and affirming manner.

Bibliography

Lewis EB, Vincent B, Brett A, Gibson S, Walsh RJ. I am your trans patient. BMJ. 2017;357:j2963. [PMID: 28667010] doi:10.1136/bmj.j2963

Item 23   Answer: D

Educational Objective: Use a discharge summary to improve patient safety at transitions of care.

Communicating with and sharing the discharge summary with the primary care physician is recommended to improve patient safety and reduce rehospitalization in this patient. The evidence to support a reduction in hospital readmissions with completion of a discharge summary is mixed, most likely because of many complex factors that are difficult to control, such as timeliness, completeness, and quality of the discharge summary. However, the Institute for Healthcare Improvement identifies the lack of a timely discharge summary as a barrier to patient safety and prevention of early hospital readmission and therefore recommends a timely discharge summary as a key element in improving the transition of care from hospital to home. A discharge summary should include the evaluations performed, medication reconciliation, pending test results, required follow-up tests, and follow-up appointments and should be shared with the follow-up clinician. Timely follow-up with the primary care clinician is also important in ensuring that the transition goes smoothly. Another approach that has been successful in reducing hospitalization is the use of multiple team members, such as a nurse and pharmacist, to provide components of care.

A systematic review found that implementation of an intensive home visitation program reduced the risk for hospital readmission for heart failure at 3 to 6 months. This intervention included a series of eight planned home visits, the first within 24 hours of discharge. A medium-intensity intervention that included one telephone call within 7 days of discharge and one planned home visit within 10 days of discharge found no

statistically significant reduction in all-cause readmissions or mortality.

Home telemonitoring of patients with heart failure had no impact on hospital readmission or mortality. Post-discharge heart failure patient education programs also failed to result in reduced readmission rates or lower mortality.

> **KEY POINT**
>
> • A discharge summary that includes the evaluations performed, medication reconciliation, pending test results, required follow-up tests, and follow-up appointments is an important tool in the communication between the hospital and the follow-up clinician.

Bibliography

Rattray NA, Sico JJ, Cox LM, Russ AL, Matthias MS, Frankel RM. Crossing the communication chasm: challenges and opportunities in transitions of care from the hospital to the primary care clinic. Jt Comm J Qual Patient Saf. 2017;43:127-137. [PMID: 28334591] doi:10.1016/j.jcjq.2016.11.007

Item 24   Answer: B

Educational Objective: Diagnose adhesive capsulitis.

This patient's clinical presentation is most consistent with adhesive capsulitis, also known as frozen shoulder. Adhesive capsulitis commonly presents as poorly localized, progressive pain described as a deep aching with an insidious onset. Pain is also frequently worse at night and in cold weather. In addition to pain, patients with adhesive capsulitis frequently develop decreased shoulder mobility as the disease progresses. Range of motion (both active and passive) is decreased in all planes of motion. Adhesive capsulitis may be idiopathic (primary adhesive capsulitis) or secondary to several conditions (secondary adhesive capsulitis). Secondary conditions include diabetes mellitus, hypothyroidism, prior surgery or trauma, prolonged immobilization, autoimmune disorders, and stroke.

Acromioclavicular joint degeneration is unlikely to be responsible for this patient's clinical presentation. Patients with acromioclavicular joint degeneration typically report pain localized to the acromioclavicular joint. Physical examination findings include tenderness to palpation of the joint, pain with shoulder abduction beyond 120 degrees, and pain with passive shoulder adduction (a positive cross-arm test).

Bicipital tendinitis typically results in pain localized to the anterior shoulder that may radiate toward the deltoid and into the arm. Pain classically worsens with overhead activity. On examination, tenderness may be elicited by palpating the bicipital groove. Pain also can be reproduced by placing the patient's ipsilateral arm at his or her side while flexing the elbow to 90 degrees and supinating against resistance (Yergason test).

Rotator cuff disease would not be expected to cause pain with both active and passive movement of the shoulder; therefore, it would not account for this patient's presentation.

KEY POINT

- Adhesive capsulitis is characterized by loss of shoulder movement accompanied by pain; examination discloses significant loss of both active and passive range of motion.

Bibliography

Le HV, Lee SJ, Nazarian A, Rodriguez EK. Adhesive capsulitis of the shoulder: review of pathophysiology and current clinical treatments. Shoulder Elbow. 2017;9:75-84. [PMID: 28405218] doi:10.1177/1758573216676786

Item 25   Answer: C

Educational Objective: Treat premature ejaculation.

Topical lidocaine is the most appropriate treatment for this patient's premature ejaculation. Premature ejaculation is defined as ejaculation that occurs sooner than desired and is distressful to either or both partners. The mainstays of therapy include counseling and pharmacotherapy (oral and topical agents). According to the American Urological Association, pharmacologic options include selective serotonin reuptake inhibitors (SSRIs), tricyclic antidepressants, and topical anesthetic agents. Oral medications (fluoxetine, paroxetine, sertraline) are effective because they tend to cause delayed ejaculation as a side effect. This patient is currently taking a tricyclic antidepressant and has had previous mood instability with an SSRI; therefore, the most appropriate treatment is a regimen of topical lidocaine to help reduce tactile stimulation and thus prolong the time to ejaculation. Topical medications (lidocaine, prilocaine) may be used with or without a condom.

Paroxetine therapy is an effective treatment strategy for premature ejaculation. However, it is not appropriate in this case because of the patient's previously reported mood instability when exposed to sertraline. Both sertraline and paroxetine are SSRIs, which can cause deleterious mood changes (a class effect). In a patient with depression that is currently well controlled, adding an additional psychoactive medication is not warranted.

Testosterone gel, which is used in the treatment of hypogonadism, is not appropriate for this patient. Hypogonadism (androgen deficiency) can lead to decreased libido and erectile dysfunction, but it has not been shown to be a causative or correlative factor in premature ejaculation. Furthermore, this patient has no examination findings that would raise concern for hypogonadism, such as body hair growth and pattern changes, reduced testicular size, or gynecomastia, and his 8:00 AM serum total testosterone level was normal.

Given that the patient's premature ejaculation is distressing to both the patient and his spouse, offering no treatment options could lead to worsening self-confidence, mood, and quality of life.

KEY POINT

- Pharmacologic options for the treatment of premature ejaculation include selective serotonin reuptake inhibitors, tricyclic antidepressants, and topical anesthetic agents.

Bibliography

Martin C, Nolen H, Podolnick J, Wang R. Current and emerging therapies in premature ejaculation: Where we are coming from, where we are going. Int J Urol. 2017;24:40-50. [PMID: 27704632] doi:10.1111/iju.13202

Item 26   Answer: D

Educational Objective: Treat a woman with stress urinary incontinence.

The most appropriate treatment for this patient is pelvic floor muscle training (PFMT; also known as Kegel exercises). This multiparous, postmenopausal woman describes classic stress urinary incontinence, which is characterized by urine leakage associated with activities that cause increased intra-abdominal pressure, such as coughing, laughing, or sneezing. The American College of Physicians (ACP) recommends PFMT as first-line therapy for women with stress incontinence. PFMT may also be of benefit in patients with mixed urge and stress incontinence. If performed correctly and diligently, PFMT exercises may strengthen the pelvic floor muscles and enhance urinary retention. The patient is advised to tighten the pelvic muscles as if trying to interrupt urination. Best results require three or four sets of 10 contractions daily, with contractions lasting 10 seconds. The regimen should be continued for a minimum of 15 to 20 weeks. The ACP recommends against pharmacotherapy for this condition.

Bladder training and suppressive therapy are recommended by the ACP for urgency and mixed incontinence. With bladder training, patients are instructed to void regularly throughout the day, regardless of urge, and progressively increase the interval between voids. Suppression techniques are used to manage urge to void outside of the schedule. The patient is instructed to contract pelvic floor muscles quickly three or four times, use a distraction technique (counting backwards from 100), and, when the urge passes, walk to the bathroom to urinate.

The risks and benefits of systemic hormone replacement therapy, such as oral estradiol, in postmenopausal women must be carefully considered. Its use should be reserved for vasomotor symptoms of menopause at the lowest effective dosage. Estrogen replacement therapy is not recommended for chronic medical problems. Trials of topical estrogen therapy for stress urinary incontinence in patients with vaginal atrophy are of mixed quality at best, and its use is not routinely recommended.

Oxybutynin is a treatment for urgency urinary incontinence when bladder training is only partially successful or has failed. It is not recommended for the treatment of stress urinary incontinence.

Answers and Critiques

The ACP recommends exercise and weight loss for all obese women with urinary incontinence. This patient is not overweight, and her incontinence would likely not benefit from exercise and weight loss.

KEY POINT

- Stress urinary incontinence is characterized by urine leakage associated with activities that cause increased intra-abdominal pressure, such as coughing, laughing, or sneezing; it is best managed with pelvic floor muscle training exercises.

Bibliography

Qaseem A, Dallas P, Forciea MA, Starkey M, Denberg TD, Shekelle P; Clinical Guidelines Committee of the American College of Physicians. Nonsurgical management of urinary incontinence in women: a clinical practice guideline from the American College of Physicians. Ann Intern Med. 2014;161:429-40. [PMID: 25222388] doi:10.7326/M13-2410

Item 27   Answer: A

Educational Objective: Manage a request for potentially inappropriate treatment.

The most appropriate management is consultation with the hospital ethics committee. A recent policy statement from the Society of Critical Care Medicine recommends that appropriate treatment goals of ICU care include treatment that provides a reasonable expectation of survival outside of the acute care setting with sufficient cognitive ability to perceive benefits of treatment, or palliative care through the dying process in the ICU. Because conflicts between the desire to provide benefit to the patient and the desire to minimize the burden of treatment can be very difficult, one of the most important skills of the physician is the ability to communicate and negotiate a reasonable treatment plan with the patient's family. If these situations become intractable, many organizations recommend initiating a process to resolve the disagreement, including notifying surrogates of the process, seeking a second medical opinion, obtaining review by an interdisciplinary ethics committee, offering the surrogate the opportunity to seek care at another institution, and implementing the decision of the resolution process. This patient's family is requesting treatment that the care team does not think will achieve reasonable goals, and an ethics consultation may lead to conflict resolution.

In some situations, the physician and the patient's family may mutually establish a time frame in which care will be withdrawn if there is no improvement; however, these decisions should not be made unilaterally by the care team.

A physician should not provide treatment that conflicts with professional obligations and will not meet the goals of care. However, often by communicating his or her concerns, a physician is able to help a family understand the burden of continued, ineffective treatment. If resolution is not possible, family members may seek transfer to another institution; however, the physician is not obliged to initiate such arrangements.

KEY POINT

- A physician should not provide treatment that conflicts with professional obligations and will not meet the goals of care; when the physician and the patient (or family members) have conflicting goals of care, an ethics consultation may be beneficial.

Bibliography

Kon AA, Shepard EK, Sederstrom NO, Swoboda SM, Marshall MF, Birriel B, et al. Defining futile and potentially inappropriate interventions: a policy statement from the Society of Critical Care Medicine Ethics Committee. Crit Care Med. 2016;44:1769-74. [PMID: 27525995] doi: 10.1097/CCM.0000000000001965

Item 28   Answer: D

Educational Objective: Treat genitourinary syndrome of menopause.

Vaginal estrogen therapy is the most appropriate treatment for this patient with genitourinary syndrome of menopause (GSM), also known as vaginal atrophy. GSM is a common condition in postmenopausal women that is characterized by dryness, inflammation, and thinning of the vaginal walls due to decreased estrogen. Other symptoms include dyspareunia, itching, and vulvovaginal irritation. The associated dyspareunia may lead to avoidance of sexual activity because of discomfort. This patient's pelvic examination features are classic for GSM, including a pale and dry vaginal lining with reduction in rugae. For severe symptoms or symptoms not responsive to moisturizers and lubricants, topical estrogen therapy has numerous beneficial effects, including restoration of the acidic vaginal pH, thickening of the epithelium, and increase in vaginal secretions. Available preparations include estradiol or conjugated estrogen in tablet, cream, or ring forms. Low-dose vaginal estradiol tablets and the estradiol vaginal ring have minimal systemic estrogen absorption. Because estradiol absorption is insufficient to cause endometrial proliferation, concurrent progestin is typically not indicated when low-dose local estrogen is used to treat GSM. The dose and duration of topical estrogen therapy are individualized according to symptom severity. Family history of breast cancer is not a contraindication to use.

A potent topical glucocorticoid, such as clobetasol, is used to treat vulvar lichen sclerosus. This inflammatory condition often presents as white, atrophic patches on the genital and perianal skin. It is associated with dyspareunia, pain, and pruritus. Prepubertal girls and postmenopausal women appear to be at highest risk. The intense itching and plaque-like involvement of the labia, introitus, and perianal region are clinical clues that distinguish vulvar lichen sclerosus from the generalized thinning and drying associated with GSM.

Ospemifene is an estrogen agonist/antagonist used to reduce the severity of moderate to severe dyspareunia in postmenopausal women. It is recommended that women with an intact uterus also take a progestin. How ospemifene compares to vaginal estrogens in terms of efficacy and safety is

Answers and Critiques

unknown. Because topical estrogen therapy has a long history of safety, experts recommend that ospemifene be reserved for women who cannot or will not use topical estrogens.

Although systemic estrogen therapy may help with symptoms of vaginal atrophy, use of vaginal estrogen is most effective for treatment of GSM in a patient with no other menopausal symptoms, such as hot flushes, night sweats, or mood concerns.

Recent evidence suggests that vaginal estrogen therapy may be as effective as vaginal lubricants for treating post-menopausal vaginal symptoms. However, in this patient with symptoms that have not responded to vaginal lubricants, vaginal estrogen is the most reasonable option.

KEY POINT

- Vaginal estrogen therapy is appropriate treatment for patients with moderate to severe genitourinary syndrome of menopause that has not responded to moisturizers and lubricants.

Bibliography

The NAMS 2017 Hormone Therapy Position Statement Advisory Panel. The 2017 hormone therapy position statement of The North American Menopause Society. Menopause. 2017;24:728-753. [PMID: 28650869] doi:10.1097/GME.0000000000000921

Item 29 Answer: D

Educational Objective: Treat generalized anxiety disorder with pharmacologic therapy.

The most appropriate long-term pharmacologic treatment for this patient with generalized anxiety disorder (GAD) is sertraline. GAD is characterized by excessive anxiety about activities or events (occupation, school) occurring more days than not for at least 6 months and causing significant functional impairment. Patients with GAD also experience difficulty concentrating, irritability, muscle tension, restlessness, and sleep disturbance. A useful tool for identifying and assessing the severity of GAD is the Generalized Anxiety Disorder 7-item scale (GAD-7), which asks patients to rate seven items on a scale of 0 to 3 based on increasing severity (https://www.integration.samhsa.gov/clinical-practice/GAD708.19.08Cartwright.pdf). A score of 5 to 9 indicates mild anxiety, 10 to 14 moderate anxiety, and 15 to 21 severe anxiety. The GAD-7 can be used to monitor symptom severity over time, allowing clinicians to monitor treatment effectiveness.

Treatment options for GAD include cognitive behavioral therapy (CBT) and pharmacologic therapy, such as with a selective serotonin reuptake inhibitor (SSRI) or serotonin-norepinephrine reuptake inhibitor (SNRI). Patients with GAD often have comorbid mood and anxiety disorders, which often make SSRIs (such as sertraline) and SNRIs (such as venlafaxine) preferred because of their broad therapeutic applicability. CBT is the most effective psychotherapy for GAD; trials have shown it is as effective as pharmacologic therapy and can be used as monotherapy or in combination with drugs. The choice between pharmacologic therapy and CBT is often based on patient preference and the presence of comorbid disorders. Another consideration may be costs of treatment, both direct and indirect (due to time away from work or school). Depending on the particular agent, antidepressant therapy costs $100 to $300 per year, with low indirect costs. On average, annual costs for CBT are three to four times higher than for antidepressant therapy and also require significant time away from work or school to attend therapy.

Tricyclic antidepressants, such as amitriptyline, are considered second-line therapy for GAD because of a higher incidence of side effects with their use.

Benzodiazepines, such as clonazepam, are useful for controlling severe anxiety symptoms, especially before the benefits of CBT or other pharmacologic therapy take effect. These agents should be used only for short periods (<4-6 weeks) because of the potential for dependency.

Lithium and other mood stabilizers are appropriate treatment for bipolar disorder but are not indicated for the treatment of anxiety disorders.

KEY POINT

- Treatment options for generalized anxiety disorder include cognitive behavioral therapy and pharmacologic therapy with a selective serotonin reuptake inhibitor or serotonin-norepinephrine reuptake inhibitor.

Bibliography

Patel G, Fancher TL. In the clinic. Generalized anxiety disorder. Ann Intern Med. 2013;159:ITC6-1–ITC6-11; quiz ITC6-12. [PMID: 24297210] doi:10.7326/0003-4819-159-11-201312030-01006

Item 30 Answer: B

Educational Objective: Implement risk-mitigation strategies for patients at high risk for opioid overdose.

The most appropriate next step before continued prescription of this patient's long-term opioid therapy is to prescribe naloxone and provide caregiver education on its use. Naloxone, a pure opioid antagonist that acts as a competitive inhibitor at opioid receptors, can be a life-saving reversal agent for patients with opioid overdose, and evidence shows that naloxone is effective in preventing opioid-related overdose death at the community level through community-based distribution. The Centers for Disease Control and Prevention Guideline for Prescribing Opioids for Chronic Pain recommends that physicians consider offering naloxone to patients with a high risk for overdose (history of overdose or substance use disorder, high opioid dosage [≥50 morphine milligram equivalents/day], or concurrent benzodiazepine use). When naloxone is prescribed, patients and patients' household members should be educated on its use and on ways to prevent overdose. This patient is currently taking approximately 75 morphine milligram equivalents/day and using a long-acting formulation; therefore, she is considered at high risk for overdose and should be considered for naloxone prescription.

H
CONT.

Coprescription of opioids and benzodiazepines is associated with an increased risk for death from overdose and should be avoided when prescribing medications for patients with chronic pain.

Close monitoring, including review of prescription monitoring databases (where available), urine drug screening, and ongoing functional assessment, are all appropriate tools in the safe prescribing of long-term opioid therapy; however, weekly nursing visits are not currently recommended as a risk-mitigation strategy.

Although current guidelines recommend avoiding the use of extended-release opioids, this patient's pain and quality of life improved with substitution of a short-acting regimen for a transdermal fentanyl patch. If the benefits outweigh the risks and the patient has provided informed consent and received appropriate education, continued extended-release opioid therapy (with implementation of appropriate safety mechanisms) could be considered in this patient with chronic, irreversible pain.

KEY POINT

- Physicians should consider offering naloxone to patients receiving long-term opioid therapy with a high risk for overdose (history of overdose or substance use disorder, high opioid dosage [≥50 morphine milligram equivalents/day], or concurrent benzodiazepine use).

Bibliography

Dowell D, Haegerich TM, Chou R. CDC guideline for prescribing opioids for chronic pain—United States, 2016. JAMA. 2016;315:1624-45. [PMID: 26977696] doi:10.1001/jama.2016.1464

Item 31   Answer: A

Educational Objective: Treat a patient with clinical atherosclerotic cardiovascular disease who has not achieved target LDL cholesterol reduction with statin therapy.

In addition to discontinuing ezetimibe, the most appropriate management of this patient with clinical atherosclerotic cardiovascular disease (ASCVD) is to initiate alirocumab. For patients with clinical ASCVD, high-intensity statin therapy is recommended, with a goal of at least 50% LDL cholesterol reduction. Nonstatin drugs, preferably ezetimibe or a proprotein convertase subtilisin/kexin type 9 (PCSK9) inhibitor, should be considered alone or in combination with statins in patients who do not achieve target LDL cholesterol reduction. PCSK9 inhibitors, such as alirocumab, are monoclonal antibodies that bind to serine protease PCSK9, a liver enzyme that degrades hepatocyte LDL receptors. Treatment with PCSK9 inhibitors produces a 50% to 60% reduction in LDL cholesterol. ASCVD risk reduction has also been demonstrated with PCSK9 inhibitors, although studies have included a relatively small number of patients with limited follow-up. A modest reduction in triglyceride level and increase in HDL cholesterol level have also been observed

with their use. Limitations include high cost and the need for subcutaneous injections every 2 to 4 weeks. Common side effects include injection-site reactions, fatigue, and limb pain. This patient with clinical ASCVD has not achieved the goal LDL cholesterol reduction on maximally tolerated statin therapy and did not tolerate ezetimibe. Therefore, alirocumab should be initiated. In addition to starting a PCSK9 inhibitor, intensification of therapeutic lifestyle changes, such as weight loss and regular exercise, should be encouraged.

A bile acid sequestrant, such as cholestyramine, may be considered as an optional alternative agent for patients with ezetimibe intolerance and a triglyceride level less than 300 mg/dL (3.39 mmol/L) or because of patient preference, but there is no evidence of a net cardiovascular risk reduction benefit with bile acid sequestrants in combination with statins.

Niacin is no longer routinely recommended for treatment of hyperlipidemia based on lack of efficacy and potential harms.

Continuing atorvastatin without additional intervention is unlikely to result in further LDL cholesterol reduction.

KEY POINT

- Proprotein convertase subtilisin/kexin type 9 (PCSK9) inhibitors and ezetimibe are the preferred nonstatin drugs for patients with clinical atherosclerotic cardiovascular disease who do not achieve goal LDL cholesterol reduction with maximally tolerated statin therapy.

Bibliography

Lloyd-Jones DM, Morris PB, Ballantyne CM, Birtcher KK, Daly DD Jr, DePalma SM, et al. 2017 focused update of the 2016 ACC expert consensus decision pathway on the role of non-statin therapies for LDL-Cholesterol lowering in the management of atherosclerotic cardiovascular disease risk: a report of the American College of Cardiology Task Force on Expert Consensus Decision Pathways. J Am Coll Cardiol. 2017;70:1785-1822. [PMID: 28886926] doi:10.1016/j.jacc.2017.07.745

Item 32   Answer: C

Educational Objective: Screen for colorectal cancer in an average-risk patient with fecal immunochemical testing.

The most appropriate screening test for this patient is a fecal immunochemical test (FIT). The U.S. Preventive Services Task Force (USPSTF) recommends screening for colorectal cancer in asymptomatic adults aged 50 to 75 years. For patients with average risk for colorectal cancer, several screening strategies are available, including fecal occult blood testing, direct endoscopic visualization, radiologic examination, and testing the blood for molecular markers of cancer. There is little head-to-head comparative evidence that any one recommended screening modality provides a greater benefit than the others. In addition, despite unequivocal evidence that colon cancer screening reduces mortality, an estimated one in three U.S. adults who are eligible for colon cancer screening has not been screened. Therefore, the USPSTF supports using the test that is most likely to result in completion of screening. Test selection should be guided by evidence, patient preferences, and local availability. Two fecal blood detection tests are available: a sensitive guaiac-based fecal occult blood test (gFOBT) and an FIT that uses antibodies to detect human hemoglobin. Sensitive gFOBT requires dietary restriction in order to reduce false-positive results, whereas FIT does not. The FDA has approved a third stool-based screening test that is combined with FIT and detects cancer DNA in the stool (the multitargeted stool DNA test). Mortality data for this screening strategy are not available. Because this patient would prefer not to modify his diet, FIT is the most appropriate screening option.

The plasma circulating methylated *SEPT9* DNA test is an FDA-approved colorectal cancer screening test that holds promise, as blood tests may result in increased screening adherence. However, its sensitivity for detecting colorectal cancer is suboptimal at 48%, and mortality data are lacking.

Endoscopic tests include flexible sigmoidoscopy and colonoscopy. The mortality benefit of flexible sigmoidoscopy is limited to cancers of the distal bowel. Colonoscopy can visualize the entire bowel but requires colon preparation, which can be a barrier to completing the study. CT colonography is a radiologic technique that also requires colon preparation, which this patient has refused.

Major guidelines differ in their recommendations regarding screening strategy and frequency. The 2016 USPSTF guideline recommends sensitive gFOBT or FIT annually or multitargeted stool DNA testing every 3 years. Flexible sigmoidoscopy is recommended every 5 years, but if combined with FIT (or possibly gFOBT), the interval can be increased to every 10 years, the same interval recommended for colonoscopy. CT colonography can be performed every 5 years.

KEY POINT

- The U.S. Preventive Services Task Force recommends screening for colorectal cancer in asymptomatic adults aged 50 to 75 years; the choice of screening test should be guided by evidence, patient preferences, and local availability.

Bibliography
Inadomi JM. Screening for colorectal neoplasia. N Engl J Med. 2017;376:149-156. [PMID: 28076720] doi:10.1056/NEJMcp1512286

Item 33   Answer: C

Educational Objective: Counsel a patient on the use of herbal supplements.

This patient should be advised to discontinue drinking kava tea. Patients take dietary supplements for various reasons, such as to prevent illness, enhance health, and correct perceived deficiencies. In the United States, approximately 50% of adults report using vitamins or dietary supplements, with total consumer spending of more than $20 billion each year. Despite their prevalent use, the U.S. Preventive Services

Task Force does not recommend multivitamins or herbal supplements for the prevention of cardiovascular disease or cancer. In addition to questionable efficacy, supplement use is associated with risk for considerable harms, including side effects; interactions with other drugs; and harms related to inclusion of unadvertised additives, compounds, or toxins. Despite the risks, many patients strongly believe in supplement use, and the role of the physician is to inform these patients of harmful supplements and suggest safer alternatives. This patient is taking kava, which is derived from *Piper methysticum*, a plant native to the western Pacific islands. It is often used to relieve stress and anxiety but has been associated with liver damage. In 2002, the FDA issued a consumer advisory regarding the potential risk for severe liver injury with kava use, especially in patients with liver disease or at risk for liver disease. Therefore, advising this patient with nonalcoholic steatohepatitis to discontinue kava tea would be the best management option.

Echinacea may be slightly effective for prevention but not treatment of the common cold. The most common side effects are gastrointestinal upset and nausea. Although this patient does not need to take echinacea, this herb has a relatively safe side effect profile, and she may continue it if she wishes.

The U.S. Preventive Services Task Force recommends daily folic acid supplementation (400 to 800 µg) for women of child-bearing age to prevent fetal neural tube defects; therefore, folic acid should be continued in this 35-year-old patient.

This patient has diagnoses of nonalcoholic steatohepatitis and obesity, and continuing an herbal supplement that is associated with known hepatotoxicity may cause harms.

KEY POINT

- Dietary and herbal supplements have questionable efficacy and may be associated with considerable harms; physicians must inform patients of harmful supplements and suggest safer alternatives.

Bibliography
Teschke R, Wolff A, Frenzel C, Schulze J, Eickhoff A. Herbal hepatotoxicity: a tabular compilation of reported cases. Liver Int. 2012;32:1543-56. [PMID: 22928722] doi: 10.1111/j.1478-3231.2012.02864.x

Item 34   Answer: B

Educational Objective: Evaluate preoperative cardiac risk using electrocardiography in a patient with known cardiovascular disease.

The most appropriate preoperative cardiac testing for this patient is electrocardiography (ECG). The 2014 American College of Cardiology/American Heart Association guideline on perioperative cardiovascular evaluation and management of patients undergoing noncardiac surgery states that preoperative ECG is reasonable for patients with known atherosclerotic cardiovascular disease (including coronary artery disease, arrhythmia,

CONT. peripheral artery disease, cerebrovascular disease, or significant structural heart disease) who are undergoing moderate- to high-risk surgeries. Preoperative ECG also may be considered for other asymptomatic patients, except for those undergoing low-risk procedures. This patient has known coronary artery disease and has not undergone ECG in 2 years. It is reasonable to obtain ECG preoperatively because certain interval findings (for example, new Q waves), additional evidence of conduction disease, or arrhythmia may result in changes in perioperative management.

Risk calculators, including the Revised Cardiac Risk Index and the American College of Surgeons National Surgical Quality Improvement Program myocardial infarction and cardiac arrest calculator, can be used to determine the risk for a perioperative major adverse cardiac event (MACE). Patients with low risk (<1% risk for perioperative MACE) may proceed to surgery without preoperative cardiac stress testing, whereas patients with elevated risk (≥1% risk for perioperative MACE) should undergo assessment of functional capacity. Metabolic equivalents (METs) are used to represent the patient's functional capacity based on the intensity of activity able to be performed. If the patient's functional capacity exceeds 4 METs, the patient may proceed to surgery without further testing. Examples of 4 METs of activity include the ability to walk 4 miles per hour on a flat surface, climb one to two flights of stairs without stopping, or perform vigorous housework such as vacuuming. Swimming for 30 minutes also exceeds this threshold. Cardiac stress testing should generally be reserved for patients at elevated risk for MACE with a functional capacity less than 4 METs, but only if the results of the test will change perioperative management. Although this patient has an elevated risk for a MACE perioperatively, his functional capacity exceeds 4 METs; therefore, he does not require preoperative cardiac stress testing with dobutamine or exercise.

KEY POINT

- Preoperative electrocardiography is reasonable for patients with known atherosclerotic cardiovascular disease, including coronary artery disease, arrhythmia, peripheral artery disease, cerebrovascular disease, or significant structural heart disease, who are undergoing moderate- to high-risk surgeries; cardiac stress testing should generally be reserved for patients at elevated risk for major adverse cardiac event with a functional capacity less than 4 metabolic equivalents, but only if the results of the test will change perioperative management.

Bibliography
Fleisher LA, Fleischmann KE, Auerbach AD, Barnason SA, Beckman JA, Bozkurt B, et al; American College of Cardiology. 2014 ACC/AHA guideline on perioperative cardiovascular evaluation and management of patients undergoing noncardiac surgery: a report of the American College of Cardiology/American Heart Association Task Force on Practice Guidelines. J Am Coll Cardiol. 2014;64:e77-137. [PMID: 25091544]

Item 35   Answer: D
Educational Objective: Diagnose ulnar nerve entrapment.

This patient has symptoms consistent with ulnar neuropathy (fourth and fifth finger numbness and, more rarely, interosseous muscle weakness), making ulnar nerve entrapment the most likely diagnosis. Ulnar nerve entrapment, also known as cubital tunnel syndrome, is caused by impingement of the ulnar nerve at the elbow by bone spurs, fibrous tissue, ganglion cysts, or ulnar nerve subluxation. Elbow pain typically worsens with flexion. The diagnosis is usually made clinically and does not require imaging. Initial treatment consists of activity modification, splinting the elbow at night to prevent prolonged elbow flexion, and use of an elbow pad during the day to avoid direct trauma. Surgery is an option when conservative measures fail in the setting of significant or progressive symptoms.

Carpal tunnel syndrome is associated with wrist pain and symptoms of median nerve dysfunction, namely numbness in the first three fingers and pain that radiates into the forearm and hand. Pain frequently worsens at night and with repetitive actions. Findings on physical examination may include weakened thumb abduction; thenar muscle atrophy suggests severe disease. These symptoms and findings are not present in this patient.

Medial epicondylitis is an important differential diagnosis in a patient presenting with medial elbow pain. Patients with this condition usually have pain and tenderness over the medial epicondyle and ventral forearm, which worsens with resisted wrist flexion rather than elbow flexion. Medial epicondylitis is not usually associated with hand symptoms.

Olecranon bursitis is associated with swelling and, depending on the cause, significant tenderness of the posterior elbow over the olecranon bursa. This patient has not had signs of elbow swelling, and olecranon bursitis does not cause neuropathic symptoms.

KEY POINT

- Ulnar nerve entrapment, also known as cubital tunnel syndrome, is caused by impingement of the ulnar nerve at the elbow by bone spurs, fibrous tissue, ganglion cysts, or ulnar nerve subluxation; characteristics include pain at the elbow that worsens with flexion, paresthesias and numbness of the fourth and fifth fingers, and weakness of the interosseous muscles.

Bibliography
Hobson-Webb LD, Juel VC. Common entrapment neuropathies. Continuum (Minneap Minn). 2017;23:487-511. [PMID: 28375915] doi:10.1212/CON.0000000000000452

Item 36   Answer: D
Educational Objective: Evaluate a patient with syncope.

The most appropriate diagnostic tests to perform next are orthostatic blood pressure measurement and electrocardiography.

The American Heart Association (AHA), the American College of Cardiology (ACC), and the Heart Rhythm Society (HRS) jointly conclude that the history and physical examination are the most important diagnostic tools in determining the underlying cause of a syncopal event. The history should focus on eliciting prodromal or postepisode symptoms, comorbid medical or psychiatric conditions, the psychosocial context of the event, and bystander information. The patient's prescription and over-the-counter medications should also be thoroughly reviewed. The physical examination should include an in-depth cardiovascular evaluation, including orthostatic (postural) blood pressure measurements, as well as a basic neurologic examination to evaluate for focal defects. Orthostatic blood pressure assessment has consistently been shown to be the most valuable diagnostic tool in the evaluation of syncope. The AHA/ACC/HRS guideline for the evaluation and management of patients with syncope additionally recommends that resting 12-lead electrocardiography (ECG) be performed in all patients with syncope to identify an underlying arrhythmia, myocardial ischemia, or QT prolongation. Further diagnostic testing should be methodically selected on the basis of the clinical circumstances.

The diagnostic yield of 24- to 48-hour electrocardiographic monitoring is low (1%-2%), unless there are frequent episodes over a short period. More prolonged rhythm monitoring with an external loop event recorder improves yield if the patient has clinical or ECG features of arrhythmia-related syncope. Clinical evidence does not support routine echocardiography in patients with syncope. Unexpected findings on echocardiogram to explain syncope are uncommon.

Laboratory testing, such as B-type natriuretic peptide and cardiac enzyme measurement, has considerably low diagnostic yield and is not recommended in the routine evaluation of patients with syncope. Rather, further diagnostic testing should be based on the findings on the history, physical examination, and ECG.

The AHA/ACC/HRS syncope guideline does not recommend MRI and CT of the head in the routine evaluation of patients with syncope in the absence of head injury or focal neurologic findings that support further evaluation. Similarly, carotid artery imaging is not recommended in the routine evaluation of patients with syncope in the absence of focal neurologic findings.

KEY POINT

- In patients with syncope, the physical examination should include an in-depth cardiovascular evaluation, including orthostatic (postural) blood pressure measurements, as well as a basic neurologic examination to evaluate for focal defects; electrocardiography is the only diagnostic study that is routinely recommended in patients with syncope.

Bibliography

Shen WK, Sheldon RS, Benditt DG, Cohen MI, Forman DE, Goldberger ZD, et al. 2017 ACC/AHA/HRS guideline for the evaluation and management of patients with syncope: executive summary: a report of the American College of Cardiology/American Heart Association Task Force on Clinical Practice Guidelines and the Heart Rhythm Society. J Am Coll Cardiol. 2017;70:620-663. doi: 10.1016/j.jacc.2017.03.002. [PMID: 28286222]

Item 37   Answer: C

Educational Objective: Identify appropriate contraceptive care for a smoker.

The most appropriate contraceptive option for this patient is a progesterone-containing intrauterine device (IUD). Hormonal contraception options include oral contraceptive pills, a transdermal patch, a vaginal ring, and long-acting reversible contraceptives. Long-acting reversible contraceptives are progestin-only forms of contraception that include depot medroxyprogesterone acetate injections, subcutaneous implants, and progestin-containing IUDs. These preparations are less reliant on user adherence than oral contraceptive pills, are highly effective, and may be ideal for this patient who has proven difficulty with adhering to a daily pill routine. Return of fertility may be delayed with these methods, with a median time to conception of 10 months after cessation of use. As with other progestin-only methods, irregular bleeding and amenorrhea are prevalent, and weight gain is a common side effect. The levonorgestrel IUD is available in two dosage formulations: one that releases 14 μg/d and is effective for 3 years and one that releases 20 μg/d and is effective for 5 years. The levonorgestrel-containing IUD releases a low dose of progestin, which causes endometrial atrophy and generally leads to decreased or absent menstrual flow. The progesterone-containing IUD may be ideal for this patient who is bothered by heavy menstrual flow, and it will simultaneously eliminate the need for daily adherence to a pill.

Oral contraceptive pills are the most common form of contraception. These include combination estrogen-progestin pills and progestin-only pills ("mini-pill"). Combination preparations differ based on the strength of estrogen and the type of progestin component. All preparations are therapeutically equivalent in preventing pregnancy. Contraindications to estrogen-containing preparations (including oral contraceptives and estrogen-progestin vaginal rings) include breast cancer, liver disease, migraine with aura, uncontrolled hypertension, and venous thromboembolism. They are also contraindicated in women older than age 35 years who smoke more than 15 cigarettes per day, such as this patient, because of an increased risk for venous thromboembolism. When estrogen-containing products are contraindicated, a progesterone-only contraceptive could safely be used. In this patient, a progestin-only pill is less preferable to a progesterone-containing IUD because a pill would require daily adherence.

KEY POINT

- Estrogen-containing hormonal contraceptives are contraindicated in women older than 35 years who smoke more than 15 cigarettes a day because of an increased risk for venous thromboembolism.

Bibliography

Tracy EE. Contraception: menarche to menopause. Obstet Gynecol Clin North Am. 2017;44:143-158. [PMID: 28499527] doi:10.1016/j.ogc.2017.02.001

Item 38   Answer: B

Educational Objective: Treat obesity with liraglutide in a patient with type 2 diabetes mellitus.

Liraglutide is the most appropriate next step in treatment. Weight-loss medications are recommended when a trial of comprehensive lifestyle modification, including reduced dietary intake, exercise, and behavioral therapy, fails to achieve a 5% to 10% reduction in weight at 3 to 6 months. This patient has appropriately adhered to dietary caloric restriction, with regular self-monitoring of calorie intake and weight, and is now exercising for more than 150 minutes per week. Her BMI is greater than 27, and she has obesity-related comorbid conditions (type 2 diabetes mellitus and uncontrolled hypertension). Liraglutide has been shown to increase satiety and aid in achieving more than 5% weight loss after 52 weeks of therapy, and it may help the patient feel less hungry.

Bariatric surgery is recommended for patients with BMI of 40 or greater, and for patients with BMI of 35 or greater who have obesity-related comorbidities and who have tried all other weight loss therapies without achieving significant weight loss or improvements in comorbid conditions.

There is no evidence that low-carbohydrate diets are more effective for reducing weight than low-fat diets. This patient is adherent to her chosen diet but has difficulty reducing her caloric intake to achieve continued weight loss. Clinicians should prescribe a diet with which the patient will adhere (that is, a diet that is palatable and affordable) and that maintains negative energy balance in order to achieve weight loss.

Very-low-calorie diets are recommended when rapid weight loss is medically indicated. This patient does not require rapid weight loss, and neither the risk nor the expense of frequent visits and laboratory monitoring are justified in this case.

KEY POINT

- Weight-loss medications are recommended when a trial of comprehensive lifestyle modification, including reduced dietary intake, exercise, and behavioral therapy, fails to achieve a 5% to 10% reduction in weight after 3 to 6 months.

Bibliography

Jensen MD, Ryan DH, Apovian CM, Ard JD, Comuzzie AG, Donato KA, et al; American College of Cardiology/American Heart Association Task Force on Practice Guidelines. 2013 AHA/ACC/TOS guideline for the management of overweight and obesity in adults: a report of the American College of Cardiology/American Heart Association Task Force on Practice Guidelines and The Obesity Society. Circulation. 2014;129:S102-38. [PMID: 24222017] doi:10.1161/01.cir.0000437739.71477.ee

Item 39   Answer: A

Educational Objective: Identify appropriate timing for palliative medicine referral in a patient with advanced cancer.

The most appropriate time for palliative medicine referral is now. Palliative medicine (or palliative care) focuses on reducing pain, nonpain symptoms, and psychosocial stress associated with advanced disease. This patient has been diagnosed with incurable lung cancer and would benefit from concurrent specialty palliative medicine in conjunction with initiation of disease-directed therapy. Studies have consistently shown improvements in various quality-of-life metrics when palliative medicine is integrated early in the course of incurable cancer, and such integration is consistent with recommendations from the American Society of Clinical Oncology.

Although referral to palliative care historically occurred at the end of life, an emerging consensus of research indicates that early initiation during a serious or life-threatening illness is associated with substantial advantages. Evidence shows that early palliative medicine referral improves mood and decreases rates of depressive symptoms; anxiety is not heightened by palliative medicine referral. Palliative medicine teams are positioned to work with oncologists and primary care physicians in treating the complex symptoms of serious illness, and an integrated approach is recommended.

Hospice is a specialized form of palliative medicine that can provide a team-based care platform in the patient's preferred setting (for example, home, skilled nursing facility, or residential hospice house). Hospice should be considered for patients with an advanced illness who are no longer candidates for further disease-directed therapy, or whose goals (such as quality of life) are not likely to be met with further disease-directed therapies. Despite significant quality-of-life benefits for patients and their caregivers, hospice referrals often happen late in a patient's illness trajectory, leading to short hospice lengths of stay.

KEY POINT

- Palliative medicine, with its focus on reducing pain, nonpain symptoms, and psychosocial stress associated with advanced disease, improves quality of life for patients and their caregivers; early initiation of palliative medicine during a life-threatening illness has substantial advantages.

Bibliography

Ferrell BR, Temel JS, Temin S, Alesi ER, Balboni TA, Basch EM, et al. Integration of palliative care into standard oncology care: American Society of Clinical Oncology Clinical Practice Guideline Update. J Clin Oncol. 2017;35:96-112. [PMID: 28034065]

Item 40   Answer: B

Educational Objective: Prevent atherosclerotic cardiovascular disease with low-dose aspirin therapy.

The most appropriate measure to reduce this patient's atherosclerotic cardiovascular disease (ASCVD) risk is low-dose aspirin. The U.S. Preventive Services Task Force (USPSTF) recommends low-dose aspirin for the primary prevention of ASCVD and colorectal cancer in adults aged 50 to 59 years with a 10-year ASCVD risk of 10% or higher who do not have an increased risk for bleeding, have a life expectancy of at least 10 years, and are willing to take low-dose aspirin daily for at least 10 years. In those aged 60 to 69 years with a 10-year ASCVD risk of 10% or higher, the benefits of aspirin use for primary prevention are smaller but still outweigh the risk for bleeding, and the decision to initiate low-dose aspirin in this population should be individualized. In contrast to the USPSTF recommendations, the American Diabetes Association recommends consideration of low-dose aspirin therapy as a primary prevention strategy in patients with type 1 or type 2 diabetes mellitus who are at increased cardiovascular risk. This group of patients includes most men and women with diabetes aged 50 years or older who have at least one additional major risk factor (family history of premature ASCVD, hypertension, dyslipidemia, smoking, or albuminuria) and are not at increased risk for bleeding. Aspirin therapy for the primary prevention of ASCVD is likely underused (approximately 40% of eligible candidates). Among patients told by a physician to take aspirin, 80% adhere to the recommendation.

For patients with ASCVD and documented aspirin allergy, the ADA recommends clopidogrel as an alternative preventive measure. This patient does not have a documented aspirin allergy, and therapy in this patient will be initiated for primary, not secondary, prevention; therefore, clopidogrel is not recommended for this patient.

The most commonly recommended dose of aspirin for primary prevention of cardiovascular events is 75 mg to 100 mg. Primary prevention trials have shown that lower doses are likely as effective as higher doses; however, observational trials and a meta-analysis have demonstrated an increased risk for bleeding with regular-dose aspirin compared with low-dose aspirin.

KEY POINT

- Low-dose aspirin for the primary prevention of atherosclerotic cardiovascular disease (ASCVD) and colorectal cancer is recommended for adults aged 50 to 59 years with a 10-year ASCVD risk of 10% or higher who do not have an increased risk for bleeding.

Bibliography
Bibbins-Domingo K; U.S. Preventive Services Task Force. Aspirin use for the primary prevention of cardiovascular disease and colorectal cancer: U.S. Preventive Services Task Force recommendation statement. Ann Intern Med. 2016;164:836-45. [PMID: 27064677] doi: 10.7326/M16-0577

Item 41   Answer: E

Educational Objective: Evaluate a patient with symptoms of chronic insomnia with a sleep diary.

The most appropriate next step in management of this patient with symptoms of chronic insomnia is to obtain a 2-week sleep diary. Symptoms of insomnia vary and may include poor sleep quality, frustration with sleep quantity, difficulty initiating sleep, or an inability to return to sleep after awakening. In patients with symptoms of insomnia, a thorough history, physical examination, and medication review may point to potentially reversible causes, such as sleep apnea or restless legs syndrome. In the absence of specific historical features that are consistent with a primary sleep disorder, the initial evaluation of insomnia additionally involves obtaining a sleep diary to identify adverse environmental factors, inappropriate exposure to electronic screens (computer, phone, tablet, television) before bedtime, and sleep patterns. If the sleep diary reveals red flags for a primary sleep disorder or another condition that may interfere with sleep, further diagnostic testing would be indicated. In this patient with daytime somnolence, fatigue, and difficulty with sleep initiation, a sleep log may facilitate collection of an accurate sleep history.

Polysomnography is indicated in patients for whom there is a strong suspicion of a primary sleep disorder based on the initial history and physical examination. Polysomnography typically involves overnight, laboratory-based testing that is monitored by a sleep technician. Similarly, multiple sleep latency testing is a labor-intensive evaluation designed to identify diagnoses of narcolepsy and idiopathic hypersomnia. Neither study is indicated in the initial evaluation of this patient, whose primary problem appears to be initiating sleep.

Overnight pulse oximetry has a high rate of false-positive and false-negative results and has not been validated as a screening tool for obstructive sleep apnea. Normal-appearing results on overnight pulse oximetry may allow for avoidance of further testing in patients with a low pretest probability. However, there is no clinical suspicion for obstructive sleep apnea in this patient, and it would not be indicated in her initial evaluation.

Low serum ferritin levels are strongly correlated with restless legs syndrome, which is characterized by discomforting sensations in the legs at rest or when falling asleep, an urge to move the legs, and immediate relief after moving the legs or walking. However, no features in the history suggest restless legs syndrome as a cause of this patient's chronic insomnia.

KEY POINT

- The initial evaluation of chronic insomnia involves obtaining a sleep diary to identify adverse environmental factors, inappropriate exposure to electronic screens before bedtime, and sleep patterns.

Bibliography
Masters PA. In the clinic. Insomnia. Ann Intern Med. 2014;161:ITC1-15; quiz ITC16. [PMID: 25285559] doi: 10.7326/0003-4819-161-7-201410070-01004

Item 42   Answer: C

Educational Objective: Manage online physician-patient communication.

The most appropriate management is to request that the patient establish care through the office. Professional

Answers and Critiques

assessments should be performed within the context of an existing physician-patient relationship. In general, relationships should be established on the basis of an in-person professional encounter. Telemedicine, or the use of electronic communication and technologies to provide health care to patients at a distance, may increase access to care, improve outcomes, enhance physician-patient collaboration, and reduce costs; however, the American College of Physicians holds the position that a valid patient-physician relationship must be established for professionally responsible telemedicine services to occur. In this situation, the physician should reply to the patient and ask him to contact the office for an appointment to establish care or provide a second opinion, if that is what the patient desires. Once a physician-patient relationship is established, online communication should ideally occur through a secure portal that meets the requirements of the Health Insurance Portability and Accountability Act of 1996 (HIPAA).

Providing specific medical advice, such as suggesting celiac disease testing, without a thorough and proper medical evaluation would be inappropriate.

A request for the patient's records and provision of advice based on review of those records should not be made until a physician-patient relationship is established. Additionally, in digital environments, the sharing of patient information must always be held to a higher level of security than standard residential Internet connections. Encrypted or virtual proxy network connections in hospital-based information technology systems should be used for all patient information exchange and review to ensure a secure digital environment.

If a member of the public contacts a physician electronically in his or her professional role, the physician should politely respond and direct the patient to seek care through suitable channels by appropriately responding to the email or other online query.

KEY POINT

- Telemedicine, or the use of electronic communication and technologies to provide health care to patients at a distance, may increase access to care, improve outcomes, enhance physician-patient collaboration, and reduce costs; however, a valid patient-physician relationship must be established for professionally responsible telemedicine services to occur.

Bibliography
Farnan JM, Snyder Sulmasy L, Worster BK, Chaudhry HJ, Rhyne JA, Arora VM; American College of Physicians Ethics, Professionalism and Human Rights Committee. Online medical professionalism: patient and public relationships: policy statement from the American College of Physicians and the Federation of State Medical Boards. Ann Intern Med. 2013;158:620-7. [PMID: 23579867] doi:10.7326/0003-4819-158-8-201304160-00100

Item 43   Answer: C
Educational Objective: Diagnose optic neuritis.

This patient with acute vision loss and eye pain unassociated with trauma has signs and symptoms suggestive of optic neuritis, including pain with eye movement, loss of color vision out of proportion to the vision loss, and an afferent pupillary defect. Two thirds of optic neuritis cases occur in women. The average age of onset is between 20 and 40 years, and it is often associated with multiple sclerosis. Most of these patients have a normal optic disc on funduscopy, but one third may have a swollen disc or papillitis. An urgent evaluation by an ophthalmologist is required; treatment usually involves high-dose intravenous glucocorticoids.

Corneal abrasion can cause sudden onset of pain and foreign-body sensation. It is classically seen in patients who sleep without taking out their contact lenses and then awaken with eye pain and photophobia. If the abrasion is in the central area of the visual axis, visual acuity may be diminished. Corneal abrasion cannot explain the loss of color discrimination and the afferent pupillary defect in this patient.

Herpes simplex keratitis typically presents with acute onset of pain, blurry vision, and watery discharge. The absence of discharge and ciliary flush in this case make keratitis unlikely. Ciliary flush is characterized by erythema that is most marked at the limbus, which is the junction of the sclera and cornea. Keratitis would not be associated with loss of color discrimination or an afferent pupillary defect.

Orbital cellulitis often presents with eye pain as well as eyelid swelling and erythema, although some cases present without erythema. In the case of inflammation of the extraocular muscles and fatty tissue in the orbit, the patient may experience pain with eye movement. When the condition is severe, visual acuity may be impaired. Orbital cellulitis, however, is more likely to be associated with fever and chemosis, which are not present in this patient, and it would not explain the patient's other findings related to optic nerve damage.

KEY POINT

- The hallmarks of optic neuritis are acute vision loss, eye pain with movement, color perception change, and afferent pupillary defect; results of a funduscopic examination may be normal.

Bibliography
Balcer LJ. Clinical practice. Optic neuritis. N Engl J Med. 2006;354:1273-80. [PMID: 16554529]

Item 44   Answer: A
Educational Objective: Recognize threats to validity with a cross-sectional study.

The most likely threat to the validity of this cross-sectional study is confounding. Cross-sectional studies evaluate the relationship between exposures and health outcomes in a population of interest. These studies are characterized by the measurement of factors and outcomes at a single point in time. The validity of cross-sectional studies is particularly susceptible to recall bias and confounding. Recall bias is a systematic error that is introduced into a study by differences in the accuracy of the recollections of study participants; participants who have unpleasant experiences may recall past events differently than those who do not have similar experiences. Because cross-sectional studies are observational and not experimental, there is also no opportunity to randomly distribute factors that might influence the relationship being studied. Although statistical techniques can be used to control for known potential confounders, unknown confounders remain a threat to the validity of the conclusions. As such, cross-sectional studies are best suited to identifying potentially significant associations that can be more rigorously tested in experimental studies. Finally, because there is no way to verify that the purported cause (statin therapy) preceded the effect (memory loss), cross-sectional studies cannot prove cause-and-effect relationships.

Selection bias occurs when the study participants do not accurately reflect the population being studied, usually because the choice to participate is influenced by the clinical question. Selection bias can compromise the validity of observational study designs; however, in this study, the random sampling according to zip code of residence minimizes the possibility of selection bias.

Although self-reported data are less robust than measured data, well-validated survey designs may use self-reported data to determine the presence or absence of conditions, risk factors, or behaviors in a population.

The conventional level of statistical significance is a P value less than or equal to 0.05, and an odds ratio of 1 implies the absence of a significant relationship. In this case, the confidence interval for the odds ratio does not include the value 1, which supports the statistical significance of the findings.

KEY POINT

- The validity of cross-sectional studies is particularly susceptible to recall bias and confounding.

Bibliography
Grimes DA, Schulz KF. Bias and causal associations in observational research. Lancet. 2002;359:248-52. [PMID: 11812579]

Item 45   Answer: D

Educational Objective: Manage postoperative urinary retention with urinary catheterization.

Bladder decompression with urinary catheterization is the most appropriate management of this patient who has developed postoperative urinary retention (POUR). POUR is a common complication in the postoperative setting and is characterized by the inability to spontaneously and adequately empty the bladder. Risk factors include type of surgery (incontinence and anorectal surgery, hernia repair, joint arthroplasty), longer surgery, use of regional anesthesia, administration of greater than 750 mL of intraoperative fluids, use of certain postoperative medications (opioids, anticholinergic agents), older age, constipation, pelvic organ prolapse, neurologic disease, history of urinary retention,

and history of pelvic surgery. POUR is a urologic emergency. Symptoms of suprapubic pain and the finding of a palpable bladder are insensitive indicators of POUR. Patients may also present with frequent urination of small volumes and overflow incontinence. Reversible causes of POUR, such as medication use, should be addressed. Whenever possible, offending medications, including opioids, anticholinergics, antihistamines, antipsychotics, and calcium-blocking drugs, should be discontinued. Early removal of indwelling urinary catheters and voiding trials are recommended. Retrograde voiding trials are preferred to spontaneous voiding trials because they are more predictive of the need for continued catheterization. A retrograde voiding trial involves infusion of sterile saline, followed by the attempt to void. For patients in whom a voiding trial is unsuccessful, intermittent urinary catheterization should be considered in place of indwelling bladder catheterization. Results of a recent randomized controlled trial in patients undergoing total hip arthroplasty and total knee arthroplasty demonstrated that a catheterization threshold of 800 mL significantly reduced the need for postoperative urinary catheterization and did not increase urologic complications.

Placement of a suprapubic catheter would require another surgical procedure and is reserved for situations in which urethral catheterization is not possible or in cases of pelvic trauma.

Suprapubic application of hot packs or warm wet gauze may stimulate spontaneous voiding but lacks proof from well-designed clinical trials. Some experts recommend consideration of this technique in patients for a limited time when residual bladder volume is 200 mL to 400 mL. Greater residual volume should be treated with bladder catheterization.

There is no role for tamsulosin in the treatment of POUR in women. Randomized studies in men have demonstrated that α_2-blockade for the treatment of acute urinary retention is associated with a reduced need for bladder catheterization. α_2-Blockers should be continued in men with benign prostatic hyperplasia.

KEY POINT

- Patients with postoperative urinary retention and residual bladder volume of 800 mL or more should be treated with bladder decompression and urinary catheterization.

Bibliography
Bjerregaard LS, Hornum U, Troldborg C, Bogoe S, Bagi P, Kehlet H. Postoperative urinary catheterization thresholds of 500 versus 800 ml after fast-track total hip and knee arthroplasty: a randomized, open-label, controlled trial. Anesthesiology. 2016;124(6):1256-64. [PMID: 27054365] doi: 10.1097/ALN.0000000000001112

Item 46   Answer: D

Educational Objective: Determine adequacy of previous cervical cancer screening in an older woman.

The most appropriate screening strategy is to obtain the results of the patient's last cervical cancer screening examination. The U.S. Preventive Services Task Force recommends against cervical cancer screening in women older than age 65 years who have had adequate prior screening and are not otherwise at high risk for cervical cancer. Adequate screening is commonly defined as three consecutive negative cytology (Pap smear) results or two consecutive negative cytology plus human papillomavirus (HPV) test results within the last 10 years, with the most recent test occurring within 5 years. Data suggest that cervical cancer screening rates decline with increasing patient age; however, a Kaiser Permanente registry study found that 13% of 65-year-old women have not been adequately screened, with higher rates in patients without a primary physician or other health care provider. Other populations that are less likely to have received adequate screening include women with limited access to care, women from racial or ethnic minority groups, and women from countries where screening is not available. The study also documented that most cases of invasive cervical cancer in women older than age 65 years occurred among those who had not met criteria for stopping screening. The decision to stop screening at age 65 years should only be made after confirming that the patient has received adequate prior screening. In patients who do not meet the criteria for adequate prior screening, screening may be clinically indicated after age 65 years.

Cervical cytology, high-risk HPV testing, or co-testing with cervical cytology and high-risk HPV testing may all be reasonable methods to screen for cervical cancer in this patient, but reviewing the adequacy of previous screening remains the first step in management.

KEY POINT

- The decision to discontinue cervical cancer screening at age 65 years should be made only after confirming that the patient has received adequate prior screening.

Bibliography

Dinkelspiel H, Fetterman B, Poitras N, Kinney W, Cox JT, Lorey T, Castle PE. Screening history preceding a diagnosis of cervical cancer in women age 65 and older. Gynecol Oncol. 2012;126:203-6. [PMID: 22561038] doi: 10.1016/j.ygyno.2012.04.037

Item 47   Answer: B

Educational Objective: Treat chronic pain with structured physical therapy.

The most appropriate next step in treatment is physical therapy. This patient has a long-standing history of chronic pain that is most consistent with a diagnosis of fibromyalgia. All patients with chronic pain should be referred to a structured physical therapy program for evaluation and treatment. Physical therapy teaches patients safe, self-guided exercises to improve functional status, and there is a clear evidence base to support its use in all patients with chronic pain. Guided/progressive physical therapy programs are associated with a reduction in pain and, perhaps most importantly, improvement in function. No evidence suggests that a specific type of

physical therapy is superior to another, and programs should be tailored to patient ability and adherence.

Clinicians should avoid prescribing opioids and benzodiazepines concurrently whenever possible. Epidemiologic studies indicate that concomitant use of benzodiazepines, such as lorazepam, and opioids may place patients at increased risk for fatal overdose. In three studies of opioid overdose deaths, there was evidence of concurrent benzodiazepine use in 31% to 61% of persons.

Trials of transcutaneous electrical nerve stimulation (TENS) for the treatment of fibromyalgia have yielded inconclusive results. Positive trials of TENS are frequently contaminated with concurrent use of an exercise program and massage. On the basis of inconclusive evidence, TENS cannot be recommended as the next treatment modality for this patient.

Opioid rotation would not be an ideal next step in this patient with a long history of chronic pain, particularly in the setting of previous unsuccessful opioid trials. Despite high opioid prescribing rates, no evidence supports the use of long-term opioid therapy in patients with chronic noncancer pain. In one study, patients receiving long-term opioids for chronic pain had more pain, poorer quality of life, and poorer function than a population of patients with chronic pain who were not taking opioids. Given the lack of evidence to support chronic opioid therapy, the continued use of opioids for chronic pain should be justified at every follow-up visit by documenting the patient's sustained functional improvement due to effective opioid therapy. In this patient with pain that has failed to improve with opioid therapy, oxycodone should be carefully withdrawn, and nonpharmacologic therapy should be instituted.

KEY POINT

- In patients with chronic noncancer pain, physical therapy reduces pain and improves function.

Bibliography

Hooten M, Thorson D, Bianco J, Bonte B, Clavel A Jr, Hora J. Institute for Clinical Systems Improvement. Pain: assessment, non-opioid treatment approaches and opioid management. Available at www.icsi.org/guidelines_more/catalog_guidelines_and_more/catalog_guidelines/catalog_neurological_guidelines/pain/. Updated August 2017. Accessed February 27, 2018.

Item 48   Answer: D

Educational Objective: Test for cognitive impairment in a symptomatic older woman.

This patient would most benefit from evaluation with the Mini-Cog test or another validated screening test for cognitive function. Cognitive impairment is a progressive decline that impairs function in at least two areas: attention, executive function, language, memory, or visual-spatial function. Patients with signs and symptoms of cognitive impairment, such as this patient who reports difficulty with both memory and executive function, should undergo evaluation. A variety of validated tools are available to assess cognitive function. Among the free tools, the Montreal Cognitive Assessment and Mini-Cog test have been validated in primary care populations; these instruments screen for impairments in executive function. Self-administered instruments, such as the Self-Administered Gerocognitive Examination and Test Your Memory examination, have been validated in memory clinic populations to detect mild cognitive impairment and early dementia. Although the Mini–Mental State Examination has been the most extensively studied screening instrument, it is now proprietary, with a cost per use.

Although numerous factors have been studied, and some have been associated with a higher risk for progression to dementia (such as baseline functional impairment, abnormal results of fluorodeoxyglucose-PET brain imaging, and the apolipoprotein E [*APOE*-ε4] genotype), no reliable clinical markers can predict the clinical likelihood that an individual patient with mild cognitive impairment will develop dementia. More importantly, these tests do not establish the diagnosis of cognitive impairment.

In clinical practice, a careful history and results of a standard mental examination are often sufficient to diagnose cognitive impairment, and extensive formal cognitive testing is not routinely required. Occasionally, a formal battery of neuropsychologic testing beyond the standard mental examination is needed to distinguish particularly mild cases of cognitive impairment from normal aging.

KEY POINT

- Cognitive impairment is a progressive decline that impairs function in at least two areas, including attention, executive function, language, memory, and visual-spatial function; it is best measured with assessment examinations, such as the Mini-Cog and the Mini–Mental State Examination, rather than laboratory testing or imaging.

Bibliography

Lin JS, O'Connor E, Rossom RC, Perdue LA, Eckstrom E. Screening for cognitive impairment in older adults: a systematic review for the U.S. Preventive Services Task Force. Ann Intern Med. 2013;159:601-12. [PMID: 24145578]

Item 49   Answer: C

Educational Objective: Diagnose cervical sprain.

This patient most likely has a cervical sprain (nonspecific or axial neck pain), which is the most common cause of neck pain. The pain associated with cervical sprain is usually an aching sensation that is isolated to the neck, but it can radiate to the posterior head or shoulders. The pain does not typically radiate into the arms. Cervical sprain symptoms can be precipitated by an unaccustomed activity or overuse. Physical examination of the neck usually shows decreased range of motion, tenderness to palpation, and reproduction of the pain with flexion or extension. The condition is also notable for the absence of abnormal neurologic findings.

Cervical myelopathy (compression of the cervical spinal cord) can also cause neck pain. Common clinical manifestations include progressive worsening of symptoms, difficulty with fine object manipulation and manual dexterity, and gait abnormalities. This patient's symptoms are not consistent with cervical myelopathy.

Cervical radiculopathy is caused by disk herniation or bony degeneration causing compression of adjacent nerve roots; it is characterized by neck pain associated with radiating arm pain and paresthesias that follow a dermatomal distribution. On examination, affected patients frequently have reproduction of their pain with the Spurling test (examiner bends the patient's head to the affected side while extending the neck and applying a downward pressure on the top of the head). Symptoms can be improved by holding the patient's hand on the affected side above the patient's head (shoulder abduction test). This patient's presentation is not consistent with cervical radiculopathy.

Whiplash-associated neck pain is a poorly understood entity that refers to cervical sprain that develops in the setting of trauma, such as a car accident, which produces an abrupt flexion/extension movement of the cervical spine. Typical symptoms include persistent severe pain, spasm, loss of range of motion in the neck, and occipital headache. Because this patient's neck pain did not result from direct abrupt flexion/extension trauma, it would be incorrect to classify it as whiplash-associated neck pain.

KEY POINT

- Pain associated with cervical sprain is usually an aching sensation that is isolated to the neck but can radiate to the posterior head or shoulders; physical examination usually shows decreased range of motion, tenderness to palpation, and reproduction of the pain with flexion or extension, but no neurologic findings.

Bibliography

Cohen SP. Epidemiology, diagnosis, and treatment of neck pain. Mayo Clin Proc. 2015;90:284-99. [PMID: 25659245] doi:10.1016/j.mayocp.2014.09.008

Item 50   Answer: C

Educational Objective: Treat trichomoniasis in a sexual partner.

The most appropriate additional management is to treat the patient's sexual partner for trichomoniasis. Trichomoniasis, which is caused by *Trichomonas vaginalis*, is the most common nonviral sexually transmitted infection (STI) worldwide. Unlike other STIs that predominate in adolescents and younger adults, rates of trichomoniasis are evenly distributed among women of all age groups. It is caused by motile flagellated protozoa that infect the urogenital tract, causing inflammatory vaginitis and urethritis. Treatment with a single 2-g dose of metronidazole is associated with a high rate of cure and should be offered to all symptomatic women, including pregnant women. Because of the high rate of reinfection among women treated for trichomoniasis (17% within 3 months in one study), retesting for *T. vaginalis* is recommended by the Centers for Disease Control and Prevention (CDC) for all sexually active women within 3 months after initial treatment, regardless of whether they believe their sexual partners were treated. Testing by nucleic acid amplification can be conducted as soon as 2 weeks after treatment. It is important that sexual partners also be treated, even if they are asymptomatic; documentation of infection is not required before treatment in any partners. Data are insufficient to support retesting men after treatment for trichomoniasis. *T. vaginalis* infection is associated with a two- to threefold increased risk for HIV acquisition. Therefore, the CDC recommends that testing for other STIs, including HIV, be performed in persons infected with *T. vaginalis*.

Pap testing is not needed for management of trichomoniasis because the infection is not associated with cervical malignancy.

Because of the high rate of partner infection with *T. vaginalis* and its association with other STIs, it would be inappropriate to not provide further testing or intervention after a primary *T. vaginalis* diagnosis.

KEY POINT

- Following diagnosis and treatment of a woman with *Trichomonas vaginalis* infection, the sexual partner should be treated and both individuals should be screened for other sexually transmitted infections; retesting of women for *T. vaginalis* infection within 3 months of treatment is also recommended.

Bibliography
Mills BB. Vaginitis: beyond the basics. Obstet Gynecol Clin North Am. 2017;44:159-177. [PMID: 28499528] doi:10.1016/j.ogc.2017.02.010

Item 51   Answer: C

Educational Objective: Diagnose a patient with a medically unexplained symptom.

This patient most likely has a medically unexplained symptom. Such symptoms cannot be attributed to a specific medical cause after a thorough medical evaluation. Symptoms that are common in these patients include fatigue, headache, abdominal pain, musculoskeletal pain (back pain, myalgia, and arthralgia), dizziness, paresthesia, generalized weakness, transient edema, insomnia, dyspnea, chest pain, chronic facial pain, chronic pelvic pain, and chemical sensitivities. Symptoms can range from a minor nuisance to functional impairment. In this case, the patient's symptom does not appear to have a pathologic basis, and she is not excessively focused on or functionally limited by her symptom. As such, this patient would most appropriately be diagnosed with a medically unexplained symptom.

Conversion disorder involves at least one symptom of neurologic dysfunction (abnormal sensation or motor function) that is unexplained by a medical condition and not

consistent with examination findings. Conversion disorder represents not fabrication of symptoms but rather unexplained symptoms that do not have a pathophysiologic basis. These symptoms, which are functionally limiting, occur during times of substantial physical, emotional, or psychological stress.

Illness anxiety disorder (formerly named hypochondriasis) is characterized by excessive concern about health and preoccupation with health-related activities (for example, measuring pulse). In patients with illness anxiety disorder, no or only mild somatic symptoms are present.

Somatic symptom disorder is characterized by one or more somatic symptoms present for at least 6 months, causing significant distress or interference with life and associated with excessive thoughts, behaviors, and feelings related to the symptoms. The diagnosis of somatic symptom disorder has replaced the previous diagnosis of somatization disorder.

KEY POINT

- Medically unexplained symptoms are diagnosed according to the presence of symptoms that cannot be attributed to a specific medical cause after a thorough medical evaluation.

Bibliography
Haller H, Cramer H, Lauche R, Dobos G. Somatoform disorders and medically unexplained symptoms in primary care. Dtsch Arztebl Int. 2015;112:279-87. [PMID: 25939319] doi: 10.3238/arztebl.2015.0279

Item 52   Answer: D

Educational Objective: Treat drug-induced lower extremity edema.

The most appropriate next step in the management of this patient is to discontinue pregabalin and initiate duloxetine. In most patients with lower extremity edema, a detailed history and physical examination will suggest the cause. The most common causes of lower extremity edema include venous obstruction or insufficiency, heart failure (including right-sided heart failure secondary to pulmonary disease), cirrhosis, and nephrotic syndrome and hypoalbuminemia of other etiologies. Certain drugs and classes of drugs are frequent causes of edema. Direct vasodilators (minoxidil, hydralazine, calcium channel blockers, α-blockers) may produce edema by several mechanisms, including arteriolar dilatation (increases intracapillary pressure) and activation of the renin-angiotensin-aldosterone system (sodium retention). The thiazolidinediones, such as pioglitazone and rosiglitazone, stimulate sodium reabsorption by the sodium channels in the cortical collecting tubule cells. NSAIDs increase renal sodium reabsorption by inhibition of renal vasodilatory prostaglandins. Pregabalin is a calcium channel blocker and likely produces edema by the same mechanism as other calcium channel blockers; it is associated with peripheral edema in up to 17% of cases. In drug-induced edema, removal of the offending agent is the treatment of choice. This patient would benefit from switching pregabalin to a different fibromyalgia drug that is not associated with peripheral edema, such as duloxetine.

This patient's lower extremity edema is associated with the vasodilatory effects of pregabalin and not volume overload (no jugular venous distension, S₃, pulmonary crackles). In this situation, the use of diuretics can lead to volume depletion, electrolyte disorders, and kidney dysfunction. Discontinuing the drug responsible for the edema is a better strategy.

Duplex Doppler ultrasonography is a useful tool in the evaluation of deep venous thrombosis (DVT). However, DVT typically produces unilateral edema. Additionally, this patient has no risk factors for DVT (prolonged immobilization, cancer, previous DVT) and lacks supporting findings, such as calf swelling, tenderness, and superficial venous dilation.

Although compression stockings may help reduce edema, removal of the offending agent will likely resolve this patient's edema and obviate the need for compression stockings. Furthermore, compression stockings have poor adherence rates because of high cost, discomfort, and the difficulty that patients experience in donning and removing the stockings.

KEY POINT

- In patients with drug-induced edema, removal of the offending agent is the treatment of choice.

Bibliography
Ratchford EV, Evans NS. Approach to lower extremity edema. Curr Treat Options Cardiovasc Med. 2017;19:16. [PMID: 28290004] doi: 10.1007/s11936-017-0518-6

Item 53   Answer: C

Educational Objective: Diagnose major depressive disorder.

This patient meets the diagnostic criteria for major depressive disorder. The DSM-5 requires at least five of the following symptoms (at least one of which must be depressed mood or anhedonia) to be present almost all of the time during the same 2-week period: depressed mood, anhedonia, insomnia or hypersomnia, significant change in weight or appetite, fatigue or decreased energy, psychomotor agitation or retardation, difficulty concentrating, feelings of worthlessness or excessive guilt, and recurrent thoughts of death or suicidal ideation. Symptoms of major depressive disorder cause work-related and social impairment and cannot be attributed to a medical condition, drug, or substance use. A tool for identifying and assessing the severity of depression is the PHQ-9 (www.integration.samhsa.gov/images/res/PHQ%20-%20Questions.pdf). The items of the PHQ-9 correlate with the DSM-5 criteria. Each item is scored from 0 (not bothered by the symptom) to 3 (bothered by the symptom every day); the maximum score is 27. A score of 5 to 9 indicates mild depression, 10 to 14 moderate depression, 15 to 19 moderately severe depression, and 20 or more severe depression.

Patients with bipolar disorder often present with major depressive disorder, and it is important for clinicians to inquire about any history of periods of elevated mood, increased energy, and decreased need for sleep. Without a history of such episodes, bipolar disorder cannot be diagnosed.

Generalized anxiety disorder (GAD) and other anxiety disorders can often be comorbid with major depressive disorder. Patients with GAD often experience sweats, dyspnea, palpitations, difficulty swallowing, nausea, chest and abdominal pain, loose stools, muscle tension, insomnia, fatigue, tachycardia, and tremor. Diagnosis should be considered in patients with multiple unexplained physical symptoms. This patient does not exhibit the excessive anxiety and restlessness typical of a patient with GAD.

Persistent depressive disorder, previously known as dysthymic disorder or dysthymia, is characterized by depressed mood most of the time for at least 2 years and with at least two of the following symptoms while depressed: appetite change (increased or decreased), fatigue or low energy, decreased self-esteem, insomnia or hypersomnia, poor concentration, and feelings of hopelessness. The symptoms are less severe than in major depressive disorder. This patient has more severe symptoms that have lasted only 6 months, with no history of depression.

KEY POINT

- Major depressive disorder is diagnosed by the presence of at least five cardinal symptoms, at least one of which is depressed mood or anhedonia, during the same 2-week period; a tool for identifying and assessing the severity of depression is the PHQ-9.

Bibliography
McCarron RM, Vanderlip ER, Rado J. Depression. Ann Intern Med. 2016;165:ITC49-ITC64. [PMID: 27699401] doi:10.7326/AITC201610040

Item 54   Answer: D

Educational Objective: Diagnose systemic exertion intolerance disease.

The most likely diagnosis is systemic exertion intolerance disease (SEID). Fatigue can be classified as fatigue secondary to another cause, secondary to multiple factors (termed chronic multifactorial fatigue), or a primary condition. In the past, the latter condition was termed chronic fatigue syndrome, myalgic encephalitis, or neurasthenia. In 2015, the Institute of Medicine recommended using the term systemic exertion intolerance disease over the other terms. The diagnosis of SEID requires the presence of (1) substantial reduction or impairment in the ability to engage in preillness levels of occupational, educational, social, or personal activities for at least 6 months, accompanied by profound fatigue that is not relieved by rest; (2) postexertional malaise (worsening of symptoms after physical, cognitive, or emotional effort); and (3) unrefreshing sleep. In addition to the three major criteria, the patient must also demonstrate cognitive impairment or orthostatic intolerance (symptoms such as lightheadedness, dizziness, fatigue, cognitive deficits, and visual difficulties that worsen when a person stands upright and improve when the person lies back down). This patient meets the validated diagnostic criteria for SEID.

Chronic multifactorial fatigue is a clinical condition defined as chronic fatigue symptoms of at least 6 months' duration in the setting of multiple fatiguing factors (medical and/or psychosocial). This patient's benign history and unrevealing evaluation argue against chronic multifactorial fatigue.

Mood disturbances are highly comorbid in patients with SEID (approximately 70% of patients), and all patients with SEID should be screened for depression and anxiety. This patient was screened appropriately and does not have findings consistent with an underlying mood disorder.

Post–Lyme disease syndrome has been reported in approximately 10% of patients after treatment of erythema migrans. Although the condition is often erroneously called chronic Lyme disease, studies have found no microbiologic evidence of chronic or latent infection after appropriate treatment. Symptoms include fatigue, arthralgia, myalgia, and impairment of memory or cognition that can last for years after treatment of the acute infection. Clinical trials have shown no benefit of prolonged antibiotic treatment for post–Lyme disease syndrome. This patient has unrefreshing sleep, postexertional malaise, and orthostatic intolerance, which are more consistent with SEID.

KEY POINT

- The diagnosis of systemic exertion intolerance disease requires the presence of fatigue of at least 6 months' duration with substantial reduction in preillness activities, postexertional malaise, unrefreshing sleep, and either cognitive impairment or orthostatic intolerance.

Bibliography
Committee on the Diagnostic Criteria for Myalgic Encephalomyelitis/Chronic Fatigue Syndrome, Board on the Health of Select Populations, Institute of Medicine. Beyond Myalgic Encephalomyelitis/Chronic Fatigue Syndrome: Redefining an Illness. Washington, DC: National Academies Press; 2015. [PMID: 25695122]

Item 55   Answer: B

Educational Objective: Diagnose epididymitis by physical examination.

This patient is most likely to have pain relief with testicular elevation (Prehn sign). His history and examination findings (erythema and swelling of the hemiscrotum; fever; tenderness to palpation near the epididymis; and lack of worsening symptoms, nausea, vomiting, and abdominal pain) suggest a diagnosis of epididymitis. Prehn sign, which is alleviation of pain with elevation of the testicle or scrotum, can clinically support this diagnosis. Although this finding can suggest a diagnosis of epididymitis, it does not rule out other possibilities, such as testicular torsion; however, testicular torsion is less likely given this patient's presentation.

An absent cremasteric reflex suggests testicular torsion. A patient with testicular torsion would have acutely worsening and severe hemiscrotal pain, hemiscrotum elevation, abdominal pain, nausea, and vomiting. These findings are not present in this patient, and the test result would likely be negative.

Varicoceles are caused by dilation of the testicular vein and pampiniform plexus. They are common, occurring in 15% of men. Scrotal examination reveals a left-sided (90%) scrotal mass with a "bag of worms" consistency that increases with standing and decreases while supine. This patient's findings are not consistent with varicocele, and examining the patient in both standing and supine positions is unlikely to support this diagnosis.

A transillumination study, which is performed to identify a hydrocele, is not likely to have a positive result in this patient with findings that suggest epididymitis. A hydrocele manifests over a longer time frame, initially causing no symptoms and then causing a dull aching scrotal discomfort. Examination can reveal a smooth though tense scrotal mass, which transilluminates when a light source is applied adjacently.

KEY POINT

- A positive Prehn sign (relief of pain with scrotal elevation) suggests a diagnosis of epididymitis, although it does not rule out other possibilities, such as testicular torsion.

Bibliography
Crawford P, Crop JA. Evaluation of scrotal masses. Am Fam Physician. 2014;89:723-7. [PMID: 24784335]

Item 56   Answer: D

Educational Objective: Treat chronic low back pain with an NSAID.

The most appropriate pharmacologic option for this patient is an NSAID, such as ibuprofen. For patients with chronic low back pain, clinicians and patients should initially select nonpharmacologic treatment with acupuncture, cognitive behavioral therapy, electromyography biofeedback, exercise, mindfulness-based stress reduction (moderate-quality evidence), low-level laser therapy, motor control exercise, multidisciplinary rehabilitation, progressive relaxation, operant therapy or spinal manipulation, tai chi, or yoga. According to a 2017 clinical practice guideline from the American College of Physicians (ACP), pharmacologic therapy can be considered in patients with chronic low back pain that has not responded to nonpharmacologic therapy. The ACP recommends NSAIDs as first-line therapy, administered in the lowest effective dosage.

There is little evidence that acetaminophen is effective in reducing pain or improving functional status in patients with acute or chronic low back pain. As such, acetaminophen should not be recommended to this patient.

The FDA recently approved duloxetine for treating chronic low back pain on the basis of evidence from randomized controlled trials that showed a small improvement in both pain and function with its use. However, the ACP guideline deems both duloxetine and tramadol as second-line pharmacologic options (weak recommendation, moderate-quality evidence), reserved for use only after first-line options have been exhausted.

In a randomized controlled trial, opioids, such as hydrocodone, were not more effective than nonopioid therapy in treating chronic low back pain. Opioids should be used only in the treatment of chronic pain when the benefits outweigh the risks (such as abuse potential) and when a clear discussion of risks and benefits has occurred with the patient. This patient is unlikely to benefit from hydrocodone therapy.

Moderate-quality evidence showed that tramadol resulted in moderate short-term pain relief in patients with chronic low back pain and a small improvement in function compared with placebo. Of note, tramadol is a weak opioid agonist that also blocks reuptake of serotonin and norepinephrine; like other opioids, it is associated with the risk for abuse. Its use is relegated to patients who achieve inadequate relief with nonpharmacologic therapy and NSAIDs, and only after a frank discussion of the harms and benefits.

KEY POINT

- For patients with chronic low back pain, clinicians and patients should initially select nonpharmacologic treatment; NSAIDs can be considered in patients who have had an inadequate response to nonpharmacologic therapy.

Bibliography
Qaseem A, Wilt TJ, McLean RM, Forciea MA; Clinical Guidelines Committee of the American College of Physicians. Noninvasive treatments for acute, subacute, and chronic low back pain: a clinical practice guideline from the American College of Physicians. Ann Intern Med. 2017;166:514-530. [PMID: 28192789] doi:10.7326/M16-2367

Item 57   Answer: D
Educational Objective: Evaluate recurrent epistaxis.

The most appropriate management is nasal endoscopy. Ninety percent of episodes of epistaxis occur in the anterior nasal septum in the Kiesselbach area. Anterior bleeding can be managed with compression for at least 15 minutes. Posterior epistaxis (behind the posterior middle turbinate, requiring a nasopharyngoscope for visualization) may be more difficult to manage and is more common in older patients. Common causes of epistaxis include topical intranasal medications (such as glucocorticoids or antihistamines), dehumidification, and self-induced digital trauma. Among patients with epistaxis serious enough to require hospitalization, almost half have a causal systemic condition, such as anticoagulation, hemophilia, hematologic malignancy, neoplasm, and acquired coagulopathies from kidney or liver disease. Recurrent unilateral epistaxis may represent a neoplasm; hence, this patient should be referred for nasal endoscopy.

Low-dose aspirin may be associated with a slight increase in the risk for epistaxis, although data have not been conclusive and do not support routine discontinuation in otherwise healthy patients with epistaxis. Notably, other NSAIDs have not been associated with epistaxis. Even if aspirin were stopped, this patient requires further assessment given the presence of unilateral bleeding.

This patient has no symptoms of anemia or history of excessive blood loss. Although epistaxis may be associated with coagulopathies, this patient is not taking an anticoagulant and is otherwise at low risk for an acquired coagulopathy that manifests only as epistaxis. Therefore, coagulation studies are not warranted.

In 80% of patients with epistaxis, results of laboratory evaluation are normal; therefore, routine laboratory testing is not required. A complete blood count, prothrombin time, and activated partial thromboplastin time might be considered in patients with symptoms or signs of a bleeding disorder and those with severe or recurrent epistaxis.

KEY POINT

- Recurrent unilateral epistaxis may be a sign of neoplasm and warrants referral for nasal endoscopy.

Bibliography
Morgan DJ, Kellerman R. Epistaxis: evaluation and treatment. Prim Care. 2014;41:63-73. [PMID: 24439881] doi:10.1016/j.pop.2013.10.007

Item 58   Answer: D
Educational Objective: Identify the Plan-Do-Study-Act cycle as an effective quality improvement method.

The most likely intervention to improve hand hygiene in this hospital is to use a Plan-Do-Study-Act (PDSA) cycle. A PDSA cycle is a four-step process involving a rapid cycle of change in which baseline data are collected, an intervention is planned and then implemented on a small scale, the results are analyzed, and an action plan is made. Additional PDSA cycles are completed until the desired results are achieved. In this case, a PDSA cycle could be used to study hand hygiene procedures and implement interventions to increase rates of hand hygiene, with the overall goal of reducing the incidence of hospital-acquired infections.

Spaghetti diagrams are used to visually display flow through a system. The flows are drawn as lines on a map and look similar to spaghetti noodles. As an example, a spaghetti diagram may be used to follow a medication order through a hospital unit from order generation to administration of the medication. The diagram can help highlight inefficiencies or redundancies in a system. Although useful in identifying areas ripe for increased efficiency, a spaghetti diagram will have no impact on improving hand hygiene rates.

The Lean model aims to maximize value and minimize waste by closely examining a system's processes and eliminating non–value-added activities within the system. Value stream mapping can be used to graphically display the steps of a process and the time required for each step, thereby

CONT.

highlighting process inefficiencies or areas of waste and allowing for their improvement. The Lean model could be used to determine inefficiencies in hospital processes (such as waiting times); however, it would not help improve hand hygiene rates.

Reiterating the importance of hand hygiene in an email to the entire staff may be a part of a planned intervention to improve hand hygiene, although it alone is unlikely to provide sustained results.

KEY POINT

- A Plan-Do-Study-Act cycle is a four-step process involving a rapid cycle of change in which baseline data are collected, an intervention is planned and then implemented on a small scale, the results are analyzed, and an action plan is made.

Bibliography

Morelli MS. Using the Plan, Do, Study, Act Model to implement a quality improvement program in your practice. Am J Gastroenterol. 2016;111: 1220-2. [PMID: 27527744]

Item 59   Answer: D

Educational Objective: Identify medications associated with increased risk for side effects in an older patient.

Quetiapine is the medication with greatest potential for adverse effects in this older patient taking multiple prescription medications. Although treatment of comorbid conditions often requires multiple medications, evidence shows that half of older adults take one or more medications that are not medically necessary (that is, not indicated, not effective, or therapeutically duplicative). Frequent review of patient medications to verify their necessity and proper dosing is an essential aspect of optimal geriatric care. Notably, certain medications carry a particularly high risk for geriatric patients. In an effort to improve the care of older adults by reducing the use of potentially inappropriate medications, the American Geriatrics Society (AGS) has compiled a list of high-risk drugs that must be carefully considered in terms of risk-to-benefit ratio in the elderly (available at http://geriatricscareonline.org/ProductAbstract/american-geriatrics-society-updated-beers-criteria-for-potentially-inappropriate-medication-use-in-older-adults/CL001). All antipsychotic medications, both first- and second-generation, have significant adverse effects, including anticholinergic effects, extrapyramidal symptoms, and sedation, and older patients are particularly susceptible to these negative effects. For this reason, the AGS 2015 Beers Criteria for Potentially Inappropriate Medication Use in Older Adults recommends avoidance of quetiapine and all antipsychotic medications.

Acetaminophen is relatively safe for older patients if not used at maximal doses for extended periods. Side effects from acetaminophen are far less likely and less severe than other commonly used systemic analgesics, including opioids and NSAIDs.

Amlodipine is not listed as a medication to avoid in the AGS 2015 Beers Criteria. Although the drug could potentially cause excessive blood pressure reduction, this patient's blood pressure is under acceptable control and without orthostatic changes.

Lisinopril can potentially cause electrolyte abnormalities, orthostatic hypotension, and kidney insufficiency. However, this patient has no evidence of these problems, and lisinopril is not included in the Beers Criteria as a potentially inappropriate medication.

KEY POINT

- Frequent review of patient medications to verify their necessity and proper dosing is an essential aspect of optimal geriatric care.

Bibliography

The American Geriatrics Society 2015 Beers Criteria Update Expert Panel. American Geriatrics Society 2015 updated Beers criteria for potentially inappropriate medication use in older adults. J Am Geriatr Soc. 2015;63:2227-46. [PMID: 26446832] doi:10.1111/jgs.13702

Item 60   Answer: B

Educational Objective: Diagnose opioid-induced hyperalgesia.

The most likely diagnosis is opioid-induced hyperalgesia. Opioid-induced hyperalgesia is thought to result from repeated exposure to systemic opioids. In patients with this pain syndrome, the character of their pain may change during the course of opioid therapy, pain may worsen with increased opioid dosages, and pain may decrease when opioid dosages are reduced. In this case, the patient has chronic pain as a sequela of her cancer diagnosis and treatment, and she has required significant dosage escalation in the absence of progressive disease. She also has evidence of cognitive slowing, hyperreflexia, and myoclonus as a result of the neuroexcitatory effects of long-term opioid use; these signs are concerning for opioid-induced toxicity. Appropriate management of opioid-induced hyperalgesia includes opioid dosage reduction in a monitored setting with close follow-up.

Malingering is characterized by the development of symptoms that lack a pathologic basis. The key feature is faking or exaggerating symptoms for an obvious external benefit, such as money, drugs, or escaping criminal prosecution. Malingering should be suspected in patients with inconsistencies in the history and physical examination; nonadherence to recommended diagnostic testing or treatments; known or suspected personality disorder; and legal difficulties. There is no indication of these traits to suggest malingering as the cause of this patient's symptoms.

Opioid withdrawal is unlikely in this patient given her constant symptoms and escalation in the dosages of hydromorphone and transdermal fentanyl.

Pseudoaddiction is a phenomenon in which patients exhibit behaviors concerning for substance use disorder or addiction that are driven by inadequate pain control in the setting of a documented progressive disease. Although this patient has a sequela of cancer therapy, her clinical status is unchanged, and there is no evidence of progressive disease on physical examination or CT scan.

KEY POINT

- In patients with opioid-induced hyperalgesia, the character of their pain may change during the course of opioid therapy, pain may worsen with increased opioid dosages, and pain may decrease when opioid dosages are reduced.

Bibliography

Yi P, Pryzbylkowski P. Opioid induced hyperalgesia. Pain Med. 2015;16 Suppl 1:S32-6. [PMID: 26461074] doi: 10.1111/pme.12914

Item 61   Answer: D

Educational Objective: Manage dual antiplatelet therapy in a patient with recent coronary stent placement who is undergoing urgent noncardiac surgery.

The most appropriate management of this patient's antiplatelet therapy is to withhold clopidogrel 5 to 7 days before surgery and continue aspirin. According to the 2016 American College of Cardiology/American Heart Association focused update on the duration of dual antiplatelet therapy (DAPT), perioperative management is based on surgical bleeding risk balanced with the risk for stent thrombosis. The risk for stent thrombosis is contingent on both the indication for coronary stent placement (stable ischemic heart disease [SIHD] or acute coronary syndrome [ACS]) and the amount of time that has passed from the time of stent placement.

For patients who have a stent placed for SIHD, DAPT (aspirin plus a $P2Y_{12}$ inhibitor) should be continued for at least 30 days after bare metal stent placement and a minimum of 6 months after drug-eluting stent placement. DAPT is recommended for 1 year in patients with ACS, regardless of medical management or cardiac stent placement, with the understanding that discontinuation may be reasonable if high bleeding risk is identified or the patient has overt bleeding on DAPT. However, in the perioperative setting, and especially if the risk of surgical delay exceeds the risk for stent thrombosis, discontinuation of the $P2Y_{12}$ inhibitor can be considered after a minimum of 30 days in the case of bare metal stent placement or 3 months after drug-eluting stent placement. It is optimal to continue DAPT for 6 months after drug-eluting stent placement, especially in the case of ACS, if the risk for surgical delay does not exceed the risk for stent thrombosis. Aspirin should be continued, if at all possible, along with restarting of DAPT as soon as bleeding risk has sufficiently diminished.

If surgery must be performed within those periods after percutaneous coronary intervention, DAPT should be maintained perioperatively unless the risk for major bleeding exceeds the risk for stent thrombosis. Communication with the surgical team and the patient regarding risks and benefits of withholding DAPT within these time frames is advised.

KEY POINT

- In patients taking dual antiplatelet therapy, if the risk of surgical delay exceeds the risk for stent thrombosis, discontinuation of the $P2Y_{12}$ inhibitor can be considered after a minimum of 30 days in the case of bare metal stent placement or 3 months after drug-eluting stent placement.

Bibliography

Levine GN, Bates ER, Bittl JA, Brindis RG, Fihn SD, Fleisher LA, et al. 2016 ACC/AHA guideline focused update on duration of dual antiplatelet therapy in patients with coronary artery disease: a report of the American College of Cardiology/American Heart Association Task Force on Clinical Practice Guidelines. J Am Coll Cardiol. 2016;68:1082-115. [PMID: 27036918]

Item 62   Answer: A

Educational Objective: Engage a patient in shared decision making for prostate cancer screening.

The most appropriate action is to first engage the patient in a discussion of the benefits and harms of prostate cancer screening. No organization recommends prostate-specific antigen (PSA) testing for prostate cancer screening without a discussion of the benefits and harms and a patient's clear expressed preference for screening. Clinicians should inform men about the limited potential benefits and substantial harms of screening for prostate cancer. Screening offers a small potential benefit of reducing the chance of dying of prostate cancer. However, many men will experience potential harms of screening, including false-positive results that require additional testing and possible prostate biopsy; overdiagnosis and overtreatment; and treatment complications, such as incontinence and impotence. All organizations recommend individualized decision making about screening for prostate cancer so that each man has an opportunity to incorporate his values and preferences into his decision. On the basis of the available evidence, it is not possible to make a definitive recommendation for or against prostate cancer screening in men with a family history of prostate cancer. Although screening may offer additional potential benefits for these men compared with the general population, screening also has the potential to increase exposure to potential harms, especially among men with relatives whose cancer was overdiagnosed.

Although some expert groups recommend performing a digital rectal examination in conjunction with PSA testing for prostate cancer screening, digital rectal examination alone is not recommended because this test has suboptimal sensitivity and very low positive predictive value.

The U.S. Preventive Services Task Force recommends that clinicians should not screen men who do not express a preference for screening and recommends against

PSA-based screening for prostate cancer in men aged 70 years and older.

KEY POINT

- The decision to pursue prostate cancer screening should be individualized so that each man has an opportunity to understand the potential benefits and harms of screening and to incorporate his values and preferences into his decision.

Bibliography

Grossman DC, Curry SJ, Owens DK, Bibbins-Domingo K, Caughey AB, Davidson KW, et al; US Preventive Services Task Force. Screening for prostate cancer: US Preventive Services Task Force recommendation statement. JAMA. 2018;319:1901-1913. [PMID: 29801017] doi:10.1001/jama.2018.3710

Item 63   Answer: E

Educational Objective: Manage audible oropharyngeal secretions in a patient at the end of life.

This patient has audible posterior oropharyngeal secretions, which are most appropriately managed with family education and reassurance. Although several studies suggest that respiratory distress is not typically associated with these secretions, caregivers are often concerned by what is commonly referred to as the "death rattle." The first steps in management include caregiver education and anticipatory guidance. Additionally, repositioning often allows secretions to drain without pharmacologic intervention. Mouth hygiene with a sponge swab may also be helpful.

Current literature does not support the routine use of antimuscarinic drugs in the treatment of death rattle. A 2014 literature review acknowledged that death rattle leads to distress in both relatives and professional caregivers; however, its impact on patients is unclear, and medical therapy is unproven. Studies involving atropine, glycopyrronium, scopolamine, hyoscine butylbromide, and/or octreotide were reviewed, and only one study used a placebo group. There is currently no evidence that the use of any antimuscarinic drug is superior to no treatment. In addition, the use of anticholinergic agents in patients who are awake can lead to undesirable symptoms, such as dry mouth and urinary retention.

Suctioning by catheter should be avoided in managing end-of-life secretions unless the secretions are causing the patient obvious respiratory distress or cough. Suction catheters can cause local trauma.

KEY POINT

- Audible posterior oropharyngeal secretions ("death rattle") are common at the end of life and are best managed with family education and reassurance.

Bibliography

Lokker ME, van Zuylen L, van der Rijt CC, van der Heide A. Prevalence, impact, and treatment of death rattle: a systematic review. J Pain Symptom Manage. 2014;47:105-22. [PMID: 23790419] doi:10.1016/j.jpainsymman.2013.03.011

Item 64   Answer: D

Educational Objective: Vaccinate an adult smoker against pneumococcal disease.

This patient should be administered the 23-valent pneumococcal polysaccharide vaccine (PPSV23). Pneumococcal vaccination is recommended in all adults aged 65 years and older and adults aged 19 to 64 years with certain high-risk conditions. Two pneumococcal vaccines are available: PPSV23 and a 13-valent conjugate vaccine (PCV13). The Advisory Committee on Immunization Practices recommends administering PPSV23 alone to select immunocompetent patients aged 19 to 64 years, including those with chronic heart, liver, or lung disease; diabetes mellitus; cochlear implants; cerebrospinal fluid leak; alcoholism; or cigarette smoking. Because this patient is a current smoker, he should be given PPSV23.

In adults aged 19 to 64 years with immunocompromise, cochlear implants, or a history of cerebrospinal fluid leaks, PCV13 should be administered in addition to PPSV23. In these patients, a single dose of PCV13 should be given first, followed by a single dose of PPSV23 at least 8 weeks later. Additionally, all adults aged 65 years and older who have not previously been vaccinated should receive PCV13, followed by a dose of PPSV23 1 year later. For immunocompetent adults aged 65 years and older who previously received one or more doses of PPSV23, a single dose of PCV13 should be given at least 1 year after the most recent PPSV23 dose. This patient does not meet the criteria for PCV13 administration.

All adults aged 50 years and older, including those with a previous episode of zoster, should receive the recombinant (inactivated) zoster vaccine to reduce the incidence of zoster and postherpetic neuralgia. The recombinant zoster vaccine is recommended in preference to the live attenuated zoster vaccine, and adults who have been previously vaccinated with the live attenuated zoster vaccine should be revaccinated with the recombinant zoster vaccine after a period of at least 8 weeks. This patient should receive the recombinant zoster vaccine in 2 years.

In persons who previously received the tetanus toxoid, reduced diphtheria toxoid, and acellular pertussis (Tdap) vaccine, revaccination with a tetanus and diphtheria toxoids (Td) booster is recommended every 10 years. Additionally, for pregnant women, one dose of the Tdap vaccine should be administered during each pregnancy between 27 weeks' and 36 weeks' gestation, regardless of when the last dose of Td or Tdap was given. This patient last received the Tdap vaccine 9 years ago and should receive a Td booster in 1 year.

Given the patient's history of cigarette smoking, offering no vaccinations at this time would not be the best strategy.

KEY POINT

- The 23-valent pneumococcal polysaccharide vaccine should be administered to select immunocompetent patients aged 19 to 64 years, including those with chronic heart, liver, or lung disease; diabetes mellitus; cochlear implants; cerebrospinal fluid leak; alcoholism; or cigarette smoking.

Bibliography

Kim DK, Riley LE, Hunter P; Advisory Committee on Immunization Practices. Recommended immunization schedule for adults aged 19 years or older, United States, 2018. Ann Intern Med. 2018;168:210-220. [PMID: 29404596] doi:10.7326/M17-3439

Item 65   Answer: B

Educational Objective: Diagnose binge eating disorder.

This patient most likely has binge eating disorder (BED), which is characterized by impulsive overeating and feeling loss of control around food. The diagnosis of this disorder requires at least three of the following characteristics occurring at least once weekly for 3 months: abnormally rapid consumption, consuming large amounts of food when not hungry, eating alone due to embarrassment, eating until uncomfortably full, and feelings of guilt related to overconsumption. BED is more common than both anorexia and bulimia nervosa and is often accompanied by other psychiatric problems. The primary treatment is cognitive behavioral therapy.

Bulimia nervosa and the binging subtype of anorexia nervosa both include episodes of binge eating like BED. The key in differentiating BED from these diseases is the lack of compensatory behaviors (such as induced vomiting and laxative abuse) to avoid weight gain. The major difference between bulimia nervosa and the binging subtype of anorexia nervosa is that patients with anorexia nervosa have a low BMI (usually <18).

Many people have episodes of overeating in which they may eat until uncomfortable or feel guilty about their eating. However, simple overeating does not meet the diagnostic criteria for BED and is not accompanied by the feelings of loss of control over food consumption.

KEY POINT

- The diagnosis of binge eating disorder requires at least three of the following characteristics occurring at least once weekly for 3 months: abnormally rapid consumption, consuming large amounts of food when not hungry, eating alone due to embarrassment, eating until uncomfortably full, and feelings of guilt related to overconsumption.

Bibliography

Attia E. In the clinic. Eating disorders. Ann Intern Med. 2012;156:ITC4-1–ITC4-15, quiz ITC4-16. [PMID: 22473445] doi:10.7326/0003-4819-156-7-201204030-01004

Item 66   Answer: B

Educational Objective: Manage cyclic mastalgia.

The most appropriate next step in this patient's management is the use of a well-fitting bra. Breast pain is common among women and is categorized primarily as cyclic or noncyclic in relation to the menstrual cycle. This patient has cyclic mastalgia, which is bilateral and diffuse and worsens in the days before menses and then abates. Cyclic mastalgia is often related to hormonal changes that occur with ovulation. Because most symptoms of cyclic mastalgia are self-limited, management usually requires only education, reassurance, and appropriate breast support.

There is no evidence from controlled studies that avoidance of caffeine in the diet or beverages relieves breast pain. Similarly, no evidence supports the use of vitamin E and evening primrose oil in reducing pain.

Cyclic mastalgia with no abnormal clinical findings, such as a breast mass or skin changes, does not warrant diagnostic imaging. Hence, ultrasonography and mammography are unnecessary in this patient.

Danazol is approved by the FDA for management of mastalgia, but because of limiting androgenic side effects, it is recommended only for management of persistent severe cyclic breast pain unrelieved by conservative management. If education, reassurance, and appropriate breast support do not sufficiently control symptoms, acetaminophen or an oral or topical NSAID may be useful and can be recommended before consideration of danazol therapy.

KEY POINT

- Cyclic mastalgia is often related to hormonal changes that occur with ovulation, resulting in diffuse premenstrual breast pain that resolves with the menstrual cycle; the most appropriate management is education, reassurance, and appropriate breast support.

Bibliography

Iddon J, Dixon JM. Mastalgia. BMJ. 2013;347:f3288. [PMID: 24336097] doi:10.1136/bmj.f3288

Item 67   Answer: D

Educational Objective: Diagnose central vertigo on the basis of Dix-Hallpike maneuver results.

The most likely diagnosis is vertebrobasilar ischemia. In patients with vertigo, it is crucial to differentiate central from peripheral causes, especially in patients with acute vertigo concerning for vertebrobasilar ischemia and other central causes. The Dix-Hallpike maneuver is an effective bedside test for this purpose. In this test, the examiner stands at the patient's side and rotates the patient's head 45 degrees; the examiner then moves the patient, whose eyes are open, from the seated to the supine ear-down position. The patient's neck is extended slightly so that the chin is pointed upward, and the patient is observed for nystagmus. During the test, the latency, duration, fatigability, and direction of nystagmus are noted. The maneuver is repeated with the patient's head turned in the opposite direction. Findings that indicate central vertigo are nystagmus with an immediate onset (no latency), longer duration (>1 minute), no fatigability, and vertical or horizontal directionality without a torsional component. With central vertigo, the direction of nystagmus may vary depending on the direction of the patient's gaze. Potentially life-threatening conditions associated with

H
CONT.

central vertigo include ischemia, infarction, or hemorrhage of the cerebellum or brainstem. Patients at high risk include those with hypertension, diabetes mellitus, hyperlipidemia, or advanced age. Vertebrobasilar stroke is usually, but not always, accompanied by dysarthria, dysphagia, diplopia, weakness, or numbness. Cerebellar infarct may present with gait or truncal ataxia or with vertigo alone. In a patient presenting with suspicion for a central cause of vertigo, brain MRI and magnetic resonance angiography of the posterior cerebral circulation are the preferred diagnostic studies.

Dix-Hallpike maneuver results that suggest peripheral vertigo include nystagmus that is delayed in onset (presence of latency), is of short duration (<1 minute), exhibits fatigability (habituation), and is primarily unidirectional (usually up-beating and torsional [rotary phenomenon]). The presence of severe symptoms also indicates peripheral vertigo. The most common cause of peripheral vertigo (and all types of vertigo) is benign paroxysmal positional vertigo. Vestibular neuronitis (or labyrinthitis, if hearing is affected), another cause of peripheral vertigo, may follow a viral syndrome that has affected the vestibular portion of cranial nerve VIII. Less common causes of peripheral vertigo are Meniere disease (triad of vertigo, hearing loss, and tinnitus), perilymphatic fistula (vertigo and hearing loss with history of straining or trauma), and acoustic neuroma (tinnitus and associated unilateral sensorineural hearing loss).

An additional bedside test that can be performed to help differentiate central from peripheral causes of vertigo is the HINTS (Head Impulse, Nystagmus, and Test of Skew) examination. Findings concerning for a central cause of vertigo are the absence of catch-up saccades on the head impulse test, bidirectional nystagmus on the nystagmus assessment, and the presence of vertical skew on the test of skew.

KEY POINT

- In patients with central vertigo, the Dix-Hallpike maneuver produces nystagmus with an immediate onset (no latency), longer duration (>1 minute), no fatigability, and vertical or horizontal directionality without a torsional component.

Bibliography

Kim JS, Zee DS. Clinical practice. Benign paroxysmal positional vertigo. N Engl J Med. 2014;370:1138-47. [PMID: 24645946] doi: 10.1056/NEJMcp1309481

Item 68   Answer: B

Educational Objective: Evaluate prepatellar bursitis.

This patient has prepatellar bursitis, and the first step in management should be fluid aspiration. Prepatellar bursitis is caused by inflammation of the prepatellar bursa that overlies the patella. Patients present with anterior knee pain and swelling. Physical examination reveals a palpable fluid collection with preserved active and passive range of motion of the knee. The most common cause of chronic prepatellar bursitis is repetitive trauma, as is likely the case in this patient, who must frequently kneel in his job as a carpet installer. Other causes include gout and infection. Most cases of acute prepatellar bursitis are infectious (typically related to skin bacteria), although trauma and gout are other potential causes. Regardless of the duration of the swelling, all patients with prepatellar bursitis should undergo fluid aspiration. Gram stain and culture of the bursal fluid should be obtained and analyzed for leukocyte count and for the presence of crystals to evaluate for the possibility of an underlying infectious cause and gout.

Prepatellar bursitis due to repetitive trauma from kneeling is managed with activity modification (avoidance of kneeling), in addition to the use of oral NSAIDs such as ibuprofen. It would be inappropriate to recommend activity modification or NSAIDs before first analyzing bursal fluid to rule out infection or gout.

Plain radiography is not usually required for the diagnosis of prepatellar bursitis. It may show soft-tissue swelling on lateral views but rarely aids in establishing the correct diagnosis. Plain radiographs should be obtained when knee osteoarthritis is suspected or there is concern for fracture, neither of which applies to this patient.

Prepatellar bursitis caused by gout is diagnosed by bursal fluid analysis and detecting monosodium urate crystals with polarized microscopy. A high serum urate level supports the potential for gout; however, most patients with hyperuricemia do not have gout, and the serum urate level may be low during some acute attacks. Therefore, it would be inappropriate to obtain a serum uric acid level in this patient.

KEY POINT

- Prepatellar bursitis can be caused by repetitive trauma, infection, or gout; fluid aspiration and subsequent analysis should be performed in all patients.

Bibliography

Hong E, Kraft MC. Evaluating anterior knee pain. Med Clin North Am. 2014;98:697-717, xi. [PMID: 24994047] doi:10.1016/j.mcna.2014.03.001

Item 69   Answer: A

H

Educational Objective: Prevent a pressure injury in a patient with limited mobility.

An advanced static mattress is the most appropriate intervention to prevent pressure injuries (also known as pressure ulcers) in this patient. Pressure injuries are common in hospitals and long-term care settings. They can result in decreased quality of life, with associated depression, impaired mobility, and social isolation. The Centers for Medicare & Medicaid Services has selected the development of pressure ulcers as a sentinel health event (unexpected and preventable occurrence that results in serious patient injury) for health care facilities. Prevention of pressure injuries starts with identifying patients at risk. There are many standardized risk assessment tools, but evidence of whether these are superior to clinical judgment is inconclusive. Risk factors include advanced age, cognitive impairment, reduced mobility, sensory impairment, and comorbid conditions that affect skin integrity (such as low body weight, incontinence, edema, poor microcirculation, and hypoalbuminemia). Pressure redistribution is the most important factor in preventing pressure injuries through the use of pressure-reducing equipment and proper patient positioning. In 2015, the American College of Physicians (ACP) published a clinical practice guideline for risk assessment and prevention of pressure ulcers. The guideline recommends regular, structured risk assessment of patients and the use of an advanced static mattress or advanced static overlay for patients who are at increased risk. An advanced static mattress is made of specialized sheepskin, foam, or gel and is immobile when a patient lies on it, whereas an advanced static overlay is a pad composed of foam or gel that is secured to the top of a regular mattress.

The ACP guideline recommends against the use of alternating air mattresses because of lack of data showing a clear advantage as well as cost considerations.

There are limited data concerning the preventive effectiveness of frequent patient repositioning, dietary supplements (such as zinc, creams, or dressings), and silicone foam dressings as isolated interventions.

KEY POINT

- An advanced static mattress or mattress overlay made of specialized sheepskin, foam, or gel provides the best protection against the development of pressure injuries in hospitalized patients.

Bibliography

Qaseem A, Mir TP, Starkey M, Denberg TD; Clinical Guidelines Committee of the American College of Physicians. Risk assessment and prevention of pressure ulcers: a clinical practice guideline from the American College of Physicians. Ann Intern Med. 2015;162:359-69. [PMID: 25732278] doi:10.7326/M14-1567

Item 70   Answer: A

Educational Objective: Screen for HIV infection in a high-risk patient.

The most appropriate interval for HIV screening in this high-risk patient is at least annually. The U.S. Preventive Services Task Force (USPSTF) recommends HIV screening for patients aged 15 to 65 years in all health care settings. The currently recommended method for initial testing is combination HIV antibody immunoassay/p24 antigen testing. An "opt-out" approach is preferred; patients are notified that testing will be performed but can decline. Special consent for testing is not required. HIV testing provides a "teachable moment" to conduct HIV/sexually transmitted infection (STI) prevention counseling and offer pre-exposure prophylaxis for high-risk patients. However, prevention counseling should not be a required activity because it can be perceived as a barrier to screening.

The USPSTF suggests that a reasonable approach is one-time screening of adolescent and adult patients and repeated

screening of high-risk persons, persons engaged in risky behaviors, and those who reside in or receive medical care in high-prevalence settings for HIV infection. Persons at high risk (as opposed to very high risk) include those who have acquired or requested testing for other STIs. High-prevalence settings include STI clinics, correctional facilities, homeless shelters, tuberculosis clinics, clinics serving men who have sex with men (MSM), and adolescent health clinics with a high prevalence of STIs. The USPSTF suggests rescreening persons at increased risk every 3 to 5 years. In the absence of reliable data, the USPSTF suggests screening very high-risk individuals (MSM and injection drug users) for new HIV infection at least annually. Risk categories may change, and the USPSTF notes that rescreening may not be necessary for persons who have not been at increased risk since they were last tested. Women screened during a previous pregnancy should be rescreened in subsequent pregnancies.

In 2015, the Centers for Disease Control and Prevention recommended that providers should offer HIV screening at least annually to all sexually active MSM. Clinicians can also consider the potential benefits of more frequent HIV screening (such as every 3 or 6 months) for some asymptomatic sexually active MSM based on their individual risk factors, local HIV epidemiology, and local policies. The CDC also recommends yearly testing for syphilis, gonorrhea, and chlamydia in MSM; in contrast, the USPSTF has found insufficient evidence to recommend screening for these diseases in men.

KEY POINT

- Sexually active gay, bisexual, and other men who have sex with men and injection drug users should be screened for HIV infection at least annually.

Bibliography

DiNenno EA, Prejean J, Irwin K, Delaney KP, Bowles K, Martin T, et al. Recommendations for HIV screening of gay, bisexual, and other men who have sex with men - United States, 2017. MMWR Morb Mortal Wkly Rep. 2017;66:830-832. [PMID: 28796758]

Item 71   Answer: D

Educational Objective: Reduce cardiovascular risk with statin therapy in a patient without known atherosclerotic cardiovascular disease.

The most appropriate therapy for primary prevention of atherosclerotic cardiovascular disease (ASCVD) in this patient is simvastatin. All patients at increased cardiovascular risk should be counseled regarding therapeutic lifestyle changes, including dietary modification, regular physical activity, weight loss, and smoking cessation. In addition to therapeutic lifestyle changes, the American College of Cardiology (ACC)/American Heart Association (AHA) cholesterol treatment guideline recommends adding moderate- or high-intensity statin therapy for primary prevention of ASCVD in adults aged 40 to 75 years without known ASCVD or diabetes mellitus if ASCVD risk is 7.5% or higher, taking into account patient preferences, adverse effects, and expected ASCVD risk reduction. The U.S. Preventive Services Task Force (USPSTF) recommends low- to moderate-intensity statin therapy in asymptomatic adults aged 40 to 75 years without ASCVD who have at least one ASCVD risk factor (dyslipidemia, diabetes, hypertension, or smoking) and a calculated 10-year ASCVD event risk of 10% or higher. This patient with a 10-year risk for ASCVD of 11.1% meets the criteria of both the ACC/AHA and USPSTF guidelines, and both guidelines support initiation of moderate-intensity statin therapy.

In the absence of familial hypercholesterolemia, proprotein convertase subtilisin/kexin type 9 (PCSK9) inhibitors, such as alirocumab and evolocumab, are not indicated in the primary prevention of ASCVD. Cost, treatment burden (injections), and minimal long-term safety data argue against their use in primary prevention.

Nonstatin drugs should be considered alone or in combination with statins in patients who do not achieve adequate LDL cholesterol reduction with statin therapy, especially in high-risk patients (those with clinical ASCVD, baseline LDL cholesterol level >190 mg/dL [4.92 mmol/L], or diabetes). This patient does not have an indication for ezetimibe therapy alone or in combination with a statin.

In patients with a fasting triglyceride level of 500 mg/dL (5.65 mmol/L) or higher, triglyceride-lowering drug therapy is useful to prevent pancreatitis. Fibrates, such as gemfibrozil, result in an average reduction in triglyceride levels of 30% to 50%, but this patient does not have an indication for fibrate therapy.

KEY POINT

- In patients aged 40 to 75 years with no atherosclerotic cardiovascular disease (ASCVD) or diabetes mellitus and a 10-year ASCVD risk of 7.5% or higher, the American College of Cardiology/American Heart Association recommend moderate- or high-intensity statin therapy for primary prevention of ASCVD.

Bibliography

Stone NJ, Robinson JG, Lichtenstein AH, Bairey Merz CN, Blum CB, Eckel RH, et al; American College of Cardiology/American Heart Association Task Force on Practice Guidelines. 2013 ACC/AHA guideline on the treatment of blood cholesterol to reduce atherosclerotic cardiovascular risk in adults: a report of the American College of Cardiology/American Heart Association Task Force on Practice Guidelines. Circulation. 2014;129:S1-45. [PMID: 24222016] doi:10.1161/01.cir.0000437738.63853.7a

Item 72   Answer: A

Educational Objective: Disclose a medical error to an affected patient.

The most appropriate management is to explain to the patient that an error was committed and the steps that will be taken to reduce the chance of recurrence. This case involves the most common type of medical error, one related to inappropriate medication dosing. Current standards recommend full disclosure of serious unanticipated outcomes, and several states mandate such disclosures. Disclosure of errors is necessary to respect the patient's autonomy,

promote trust through honesty, and promote justice through appropriate compensation. Error disclosure should include an explanation of the course of events and how the error occurred, an apology by the physician, a description of how the effects of the error will be minimized or rectified, and steps the physician or system will take to reduce recurrences. In this case, the physician should inform his or her colleague of the error, and they should work within the practice to explore factors that caused the error and determine ways to reduce errors in the future.

The pharmacy may have played a role in commission of the error; however, it would be inappropriate to deflect blame to another source. Communication with the pharmacy regarding the correct dosage would be important in rectifying the situation.

The National Practitioner Data Bank is a federal repository of reports regarding serious professional or safety concerns, including medical malpractice payments or serious actions taken against physicians (such as suspension of licensure or clinical privileges). The error in this case should be disclosed and investigated; however, it would not be appropriate to report to the National Practitioner Data Bank.

Although addressing this patient's symptom without disclosing that an error occurred is an attractive option, disclosure respects the patient's autonomy by providing her with information necessary to make an informed decision about her care. Furthermore, the disclosure may enhance physician-patient communication and trust. Data from health systems that implement medical error disclosure policies suggest that disclosure decreases malpractice lawsuits and litigation costs.

KEY POINT

- Error disclosure should include an explanation of the course of events and how the error occurred, an apology by the physician, a description of how the effects of the error will be minimized or rectified, and steps the physician or system will take to reduce recurrences.

Bibliography

Snyder L; American College of Physicians Ethics, Professionalism, and Human Rights Committee. American College of Physicians ethics manual: sixth edition. Ann Intern Med. 2012;156:73-104. [PMID: 22213573] doi: 10.7326/0003-4819-156-1-201201031-00001

Item 73   Answer: C

Educational Objective: Evaluate a patient with probable overflow incontinence.

Obtaining a postvoid residual urine volume is the most appropriate next step in the management of this patient. This patient likely has neurogenic bladder with overflow incontinence, characterized by constant urine leaking and dribbling and a palpable bladder. Overflow incontinence is more commonly found in men with prostatic hyperplasia and bladder outlet obstruction. However, this patient has long-standing diabetes mellitus and evidence of autonomic neuropathy (resting tachycardia, dry feet, distended bladder) on physical examination. Postvoid residual bladder volume measurement with ultrasonography can confirm the presence of large volumes of urine in the bladder, supporting the clinical diagnosis.

Botulinum toxin injection is used in the treatment of urgency urinary incontinence that persists despite behavioral and pharmacologic therapies. A systematic review concluded that botulinum toxin injection was superior to placebo in reducing incontinence in patients with urgency incontinence unresponsive to more conservative measures. Symptoms are typically reduced for 3 to 6 months, and then reinjection is required. Such injections can worsen overflow incontinence and would be contraindicated in this patient.

Oxybutynin is an anticholinergic agent used in the treatment of urgency incontinence. Anticholinergic drugs (oxybutynin, darifenacin, fesoterodine, solifenacin, tolterodine, trospium) block the muscarinic cholinergic receptors and decrease bladder contractility. The use of oxybutynin would worsen overflow incontinence due to neurogenic bladder and would be contraindicated in this patient.

Urodynamic testing is not recommended in the initial evaluation of urinary incontinence. Urodynamic testing consists of measuring bladder pressure during bladder filling, urine flow rate, and pressure-flow correlations and testing for sphincter deficiency. Urodynamic studies are required only for complex cases in which neurologic disease is suspected or surgical intervention is being considered.

KEY POINT

- A postvoid residual urine volume, determined by ultrasonography, can confirm a suspected case of overflow urinary incontinence.

Bibliography

Kadow BT, Tyagi P, Chermansky CJ. Neurogenic causes of detrusor underactivity. Curr Bladder Dysfunct Rep. 2015;10:325-331. [PMID: 26715948]

Item 74   Answer: B

Educational Objective: Treat chronic pelvic pain syndrome.

A trial of pregabalin is the most appropriate treatment for this patient with chronic pelvic pain syndrome (CPPS). CPPS is characterized by chronic pelvic pain and intermittent voiding symptoms without evidence of infection. Subtypes of this condition include inflammatory and noninflammatory forms. Treatment involves a multimodal approach; options include pharmacologic therapies (antibiotics, anti-inflammatory agents, α-blocking agents, 5α-reductase inhibitors, and neuromodulating agents) and nonpharmacologic strategies (biofeedback, cognitive behavioral therapy, and physical therapy). There is limited and conflicting evidence for thermal ablation therapies and direct surgical interventions. Despite these options, treatment can be challenging, with minimal rates of improvement. This patient has already attempted numerous medication regimens without

symptomatic improvement. At this time, it would be most prudent to proceed with a neuromodulatory approach, with medications such as pregabalin, gabapentin, or nortriptyline. Nonpharmacologic options could also be recommended at this juncture.

No evidence supports the use of lidocaine-hydrocortisone suppositories in the treatment of CPPS.

This patient has already attempted numerous trials of antibiotics, anti-inflammatory agents, and α-blocking agents without any appreciable symptomatic improvement. Furthermore, the laboratory results do not reflect any evidence for an underlying active infection, systemic inflammation, or urinary retention. Consequently, a trial of tamsulosin or trimethoprim-sulfamethoxazole would not be appropriate.

KEY POINT

- Treatment of chronic pelvic pain syndrome demands a multimodal approach, with options including both pharmacologic and nonpharmacologic strategies; among the pharmacologic options are neuromodulatory agents, such as pregabalin, gabapentin, and nortriptyline.

Bibliography

Bharucha AE, Lee TH. Anorectal and pelvic pain. Mayo Clin Proc. 2016; 91:1471-1486. [PMID: 27712641] doi:10.1016/j.mayocp.2016.08.011

Item 75   Answer: A

Educational Objective: Treat somatic symptom disorder.

Cognitive behavioral therapy (CBT) is the most appropriate next step in management. This patient meets the diagnostic criteria for somatic symptom disorder: one or more somatic symptoms causing distress or interference with daily life; excessive thoughts, feelings, and behaviors related to the somatic symptoms; and persistence of somatic symptoms for at least 6 months. Furthermore, after thorough investigation, her symptoms have no identifiable organic source. In addition to acknowledging the patient's symptoms and establishing rapport through frequent scheduled follow-up visits, CBT is the best next step in management. Several studies have shown that CBT is superior to usual care, and the benefits are maintained after completion of therapy.

Familial Mediterranean fever (FMF) is the classic autoinflammatory disease associated with mutation of the *MEFV1* gene, which codes for pyrin (a regulator of interleukin-1β production). Attacks last 1 to 3 days and are characterized by polyserositis, arthritis, erysipeloid rash around the ankles, and elevation of acute phase reactants. Most cases (90%) present before age 20 years, and a family history of similar symptoms is common. This patient's age of onset, chronic symptoms, and negative evaluation results, including acute phase reactant measurement, argue strongly against the diagnosis of FMF and the need to analyze the *MEFV* gene.

Pregabalin is an FDA-approved treatment for fibromyalgia and other conditions associated with neuropathic pain, such as diabetic peripheral neuropathy and postherpetic neuralgia. However, this patient does not have the fatigue and widespread musculoskeletal symptoms typical of fibromyalgia. Pregabalin has no role in the treatment of somatic symptom disorder.

Whole-body PET is not indicated in a patient without clinical evidence of malignancy. Furthermore, advanced diagnostic testing is not recommended in patients with somatic symptom disorder to provide technological reassurance. In addition to being cost ineffective, such testing may lead to false-positive results, triggering further unnecessary testing and patient stress.

KEY POINT

- Treatment of somatic symptom disorder focuses on acknowledging the patient's symptoms, building a therapeutic relationship with the patient through frequent scheduled visits, implementing cognitive behavioral therapy, and avoiding further testing.

Bibliography

Schröder A, Rehfeld E, Ornbøl E, Sharpe M, Licht RW, Fink P. Cognitive-behavioural group treatment for a range of functional somatic syndromes: randomised trial. Br J Psychiatry. 2012;200:499-507. [PMID: 22539780] doi:10.1192/bjp.bp.111.098681

Item 76   Answer: B

Educational Objective: Diagnose central retinal artery occlusion.

The most likely diagnosis for this patient's painless visual loss is central retinal artery occlusion (CRAO). This patient has several risk factors for this condition, including advanced age; male sex; and associated cardiovascular risk factors, such as hypertension and hyperlipidemia. Examination reveals an afferent pupillary defect and cherry red fovea (*blue arrow*) that is accentuated by a pale retinal background. Interruption of the venous blood columns may be recognized with the appearance of "boxcarring" rows of corpuscles separated by clear intervals seen in the vein just superior to the optic disc (*white arrow*). The most likely cause in this case is carotid atherosclerosis, but CRAO may also be caused by cardiogenic emboli; carotid artery dissection; hematologic conditions, such as sickle cell disease; or hypercoagulable states. The occlusion may be preceded by transient visual loss or a stuttering course. Retinal examination may demonstrate emboli. In an older patient who lacks emboli on examination, erythrocyte sedimentation rate and C-reactive protein level should be obtained to rule out giant cell arteritis, which is a rare but important cause of CRAO. Prognosis is based on visual acuity at presentation. Ischemia that lasts 4 hours or longer tends to result in irreversible vision loss. Treatment may include measures to lower intraocular pressure. Emergent ophthalmology consultation is required.

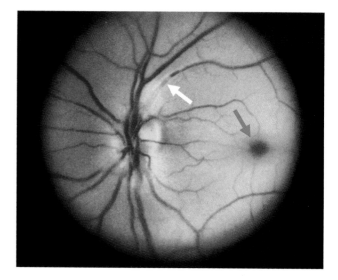

Acute angle-closure glaucoma typically presents with severe eye pain and visual loss. It may involve headache, nausea, and vomiting. Ophthalmoscopic examination reveals a mid-dilated (4-6 mm), nonreactive pupil and intraocular pressure greater than 50 mm Hg. This patient's clinical picture is not consistent with acute angle-closure glaucoma.

Idiopathic intracranial hypertension (previously known as pseudotumor cerebri) may present with diplopia, headache, and, most often, bilateral visual symptoms. These may include transient visual obscurations, which can be brief and triggered by body position change or the Valsalva maneuver. Papilledema is almost always present on examination.

Retinal detachment most commonly presents with photopsias (flashes of light); patients may also report seeing cobwebs and large floaters. Painless complete visual loss is possible, but retinal detachment is more often associated with progressive vision compromise that may involve partial visual fields. A horseshoe-shaped retinal tear may be observed on funduscopic examination.

KEY POINT

- Central retinal artery occlusion presents as acute, profound, and painless loss of monocular vision associated with an afferent pupillary defect and cherry red fovea.

Bibliography

Georgalas I, Pagoulatos D, Koutsandrea C, Pavlidis M. Sudden unilateral painless loss of vision. BMJ. 2014;349:g4117. [PMID: 24986885] doi: 10.1136/bmj.g4117

Item 77   Answer: B   🅷

Educational Objective: Treat dyspnea refractory to medical therapy in a patient with heart failure and COPD.

The most appropriate treatment is oral hydromorphone. This patient has severe chronic dyspnea that is refractory to maximal therapy for his underlying heart failure and COPD. Oral opioids, dosed appropriately, have been found to be both safe and efficacious in the treatment of dyspnea. Treatment efficacy is thought to be related to modulation of shared neural structures that are involved in the pathogenesis of both pain and dyspnea, as there are numerous μ-opioid receptors throughout the respiratory centers in the central nervous system. No evidence suggests that one opioid is superior to another in the treatment of dyspnea, and agent selection should be based on individual patient considerations, such as avoidance of morphine products in patients with reduced kidney function.

Furosemide would be a reasonable selection in a patient with volume overload as the driver of dyspnea; however, this patient has no evidence to suggest this cause (such as an elevated central venous pressure, an S_3, crackles, or peripheral edema).

Benzodiazepines, such as lorazepam, are effective for short-term control of anxiety symptoms. However, this patient's anxiety is a result of his shortness of breath, and as such, treatment should focus on relieving the dyspnea, not on treating the associated anxiety. For this reason, benzodiazepines should be considered only when adjunctive therapy is indicated.

Although systemic opioids have shown clear benefit in treating refractory dyspnea, inhaled opioids, such as nebulized morphine, have not shown significant efficacy in several placebo-controlled trials.

KEY POINT

- In patients with severe refractory dyspnea, appropriately dosed oral opioids are first-line therapy for symptomatic relief.

Bibliography

Kamal AH, Maguire JM, Wheeler JL, Currow DC, Abernethy AP. Dyspnea review for the palliative care professional: treatment goals and therapeutic options. J Palliat Med. 2012;15:106-14. [PMID: 22268406] doi:10.1089/jpm.2011.0110

Item 78   Answer: D

Educational Objective: Avoid aspirin therapy for primary prevention of atherosclerotic cardiovascular disease in a patient at high risk for bleeding.

No further intervention is the most appropriate management of this patient. Although he has a 10-year risk for atherosclerotic cardiovascular disease (ASCVD) of 14.6%, he is at high risk for bleeding with the addition of aspirin therapy. The U.S. Preventive Services Task Force recommends low-dose aspirin for the primary prevention of ASCVD and colorectal cancer in adults aged 50 to 59 years with a 10-year ASCVD risk of 10% or higher who do not have an increased risk for bleeding, have a life expectancy of at least 10 years, and are willing to take low-dose aspirin daily for at least 10 years. Patients aged 60 to 69 years may also benefit from aspirin; however, the net benefit is smaller because of the increased risk for bleeding in this population. In addition to increasing

age, male sex and use of anticoagulants or NSAIDs increase the risk for bleeding. Many patients with cardiovascular disease who are eligible for secondary prevention with aspirin therapy also require long-term oral anticoagulant therapy for atrial fibrillation. In these patients, the addition of aspirin to anticoagulant therapy provides some additional protection against cardiovascular events, but the risk for major bleeding is significantly increased. Therefore, aspirin is not generally recommended in these patients. Although this patient's risk for ASCVD is higher than 10%, he is already receiving anticoagulant therapy with rivaroxaban; therefore, the potential benefits of aspirin therapy for primary prevention of ASCVD are likely outweighed by the increased risk for bleeding.

High doses of fish oil increase bleeding time in vitro by suppressing platelet-activating factor, but this mechanism has not been associated with higher rates of clinical bleeding, even when the supplement is combined with aspirin or warfarin. However, a 2018 systematic review concluded that omega-3 fatty acid supplementation does not reduce heart disease, stroke, or death; therefore, fish oil supplementation cannot be recommended.

Switching rivaroxaban to low-dose aspirin is not recommended because this patient is at high risk for atrial fibrillation–related stroke. For this patient, anticoagulant therapy is significantly superior to aspirin in reducing his risk for stroke.

KEY POINT

- In the primary and secondary prevention of cardiovascular events, the addition of aspirin to long-term anticoagulation is associated with significantly increased bleeding events and is not routinely recommended.

Bibliography

Whitlock EP, Burda BU, Williams SB, Guirguis-Blake JM, Evans CV. Bleeding risks with aspirin use for primary prevention in adults: a systematic review for the U.S. Preventive Services Task Force. Ann Intern Med. 2016;164(12):826-35. [PMID: 27064261] doi: 10.7326/M15-2112

Item 79   Answer: C

Educational Objective: Diagnose high ankle sprain.

The most likely diagnosis is a high ankle sprain. High ankle sprains result from excessive dorsiflexion or eversion that causes injury to the tibiofibular syndesmotic ligaments connecting the distal tibia and fibula. Pain can be elicited by compressing the leg at mid-calf (squeeze test), by having the patient cross the legs with the lateral malleolus of the injured leg resting on the other knee (crossed-leg test), or by dorsiflexing and externally rotating the foot with the knee flexed (dorsiflexion-external rotation test). The most common mechanism of injury involves an externally rotated force applied to a dorsiflexed ankle, as is the case with this patient. Patients with high ankle sprains report the acute onset of pain proximal to the ankle. Pain is often accompanied by swelling and ecchymosis. Treatment is similar to that used for other ankle sprains and includes cryotherapy (ice or cold water), mobilization, and analgesics for pain control, but recovery is usually delayed.

Achilles tendon rupture most commonly results from sudden, forceful plantar flexion, such as occurs with jumping and sprinting. Patients report sudden onset of heel pain and often hear a popping sound at the time of the injury. On examination, patients have weak or absent plantar flexion. Absent plantar flexion with calf squeezing (Thompson test) also suggests the diagnosis. This patient's clinical presentation is not consistent with Achilles tendon rupture.

The Ottawa ankle and foot rules are useful in excluding ankle fractures, with an extremely high sensitivity (>95%). According to these validated rules, radiography should be obtained when a patient is unable to walk four steps both immediately after the injury and during evaluation, and when focal tenderness is present at the posterior aspect of the malleolus, the navicular bone, or the fifth metatarsal base. If these criteria are not met, obtaining radiography is not necessary because the probability of an ankle fracture is exceedingly low, as in this patient.

Lateral ankle sprains typically result from inversion injuries to the lateral ankle ligaments (the anterior and posterior talofibular ligaments and the calcaneofibular ligament). Physical examination reveals ecchymosis, lateral ankle tenderness, and swelling, which was not the case with this patient. This patient's symptoms and findings were located above the ankle.

KEY POINT

- Patients with high ankle sprains report the acute onset of pain proximal to the ankle, accompanied by swelling and ecchymosis.

Bibliography
Vopat ML, Vopat BG, Lubberts B, DiGiovanni CW. Current trends in the diagnosis and management of syndesmotic injury. Curr Rev Musculoskelet Med. 2017;10:94-103. [PMID: 28101828] doi:10.1007/s12178-017-9389-4

Item 80   Answer: A

Educational Objective: Treat vulvovaginal candidiasis.

The most appropriate treatment for this patient with symptoms of vulvovaginal candidiasis is intravaginal clotrimazole. Vulvovaginitis describes infectious and noninfectious conditions that cause vulvovaginal symptoms, including abnormal vaginal discharge, vulvar itching, burning, irritation, and malodor. When discharge is associated with abnormal findings, the differential diagnoses most commonly include bacterial vaginosis, trichomoniasis, and vulvovaginal candidiasis. Vaginal irritation also may be caused by dermatologic conditions or allergic reactions, cervical infections, or genitourinary syndrome of menopause. A woman may have more than one type of infection at a time. The diagnosis of vulvovaginal candidiasis is suggested by the presence of vaginal discharge and vulvar pruritus, pain, irritation, and

redness. Signs include vulvar edema; fissures; excoriations; and thick, white, curdy vaginal discharge. The diagnosis can be made when a saline or 10% potassium hydroxide wet mount of vaginal discharge shows hyphae, pseudohyphae, or yeast. Because the sensitivity of microscopy is low, empiric treatment of vulvovaginal candidiasis can be considered if symptoms are accompanied by characteristic findings. Several therapeutically equivalent topical and oral drugs are available; among the topically applied drugs, imidazoles (fluconazole, miconazole, clotrimazole) are the most effective. Evidence suggests that topical and oral agents have similar efficacy and that treatment preference should be based on cost, convenience, and patient preference.

Intravaginal nystatin, a topical antifungal drug, lacks good supporting evidence for the treatment of vulvovaginal candidiasis and currently is not recommended.

Oral metronidazole is used to treat bacterial vaginosis, the most common cause of vaginal discharge, as well as to treat trichomoniasis. Accepted clinical criteria for diagnosing bacterial vaginosis include the presence of three of four characteristics: vaginal pH greater than 4.5, amine ("fishy") odor on the application of 10% potassium hydroxide to vaginal secretions (whiff test), the presence of a thin homogeneous vaginal discharge, and the finding of at least 20% clue cells on a microscopic saline wet mount examination. Although the presentation of trichomoniasis varies, many women develop a copious, malodorous, pale yellow or gray frothy discharge with vulvar itching, burning, and postcoital bleeding. Point-of-care vaginal swab rapid immunoassays and nucleic acid amplification tests for detection of *Trichomoniasis vaginalis* have replaced microscopy or culture as the gold standard for diagnosis. This patient does not have findings of bacterial vaginosis or trichomoniasis; hence, metronidazole is not indicated.

Oral voriconazole should not be used to treat vulvovaginal candidiasis because no data support its use. Case reports suggest that it is ineffective, and there is the added potential for toxicity.

KEY POINT

- Topical antifungal imidazole therapy, such as intravaginal clotrimazole, is an effective treatment for uncomplicated vulvovaginal candidiasis, which is usually caused by *Candida albicans*.

Bibliography
Mills BB. Vaginitis: beyond the basics. Obstet Gynecol Clin North Am. 2017;44:159-177. [PMID: 28499528] doi:10.1016/j.ogc.2017.02.010

Item 81   Answer: A

Educational Objective: Implement appropriate monitoring strategies before and during opioid therapy in a patient with chronic pain.

Baseline urine drug screening is recommended before starting opioid therapy in this patient. Many guidelines, including the Centers for Disease Control and Prevention

(CDC) Guideline for Prescribing Opioids for Chronic Pain, recommend initial and ongoing urine drug screening. Urine drug screening is used to test for adherence to current therapy, identify potential opioid diversion (by assessing whether the expected metabolite is present within an appropriate time frame), and evaluate for the presence of other controlled prescription and nonprescription drugs. Urine drug screening should be performed before opioids are prescribed for chronic pain and at least yearly during therapy. More frequent screening may be necessary in the setting of therapy changes or the presence of red flags (lost prescriptions, early refill requests, multiple concurrent opioid providers or "doctor shopping," consistently missed appointments, or erratic follow-up).

The CDC guideline and other opioid prescribing guidelines recommend that opioid therapy be considered only if expected benefits for both pain and function are anticipated to outweigh the risks. If opioids are used, they should be combined with nonpharmacologic and nonopioid pharmacologic therapies as appropriate. Discontinuing this patient's current nonpharmacologic and pharmacologic therapies is not indicated.

Chronic pain is often associated with comorbid psychological issues. Patients who meet the criteria for diagnosis of a psychological comorbidity, such as depression or anxiety, should be treated accordingly. However, routine referral for a psychiatric evaluation is not mandatory and is based on the presence and severity of comorbid mental health disorders.

KEY POINT

- In patients in whom opioid therapy is being considered for the treatment of chronic pain, urine drug screening should be performed before opioid prescription and at least yearly during therapy to evaluate for adherence to therapy and to identify the presence of other controlled drugs.

Bibliography

Dowell D, Haegerich TM, Chou R. CDC guideline for prescribing opioids for chronic pain—United States, 2016. JAMA. 2016;315:1624-45. [PMID: 26977696]

Item 82   Answer: C

Educational Objective: Evaluate preoperative cardiac risk using transthoracic echocardiography in a patient with moderate aortic stenosis.

In addition to electrocardiography, the most appropriate preoperative testing for this patient is transthoracic echocardiography (TTE). The patient was diagnosed with moderate aortic stenosis several years ago and has occasional dizziness with physical exertion, a potential symptom of severe aortic stenosis. Preoperative TTE should not be ordered routinely but is recommended in certain cases. Indications for preoperative echocardiography include dyspnea of unknown origin, heart failure with change in clinical status, and known left ventricular dysfunction in the absence of an assessment in the previous 12 months. Relevant to this patient, TTE is indicated in patients with known or suspected moderate or greater degrees of valvular stenosis or regurgitation if TTE has not been performed within 1 year or in those whose clinical status has changed or who have referable symptoms. It is reasonable to perform elevated-risk elective noncardiac surgery in patients with severe asymptomatic aortic stenosis, with appropriate intraoperative and postoperative hemodynamic monitoring. For patients who are candidates for valvular intervention because of symptoms or severity of disease, valvular intervention before elective noncardiac surgery is effective at reducing risk.

In a systematic review, a preoperative B-type natriuretic peptide (BNP) level greater than 92 pg/mL (92 ng/L) predicted the composite outcome of death or nonfatal myocardial infarction at 30 days, at 180 days, and beyond. Despite the improvement in predicting poor surgical outcomes, it is unclear what role BNP measurement should play in perioperative cardiovascular care; this test is currently not recommended by American College of Cardiology/American Heart Association guidelines. The Canadian Cardiovascular Society guidelines on perioperative cardiac risk assessment and management for patients who undergo noncardiac surgery strongly recommend that a BNP level be obtained to enhance perioperative cardiac risk estimation in patients with a Revised Cardiac Risk Index score of 1 or more, patients aged 65 years and older, and patients aged 45 to 64 years who have significant cardiovascular disease.

This patient is scheduled to undergo surgery (total knee arthroplasty) and has good functional capacity (able to swim for 30 minutes), and she does not have coronary artery disease or its equivalents (chronic kidney disease, cerebrovascular disease, heart failure, or diabetes mellitus). This patient's risk for major ischemic events is low; therefore, dobutamine stress echocardiography is not indicated.

KEY POINT

- Transthoracic echocardiography to evaluate preoperative cardiac risk is appropriate for patients with moderate to severe valvular stenosis or regurgitation in the absence of an assessment in the previous year or for those whose clinical status has changed or who have referable symptoms.

Bibliography

Fleisher LA, Fleischmann KE, Auerbach AD, Barnason SA, Beckman JA, Bozkurt B, et al; American College of Cardiology. 2014 ACC/AHA guideline on perioperative cardiovascular evaluation and management of patients undergoing noncardiac surgery: a report of the American College of Cardiology/American Heart Association Task Force on practice guidelines. J Am Coll Cardiol. 2014;64:e77-137. [PMID: 25091544]

Item 83   Answer: D

Educational Objective: Evaluate serum lipid levels in an obese patient.

This patient with obesity should undergo serum lipid screening. The American Heart Association, American College of Cardiology, and The Obesity Society guideline for the management of overweight and obesity recommends measurement of height and weight; calculation of BMI; measurement of waist circumference; and measurement of cardiovascular disease risk factors, including blood pressure, fasting blood glucose (or hemoglobin A_{1c}), and serum lipid levels. Obesity is associated with insulin resistance and dyslipidemia characterized by elevations of total cholesterol, LDL cholesterol, VLDL cholesterol, and triglycerides and a reduction in HDL cholesterol. The history should address symptoms of obesity-related comorbid conditions, but no additional screening is recommended in the absence of suggestive symptoms or findings.

Exercise stress testing is recommended for patients with symptoms of cardiac ischemia. Overweight and obese patients are at increased risk for cardiovascular disease and should be questioned about symptoms and referred for testing if symptoms are present. Routine screening of asymptomatic patients is not recommended.

Hepatic ultrasonography is not necessary for this patient. The risk for nonalcoholic steatohepatitis is increased in overweight and obese patients. A presumptive diagnosis can be made in a patient with mild abnormalities in aminotransferase levels, risk factors for nonalcoholic fatty liver disease (such as diabetes mellitus, obesity, and hyperlipidemia), and ultrasonographic features consistent with hepatic steatosis. The recommended treatment of nonalcoholic steatohepatitis is weight loss, but no screening for this condition is recommended.

Risk for obstructive sleep apnea is increased among overweight and obese patients, particularly those with neck circumference greater than 38 cm (15 in) in women and greater than 43 cm (17 in) in men. The patient should be referred for overnight polysomnography only if symptoms of the disorder are present. He does not report nonrestorative sleep or daytime hypersomnolence, which would suggest obstructive sleep apnea.

The prevalence of an endocrine cause of obesity is very low. Thyroid function testing should be reserved for patients with symptoms and findings indicating thyroid disease.

KEY POINT

- Management guidelines for overweight and obese patients recommend measurement of height and weight; calculation of BMI; measurement of waist circumference; and measurement of cardiovascular disease risk factors, including blood pressure, fasting blood glucose (or hemoglobin A_{1c}), and serum lipid levels.

Bibliography

Jensen MD, Ryan DH, Apovian CM, Ard JD, Comuzzie AG, Donato KA, et al; American College of Cardiology/American Heart Association Task Force on Practice Guidelines. 2013 AHA/ACC/TOS guideline for the management of overweight and obesity in adults: a report of the American College of Cardiology/American Heart Association Task Force on Practice Guidelines and The Obesity Society. Circulation. 2014;129:S102-38. [PMID: 24222017] doi:10.1161/01.cir.0000437739.71477.ee

Item 84 Answer: D

Educational Objective: Treat unexplained chronic cough.

Multimodal speech therapy is an appropriate treatment for this patient with unexplained chronic cough (UCC). UCC is defined as cough persisting for more than 8 weeks with no identifiable cause despite comprehensive evaluation. The evidence supporting the diagnosis and management of UCC is limited and generally weak. The American College of Chest Physicians (ACCP) expert panel recommends multimodal speech therapy consisting of two to four sessions of education, cough suppression techniques, breathing exercises, and counseling. This intervention helps reduce cough frequency and severity and improve cough-related quality of life. The ACCP also recommends a therapeutic trial of the neuromodulator gabapentin as long as the potential side effects and the risk-benefit profile are discussed with patients before use of the medication and the risk-benefit profile is reassessed at 6 months before continuation of the drug. Neuromodulators may diminish neural sensitization, which is a key driver of unexplained cough.

Levels of neutrophils are frequently increased in patients with chronic cough. Macrolide antibiotics are effective in the treatment of exacerbations of COPD and bronchiectasis, possibly because of their anti-inflammatory and antineutrophil effects that are independent of antimicrobial effects. However, trials with macrolide antibiotics, such as azithromycin and erythromycin, have not demonstrated benefit in patients with UCC.

Inhaled ipratropium bromide was found to be beneficial in patients with chronic cough after an upper respiratory tract infection. The ACCP does not recommend ipratropium for the treatment of UCC because the findings related to ipratropium were from an older study with a small sample size and limited reporting of methods, and the results have not been replicated.

Like gabapentin, morphine was found to be effective in reducing cough severity and frequency, but the ACCP expert panel has declined to recommend morphine as an intervention for chronic cough. The danger of overdose and addiction potential of morphine have been well described.

KEY POINT

- Recommended treatments for unexplained chronic cough include multimodality speech pathology therapy and neuromodulators, such as gabapentin.

Bibliography

Gibson P, Wang G, McGarvey L, Vertigan AE, Altman KW, Birring SS; CHEST Expert Cough Panel. Treatment of unexplained chronic cough: CHEST guideline and expert panel report. Chest. 2016;149:27-44. [PMID: 26426314] doi:10.1378/chest.15-1496

Item 85 Answer: B

Educational Objective: Manage sexual side effects in a patient taking a selective serotonin reuptake inhibitor for major depressive disorder.

The most appropriate next step in management is to discontinue sertraline and initiate bupropion, which has a lower rate of sexual side effects. Cognitive behavioral therapy (CBT) or a second-generation antidepressant is an appropriate first choice for the treatment of major depressive disorder. Side effects, comorbid conditions, and cost are important considerations in the selection of therapy for a patient with depression. The most widely prescribed antidepressant drugs are selective serotonin reuptake inhibitors (SSRIs). SSRIs have excellent safety profiles compared with tricyclic antidepressants, but adverse sexual side effects (such as reduced libido, anorgasmia, or delayed orgasm) are common. Bupropion is an appropriate substitute agent for patients experiencing sexual side effects with an SSRI because it is an effective treatment with a low rate of sexual side effects. Bupropion can also be added to SSRI therapy to reduce SSRI-induced sexual side effects, but it is important to note that bupropion is contraindicated in patients with seizure disorders. Substituting CBT for antidepressant therapy in a patient experiencing sexual side effects of an SSRI is also an acceptable alternative.

The addition of CBT to antidepressant therapy is a reasonable approach for depression that does not respond to first-line therapy. This patient's depression is responsive to treatment, and the addition of CBT without stopping sertraline will not affect the patient's sexual side effects.

In patients who develop sexual side effects with one SSRI, there is substantial risk for similar problems with all SSRIs. This patient experienced anorgasmia with sertraline, and paroxetine has the highest rate of sexual side effects of all SSRIs, making it a poor choice for this patient.

Electroconvulsive therapy is appropriate for the management of treatment-resistant depression. This patient's depression is responding to first-line therapy; therefore, electroconvulsive therapy would not be the best treatment choice.

KEY POINT

- Selective serotonin reuptake inhibitors are generally well tolerated among patients with major depressive disorder, but sexual side effects (such as anorgasmia, delayed orgasm, and reduced libido) are common; for these patients, bupropion is an appropriate alternative, as is cognitive behavioral therapy.

Bibliography

Lorenz T, Rullo J, Faubion S. Antidepressant-induced female sexual dysfunction. Mayo Clin Proc. 2016;91:1280-6. [PMID: 27594188] doi:10.1016/j.mayocp.2016.04.033

Item 86   Answer: C

Educational Objective: Treat medically unexplained symptoms.

The most appropriate management strategy in this patient with medically unexplained symptoms (MUS) is to recommend cognitive behavioral therapy (CBT). The foundation of management of patients with MUS is an open, honest, and effective therapeutic relationship. Patients should be treated respectfully and cared for in a nonjudgmental manner. It is important to not only expect but to accept the patient's feelings of frustration; acknowledging these feelings early in the patient's management course can help to build and strengthen the therapeutic alliance. Management of MUS requires a patient-focused, holistic, and multimodal approach. The goals of management are functional restoration, decreased symptom focus, and acquisition of coping mechanisms rather than abatement of symptoms. Office visits should be scheduled at regular intervals, allowing for additional discussion, educational opportunities, and longitudinal reassessment. It should be made clear to patients that the treatment of MUS will not likely be curative and that symptoms may persist. Interventions that may benefit patients with MUS include CBT, physical therapy, occupational therapy, individual or group psychotherapy, social support, biofeedback, graded exercise therapy, stress management activities, and training in coping mechanisms. A systematic review of 29 randomized controlled trials comparing CBT with various control treatments found that CBT was an effective treatment for somatization or symptom syndromes and that physical symptoms were more responsive to treatment than were psychological symptoms. At least one randomized controlled trial found that CBT improves outcomes and decreases clinic visits in patients with several unexplained symptoms. A systematic review of four randomized controlled trials of psychodynamic therapy in patients with chronic pain found that the treatment reduced pain, improved function, and decreased the use of health services.

Anti-Hu paraneoplastic syndrome can cause temporal lobe, brainstem, and cerebellar dysfunction and may also involve the dorsal roots and autonomic nervous system. This syndrome is most commonly associated with small cell lung cancer. The long duration and nature of this patient's symptoms make this an unlikely diagnosis, and antibody measurement is not indicated.

Anti-N-methyl-D-aspartate receptor (anti-NMDAR) antibody encephalitis has emerged as an increasingly common cause of encephalitis. The diagnosis is suggested by the presence of choreoathetosis, psychiatric symptoms, seizures, and autonomic instability and is confirmed by detection of anti-NMDAR antibodies in the serum. This patient has no symptoms compatible with this syndrome, and testing is not indicated.

Given the likely diagnosis of MUS, the patient's ongoing symptoms, and numerous available treatment strategies, providing no further treatment is not appropriate.

KEY POINT

- Patients with medically unexplained symptoms may benefit from cognitive behavioral therapy, physical therapy, occupational therapy, individual or group psychotherapy, social support, biofeedback, graded exercise therapy, stress management activities, and training in coping mechanisms.

Bibliography

Evens A, Vendetta L, Krebs K, Herath P. Medically unexplained neurologic symptoms: a primer for physicians who make the initial encounter. Am J Med. 2015;128:1059-64. [PMID: 25910791]

Item 87   Answer: E

Educational Objective: Evaluate a patient with nonspecific low back pain.

No additional diagnostic testing is needed in this patient with acute, nonspecific low back pain. He lacks any concerning features, such as bowel or bladder dysfunction, constitutional symptoms, leg weakness, or saddle anesthesia. Indications to perform immediate imaging include severe and/or progressive neurologic deficits on examination or suspected serious underlying pathology, neither of which are present in this patient.

According to a joint clinical practice guideline released by the American College of Physicians and the American Pain Society, clinicians should not routinely perform diagnostic testing, such as CT, erythrocyte sedimentation rate measurement, MRI, or plain radiography, in patients with nonspecific low back pain. Even in patients with acute radiculopathy or spinal stenosis, routine imaging or testing has not been shown to improve outcomes. Most patients with acute low back pain recover quickly, regardless of the therapeutic intervention used. Whenever possible, maintaining daily activities should be encouraged. Nonpharmacologic treatment with acupuncture, massage, superficial heat, or spinal manipulation is preferred. If pharmacologic treatment is desired for acute low back pain, clinicians and patients should select NSAIDs or skeletal muscle relaxants.

KEY POINT

- Diagnostic studies should not be routinely obtained in patients with nonspecific low back pain; such testing should be reserved for patients with severe or progressive neurologic deficits and patients for whom a serious underlying condition is suspected.

Bibliography
Chou R. In the clinic. Low back pain. Ann Intern Med. 2014;160:ITC6-1. [PMID: 25009837]

Item 88   Answer: D

Educational Objective: Manage a patient with a family history suggestive of an inherited disorder with genetic counseling.

This patient with a family history concerning for familial adenomatous polyposis (FAP) should be referred for genetic counseling. FAP is most commonly inherited in an autosomal-dominant pattern and is caused by a mutation in the adenomatous polyposis coli (*APC*) gene, which functions as a tumor suppressor gene. Nearly 100% of patients with the autosomal-dominant *APC* gene mutation develop colon cancer, with most developing cancer before age 40 years. Because this patient has a strong family history of colon cancer and his brother was recently diagnosed as a carrier of the genetic mutation for FAP, genetic testing is warranted if the patient desires it, and he should undergo genetic counseling first to help guide his decision on whether to pursue

genetic testing. Components of genetic counseling include assessment of the patient's risk for the condition of interest and education on the condition, risks and benefits of testing, alternative options to testing, and implications of testing for the patient and family members. Genetic counseling should be performed by individuals with appropriate training. Clinicians can use a searchable database provided by the American College of Medical Genetics to locate a genetic counselor in their area.

Aspirin and NSAIDs have been touted as a means to reduce the appearance and growth of polyps in patients with FAP. In particular, sulindac has been shown to cause regression of colorectal adenomas in FAP; however, the response is incomplete, and the degree of protection is uncertain. Chemoprevention is not a recommended strategy for patients at risk for or diagnosed with FAP.

Classic FAP results in the development of hundreds to thousands of colorectal adenomas that often manifest by the second decade of life. Gastric fundic gland polyposis and duodenal adenomas are also present in most patients. Gastric cancer is rare, but duodenal and periampullary cancers are the second leading cause of cancer death in this group. Papillary carcinoma of the thyroid is increasingly recognized as accompanying FAP. If this patient is diagnosed as a carrier of the FAP mutation, screening for colon, duodenal and periampullary, and thyroid cancers should be initiated now.

All patients in whom genetic testing is being considered should first be referred for genetic counseling.

KEY POINT

- All patients for whom genetic testing is being considered should undergo genetic counseling.

Bibliography
Hampel H, Bennett RL, Buchanan A, Pearlman R, Wiesner GL; Guideline Development Group, American College of Medical Genetics and Genomics Professional Practice and Guidelines Committee and National Society of Genetic Counselors Practice Guidelines Committee. A practice guideline from the American College of Medical Genetics and Genomics and the National Society of Genetic Counselors: referral indications for cancer predisposition assessment. Genet Med. 2015;17:70-87. [PMID: 25394175] doi:10.1038/gim.2014.147

Item 89   Answer: C

Educational Objective: Evaluate decision-making capacity.

The most appropriate management is to discharge this patient home with home care services. Patients should be presumed legally competent to make medical decisions unless found otherwise by judicial determination. However, in the clinical setting, physicians must frequently determine a patient's decision-making capacity by assessing the patient's ability to understand the relevant information, appreciate the medical consequences of the situation, consider various treatment options, and communicate a choice. Decision-making capacity should be evaluated for each decision to be made, and frequent reassessment is necessary to confirm prior determinations of capacity. Patients with depression or mild dementia may retain decision-making capacity; however, in such circumstances, the capacity assessment should be performed more cautiously, particularly when a decision may result in serious consequences. Validated tools, such as the Aid to Capacity Evaluation (www.aafp.org/afp/2001/0715/afp20010715p299-f2.pdf), may be useful for capacity assessment in the clinical setting. In this situation, the assessment reveals that the patient demonstrates sufficient capacity to make decisions; thus, he should be discharged home with appropriate services to ensure his safety. This patient's choice is also consistent with his previously expressed wishes, which lends validity to his decision.

Cognitive evaluations, such as the Mini–Mental State Examination, do not assess capacity; rather, they are used to detect cognitive impairment.

This competent and autonomous patient is able to make his own choices; therefore, the patient's daughter should not be asked to make a decision on his behalf.

Formal assessments of competence require judicial determination, although a competency hearing is not usually required for clinical decision making. In this case, a court order for the patient to be discharged to a rehabilitation facility is not required because he demonstrates decision-making capacity.

A psychiatric consultation is unnecessary to determine a patient's decision-making capacity; any physician can perform this assessment. However, some hospitals may suggest a psychiatric evaluation in high-stakes situations, such as when a patient requests to leave against medical advice.

KEY POINT

- In the clinical setting, physicians must determine a patient's decision-making capacity by assessing the patient's ability to understand the relevant information, appreciate the medical consequences of the situation, consider various treatment options, and communicate a choice.

Bibliography
Porrino P, Falcone Y, Agosta L, Isaia G, Zanocchi M, Mastrapasqua A, et al. Informed consent in older medical inpatients: assessment of decision-making capacity. J Am Geriatr Soc. 2015;63:2423-4. [PMID: 26603072]

Item 90   Answer: D

Educational Objective: Treat tobacco dependence with pharmacologic therapy in a patient with a recent cardiovascular event.

The most effective treatment is varenicline. Although bupropion and nicotine replacement therapy (NRT) monotherapy are effective for tobacco cessation, varenicline has been shown to be more effective. Some studies, including a large meta-analysis, have raised concerns of an increased risk for cardiovascular events in patients taking varenicline compared with those taking placebo. However, a recent double-blind, randomized, placebo and active-controlled trial of varenicline, bupropion, and nicotine replacement therapy showed no evidence that the use of smoking cessation pharmacotherapies increased the risk of serious cardiovascular adverse events during or after treatment. FDA drug labeling information does not list recent cardiovascular events as a contraindication to varenicline therapy. The FDA recently removed the black box warning related to serious mental health adverse reactions with varenicline use after the risk for mental health effects was found to be lower than previously reported. Varenicline should be used with caution in patients with kidney failure.

Bupropion, a norepinephrine and dopamine reuptake inhibitor with nicotinic receptor activity, effectively increases smoking cessation rates. Bupropion should not be used in patients with a history of seizure disorders, stroke, brain tumor, brain surgery, or head trauma. Blood pressure should be monitored carefully, as severity of hypertension may increase with bupropion treatment. In direct comparison trials, bupropion was less effective in achieving smoking cessation than was varenicline.

Electronic cigarettes hold promise as a harm reduction tool that may help patients quit smoking; however, the evidence regarding their efficacy, risks, and benefits is still emerging. Therefore, current FDA-approved, evidence-based agents for tobacco cessation, such as varenicline, would be more appropriate in this patient.

Effectiveness of NRT is similar to that of bupropion for smoking cessation. Options for NRT include patch, gum, lozenges, oral inhaler, and nasal spray. Concomitant use of more than one form of NRT enhances efficacy. NRT should be used with caution in patients with unstable cardiac disease, life-threatening arrhythmias, or a recent cardiac event. In these patients, the decision to initiate NRT should involve a cardiologist. Patients should also be discouraged from smoking during use of NRT. In this patient with recent non–ST-elevation myocardial infarction, NRT would not be the most appropriate smoking cessation therapy.

KEY POINT

- Varenicline is an effective therapy for smoking cessation and should be considered in smokers with a recent cardiac event.

Bibliography
Patel MS, Steinberg MB. In the clinic. Smoking cessation. Ann Intern Med. 2016;164:ITC33-ITC48. [PMID: 26926702]

Item 91   Answer: A

Educational Objective: Screen for abdominal aortic aneurysm in a man with a history of smoking.

The most appropriate screening test to perform in this former smoker is abdominal duplex ultrasonography to screen for abdominal aortic aneurysm (AAA). The most important risk factors for AAA are advancing age, male sex (6:1 male-to-female incidence ratio), and smoking. The U.S. Preventive Services Task Force (USPSTF) recommends one-time abdominal ultrasonography to screen for AAA in all men aged 65 to 75 years who have ever smoked. Ever-smokers are usually defined as those who have smoked more than 100 cigarettes in their lifetime. The USPSTF recommends that clinicians selectively offer screening for AAA in men aged 65 to 75 years who have never smoked, based on the patient's medical history, family history, other risk factors, and preferences. A recently published meta-analysis concluded that screening significantly reduces AAA-related mortality. Abdominal duplex ultrasonography is the preferred screening modality, with a sensitivity of 94% to 100% and specificity of 98% to 100% for detecting AAA.

Chest radiography and sputum cytologic evaluation have not shown adequate sensitivity or specificity as screening tests for lung cancer and are not recommended.

Although the USPSTF concludes that there is insufficient evidence to recommend routine screening for osteoporosis in men, the National Osteoporosis Foundation recommends osteoporosis screening in men aged 70 years or older. Screening may also be considered in men at high risk for osteoporosis (men with low body weight, recent weight loss, physical inactivity, use of oral glucocorticoids, previous fragility fracture, alcohol use, or androgen deprivation via pharmacologic agents or orchiectomy). The American College of Physicians recommends periodic individualized assessment of risk factors for osteoporosis in older men.

The USPSTF and the American College of Chest Physicians (ACCP) recommend lung cancer screening with annual low-dose CT in persons aged 55 to 80 years (or aged 55 to 77 years, according to the ACCP) with a 30-pack-year smoking history, including former smokers who have quit in the last 15 years. Screening should be discontinued once a person has not smoked for 15 years or develops a health problem that substantially limits life expectancy or the willingness to have curative lung surgery. This patient has a 10-pack-year smoking history and quit almost 30 years ago; therefore, he does not meet the criteria for lung cancer screening.

KEY POINT

- All men aged 65 to 75 years who have ever smoked should undergo one-time abdominal ultrasonography to screen for abdominal aortic aneurysm.

Bibliography

Takagi H, Ando T, Umemoto T; ALICE (All-Literature Investigation of Cardiovascular Evidence) Group. Abdominal aortic aneurysm screening reduces all-cause mortality. Angiology. 2017:3319717693107. [PMID: 28193091] doi:10.1177/0003319717693107

Item 92   Answer: D

Educational Objective: Prevent medication errors with medication reconciliation.

Medication reconciliation would have most likely prevented this medication error. Medication reconciliation is the process of creating an accurate, comprehensive list of the patient's prescription and nonprescription medications (including the dose, frequency, and route of administration) and comparing the list to medication orders (at admission, transfer, or discharge) to resolve inconsistencies. Completion of medication reconciliation decreases adverse drug events, and although the effect on hospital readmissions, morbidity, and mortality is less clear, medication reconciliation should occur at all care transitions to prevent medication errors. In this case, tamoxifen was withheld upon admission but should have been restarted at the time of the patient's discharge from the hospital. Medication reconciliation at the time of discharge would have prevented this error, which resulted in a lapse in the patient's breast cancer treatment.

Computerized physician order entry (CPOE) systems are designed to improve the medication ordering process and prevent medication errors and medication adverse events. Some CPOE systems are integrated with decision support systems. CPOE has resulted in many practice improvements, including standardization of care, improved legibility of orders, and implementation of medication alerts (such as allergy and drug interaction alerts). However, CPOE cannot replace medication reconciliation and would not have prevented this medication error at a transition of care.

Manually transcribing physician medication orders into a paper-based medication administration record, even if originated by using the CPOE process, can lead to medication administration errors and adverse events. However, using a system that features a direct electronic interface between CPOE and the electronic medication administration record can eliminate transcription errors and errors in reading and interpreting hand-written, paper-based medication administration records. Such a system does not replace medication reconciliation and would not have prevented this medication error at the time of discharge.

Improved medication labeling, including the use of "tall man" lettering (for example, **DOBUT**amine versus **DOP**amine), helps minimize confusion surrounding look-alike and sound-alike medications, thereby reducing medication errors. However, improved medication labeling would not have prevented this medication error resulting from a transition of care.

KEY POINT

- Medication reconciliation should occur at all transitions of care to prevent medication errors.

Bibliography

Mueller SK, Sponsler KC, Kripalani S, Schnipper JL. Hospital-based medication reconciliation practices: a systematic review. Arch Intern Med. 2012;172:1057-69. [PMID: 22733210]

Item 93   Answer: A

Educational Objective: Diagnose frailty.

Frailty is a multifactorial geriatric syndrome that may predict a patient's response to certain treatments as well as morbidity and mortality in light of chronic illness. This patient demonstrates unintentional weight loss, low energy and activity levels, slow walking speed, and weakness, all of which are associated with frailty. Indices such as the Frailty Index, the FRAIL (Fatigue, Resistance, Ambulation, Illness, and Loss of weight) scale, and the Osteoporotic Fractures Frailty Scale have been validated for use in primary care. The Frailty Index has been in use for a longer time than other indices; however, its length and complexity limit its usefulness in routine care. The FRAIL scale consists of five self-reported measures and is easy to administer and score in an office setting.

Pharmacologic cardiac stress testing is recommended for patients who cannot exercise and are experiencing symptoms suggestive of cardiac ischemia. There is no established role for pharmacologic stress testing as a predictor of response to cancer treatment.

Lung function during exertion using the 6-minute walk test is helpful to assess disability and prognosis in chronic lung conditions. Simple pulse oximetry and oxygen desaturation studies performed at rest and with exertion assess the need for oxygen supplementation. During a 6-minute walk test, oxygen saturation, heart rate, dyspnea and fatigue levels, and distance walked in 6 minutes are recorded. The 6-minute walk test has no established role in predicting response to cancer chemotherapy in frail older adults.

The Timed Up and Go test is used to identify patients at risk for falls. The individual components of the test (rising from the chair, gait, walking speed, balance maintenance while turning, and sitting) offer insight into the various mechanics of mobility and can guide a more focused evaluation and intervention. Results of the Timed Up and Go test do not predict response to cancer treatment.

KEY POINT

- Frailty is a quantifiable geriatric syndrome that may predict a patient's response to medical treatment.

Bibliography
Puts MT, Santos B, Hardt J, Monette J, Girre V, Atenafu EG, et al. An update on a systematic review of the use of geriatric assessment for older adults in oncology. Ann Oncol. 2014;25:307-15. [PMID: 24256847] doi:10.1093/annonc/mdt386

Item 94   Answer: C

Educational Objective: Treat attention-deficit/hyperactivity disorder.

In addition to cognitive behavioral therapy, methylphenidate is the best initial treatment for this patient with attention-deficit/hyperactivity disorder (ADHD). ADHD is characterized by persistent inattention and/or hyperactivity-impulsivity that disrupts functioning or development in at least two areas of a patient's life (such as work, home, or peer relationships). Some symptoms must be present since age 12 years; however, many patients are not formally diagnosed until adulthood, and up to 60% of children with ADHD continue to have symptoms as an adult. Although

symptoms of hyperactivity and impulsivity often lessen over time, adults with ADHD may be easily distracted, disorganized, and restless. Many adults have comorbid psychiatric problems, such as anxiety, depression, sleep disorders, and substance use. Cognitive behavioral therapy alone or in combination with pharmacotherapy is effective for improving executive functioning in patients with ADHD. Stimulants, such as methylphenidate, are first-line pharmacologic therapy for ADHD. However, these drugs should not be prescribed to patients with recent substance use or at high risk for serious adverse effects (arrhythmia, hypertension). Atomoxetine, bupropion, and tricyclic antidepressants can be used when stimulants are contraindicated.

Benzodiazepines, such as clonazepam, can be used for short-term treatment of severe, acute anxiety disorders. Their use is limited by the potential for abuse, and they are not indicated for the treatment of ADHD.

Escitalopram and other selective serotonin reuptake inhibitors are highly effective for the treatment of various mood and anxiety disorders. However, they have no established role in the treatment of ADHD unless there is a comorbid disorder responsive to this class of drugs.

Ropinirole is an effective therapy for restless legs syndrome. This patient is experiencing restlessness but does not report restless legs or sleep disturbance; therefore, ropinirole would not be indicated.

KEY POINT

- Stimulants, such as methylphenidate, are first-line pharmacologic therapy for attention-deficit/hyperactivity disorder; when stimulants are contraindicated, atomoxetine, bupropion, and tricyclic antidepressants can be used.

Bibliography
Volkow ND, Swanson JM. Clinical practice: adult attention deficit-hyperactivity disorder. N Engl J Med. 2013;369:1935-44. [PMID: 24224626] doi:10.1056/NEJMcp1212625

Item 95   Answer: A

Educational Objective: Diagnose iliotibial band syndrome.

The most likely diagnosis is iliotibial band syndrome (ITBS). ITBS is a common cause of lateral knee pain in runners and can also occur in patients with significant leg length difference, an excessively pronated foot, genu varum, or gluteal muscle weakness. Patients with ITBS have pain that is poorly localized to the lateral knee and distal thigh. Initially, the pain is present only after prolonged activity (such as running) that involves repeated knee flexion and extension. As the condition progresses, the pain occurs earlier in the course of activity and may eventually be present at rest. On examination, there is often tenderness to palpation 2 to 3 cm proximal to the lateral femoral condyle. Patients also frequently have weakness with hip abduction. Reproduction of the pain with knee extension from 90 degrees to 30 degrees with the examiner's thumb exerting pressure on the lateral femoral epicondyle (Noble test) supports the diagnosis of ITBS. Initial treatment consists of activity modification, ice application, and NSAIDs to reduce inflammation. Once inflammation subsides, stretching and then strengthening exercises are indicated.

This patient lacks history of trauma, joint instability, lateral joint line tenderness, or increased laxity with varus force. Lack of these features argues against the presence of a lateral collateral ligament tear.

The lack of prior trauma and absence of catching, grinding, and locking all argue against a meniscal tear, as does the absence of an effusion on examination.

Meralgia paresthetica is due to entrapment of the lateral femoral cutaneous nerve and causes paresthesias on the anterolateral thigh. Risk factors include diabetes mellitus, obesity, pregnancy, and tight clothing or belts around the waist. This patient's findings are not consistent with meralgia paresthetica.

KEY POINT

- Patients with iliotibial band syndrome report diffuse, poorly localized lateral knee and distal thigh pain; there is often tenderness to palpation 2 to 3 cm proximal to the lateral femoral condyle.

Bibliography

Baker RL, Fredericson M. Iliotibial band syndrome in runners: biomechanical implications and exercise interventions. Phys Med Rehabil Clin N Am. 2016;27:53-77. [PMID: 26616177] doi:10.1016/j.pmr.2015.08.001

Item 96   Answer: B

Educational Objective: Evaluate noncyclic mastalgia.

The most appropriate initial management of this patient is breast ultrasonography. Breast pain (mastalgia) is common and may be cyclic or noncyclic. Many younger women experience cyclic breast discomfort with the onset of menses. The discomfort is typically bilateral, lasts for several days, and varies in intensity. Noncyclic breast pain is more likely to be unilateral and may be caused by trauma, cysts, duct ectasia, mastitis, ligamentous stretching secondary to large breasts, or a breast mass. A thorough history with attention to type of pain, location, and relationship to menses and a careful physical examination are essential to rule out palpable masses or anatomic causes. All women should be up to date with screening mammography. Women with a palpable breast mass should be referred for diagnostic imaging. Women with noncyclic breast pain and no evidence of a breast mass should undergo targeted breast ultrasonography because approximately 1% of such patients may have breast cancer at the site of pain.

Despite common perception, there is no evidence that avoiding caffeine will relieve breast hypersensitivity or pain.

Danazol is approved by the FDA for management of mastalgia but is recommended only for management of persistent severe cyclic breast pain unrelieved by conservative management. Because this patient has noncyclic breast pain and danazol is associated with the side effects of acne, hirsutism, weight gain, and irregular vaginal bleeding, danazol is not a therapeutic option for this patient.

The addition of mammography to ultrasonography does not appear to improve diagnostic accuracy in young women with mammographically dense breasts.

Reassurance, coupled with the regular use of a fitted support bra, would be appropriate management for a patient with cyclic mastalgia and a normal physical examination. This patient has focal noncyclic mastalgia necessitating diagnostic imaging as the first step in management.

KEY POINT

- Patients with noncyclic mastalgia with focal breast pain but no palpable mass should undergo targeted breast ultrasonography because approximately 1% of such patients may have breast cancer at the site of pain.

Bibliography

Iddon J, Dixon JM. Mastalgia. BMJ. 2013;347:f3288. [PMID: 24336097] doi:10.1136/bmj.f3288

Item 97   Answer: D

Educational Objective: Estimate posttest probability using likelihood ratios.

This patient's posttest probability of ischemic coronary artery disease is approximately 95%. His pretest probability of ischemic coronary artery disease is estimated to be 50% based on clinical variables (including the nature of the chest pain, age, and sex). Likelihood ratios (LRs) are a statistical indicator of how much the result of a diagnostic test will increase or decrease the pretest probability of a disease in a specific patient. LRs may be determined from the sensitivity and specificity of a diagnostic test, and separate LRs are calculated for use when a test result is positive (LR+) or when a test result is negative (LR–). This patient has a positive result on a treadmill stress echocardiographic study, and the LR for a positive result on this test is approximately 10. Although very specific posttest probabilities may be calculated or estimated by using a nomogram, a clinical rule of thumb is that LR+ values of 2, 5, and 10 correspond to an increase in disease probability of 15%, 30%, and 45%, respectively. With a pretest probability of 50%, a positive result on treadmill stress echocardiography would increase the likelihood of disease by approximately 45%, leading to a posttest probability in the range of 95%; this information would be very useful clinically in making further treatment decisions.

If the stress test result had been negative, LR– values of 0.5, 0.2, and 0.1 correspond to a decrease in disease probability of 15%, 30%, and 45%, respectively. Tests with LRs between 0.5 and 2 do not alter the pretest probability significantly if they are positive or negative. Evaluating the LRs of a particular test may help in selecting an appropriate study to obtain useful clinical information in the diagnostic process.

Answers and Critiques

KEY POINT

- Likelihood ratios (LRs) are a statistical indicator of how much the result of a diagnostic test will increase or decrease the pretest probability of a disease in a specific patient; a clinical rule of thumb is that positive LRs of 2, 5, and 10 correspond to an increase in disease probability of 15%, 30%, and 45%, respectively.

Bibliography

Kent P, Hancock MJ. Interpretation of dichotomous outcomes: sensitivity, specificity, likelihood ratios, and pre-test and post-test probability. J Physiother. 2016;62:231-3. [PMID: 27637768] doi:10.1016/j.jphys.2016.08.008

KEY POINT

- For patients undergoing nonorthopedic surgery who are at high risk for postoperative venous thromboembolism as defined by the Caprini score, pharmacologic prophylaxis with low-molecular-weight heparin or low-dose unfractionated heparin and the addition of mechanical prophylaxis are recommended.

Bibliography

Gould MK, Garcia DA, Wren SM, Karanicolas PJ, Arcelus JI, Heit JA, et al. Prevention of VTE in nonorthopedic surgical patients: antithrombotic therapy and prevention of thrombosis, 9th ed: American College of Chest Physicians evidence-based clinical practice guidelines. Chest. 2012;141:e227S-e277S. [PMID: 22315263]

Item 98   Answer: E

Educational Objective: Prevent postoperative venous thromboembolism in a patient at high risk for venous thromboembolism.

Mechanical prophylaxis with intermittent pneumatic compression (IPC) and pharmacologic prophylaxis with low-molecular-weight heparin (LMWH) are appropriate for prevention of postoperative venous thromboembolism (VTE) in this patient undergoing nonorthopedic surgery. The American College of Chest Physicians (ACCP) antithrombotic guideline provides VTE prophylaxis recommendations for both orthopedic and nonorthopedic surgery populations. The ACCP guideline recommends using the Caprini score (https://venousdisease.com/dvt-risk-assessment-online/) to estimate risk for postoperative thrombosis in those undergoing general surgery, gastrointestinal surgery, urologic surgery, gynecologic surgery, bariatric surgery, vascular surgery, and plastic/reconstructive surgery (but not other types of surgeries). It includes weighted patient and surgery-related risk factors for VTE. A score of 0 defines very low risk for VTE (estimated VTE risk in the absence of prophylaxis, <0.5%); scores of 1 to 2 define low risk (VTE risk, 1.5%); scores of 3 to 4 define moderate risk (VTE risk, 3%); and scores of 5 or more define high risk (VTE risk, 6%). For patients at high risk for VTE, pharmacologic prophylaxis with LMWH or low-dose unfractionated heparin and the addition of mechanical prophylaxis are recommended. This patient has a high perioperative risk for VTE, with a Caprini score of 6 (1 point for history of inflammatory bowel disease, 2 points for major surgery >45 minutes, and 3 points for personal history of VTE). Therefore, IPC and LMWH are appropriate.

Evidence on clinical outcomes from randomized controlled trials evaluating graduated compression stockings is sparse. Available evidence shows no statistically significant difference in risk for mortality, symptomatic deep venous thrombosis, or pulmonary embolism. However, risk for lower extremity skin damage significantly increases among patients treated with compression stockings.

The addition of LMWH to graduated compression stockings is believed not to provide additional benefit to LMWH alone. In this patient, the recommended prophylaxis of IPC and heparin is most appropriate.

Item 99   Answer: C

Educational Objective: Treat radiation-induced nausea and vomiting in a patient with cancer.

The most appropriate treatment of this patient's nausea and vomiting in the setting of chemoradiation therapy is ondansetron. Nausea and vomiting are common complications of radiotherapy. Gastrointestinal mucosal injury and subsequent serotonin release are likely the driving mechanisms of this patient's nausea, and treatment targeting the neurotransmitter suspected of causing the nausea is a 5-hydroxytryptamine-3 (5-HT$_3$) antagonist, such as ondansetron. Dexamethasone may be added as an additional antiemetic therapy.

Haloperidol is a potent dopamine antagonist with robust antiemetic properties. Its numerous forms (intravenous, oral, sublingual concentrate) make it a versatile partner and commonly used medication to treat nausea in multiple settings, including hospice. However, given that the cause of this patient's nausea is suspected to be 5-HT$_3$ release in the setting of radiotherapy, ondansetron would be a preferred agent.

Olanzapine is a potent antiemetic with a diverse neurotransmitter profile, targeting dopamine, 5-HT$_3$, histaminic, and muscarinic receptors. It is effective in reducing chemotherapy-induced nausea and vomiting, but its efficacy in treating radiation-induced nausea has not yet been studied. However, olanzapine would be a reasonable choice for nausea refractory to other agents given its ability to affect multiple receptors implicated in nausea and vomiting.

Synthetic oral cannabinoids are not recommended as initial antiemetic therapy for any cancer-related condition. Experts recommend their use be limited to breakthrough symptoms caused by chemotherapy. Guidelines from the National Comprehensive Cancer Network, American Society of Clinical Oncology, and Multinational Association of Supportive Care in Cancer do not recommend the use of medical marijuana for the treatment of cancer-related nausea and vomiting.

KEY POINT

- A 5-hydroxytryptamine-3 (5-HT$_3$) antagonist, such as ondansetron, is the preferred initial agent for radiation-induced nausea and vomiting.

Bibliography

Berger MJ, Ettinger DS, Aston J, Barbour S, Bergsbaken J, Bierman PJ, et al. NCCN guidelines insights: antiemesis, version 2.2017. J Natl Compr Canc Netw. 2017;15:883-893. [PMID: 28687576] doi:10.6004/jnccn.2017.0117

Item 100   Answer: C

Educational Objective: Treat viral pharyngitis with symptom control.

The most appropriate management of this patient with pharyngitis is symptom control that might include an analgesic agent (such as an NSAID or acetaminophen), lozenges or topical sprays, and increased environmental humidity. Pharyngitis most commonly has viral causes; only 5% to 15% of pharyngitis cases are caused by bacteria, most often group A *Streptococcus pyogenes* (GAS). Clinicians must use clinical features to determine whether the patient meets the threshold for using a streptococcal rapid antigen detection test or throat culture. Several features are more predictive of a viral syndrome, and patients who present with a sore throat with accompanying features, such as conjunctivitis, cough, hoarseness, nasal congestion, and rhinorrhea, should not be tested for GAS pharyngitis. Additionally, the High Value Task Force of the American College of Physicians recommends that patients who meet fewer than three Centor criteria (fever by history, tonsillar exudates, tender anterior cervical lymphadenopathy, and absence of cough) need not be tested for GAS pharyngitis; these patients should be treated conservatively with symptom control.

Antibiotic treatment of pharyngitis is reserved for patients with a positive result on a rapid antigen detection test or throat culture; amoxicillin and penicillin are first-line therapy. In this case, the patient has features suggesting a viral cause, including cough and rhinorrhea. She also has only two Centor criteria: fever and tonsillar exudates. Therefore, she should not be treated with amoxicillin or other antibiotics or tested for GAS through rapid antigen detection testing or throat culture. She should be advised that her sore throat may last as long as 1 week.

Patients with severe pharyngitis should be assessed for more serious complications, including peritonsillar abscesses, epiglottitis, and Lemierre syndrome (thrombophlebitis of the internal jugular vein). *Fusobacterium necrophorum* has emerged as a cause of endemic pharyngitis in adolescents and young adults and is associated with Lemierre syndrome. Further study is needed to determine how to best distinguish *F. necrophorum* from other bacteria as the cause of pharyngitis.

KEY POINT

- Hallmark signs of viral pharyngitis include conjunctivitis, cough, nasal congestion, and rhinorrhea; viral pharyngitis should be treated symptomatically.

Bibliography

Harris AM, Hicks LA, Qaseem A; High Value Care Task Force of the American College of Physicians and for the Centers for Disease Control and Prevention. Appropriate antibiotic use for acute respiratory tract infection in adults: advice for high-value care from the American College of Physicians and the Centers for Disease Control and Prevention. Ann Intern Med. 2016;164:425-34. [PMID: 26785402] doi:10.7326/M15-1840

Item 101   Answer: B

Educational Objective: Diagnose neurally mediated syncope.

The most likely diagnosis is neurally mediated syncope. Neurally mediated syncope (also known as neurocardiogenic or reflex syncope) is the most common form of syncope and is seen primarily in younger adults. The underlying syncopal mechanism, termed the neurocardiogenic or vasodepressor reflex, is a response of vasodilation, bradycardia, and systemic hypotension, which leads to transient hypoperfusion of the brain. Neurally mediated syncope includes vasovagal syncope, which may be provoked by noxious stimuli, fear, stress, or heat overexposure; situational syncope, which is triggered by cough, micturition, defecation, or deglutition; and carotid sinus hypersensitivity, which is sometimes experienced during head rotation, shaving, or use of a tight-fitting neck collar. Prodromal symptoms, including nausea and diaphoresis, are classically present before the syncopal event, and fatigue and generalized weakness are typically present afterward.

Hypoglycemia in patients without diabetes mellitus is rare; therefore, evaluation for pathologic hypoglycemia should occur only in the presence of the Whipple triad: symptomatic hypoglycemia, documented plasma glucose level of 55 mg/dL (3.1 mmol/L) or lower, and prompt symptomatic relief with correction of hypoglycemia. This patient's quick recovery from the syncopal episode without any intervention is not compatible with hypoglycemia-induced syncope.

Orthostatic syncope is classically associated with rapid onset of syncope after positional changes. Prodromal symptoms (such as lightheadedness) are often present. Orthostatic syncope is most commonly caused by hypovolemia, medications, and alcohol intoxication. Less commonly, primary autonomic failure (Parkinson disease, multiple system atrophy, multiple sclerosis) or secondary autonomic failure (diabetes, amyloidosis, connective tissue disease, spinal cord injury) can lead to orthostatic syncope. The diagnosis is confirmed by a sustained reduction of 20 mm Hg or more in systolic blood pressure (or ≥10-mm Hg drop in diastolic blood pressure) within 3 minutes of assuming upright posture, which is not present in this patient.

Postural orthostatic tachycardia syndrome is characterized by (1) frequent symptoms that occur with standing (such as lightheadedness, palpitations, generalized weakness, blurred vision, and fatigue), (2) an increase in heart rate of more than 30/min during a positional change from supine to standing, and (3) the absence of orthostatic hypotension. The standing heart rate is often higher than 120/min. This patient's findings are not compatible with postural orthostatic tachycardia syndrome.

Answers and Critiques

KEY POINT

- Neurally mediated syncope is the most common form of syncope and is seen primarily in younger adults; prodromal symptoms (nausea, diaphoresis) are classically present before the syncopal event, and fatigue and generalized weakness are typically present afterward.

Bibliography

Runser LA, Gauer RL, Houser A. Syncope: evaluation and differential diagnosis. Am Fam Physician. 2017;95:303-312. [PMID: 28290647]

Item 102　Answer:　C

Educational Objective:　Treat a man with urgency urinary incontinence.

This patient reports symptoms consistent with urgency urinary incontinence, which can be best addressed with behavioral training and the use of anticholinergic agents or mirabegron. Urgency incontinence is characterized by loss of urine accompanied by a sense of urgency. The treatment of urinary incontinence generally progresses in a stepwise manner. Lifestyle changes and behavioral therapy should be initiated first, followed by pharmacologic therapy and devices, and finally surgery if all other therapies have failed. The patient is already appropriately using behavioral therapy in the form of bladder training and scheduled voiding. The addition of pharmacologic therapy is now appropriate. Anticholinergic drugs (darifenacin, fesoterodine, oxybutynin, solifenacin, tolterodine, trospium) reduce involuntary bladder contractions by blocking the muscarinic cholinergic receptors. Anticholinergic medications are appropriate for both men and women with urgency urinary incontinence, but caution should be exercised when initiating them in men with benign prostatic hyperplasia due to risk for urinary retention. The β-agonist mirabegron, another pharmacologic option for treatment of urgency urinary incontinence, enhances the inhibitory adrenergic signals to the detrusor muscle. Clinicians should base the choice of pharmacologic agents on tolerability, adverse effect profile, ease of use, and cost of medication.

Dutasteride is a 5α-reductase inhibitor used to treat benign prostatic hyperplasia. In this patient who is already being treated with tamsulosin and in whom postvoid residual bladder volume suggests that bladder outlet obstruction has been adequately addressed, there is no additional benefit from adding another therapy for benign prostatic hyperplasia; this therapy will not address the urgency and incontinence problems.

Intermittent self-catheterization might be a useful strategy for a patient with overflow incontinence due to bladder outlet obstruction. However, that is not the case, as demonstrated by this patient's bladder ultrasound, which shows a postvoid residual urine volume of only 30 mL.

Sacral nerve root stimulation is an acceptable treatment for urgency urinary incontinence in patients in whom behavioral and pharmacologic therapies fail. Placement of a sacral nerve root stimulator typically involves conscious sedation and may require general anesthesia.

KEY POINT

- Male patients with urgency urinary incontinence who have not achieved satisfactory relief of symptoms with behavioral therapy may benefit from the use of anticholinergic agents or mirabegron.

Bibliography

Gormley EA, Lightner DJ, Burgio KL, Chai TC, Clemens JQ, Culkin DJ, et al; American Urological Association. Diagnosis and treatment of overactive bladder (non-neurogenic) in adults: AUA/SUFU guideline. J Urol. 2012;188:2455-63. [PMID: 23098785] doi:10.1016/j.juro.2012.09.079

Item 103　Answer:　A

Educational Objective:　Screen for cervical cancer in a woman vaccinated against human papillomavirus infection.

This patient should be screened for cervical cancer with cytology (Pap testing) alone. Nearly all cases of cervical cancer are precipitated by persistent human papillomavirus (HPV) infection, and HPV (most commonly subtypes 16 and 18 [high-risk HPV]) is detected in most patients with cervical cancer. Immunization against HPV is thought to protect against 70% to 90% of cervical cancers depending on the type of vaccine received. However, in patients who have received the HPV vaccine series, routine cervical cancer screening is still strongly recommended. Recipients of the vaccine series may have been infected with HPV prior to immunization. Furthermore, HPV vaccination is not effective in clearing HPV infection and does not protect against all HPV types. The U.S. Preventive Services Task Force (USPSTF) has concluded that the benefits of screening for cervical cancer in women aged 21 to 29 years every 3 years with cytology alone substantially outweigh the harms.

HPV testing is not indicated in women younger than 30 years because of the higher prevalence of transient HPV in this age group. Therefore, this patient should receive Pap testing alone and not dual testing with cytology and HPV detection, or high-risk HPV testing.

In the 2018 recommendation statement, the USPSTF concluded that in women aged 30 to 65 years, the benefits of screening every 3 years with cytology alone or every 5 years with high-risk HPV testing alone outweigh the harms. Decision analysis modeling suggests that screening every 5 years with high-risk HPV testing alone in women aged 30 to 65 years results in a slightly lower mortality rate than with screening every 3 years with cytology alone but much higher rates of follow-up testing and colposcopy. Four HPV screening tests are approved by the FDA for HPV screening. The tests screen for up to 14 HPV types, but only one test specifically identifies the presence of high-risk HPV types (16 and 18); the other tests report a positive result if any HPV type is present. According to the American Society for Colposcopy and Cervical Pathology and the Society of Gynecologic Oncology, high-risk HPV testing alone can be considered as a primary cervical cancer screening modality in women aged 25 years and older; however, the American College of Obstetricians and Gynecologists has affirmed that cytology alone or cytology plus HPV testing are still specifically recommended in current guidelines from most major societies.

KEY POINT

- Routine cervical cancer screening with cytology alone is indicated in women aged 21 to 29 years, including those vaccinated against human papillomavirus.

Bibliography

Koliopoulos G, Nyaga VN, Santesso N, Bryant A, Martin-Hirsch PP, Mustafa RA, Schünemann H, Paraskevaidis E, Arbyn M. Cytology versus HPV testing for cervical cancer screening in the general population. Cochrane Database Syst Rev. 2017;8:CD008587. doi: 10.1002/14651858.CD008587.pub2. [PMID:28796882]

Item 104   Answer: B

Educational Objective: Treat symptomatic left-sided varicocele.

This patient's history and physical examination findings support a clinical diagnosis of symptomatic varicocele, and the appropriate treatment is analgesic therapy (ibuprofen) and scrotal support. Varicoceles are common, occurring in 15% of men. Notably, they are believed to be a leading cause of infertility; 40% of men who are infertile have varicoceles. They are the result of dilation of the pampiniform plexus of spermatic veins and can have a presentation ranging from no symptoms to dull aching scrotal fullness. Examination reveals a left-sided (90%) soft scrotal mass with a "bag of worms" consistency that increases with standing and decreases while supine. Ultrasonography is used for confirmation. Management is usually conservative, including analgesic agents; scrotal support should be pursued in all patients and is considered first-line therapy. Unilateral right-sided varicoceles are uncommon and may be associated with a significant underlying abnormality, such as inferior vena cava obstruction due to tumor or thrombosis because the right gonadal vein directly empties into the inferior vena cava. Many experts recommend advanced imaging with CT for patients with right-sided varicoceles.

Treatment with ceftriaxone plus doxycycline is recommended for infectious epididymitis. The chronic nature of this patient's symptoms, lack of fever, and a scrotal mass that increases with standing do not support a diagnosis of infectious epididymitis.

Surgical consultation for possible ligation or embolization of the gonadal vein would be appropriate in certain patients with symptomatic varicocele. Ligation or embolization of the gonadal vein prevents retrograde flow of blood to the pampiniform in the scrotum. Surgery may be considered in cases of testicular atrophy or infertility, or in cases refractory to first-line therapies. However, surgical repair may increase sperm counts without improving fertility. In this case, the patient has

no evidence of testicular atrophy, and he has not previously received treatment. Although a semen analysis would be reasonable to obtain, conservative therapies should still be offered at this time.

Topical lidocaine can provide local analgesia; however, its use in cases of varicocele has not been thoroughly investigated. Rather, a systemic analgesic agent with anti-inflammatory properties would be preferable.

KEY POINT

- In adult patients, first-line therapy for symptomatic left-sided varicocele that is not associated with testicular atrophy or infertility is analgesic agents and scrotal support.

Bibliography

Baigorri BF, Dixon RG. Varicocele: a review. Semin Intervent Radiol. 2016;33:170-6. [PMID: 27582603] doi:10.1055/s-0036-1586147

Item 105   Answer: C

Educational Objective: Treat carpal tunnel syndrome.

The most appropriate management is splinting of the wrist. This patient has symptoms strongly suggestive of carpal tunnel syndrome (CTS). CTS is caused by median nerve compression at the wrist; it presents with wrist pain that may radiate to the fingers or forearm and is often worse at night and with repetitive motion. Risk factors include female sex, pregnancy, connective tissue disorders, diabetes mellitus, hypothyroidism, and obesity. Examination findings are often minimal early in the disease but may include hypalgesia of the median nerve distribution (thumb and first three fingers) and weakened thumb abduction. Thenar muscle atrophy suggests severe disease. For patients with mild to moderate symptoms, initial therapy consists of avoiding repetitive hand and wrist motions; for persistent or more severe symptoms, neutral-position wrist splinting can be helpful. Splinting appears to be more effective when used full time rather than only at night.

CTS can be diagnosed on the basis of history and clinical examination findings. Electromyography is not necessary unless a patient's clinical presentation is atypical, other conditions (such as polyneuropathy, plexopathy, and radiculopathy) need to be excluded, or surgical intervention is being considered.

Local glucocorticoid injection can improve symptoms over the short term (up to 10 weeks). Although generally safe, injection therapy has known harms, including worsening of median nerve compression, accidental injection into nerves or vessels, and flexor tendon rupture. For these reasons, many experts recommend glucocorticoid injection as second-line therapy for CTS.

Surgical decompression of the median nerve is reserved for patients with symptoms that do not respond to conservative therapy or with evidence of severe neuropathy (such as weakened thumb abduction, thenar muscle atrophy, and an abnormal nerve conduction study). Electrodiagnostic studies are typically performed before surgery to confirm the presence of moderate to severe median nerve injury and to provide prognostic information.

KEY POINT

- Initial therapy for carpal tunnel syndrome consists of avoiding repetitive hand and wrist motions and neutral-position wrist splinting.

Bibliography
Hobson-Webb LD, Juel VC. Common entrapment neuropathies. Continuum (Minneap Minn). 2017;23:487-511. [PMID: 28375915] doi:10.1212/CON.0000000000000452

Item 106   Answer: B

Educational Objective: Diagnose scleritis in a patient with rheumatoid arthritis.

The most likely diagnosis in this patient with rheumatoid arthritis (RA) is scleritis. RA is one of the most common diseases associated with scleritis. Typical features include eye pain, pain with gentle palpation of the globe, and photophobia. The deep scleral vessels are involved and may lead to scleromalacia, which is characterized by thinning of the sclera and is seen as a dark area in the white sclera. Scleromalacia may lead to perforation of the sclera, called scleromalacia perforans. Scleritis can be vision-threatening and lead to blindness; it is therefore important to urgently refer the patient to an ophthalmologist for care.

Episcleritis is an abrupt inflammation of the superficial vessels of the episclera, a thin membrane that lies just beneath the conjunctiva. The cause is often unclear; rarely, it is associated with systemic rheumatologic disease. Patients with episcleritis frequently present without pain or decreased visual acuity. On examination, the inflammation appears localized. White sclera can be seen between superficial dilated blood vessels. Episcleritis typically resolves spontaneously. The presence of severe pain, diffuse redness, and decreased visual acuity make episcleritis an unlikely diagnosis.

Subconjunctival hemorrhage is a common disorder and typically benign in origin. It is caused by painless bleeding into the superficial portion of the eye. Examination reveals a blotchy redness (from extravascular blood) that is typically confined to one area of the conjunctiva. Subconjunctival hemorrhage is painless and not associated with loss of vision. Most cases resolve within several weeks without intervention. The patient's findings are not compatible with subconjunctival hemorrhage.

Viral conjunctivitis also causes a red eye. Typically, the underlying vessels are visible, a watery discharge may be seen, and the eyelids are matted in the morning. The eye may feel irritated, but there is no pain or loss of visual acuity. In general, conjunctivitis is a diagnosis of exclusion. The presence of pain and decreased visual acuity exclude viral conjunctivitis in this patient.

KEY POINT

- Rheumatoid arthritis is one of the most common diseases associated with scleritis, which can be vision-threatening and lead to thinning of the sclera and perforation.

Bibliography
Artifoni M, Rothschild PR, Brézin A, Guillevin L, Puéchal X. Ocular inflammatory diseases associated with rheumatoid arthritis. Nat Rev Rheumatol. 2014;10:108-16. [PMID: 24323074] doi:10.1038/nrrheum.2013.185

Item 107   Answer: C

Educational Objective: Select appropriate preoperative testing in a patient with chronic kidney disease.

This patient should undergo preoperative assessment of serum creatinine and electrolyte levels. Preoperative testing should be ordered selectively according to the patient's symptoms, medical history, medications, and physical examination findings. Serum creatinine and electrolyte levels should be measured preoperatively in patients with kidney disease and those who are taking medications that may affect kidney function or predispose them to electrolyte abnormalities, such as this patient, who has chronic kidney disease and is taking an ACE inhibitor (lisinopril) and diuretic (hydrochlorothiazide). In patients with chronic kidney disease undergoing surgery, electrolyte abnormalities should be corrected, and volume status should be optimized.

Serum aminotransferases (alanine aminotransferase and aspartate aminotransferase) should not be routinely ordered in the absence of known liver disease, symptoms suggestive of underlying liver disease, physical examination findings suspicious for liver disease, or history of abnormal liver chemistry results.

Coagulation testing is reserved for patients with a history of abnormal bleeding, those taking anticoagulants, and patients with medical conditions that predispose to coagulopathy (such as liver disease or hemophilia). For the patient with a history suggesting a bleeding disorder, preoperative prothrombin time, activated partial thromboplastin time, and platelet count measurements are indicated.

Routine preoperative laboratory panels are not recommended because they expose patients to unnecessary testing, risk for incidental findings that are lost to follow-up evaluation, and increased anxiety. However, given this patient's comorbidities and medication use, forgoing preoperative testing would be inappropriate.

KEY POINT

- Preoperative measurement of serum electrolyte and creatinine levels is recommended in patients with kidney disease and those who are taking medications that may affect kidney function or predispose them to electrolyte abnormalities.

Bibliography

Apfelbaum JL, Connis RT, Nickinovich DG, Pasternak LR, Arens JF, Caplan RA, et al; Committee on Standards and Practice Parameters. Practice advisory for preanesthesia evaluation: an updated report by the American Society of Anesthesiologists Task Force on Preanesthesia Evaluation. Anesthesiology. 2012;116:522-38. [PMID: 22273990] doi:10.1097/ALN.0b013e31823c1067

Item 108   Answer: B

Educational Objective: Avoid NSAID therapy in a patient who has undergone bariatric surgery.

Ibuprofen should be discontinued in this patient. This patient likely has patellofemoral pain syndrome, which is characterized by anterior knee pain that is usually gradual in onset and worsens with running, prolonged sitting, and climbing stairs. Applying direct pressure to the patella with the knee extended may reproduce the pain. Treatment generally includes activity modification and physical therapy. NSAIDs, acetaminophen, bracing, and patellar taping all have limited efficacy. Additionally, the use of NSAIDs in patients who have undergone bariatric surgery is associated with increased risk for internal bleeding; bleeding risk is increased at the sites of anastomoses and staple or suture lines in the early postoperative period, with increased risk of marginal or gastric ulceration in the later postoperative period. Therefore, ibuprofen and other NSAIDs should be avoided after bariatric surgery.

This patient with known risk factors for atherosclerotic cardiovascular disease meets the criteria for moderate- to high-intensity statin therapy and should continue atorvastatin. There is no association between statin therapy and adverse events after bariatric surgery.

Patients who have undergone bariatric surgery may experience a decline in blood pressure such that antihypertensive agents need to be reduced or discontinued. Close monitoring of blood pressure in the postoperative period is recommended. This patient's blood pressure is appropriate on the current dose of lisinopril and this drug does not need to be discontinued.

Similarly, patients who have undergone bariatric surgery may experience reduced need for medications for type 2 diabetes mellitus. Close monitoring for the development of hypoglycemia in the postoperative period is recommended. Hypoglycemia is unlikely with metformin therapy alone and does not need to be discontinued.

KEY POINT

- The use of NSAIDs in patients who have undergone bariatric surgery is associated with increased risk for internal bleeding; therefore, ibuprofen and other NSAIDs should be avoided after bariatric surgery because their use is associated with increased risk for internal bleeding.

Bibliography

Marcotte E, Chand B. Management and prevention of surgical and nutritional complications after bariatric surgery. Surg Clin North Am. 2016;96:843-56. [PMID: 27473805] doi:10.1016/j.suc.2016.03.006

Item 109   Answer: B

Educational Objective: Diagnose borderline personality disorder.

This patient demonstrates a behavioral pattern consistent with borderline personality disorder. A personality disorder is characterized by persistent patterns of inner experiences and behaviors that digress substantially from the expectations of the affected person's culture. These disorders are entrenched, rigid, and stable over time and lead to substantial impairment and distress. Onset is usually during adolescence or early adulthood. Persons with personality disorders usually do not recognize their interactions with others as abnormal. In borderline personality disorder, patients have chaotic interpersonal relationships, emotional lability, and impulsive and self-destructive behaviors (such as suicide attempts). Patients have exaggerated responses to social stressors and often perceive people as "all good" or "all bad." Comorbid psychiatric illness is common in patients with borderline personality disorder. The initial management focuses on establishing rapport and boundaries with the patient, which can improve the patient's acceptance of psychiatry referral. Psychotherapy can be effective at improving coping mechanisms. No pharmacologic therapies are approved for treating personality disorders directly, but medications can be prescribed for specific symptoms (such as mood stabilizers for impulsivity).

Bipolar disorder is characterized by manic episodes (in which patients have decreased need for sleep, greater distractibility, and increased energy) and major depressive episodes. Although patients with bipolar disorder may engage in self-destructive behavior, it is not related to interpersonal discord.

Patients with generalized anxiety disorder have excessive anxiety and worry about multiple aspects of their lives. This leads to insomnia, irritability, and fatigue. Patients with generalized anxiety disorder do not typically have impulsivity, relationship instability, or the tendency to idealize and devalue individuals as do patients with borderline personality disorder.

Histrionic personality disorder is characterized by excessive need for approval and attention-seeking behaviors. Patients with this disorder are emotionally vulnerable, and their behaviors focus on obtaining approval from others. Patients with histrionic personality disorders are uncomfortable if not the center of attention and typically use physical appearance to draw attention to self. Interaction with others may be inappropriately sexually seductive or provocative. Histrionic personality disorder is not accompanied by the same degree of emotional lability and risk for suicidality as borderline personality disorder, as exhibited in this patient.

KEY POINT

- Patients with borderline personality disorder have chaotic interpersonal relationships, emotional lability, impulsive and self-destructive behaviors, and exaggerated responses to social stressors; comorbidity with other psychiatric illnesses is high.

Answers and Critiques

Bibliography

Gunderson JG. Clinical practice. Borderline personality disorder. N Engl J Med. 2011;364:2037–42. [PMID: 21612472] doi:10.1056/NEJMcp1007358

Item 110   Answer: A

Educational Objective: Treat systemic exertion intolerance disease with cognitive behavioral therapy.

The most appropriate treatment for this patient with systemic exertion intolerance disease (SEID) is cognitive behavioral therapy. According to the Institute of Medicine (now the National Academy of Medicine), SEID is diagnosed by the presence of fatigue of at least 6 months' duration with substantial reduction in preillness activities, postexertional malaise, unrefreshing sleep, and either cognitive impairment or orthostatic intolerance (symptoms such as lightheadedness, dizziness, fatigue, cognitive deficits, and visual difficulties that worsen with upright posture and improve with recumbency). Patients with SEID benefit most from a structured, well-defined, multimodal approach that includes regularly scheduled office visits, which allow for discussion, educational opportunities, and longitudinal reassessment. There is evidence that cognitive behavioral therapy and graded exercise therapy may decrease fatigue and improve function, and these therapies should be offered to patients. Additionally, all patients should receive instruction on effective sleep hygiene. Other modalities that may be of benefit include physical therapy, occupational therapy, biofeedback therapy, massage therapy, acupuncture, yoga, tai chi, and stress management activities. Considering this patient's depression (which is likely a consequence of her chronic symptoms), cognitive behavioral therapy is an ideal treatment.

Although methylphenidate, prednisone, opioids, antiinflammatory agents, and antimicrobial agents are commonly requested in clinical practice for the treatment of chronic fatigue symptoms, there is no consistent evidence that these agents improve symptoms or prognosis in patients with SEID. Given the lack of benefit, risk for abuse, addictive potential, and array of adverse effects, these options are not recommended.

Mirtazapine (an α_2-agonist) and sertraline (a selective serotonin reuptake inhibitor) are used to treat depression. In general, selective antidepressant therapy may be useful in treating associated depression; however, it is not a direct treatment for SEID. Mirtazapine and sertraline might improve this patient's symptoms of depression, but it will not address the other symptoms associated with SEID.

KEY POINT

- The treatment of systemic exertion intolerance disease involves a structured, multimodal, nonpharmacologic approach that includes regularly scheduled office visits, cognitive behavioral therapy, graded exercise therapy, and sleep hygiene education.

Bibliography

Janse A, Nikolaus S, Wiborg JF, Heins M, van der Meer JWM, Bleijenberg G, Tummers M, Twisk J, Knoop H. Long-term follow-up after cognitive behaviour therapy for chronic fatigue syndrome. J Psychosom Res. 2017;97:45–51. [PMID: 28606498] doi:10.1016/j.jpsychores.2017.03.016

Item 111   Answer: D

Educational Objective: Manage hormonal contraception prescribing by first excluding pregnancy.

Pregnancy testing is the next step in this patient's management. Strategies to reduce unintended pregnancy require assessing pregnancy risk, counseling patients regarding contraceptive options, and ensuring correct and consistent use of contraceptives. Most women can start most contraceptive methods at any time. Available contraceptive methods include hormonal contraception; long-acting reversible preparations, including intrauterine devices; barrier contraceptives; and sterilization. Other than a thorough history and blood pressure and BMI measurements, few examinations or tests, if any, are needed before starting a contraceptive method. A pregnancy test should be obtained if more than 7 days have elapsed since the start of the last menses.

Hormonal contraceptive options include oral contraceptive pills (combination estrogen-progesterone or progesterone-only pills), long-acting reversible contraceptives, transdermal patches, and vaginal rings. Contraindications to combination products include breast cancer, liver disease, migraine with aura, uncontrolled hypertension, and venous thromboembolism. Estrogen-containing preparations are contraindicated in women older than 35 years who smoke more than 15 cigarettes a day. A family history of breast cancer is not a contraindication for hormonal contraception.

In healthy women of reproductive age, a breast examination, pelvic examination, or mammography are not needed before beginning hormonal contraception. Breast cancer and cervical cancer screenings should be performed according to established guidelines. In 2016, the U.S. Preventive Services Task Force (USPSTF) reaffirmed its recommendation for biennial screening mammography in all women aged 50 to 74 years. The USPSTF recommends individualized screening decisions for women aged 40 to 49 years based on patient context and values regarding specific benefits and harms. The patient has no indications for mammography at this time.

According to the USPSTF, cervical cancer screening in women aged 21 to 65 years may be accomplished with cytology (Pap test) every 3 years. This patient's last Pap smear was normal 2 years ago, and she does not need to undergo repeat Pap testing for another 12 months.

KEY POINT

- Before initiating hormonal contraception, a negative pregnancy test result must be documented if 7 days have passed since the onset of the last menstrual period.

Bibliography

Curtis KM, Jatlaoui TC, Tepper NK, Zapata LB, Horton LG, Jamieson DJ, Whiteman MK. U.S. Selected practice recommendations for contraceptive use, 2016. MMWR Recomm Rep. 2016;65:1–66. [PMID: 27467319] doi:10.15585/mmwr.rr6504a1

Item 112   Answer: C

Educational Objective: Treat a patient with acute low back pain with nonpharmacologic modalities.

The most appropriate initial treatment of this patient's low back pain is nonpharmacologic therapy. According to a 2017 clinical practice guideline issued by the American College of Physicians, clinicians should choose nonpharmacologic treatments as first-line therapy for acute low back pain. Options include superficial heat, acupuncture, massage, and spinal manipulation. The quality of evidence supporting individual nonpharmacologic measures is moderate or low. Recommendations for their use are based on the fact that most patients with acute low back pain will improve over time (most within 4 weeks), regardless of the treatment chosen. Harms of nonpharmacologic interventions were seldom and minor. Superficial heat was associated with increased risk for skin flushing, and massage and spinal manipulation were associated with muscle soreness.

Recent evidence, including a Cochrane review, has demonstrated that acetaminophen is not effective in treating acute low back pain. As such, it would be inappropriate to recommend its use in this patient.

The FDA has approved the use of duloxetine in chronic back pain (pain lasting >12 weeks), as studies have demonstrated its effectiveness. However, no evidence supports its use for acute low back pain.

Guidelines recommend that opioids should be the last treatment option considered for chronic back pain and should be considered only in patients in whom other therapies have failed, as these drugs are associated with substantial harms. Harms of short-term opioid therapy include increased constipation, dizziness, dry mouth, nausea, somnolence, and vomiting. Studies assessing opioids for the treatment of chronic low back pain did not address the risk for addiction, abuse, or overdose, although observational studies have shown a dose-dependent relationship between opioid use for chronic pain and serious harms. A 2018 randomized trial demonstrated that treatment with opioids was not superior to treatment with nonopioid medications for improving pain-related function for chronic back pain. In addition, pain intensity was significantly improved in the nonopioid group. There are no studies of opioids for the treatment of acute back pain, but given their questionable effect and substantial harms as well as the self-limited nature of acute nonspecific back pain, opioids should likely be avoided entirely.

KEY POINT

- First-line treatment of acute low back pain is non-pharmacologic therapy, including acupuncture, massage, spinal manipulation, and superficial heat; most patients will improve over time, regardless of the treatment chosen.

Bibliography

Qaseem A, Wilt TJ, McLean RM, Forciea MA; Clinical Guidelines Committee of the American College of Physicians. Noninvasive treatments for acute, subacute, and chronic low back pain: a clinical practice guideline from the American College of Physicians. Ann Intern Med. 2017;166:514-530. [PMID: 28192789] doi:10.7326/M16-2367

Item 113   Answer: C

Educational Objective: Prevent atherosclerotic cardiovascular disease in a patient with type 2 diabetes mellitus with statin therapy.

The most appropriate treatment for primary prevention of atherosclerotic cardiovascular disease (ASCVD) in this patient is moderate- or high-intensity atorvastatin. Intensity of statin therapy is defined by the expected decrease in LDL cholesterol levels; high-intensity statin therapy should decrease LDL cholesterol levels by at least 50% from baseline levels, whereas moderate-intensity statin therapy should decrease LDL cholesterol levels by 30% to 50%. High-intensity statin regimens recommended by the 2013 American College of Cardiology (ACC)/American Heart Association (AHA) cholesterol treatment guideline include atorvastatin, 40 mg/d to 80 mg/d, and rosuvastatin, 20 mg/d to 40 mg/d. For primary prevention of ASCVD in patients with diabetes mellitus, the decision to initiate high-intensity statin therapy or moderate-intensity statin therapy is based on the patient's estimated 10-year ASCVD risk. According to the ACC/AHA guideline, patients with diabetes with an estimated 10-year ASCVD risk of 7.5% or higher should receive high-intensity statin therapy, whereas those with an estimated 10-year ASCVD risk less than 7.5% should receive moderate-intensity statin therapy. In contrast to the ACC/AHA recommendations, the U.S. Preventive Services Task Force recommends initiating low- to moderate-intensity statin therapy in adults aged 40 to 75 years without a history of ASCVD who have one or more ASCVD risk factors (dyslipidemia, diabetes, hypertension, or smoking) and a calculated 10-year ASCVD event risk of 10% or higher.

Nonstatin drugs are not considered first-line therapy for the prevention of ASCVD in patients with or without diabetes. Fibrates, such as fenofibrate, would be first-line therapy for hypertriglyceridemia (typically, when the triglyceride level is >500 mg/dL [5.65 mmol/L]) for prevention of triglyceride-induced acute pancreatitis.

A 2017 systematic review concluded that among randomized controlled trials and observational studies, evidence of variable strength showed no association between increased fish oil intake and lower cardiovascular disease event risk. Expert opinion recommends that the use of fish oil supplementation be restricted to patients with refractory hypertriglyceridemia.

All patients should receive education on therapeutic lifestyle changes, including regular exercise, weight loss, and dietary changes. However, lifestyle modifications alone are not considered adequate for cardiovascular risk reduction in many patient groups, including patients with diabetes.

KEY POINT

- Patients with diabetes mellitus are at significantly increased lifetime risk for cardiovascular events and should receive statin therapy for primary prevention.

Bibliography
Stone NJ, Robinson JG, Lichtenstein AH, Bairey Merz CN, Blum CB, Eckel RH, et al; American College of Cardiology/American Heart Association Task Force on Practice Guidelines. 2013 ACC/AHA guideline on the treatment of blood cholesterol to reduce atherosclerotic cardiovascular risk in adults: a report of the American College of Cardiology/American Heart Association Task Force on Practice Guidelines. Circulation. 2014;129:S1-45. [PMID: 24222016] doi:10.1161/01.cir.0000437738.63853.7a

Item 114   Answer: A

Educational Objective: Treat insomnia with cognitive behavioral therapy.

The most appropriate next step in management would be to pursue targeted cognitive behavioral therapy for this patient. The American College of Physicians recommends cognitive behavioral therapy for insomnia (CBT-I) as first-line therapy for insomnia. CBT-I combines components of sleep hygiene with cognitive therapeutic interventions (to understand and identify appropriate sleep expectations) and behavioral interventions (such as relaxation techniques). Elements of sleep hygiene include avoiding strenuous exercise, large meals, caffeine, alcohol, and nicotine close to bedtime; establishing a relaxing prebedtime routine; keeping the room dark and quiet; avoiding reading, television, and use of electronic devices while in bed; and keeping a stable bedtime and arising time. CBT-I may be delivered in various formats, such as individual or group therapy, web-based modules, or written materials. It provides significant value over pharmacologic-driven approaches and carries little risk for adverse effects.

Although diphenhydramine and melatonin are popular over-the-counter remedies for insomnia, there is insufficient evidence to recommend their use before a trial of CBT-I. Additionally, sedating antihistamines (such as diphenhydramine) are associated with anticholinergic side effects and carry-over daytime sleepiness.

Some antidepressants, such as mirtazapine, are sedating and may improve sleep. Doxepin, in low doses, is the only antidepressant approved for the treatment of insomnia. Most expert opinion recommends against using antidepressants for treating insomnia in patients without depression; however, doxepin, trazodone, and mirtazapine can be useful if a sedating antidepressant is indicated.

Benzodiazepines (flurazepam, triazolam, temazepam) are effective for short-term insomnia treatment. However, their use is limited by tolerance; side effects of daytime somnolence, falls, cognitive impairment, and anterograde amnesia; and the potential for dependence. Rebound insomnia may occur upon discontinuation, especially if discontinuation is abrupt. The selective nature and shorter half-life of nonbenzodiazepines (zolpidem, zaleplon, eszopiclone) lead to fewer side effects (including rebound insomnia), making these drugs better initial choices if pharmacotherapy is warranted. However, sedation, disorientation, and agitation may still occur; rare side effects include sleep driving, sleep walking, and sleep eating. In this patient, CBT-I should be tried before pharmacologic therapy with zolpidem is considered.

KEY POINT

- Cognitive behavioral therapy for insomnia, which combines components of sleep hygiene with cognitive therapy and behavioral interventions, is first-line therapy for insomnia.

Bibliography
Qaseem A, Kansagara D, Forciea MA, Cooke M, Denberg TD; Clinical Guidelines Committee of the American College of Physicians. Management of chronic insomnia disorder in adults: a clinical practice guideline from the American College of Physicians. Ann Intern Med. 2016;165:125-33. [PMID: 27136449] doi: 10.7326/M15-2175

Item 115   Answer: C

Educational Objective: Effectively manage termination of a physician-patient relationship.

The most appropriate management is to send the patient a formal, written warning informing him that the patient-physician relationship may be terminated unless he is able to meaningfully participate in the plan of care. Physician-patient relationships are formed on the basis of mutual agreement. Rarely, the relationship fails to reach mutual goals and becomes unproductive. In some cases, the patient may not adhere to recommended therapies or may demonstrate inappropriate behavior with the physician or staff members, and it may be appropriate for the physician to terminate the relationship. After reasonable attempts to resolve differences have failed, the patient should be notified in writing that the relationship has been terminated and that care should be obtained from a different provider, usually with a several-week time frame for the patient to continue receiving urgent care. Terminations should occur only if the patient is medically stable and when alternative care is available. If a patient threatens a physician or staff member, the termination may be immediate.

Although a psychiatrist might provide interventions to help this patient better adhere to care recommendations, such a referral is unnecessary in making a decision to terminate an ineffective physician-patient relationship.

This patient has not demonstrated signs of an unstable mental health condition that warrants intervention by a crisis team.

Patient abandonment is unethical and may be a cause for legal action. In this case, the patient has not yet received a formal warning that his failure to adhere to treatment goals may result in his termination from the practice. Therefore, he should not be released from the practice immediately.

KEY POINT

- If the physician-patient relationship becomes irreparably compromised because of lack of trust, lack of mutual goals, or failure to maintain an effective working relationship despite efforts to resolve differences, the relationship can be terminated.

Bibliography

Snyder L; American College of Physicians Ethics, Professionalism, and Human Rights Committee. American College of Physicians ethics manual: sixth edition. Ann Intern Med. 2012;156:73-104. [PMID: 22213573] doi: 10.7326/0003-4819-156-1-201201031-00001

Item 116 Answer: C

Educational Objective: Treat neurogenic thoracic outlet syndrome.

Physical therapy aimed at shoulder girdle muscle strengthening and improving posture would be the best therapeutic option for this patient with thoracic outlet syndrome (TOS). TOS is caused by compression of the brachial plexus, subclavian artery, or subclavian vein as these structures pass through the thoracic outlet. There are three main clinical subtypes of TOS, defined by the primary structure involved (nerve, artery, vein). Neurogenic TOS is the most common subtype and is caused by compression of the brachial plexus nerve roots as they exit the triangle formed by the first rib and the scalenus anticus and medius muscles. Symptoms include paresthesias and pain that typically worsen with activities that involve continued use of the arm or hand, especially those that include elevation of the arm. This patient's presentation is most consistent with neurogenic TOS. In most patients, there are no abnormal neurologic findings. Electrodiagnostic studies frequently fail to reveal any abnormalities. Although imaging studies are often obtained, they are not required to make the diagnosis; they may, however, reveal the presence of a structural abnormality, such as an anomalous cervical rib. First-line therapy for neurogenic TOS includes improving posture and strengthening shoulder girdle muscles.

Although neurogenic TOS is caused by intermittent compression of the brachial plexus within the thoracic outlet, the role of gabapentin in managing this condition has not been well studied. Gabapentin is not considered to be first-line therapy.

Observational studies have supported the use of interscalene injection of anesthetic agents, glucocorticoids, or botulinum toxin type A in patients with neurogenic TOS. However, in a randomized, double-blind clinical trial, patients treated with botulinum toxin did not show improvement in function, pain, or paresthesias compared with patients treated with placebo.

Surgical decompression is not considered to be first-line therapy for neurogenic TOS, especially in patients who lack neurologic abnormalities. The procedure is reserved for patients who do not respond to conservative measures or for those with progressive or disabling neurologic symptoms.

KEY POINT

- Symptoms of neurogenic thoracic outlet syndrome include paresthesias and pain that typically worsen with activities that involve continued use of the arm or hand, especially those that include elevation of the arm; first-line therapy includes improving posture and strengthening the shoulder girdle muscles.

Bibliography

Buller LT, Jose J, Baraga M, Lesniak B. Thoracic outlet syndrome: current concepts, imaging features, and therapeutic strategies. Am J Orthop (Belle Mead NJ). 2015;44:376-82. [PMID: 26251937]

Item 117 Answer: D

Educational Objective: Diagnose sudden sensorineural hearing loss.

The most likely diagnosis for this patient's acute, unilateral hearing loss is sudden sensorineural hearing loss (SSHL). The right-sided hearing loss and the finding of lateralization to the left ear on Weber testing support the diagnosis. Approximately 90% of cases of SSHL are idiopathic; however, viral infection, drug reactions, acoustic neuroma, multiple sclerosis, head injury, vascular issues, systemic immune-mediated conditions, and Meniere disease can all be causes. SSHL most commonly presents as unilateral tinnitus and ear fullness; vertigo occurs less often. Because this patient lacks other features to explain the acute hearing loss, she should undergo urgent referral to an otolaryngologist for audiometry, clinical assessment, and MRI to exclude tumors, multiple sclerosis, or vascular causes. Treatment involves oral glucocorticoids, although strong evidence of efficacy is lacking.

Meniere disease, which is associated with endolymphatic hydrops (excess fluid in the endolymphatic spaces), can cause unilateral sensorineural hearing loss, but its presentation is characterized by episodic vertigo (lasting between 20 minutes and 24 hours) and tinnitus, which is often low pitched. The hearing loss may be described as fluctuating, and early in the disease it often involves low frequencies. Meniere disease may also present with a sensation of ear fullness.

Otosclerosis involves bony overgrowth on the footplate of the stapes, leading to a lack of functioning of the ossicles. This middle ear process typically causes gradual, painless, bilateral conductive hearing loss, not sensorineural hearing loss, as seen in this patient. Otosclerosis occurs more often in women, and there is often a family history of the condition.

Ototoxicity also can result in sensorineural hearing loss; it may be caused by a variety of medications, including antibiotics (particularly aminoglycosides), chemotherapeutic agents, loop diuretics, and aspirin or other NSAIDs. Often occurring gradually and bilaterally, ototoxicity may be reversible or permanent, depending on the agent involved. This patient is not taking and has not been exposed to drugs known to be ototoxic.

KEY POINT

- All patients with sudden sensorineural hearing loss should undergo audiometric evaluation, and most patients will require MRI.

Bibliography

Chin CJ, Dorman K. Sudden sensorineural hearing loss. CMAJ. 2017; 189:E437-E438. [PMID: 28385715] doi:10.1503/cmaj.161191

Item 118   Answer: A

Educational Objective: Treat a pressure injury with a hydrocolloid dressing.

This patient's pressure injury would be best managed with hydrocolloid or foam dressings, which have been found to be superior to standard gauze dressings in reducing ulcer size in low-quality studies. Pressure injuries (also known as pressure ulcers) are characterized by localized injury to the skin or soft tissue as a result of pressure and shear forces. They may be classified by use of a staging system, with each stage distinguished by the amount of tissue loss. In 2015, the American College of Physicians (ACP) published a clinical practice guideline for the treatment of pressure ulcers. The ACP recommends that clinicians use hydrocolloid or foam dressings in patients with pressure ulcers to reduce wound size. Hydrocolloid dressings consist of a mixture of adhesive absorbent polymers and a gelling agent, with a film covering to make them water and gas permeable. The dressing interacts with the wound fluid to form a gel. Hydrocolloids may promote wound healing by enhancing fibrinolytic activity and growth of granulation tissue and inhibiting bacterial overgrowth through their physical barrier properties. Hydrocolloids are convenient to use because they require infrequent dressing changes and are easy to apply. Foam dressings are sheets of foam polymers and are used primarily for heavily exudative wounds. Other treatment options include managing the conditions that caused the pressure injury, wound protection, surgical debridement and repair, and vacuum-assisted closure. There is moderate-quality evidence that air-fluidized beds reduce the size of pressure injuries compared with other support surfaces. The ACP also recommends protein or amino acid supplements (low-quality evidence) and electrical stimulation (moderate-quality evidence) as adjunctive therapy to accelerate wound healing.

There is insufficient evidence to recommend for or against platelet-derived growth factor dressings in the treatment of pressure injuries, and no studies have explored the benefits of vitamin- or mineral-infused dressings (such as a zinc-infused dressing). In addition, insufficient evidence was found to recommend for or against hydrotherapy, hyperbaric oxygen therapy, or maggot therapy.

KEY POINT

- Hydrocolloid or foam dressings are superior to standard gauze dressings in the treatment of pressure injuries; protein supplements and the use of electrical stimulation to accelerate wound healing are also recommended treatment strategies.

Bibliography

Qaseem A, Humphrey LL, Forciea MA, Starkey M, Denberg TD; Clinical Guidelines Committee of the American College of Physicians. Treatment of pressure ulcers: a clinical practice guideline from the American College of Physicians. Ann Intern Med. 2015;162:370–9. [PMID: 25732279] doi:10.7326/M14-1568

Item 119   Answer: C

Educational Objective: Treat obsessive–compulsive disorder with cognitive behavioral therapy.

The preferred initial treatment for this patient with obsessive-compulsive disorder (OCD) is cognitive behavioral therapy (CBT). OCD is an anxiety disorder in which patients experience obsessions (recurrent, intrusive thoughts, images, or impulses causing distress) and compulsions (repetitive behaviors done to alleviate obsession-related anxiety). Loss of time and disrupted social interactions from these thoughts and behaviors cause significant functional impairment. CBT is first-line treatment because it is more effective than pharmacotherapy alone. However, a combination of CBT and selective serotonin reuptake inhibitor (SSRI) therapy is useful for patients with severe symptoms or inadequate response to CBT. Although evidence is strongest for adjunctive therapy with SSRIs, more recent data support the adjunctive use of neuroleptics, deep-brain stimulation, and neurosurgical ablation for treatment-resistant OCD.

Buspirone is beneficial in the treatment of generalized anxiety disorder without comorbid anxiety or mood disorders but has no demonstrated benefit in patients with OCD.

Benzodiazepines, such as clonazepam, are used for short-term treatment of debilitating symptoms from severe generalized anxiety disorder and panic disorder, but they are not effective in the treatment of OCD.

Risperidone is an antipsychotic medication that can be used in the treatment of schizophrenia or other psychiatric conditions with psychotic features. Patients with OCD have obsessions and compulsions but do not have hallucinations, delusions, or disorganized thoughts that would warrant antipsychotic therapy.

KEY POINT

- Obsessive-compulsive disorder should be treated with cognitive behavioral therapy (CBT); a combination of CBT and selective serotonin reuptake inhibitor therapy is useful for patients with severe symptoms or inadequate response to CBT.

Bibliography

Hirschtritt ME, Bloch MH, Mathews CA. Obsessive-compulsive disorder: advances in diagnosis and treatment. JAMA. 2017;317:1358–1367. [PMID: 28384832] doi:10.1001/jama.2017.2200

Item 120   Answer: C

Educational Objective: Treat a patient with acute epididymitis.

The most appropriate treatment is ceftriaxone and levofloxacin. This patient's history and physical examination findings (fever, erythema, and swelling of the hemiscrotum; tenderness to palpation near the epididymis; and urinary symptoms) are concerning for a diagnosis of acute epididymitis. Prehn sign, which is alleviation of pain with elevation of the testicle or scrotum, can clinically support this diagnosis. Infectious epididymitis has a bimodal distribution: men younger than 35 years and older than 55 years. In younger patients, sexually transmitted infections (chlamydia and gonorrhea) are the most likely cause. In older patients and those who practice insertive anal intercourse, *Escherichia coli*, Enterobacteriaceae, and *Pseudomonas* species should be considered. In older men and persons who practice insertive anal intercourse, infectious epididymitis should be treated with ceftriaxone and a fluoroquinolone, such as levofloxacin.

Empiric treatment with ceftriaxone alone would provide adequate coverage for *Chlamydia trachomatis* infection but would be inadequate therapy. This older patient, who has risk factors for gram-negative infection, should be treated with ceftriaxone and a fluoroquinolone.

In younger patients (age <35 years), the most common infectious etiologies of acute epididymitis include *C. trachomatis* and *Neisseria gonorrhoeae*. In these men, and in the absence of risk factors for gram-negative infection (anal intercourse, urologic instrumentation), empirically treating with ceftriaxone and doxycycline (or azithromycin, if the patient is intolerant to doxycycline) would be appropriate.

Epididymitis can also have noninfectious causes (for example, trauma, autoimmune disease, or vasculitis). Treatment includes scrotal support, ice, and NSAIDs. Analgesic agents and scrotal support are supportive measures that can be offered to all patients presenting with acute epididymitis. However, the most appropriate treatment for this patient with risk factors for bacterial epididymitis and no history of trauma or findings supporting autoimmune disease or vasculitis would be initiation of an antimicrobial regimen rather than supportive therapies alone.

KEY POINT

- In older men and persons who practice insertive anal intercourse, infectious epididymitis should be treated with ceftriaxone and a fluoroquinolone, such as levofloxacin.

Bibliography

McConaghy JR, Panchal B. Epididymitis: an overview. Am Fam Physician. 2016;94:723-726. [PMID: 27929243]

Item 121   Answer: C

Educational Objective: Evaluate a breast mass in a woman aged 30 years and older.

This patient's breast mass should be evaluated with both diagnostic mammography and ultrasonography. Any dominant mass in the breast warrants diagnostic imaging to determine the nature of the mass and the appropriate management. A clinical examination alone cannot differentiate between a cyst and a solid mass. In a woman aged 30 years or older, diagnostic mammography is recommended for evaluation of a palpable mass, to assess for a spiculated density or associated pleomorphic calcifications that may indicate malignancy. Diagnostic mammography may also include magnification views of the focal area of concern. In

addition, targeted ultrasonography is needed to determine whether the mass is cystic or solid; however, ultrasonography is unnecessary in cases in which mammography shows a clearly benign correlate or a normal, fatty area of breast tissue in the location of the palpable finding. This diagnostic evaluation can help determine a benign finding from an indeterminate or suspicious finding requiring needle biopsy. For women aged 40 years or older, mammography, followed in most cases by ultrasonography, is recommended. For women aged 30 to 39 years old, ultrasonography or mammography may be performed first at the discretion of the radiologist or referring clinician.

Breast MRI and other advanced imaging have little to no role in the routine diagnostic evaluation of palpable breast abnormalities. Breast MRI is not an appropriate imaging technique for evaluation of palpable symptoms because it provides little added information to careful evaluation with mammography and ultrasonography.

Definitive diagnosis of a breast mass is obtained by tissue sampling using fine-needle aspiration, core-needle biopsy with or without stereotactic or ultrasound guidance, or excisional biopsy. Fine-needle aspiration is generally reserved for ultrasound-confirmed cystic lesions. Core-needle biopsy is the test of choice for most solid lesions, as it provides more tissue for histology and tissue markers. Excisional biopsy is used when core-needle biopsy findings are nondiagnostic or when biopsy and imaging studies do not concur. Further management of abnormal pathologic findings requires consultation with a breast surgeon and oncologist. Needle aspiration, core-needle biopsy, and excision are all premature until the imaging evaluation is completed.

Ultrasonography is often preferred in women younger than age 30 years because the increased density of breast tissue in younger women limits the usefulness of mammography. Ultrasonography may also be a better choice for pregnant patients in order to avoid radiation exposure.

KEY POINT

- For evaluation of palpable breast abnormalities in women aged 40 years or older, mammography, followed in most cases by ultrasonography, is recommended.

Bibliography

Lehman CD, Lee AY, Lee CI. Imaging management of palpable breast abnormalities. AJR Am J Roentgenol. 2014;203:1142-53. [PMID: 25341156] doi:10.2214/AJR.14.12725

Item 122   Answer: C

Educational Objective: Identify medications to avoid during pregnancy.

This patient should discontinue the ACE inhibitor lisinopril. Medication adjustments are an important component of preconception counseling in women who are planning pregnancy. All antihypertensive medications cross the placenta. Some antihypertensive medications are absolutely contraindicated during pregnancy, including ACE inhibitors, angiotensin receptor blockers (ARBs), and, likely, renin inhibitors. Women taking ACE inhibitors or ARBs should be counseled about the associated teratogenicity throughout all trimesters, and these medications should be stopped if pregnancy is anticipated or possible. Blood pressure goals with medical therapy in patients with chronic hypertension during pregnancy are 120 to 160/80 to 105 mm Hg. However, treatment of hypertension during pregnancy is controversial. If blood pressure control is not adequate after stopping lisinopril, methyldopa and labetalol have been used safely. Calcium channel blockers (such as long-acting nifedipine) can also be used during pregnancy. Diuretics may induce oligohydramnios if initiated during pregnancy but generally can be continued if the patient was taking a diuretic preconception. Spironolactone and eplerenone should be avoided because their safety has never been proven.

Although acetaminophen is generally considered safe during pregnancy, caution is needed with the use of NSAIDs due to their effect on organogenesis during pregnancy.

A goal for preconception wellness is the absence of uncontrolled depression. Evidence shows that women who are depressed during pregnancy have worse birth outcomes. Selective serotonin reuptake inhibitors, including citalopram, fluvoxamine, and sertraline, are pregnancy category C agents that can be continued during pregnancy. An alternative to antidepressant therapy is psychotherapy, specifically cognitive behavioral therapy, which is equally as efficacious as pharmacologic therapy. In this patient who is already taking an antidepressant, it would be more important to continue therapy than to discontinue treatment.

Optimal glycemic control with a goal hemoglobin A_{1c} value of less than 6.5% is recommended for women with diabetes mellitus who are contemplating pregnancy. Metformin is a diabetes medication deemed safe during pregnancy, as it is FDA category B. Category B denotes that animal reproduction studies have not demonstrated a fetal risk, and no controlled studies in pregnant women have shown adverse effects.

KEY POINT

- Antihypertensive medications absolutely contraindicated during pregnancy include ACE inhibitors, angiotensin receptor blockers, and, likely, renin inhibitors.

Bibliography

Frayne DJ, Verbiest S, Chelmow D, Clarke H, Dunlop A, Hosmer J, et al. Health care system measures to advance preconception wellness: consensus recommendations of the Clinical Workgroup of the National Preconception Health and Health Care Initiative. Obstet Gynecol. 2016;127:863-72. [PMID: 27054935] doi:10.1097/AOG.0000000000001379

Item 123   **Answer: D**

Educational Objective: Manage perioperative anticoagulation in a patient receiving warfarin.

The most appropriate management of this patient's preoperative anticoagulation is to withhold warfarin without bridging anticoagulation. Anticoagulant therapy increases the risk for perioperative hemorrhage and should be discontinued in most patients before surgery. Bridging anticoagulation is the administration of therapeutic doses of short-acting parenteral therapy, usually heparin, when anticoagulant therapy is being withheld during the perioperative period in patients with elevated thrombotic risk. This patient is undergoing a procedure associated with elevated bleeding risk, and she has no history of stroke, transient ischemic attack (TIA), or intracardiac thrombus. Therefore, the risks of bridging anticoagulation outweigh the thrombotic risk, and the warfarin should be withheld without bridging anticoagulation.

There is no role for aspirin in bridging anticoagulation. In patients with normal kidney function who require bridging anticoagulation, low-molecular-weight heparin is the agent of choice.

The American College of Chest Physicians (ACCP) and the American College of Cardiology (ACC)/American Heart Association (AHA) have made recommendations regarding bridging anticoagulation in patients with atrial fibrillation. Most recently in 2017, the ACC published an expert consensus decision pathway for periprocedural management of anticoagulation in patients with nonvalvular atrial fibrillation. The ACCP recommends bridging anticoagulation in patients with a $CHADS_2$ score of 3 or higher or with a history of stroke or transient ischemic attack (TIA). However, according to the ACCP guideline, bridging anticoagulation is not indicated if bleeding risk is elevated in patients with a $CHADS_2$ score of 3 or 4 and no history of stroke or TIA. The 2017 ACC decision pathway suggests forgoing bridging anticoagulation in patients with CHA_2DS_2-VASc scores of 5 and 6 or lower without a history of stroke, TIA, or systemic embolism. Because this patient has a $CHADS_2$ score of 2 and a CHA_2DS_2-VASc score of 4, bridging anticoagulation is not necessary.

KEY POINT

- In patients taking warfarin, bridging anticoagulation may be deferred if thrombotic risk is low.

Bibliography

Doherty JU, Gluckman TJ, Hucker WJ, Januzzi JL Jr, Ortel TL, Saxonhouse SJ, et al. 2017 ACC expert consensus decision pathway for periprocedural management of anticoagulation in patients with nonvalvular atrial fibrillation: a report of the American College of Cardiology Clinical Expert Consensus Document Task Force. J Am Coll Cardiol. 2017;69:871-898. [PMID: 28081965]

Item 124   **Answer: C**

Educational Objective: Screen for genital and extragenital gonorrhea and chlamydia in a man who has sex with men.

The most appropriate screening strategy in this patient is nucleic acid amplification testing (NAAT) of urine, rectal, and pharyngeal specimens for *Neisseria gonorrhoeae* and *Chlamydia trachomatis*. Multiple studies have demonstrated an increased prevalence of genital and extragenital chlamydial and gonorrheal infections in men who have sex with men (MSM). In one study, prevalence rates of *N. gonorrhoeae* in MSM were 6.9% (rectal), 6% (urethral), and 9.2% (pharyngeal); for *C. trachomatis*, prevalence rates in MSM were 7.9% (rectal), 5.2% (urethral), and 1.4% (pharyngeal). Most infections are asymptomatic. The Centers for Disease Control and Prevention (CDC) recommends at least annual gonorrhea screening with NAAT of urethral, pharyngeal, and rectal specimens and at least annual screening for chlamydia with NAAT of urethral and rectal specimens. The CDC notes that commercially available NAATs have not been cleared by the FDA for some of these indications; however, these tests can be used by laboratories that have met all regulatory requirements for an off-label procedure. The CDC also recommends screening for syphilis and HIV at least annually in MSM. In contrast to the CDC, the U.S. Preventive Services Task Force has found insufficient evidence to recommend screening for chlamydia and gonorrhea in men.

Human papillomavirus (HPV)–associated conditions (such as anogenital warts and anal squamous intraepithelial lesions) are common among MSM. However, data are insufficient to recommend routine anal cancer screening with anal cytology in MSM. The quadrivalent HPV vaccine is recommended for MSM through age 26 years.

Sexual transmission of hepatitis C infection can occur in MSM with HIV infection. The CDC recommends that screening should be performed at least yearly for hepatitis C in this population. Hepatitis C screening is also indicated in all past and current injection drug users. Because the patient does not use drugs and his HIV status is unknown, screening for hepatitis C is not indicated at this time.

All MSM should also be tested for hepatitis A and B. Vaccination against hepatitis A and B is recommended for all MSM in whom previous infection or vaccination cannot be documented.

KEY POINT

- The Centers for Disease Control and Prevention recommends that men who have sex with men should be screened at least annually for genital and extragenital chlamydial and gonorrheal infections, syphilis, and HIV infection.

Bibliography
Wilkin T. Clinical practice. Primary care for men who have sex with men. N Engl J Med. 2015;373:854-62. [PMID: 26308686] doi:10.1056/NEJMcp1401303

Item 125   Answer: C

Educational Objective: Treat recurrent major depressive disorder.

Long-term continuation of fluoxetine at the current dosage is appropriate for this patient with recurrent depression. Guidelines from the American Psychiatric Association (APA) recommend long-term maintenance therapy for patients with three or more episodes of major depressive disorder, persistent depressive disorder, or residual depressive symptoms.

The same antidepressant and dosage that were effective in the treatment of acute depression should be continued for long-term maintenance.

Fluoxetine therapy for 8 months should be sufficient for the treatment of the patient's major depressive disorder, but the medication should not be tapered. Because he has had two other episodes of depression, he should be maintained on antidepressant therapy to prevent recurrence.

Switching to another antidepressant medication (such as bupropion) for long-term maintenance is not indicated unless the patient develops intolerable adverse effects from the initial medication.

Discontinuing fluoxetine is not recommended, even if the patient were not a candidate for long-term therapy. APA guidelines recommend continuing treatment for at least 4 to 9 months after resolution of major depressive disorder, followed by gradual tapering of the antidepressant dosage. Antidepressant drugs should not be stopped abruptly because of the risk for discontinuation syndrome, which is most frequently seen in patients who abruptly stop selective serotonin reuptake inhibitors. The most common discontinuation symptoms include dizziness, fatigue, headache, and nausea. Other symptoms include agitation, anxiety, dysphoria, and irritability. Onset of the syndrome is within 1 to 4 days of abruptly stopping antidepressant therapy or after a rapid taper. Although fluoxetine has the lowest incidence of discontinuation syndrome, therapy should be tapered rather than abruptly stopped.

KEY POINT

- The American Psychiatric Association recommends long-term maintenance therapy for patients with three or more episodes of major depressive disorder, persistent depressive disorder, or residual depressive symptoms; the antidepressant dosage that was effective in acute treatment should be continued for long-term maintenance.

Bibliography
American Psychiatric Association. Practice Guideline for the Treatment of Patients With Major Depressive Disorder. 3rd edition. Arlington, VA: American Psychiatric Association; 2010. Available at https://psychiatryonline.org/pb/assets/raw/sitewide/practice_guidelines/guidelines/mdd.pdf. Accessed July 25, 2018.

Item 126   Answer: C

Educational Objective: Evaluate a patient with medically unexplained symptoms.

The most appropriate management of this patient with medically unexplained symptoms (MUS) is to avoid testing and obtain previous medical records. The most common symptoms in patients presenting with MUS are chest pain, fatigue, dizziness, headache, swelling, back pain, shortness of breath, insomnia, abdominal pain, and numbness. Frequently, patients have seen many primary care and subspecialty physicians over the course of many years and have undergone extensive laboratory testing, imaging studies, and procedures. Because patients with MUS present on a continuum of physical and mental health, a comprehensive, holistic approach is essential. Each presenting symptom merits a relevant history and physical examination. In most cases, prior records should be reviewed before repeating or extending the evaluation unless the patient's condition has changed substantially. Physicians must possess excellent patient-centered communication skills and listen carefully to the patient, validating concerns and responding to emotions. Additionally, the initial assessment should include specific questions to elicit the patient's concerns, underlying psychological status, and the degree of distress and disability attributable to the symptoms. Long-term management of the patient with MUS is challenging. A therapeutic alliance and a mutually respectful physician-patient relationship are key features in the successful management of the patient with MUS. In keeping with a patient-centered approach, the patient should be engaged fully in the plan, focusing on physical, psychological, and social aspects of health. The physician and patient should work together to create and maintain an atmosphere of mutual trust.

Physicians often find it difficult to limit further testing, prescribing, or referral because they fear missing an elusive diagnosis. The evidence that more testing helps reassure patients with MUS or improves outcomes is limited. Additional testing, such as a comprehensive metabolic profile, C-reactive protein level, rheumatoid factor, and antinuclear antibody titer, should not occur without an initial thorough investigation of the results of previous evaluations and determining whether symptoms have changed.

Familial Mediterranean fever (FMF) is the classic autoinflammatory disease, characterized by discrete attacks of pain lasting up to 72 hours associated with serosal inflammation (joints, chest, abdomen), rash, and abnormalities on *MEFV1* genetic testing. This patient's presentation does not match that of FMF. More importantly, additional testing should be avoided until after a review of previous medical records.

It is possible that the patient may ultimately benefit from a psychiatric consultation. However, before that occurs, the physician should review the patient's medical records; evaluate the current status of his symptoms; elicit his concerns, psychological status, and degree of distress and disability attributable to the symptoms; and establish a trusting relationship with the patient.

KEY POINT

- In patients with medically unexplained symptoms, clinicians must approach each symptom in a focused manner and diligently review any previous diagnostic evaluations.

Bibliography
Evens A, Vendetta L, Krebs K, et al. Medically unexplained neurologic symptoms: a primer for physicians who make the initial encounter. Am J Med. 2015;128:1059-64. [PMID: 25910791]

Item 127   Answer: E

Educational Objective: Treat a patient with cervical radiculopathy with neck exercises.

The most appropriate management of this patient with symptoms consistent with cervical radiculopathy is neck exercises. Stretching and strengthening exercises provide intermediate-term relief of symptoms and should be part of a multimodal approach. Other nonpharmacologic options include acupuncture, early mobilization, and spinal manipulation. Cervical traction appears to be of limited benefit. Patients should also be informed that most patients with neck pain have resolution or near-resolution of symptoms within 2 to 3 months of onset by using conservative measures.

The use of a cervical collar in patients with neck pain should be avoided because it can lead to neck muscle atrophy, especially when used for longer than 1 to 2 weeks. Shorter-term use appears to be no more effective for symptom relief than sham interventions.

This patient lacks any "red flag" findings that would warrant imaging, whether in the form of plain radiography or MRI. Features that would prompt imaging include constitutional symptoms; personal history of or concern for malignancy; progressive neurologic symptoms; or myelopathic findings, such as difficulty writing, gait disturbance, hypertonia, hyperflexia, or problems with fine manipulation.

Electrodiagnostic testing is most helpful to diagnose peripheral nerve entrapment syndromes or peripheral neuropathy as the cause of arm symptoms. Both of these conditions should be considered when arm symptoms are more prominent than neck symptoms. Electrodiagnostic testing can also identify cervical radiculopathy as the cause of neck pain but only when motor axonal injury is present; cervical radicular pain can exist in the absence of axonal injury. Therefore, the best course of action for this patient is conservative treatment without diagnostic testing.

NSAIDs are considered first-line pharmacologic therapy for acute neck pain, including acute cervical radiculopathy. Cyclobenzaprine, when used at doses greater than 15 mg/d, has been shown to be effective for treating acute neck pain when muscle spasm is present, although it should be used with caution in older patients. Gabapentin, a neuromodulator, can be used to treat chronic radicular pain; however, it does not have a role in the management of acute radicular symptoms.

KEY POINT

- Cervical radiculopathy, caused by nerve root compression, usually resolves within 2 to 3 months by using conservative measures; stretching and strengthening exercises of the neck muscles provide the best intermediate-term relief.

Bibliography
Iyer S, Kim HJ. Cervical radiculopathy. Curr Rev Musculoskelet Med. 2016;9:272-80. [PMID: 27250042] doi:10.1007/s12178-016-9349-4

Item 128   Answer: A

Educational Objective: **Prevent human papillomavirus infection with appropriate immunization.**

This healthy 25-year-old woman should be offered the human papillomavirus (HPV) vaccine. HPV vaccination prevents persistent HPV infection, which can lead to cervical, anogenital, and nasopharyngeal cancers. HPV genotypes 16 and 18 are responsible for causing most cases of cervical cancer and many cases of vulvar, vaginal, anal, penile, and oropharyngeal cancers. HPV genotypes 6 and 11 cause most cases of genital warts. The HPV vaccine series is recommended for all females aged 11 or 12 years or between the ages of 13 and 26 years if not given previously. In males, the series should be administered at age 11 or 12 years, between the ages of 13 and 21 years if not previously administered, or through age 26 years for immunocompromised men (including those with HIV infection) or men who have sex with men. Three different HPV vaccines are licensed for use in females (bivalent, quadrivalent, and nine-valent), and two HPV vaccines are licensed for use in males (quadrivalent and nine-valent). All vaccines target genotypes 16 and 18, and the quadrivalent vaccine also targets genotypes 6 and 11. The nine-valent vaccine protects against five additional genotypes that cause cervical cancer, resulting in the potential prevention of 90% of cervical, vulvar, vaginal, and anal cancers. If administered after age 15 years, a three-dose series is recommended, whereas a two-dose series is recommended in younger individuals.

Vaccination against meningococcal serogroups A, C, W135, and Y with the quadrivalent meningococcal conjugate vaccine is recommended in all persons by age 18 years. Revaccination with a single dose of the quadrivalent meningococcal conjugate vaccine is indicated in adult patients who are considered to be at increased risk, including those with asplenia (functional or anatomic), those with persistent complement deficiencies, first-year college students living in a dormitory, travelers to endemic areas, microbiologists exposed to *Neisseria meningitidis*, military recruits, persons at increased risk during an outbreak, and persons infected with HIV. Revaccination is indicated every 5 years in those who remain at increased risk. This patient does not have any indications for quadrivalent meningococcal conjugate revaccination.

Adults aged 19 years and older who did not receive the tetanus, diphtheria, and acellular pertussis (Tdap) vaccine during adolescence should receive a dose of the Tdap vaccine, followed by tetanus and diphtheria toxoids (Td) boosters every 10 years. Because this patient received a Tdap vaccine 7 years ago, she should receive a Td booster in 3 years.

Pneumococcal vaccination is recommended in all adults aged 65 years and older and adults aged 19 to 64 years with certain high-risk conditions. This young patient does not smoke or have any immunocompromising or chronic medical conditions; therefore, the 23-valent pneumococcal polysaccharide vaccine is not indicated.

KEY POINT

- Vaccination against human papillomavirus is recommended for all females aged 11 or 12 years or between the ages of 13 and 26 years if not previously vaccinated and for all males aged 11 or 12 years, between the ages of 13 and 21 years if not previously vaccinated, or through age 26 years for immunocompromised men and men who have sex with men.

Bibliography

Petrosky E, Bocchini JA Jr, Hariri S, Chesson H, Curtis CR, Saraiya M, et al; Centers for Disease Control and Prevention (CDC). Use of 9-valent human papillomavirus (HPV) vaccine: updated HPV vaccination recommendations of the advisory committee on immunization practices. MMWR Morb Mortal Wkly Rep. 2015;64:300-4. [PMID: 25811679]

Item 129   Answer: B

Educational Objective: **Treat vasomotor symptoms of menopause.**

The most appropriate management is hormone replacement therapy with estrogen and progesterone. The hallmark symptoms of menopause vary greatly in duration, frequency, and severity, but they may include vasomotor symptoms (hot flushes, night sweats) and urogenital symptoms (dyspareunia, vaginal dryness). Symptoms generally resolve spontaneously within a few years, and treatment should be based on symptom severity. Hormone therapy is effective treatment for relief of vasomotor symptoms of menopause, and for women who are younger than 60 years and are within 10 years of menopause onset, the low absolute risk of adverse events supports the option to prescribe hormone therapy for women with moderate to severe vasomotor or urogenital symptoms who are at low risk for breast cancer, coronary heart disease, stroke, and thromboembolic disease. The clinician should prescribe the lowest effective dosage, titrating up if needed, for the shortest period of time needed to control symptoms. Use of hormone therapy in menopause should be reassessed every year; treatment duration is based on the continued presence of vasomotor symptoms. Estrogen-progesterone therapy taken for more than 5 years is associated with increased risk for breast cancer and requires that women receive individualized breast cancer risk evaluation. For this patient with an intact uterus and no contraindications, combination estrogen-progesterone therapy is the best choice.

Long-term unopposed endometrial estrogen exposure increases the risk for endometrial hyperplasia or malignancy, and for women who experience menopausal symptoms and have an intact uterus, estrogen should be combined with progestin to avoid unopposed estrogen-related endometrial proliferation. For women who have had a hysterectomy, estrogen alone would be the preferred hormone therapy but would be inappropriate for this patient.

Ospemifene is an estrogen agonist/antagonist that is used in postmenopausal women to reduce the severity of moderate to severe dyspareunia associated with genitourinary symptoms of menopause; however, it is not indicated for vasomotor symptom management.

Vaginal estrogen therapy is effective for managing genitourinary syndrome of menopause, although vaginal estrogen alone will not be adequate therapy for vasomotor symptoms of menopause, as experienced by this patient.

KEY POINT

- Hormone therapy is an option for women with moderate to severe vasomotor symptoms of menopause who are younger than 60 years and within 10 years of menopause onset, provided they are at low risk for breast cancer, coronary heart disease, stroke, and thromboembolic disease.

Bibliography

The NAMS 2017 Hormone Therapy Position Statement Advisory Panel. The 2017 hormone therapy position statement of The North American Menopause Society. Menopause. 2017;24:728-753. [PMID: 28650869] doi:10.1097/GME.0000000000000921

Item 130   Answer: B

Educational Objective: Diagnose labyrinthitis.

The most likely diagnosis in this patient with vertigo is labyrinthitis. Patients with vertigo often describe a spinning or whirling sensation, which is frequently associated with concomitant nausea, vomiting, and sudden-onset fatigue. Once vertigo is suspected, the next important step is to distinguish central from peripheral causes. The Dix-Hallpike maneuver can help with this task but could not be performed in this patient. The identification of central vertigo is important because it can be associated with ischemia, infarction, or hemorrhage of the cerebellum or brainstem and may be life threatening. More than 80% of patients with central vertigo have focal neurologic signs, and many have experienced recurrent symptoms over days to weeks. In this patient's case, he has no risk factors for stroke (hypertension, diabetes mellitus), no focal signs, and a preceding upper respiratory tract infection, making central vertigo unlikely. Common causes of peripheral vertigo include benign paroxysmal positional vertigo (BPPV), vestibular neuronitis, labyrinthitis, and Meniere disease. Labyrinthitis is caused by postviral inflammation of both branches of the vestibulocochlear nerve (cranial nerve VIII), resulting in sudden-onset, severe, persistent vertigo and hearing loss. This patient has signs and symptoms consistent with labyrinthitis preceded by an acute viral infection, making it the most likely diagnosis.

BPPV is the most common cause of peripheral vertigo. It is characterized by sudden-onset, recurrent, and brief (usually <1 minute) vertiginous symptoms, which are provoked and worsened with positional changes of the head. Although prolonged head positioning can trigger BPPV,

BPPV is not associated with auditory changes, as seen in this patient.

Meniere disease presents with recurrent, spontaneous, and brief episodes of vertigo, tinnitus, and hearing loss. Nystagmus may be present. Symptoms resolve completely between episodes. In patients with Meniere disease, episodes of vertigo typically last hours, whereas this patient has experienced unremitting symptoms for the past 2 days.

Vestibular neuronitis is a peripheral vestibular condition caused by inflammation of the vestibular branch of the vestibulocochlear nerve, leading to vertiginous symptoms and nystagmus. It is most often preceded by a viral infection. Symptoms are sustained, ranging from days to weeks; however, auditory symptoms are not present, which is the key distinction between vestibular neuronitis and labyrinthitis.

KEY POINT

- Labyrinthitis is characterized by sudden-onset, severe, persistent peripheral vertigo accompanied by hearing loss; it is most often preceded by a viral infection affecting both branches of the vestibulocochlear nerve (cranial nerve VIII).

Bibliography

Kim JS, Zee DS. Clinical practice. Benign paroxysmal positional vertigo. N Engl J Med. 2014;370:1138-47. [PMID: 24645946] doi: 10.1056/NEJMcp1309481

Item 131   Answer: D

Educational Objective: Treat cough due to acute rhinosinusitis.

This patient with acute cough due to acute rhinosinusitis should be treated with an intranasal glucocorticoid, such as fluticasone. Most upper respiratory tract infections (URIs) are caused by viral infections and resolve spontaneously within a few days. Patients without clear evidence of bacterial infection should be treated symptomatically. A meta-analysis of patients with acute rhinosinusitis found that use of intranasal glucocorticoids increased the rate of symptom response compared with placebo; there was a dose-response curve, with higher doses offering greater relief. Analgesics, such as NSAIDs and acetaminophen, may relieve pain. Only limited evidence supports saline irrigation in the relief of nasal symptoms; careful attention should be paid to the use of sterile or bottled water. Instructions for nasal saline irrigation are available online (www.fda. gov/ForConsumers/ConsumerUpdates/ucm316375.htm). First-generation antihistamines may help dry nasal secretions; however, evidence supporting their efficacy is lacking, and sedation is a common side effect. Decongestants are of possible benefit in patients with evidence of eustachian tube dysfunction but should be used with caution in elderly patients and those with cardiovascular disease, hypertension, angle-closure glaucoma, or bladder neck obstruction. Antitussive agents are generally ineffective.

Answers and Critiques

Empiric treatment of URI symptoms with antibiotics (such as amoxicillin) is ineffective, increases bacterial antibiotic resistance, and may cause multiple adverse effects, including *Clostridium difficile* colitis. Antibiotics should be reserved for patients with symptoms lasting more than 10 days, worsening symptoms after initially improving viral illness, or severe symptoms or signs of high fever (>39 °C [102.2 °F]) with purulent nasal discharge or facial pain for at least 3 consecutive days.

A systematic review concluded that centrally acting (codeine, dextromethorphan) or peripherally acting (moguisteine) antitussive therapy results in little improvement in acute cough and is not recommended.

Inhaled albuterol is indicated for patients with evidence of wheezing, which this patient does not have. For patients who develop postinfectious airway hyperreactivity with a subacute or chronic cough, albuterol and other asthma therapies are beneficial.

KEY POINT

- Acute rhinosinusitis may be treated symptomatically with analgesics and intranasal glucocorticoids; antibiotics are not recommended without clearly established bacterial infection.

Bibliography

Harris AM, Hicks LA, Qaseem A; High Value Care Task Force of the American College of Physicians and for the Centers for Disease Control and Prevention. Appropriate antibiotic use for acute respiratory tract infection in adults: advice for high-value care from the American College of Physicians and the Centers for Disease Control and Prevention. Ann Intern Med. 2016;164:425-34. [PMID: 26785402] doi:10.7326/M15-1840

Item 132   Answer: C

Educational Objective: Treat pain in a patient with advanced serious illness and chronic kidney disease with hydromorphone.

The most appropriate treatment of this patient's pain is hydromorphone. This patient's back pain is caused by progressive myeloma, and she requires rapid treatment of her pain with oral opioids initially. Given the concern for worsening back pain in the setting of malignancy, she requires an urgent MRI of her spine to rule out impending malignant spinal cord compression, and aggressive pain treatment while pursuing a diagnostic strategy is critical. Hydromorphone is a potent opioid agonist that is thought to be safer in patients with severe kidney impairment, such as this patient on hemodialysis.

A transdermal fentanyl patch is an effective analgesic for opioid-tolerant patients. It does not have clinically relevant active metabolites that would accumulate in the setting of end-stage kidney disease; however, it should be used only in opioid-tolerant patients. This patient is opioid naïve, and she should not be started on a long-acting agent until her total daily opioid needs are identified and an appropriate equianalgesic dose of fentanyl is calculated.

Gabapentin binds to the $\alpha_2\delta$ subunit of voltage-gated calcium channels; it can be an effective nonopioid adjuvant in the treatment of various pain types, including neuropathic pain. Titration of gabapentin can be prolonged to avoid adverse effects; therefore, it would not be helpful in this patient in need of more rapid analgesia.

Morphine is a prototypical opioid agonist, but its active metabolites accumulate in the setting of kidney failure and increase the risk for adverse neuroexcitatory effects with aggressive titration. Morphine, codeine, and meperidine are all contraindicated in patients with kidney failure (glomerular filtration rate <30 mL/min/1.73 m²).

Tramadol is a weak opioid agonist whose analgesic activity is influenced by its inhibition of serotonin and norepinephrine reuptake. It is a poor analgesic in the setting of cancer-related pain and should not be used in patients with kidney failure due to accumulation of active metabolites. In addition, tramadol has the potential for significant drug interactions.

KEY POINT

- Hydromorphone is the preferred opioid to treat cancer-related pain in patients with chronic kidney disease.

Bibliography

Swetz KM, Kamal AH. Palliative care. Ann Intern Med. 2018;168:ITC33-ITC48. [PMID: 29507970] doi:10.7326/AITC201803060

Item 133   Answer: A

Educational Objective: Evaluate for coronary artery disease preoperatively in a patient with elevated cardiac risk and poor functional capacity.

Dobutamine stress echocardiography is indicated in this patient undergoing elective noncardiac surgery with an elevated cardiac risk, poor functional capacity, symptoms, and electrocardiographic findings concerning for possible silent ischemia. In patients undergoing noncardiac surgery, risk calculators, including the Revised Cardiac Risk Index (RCRI) and American College of Surgeons National Surgical Quality Improvement Program myocardial infarction and cardiac arrest calculator, can be used to determine the risk for a perioperative major adverse cardiac event (MACE). Asymptomatic patients at low risk (<1% risk for perioperative MACE) may proceed to surgery without preoperative cardiac stress testing, whereas patients with elevated risk (>1% risk for perioperative MACE) should undergo assessment of functional capacity. Metabolic equivalents (METs) are used to represent the patient's functional capacity based on the intensity of activity able to be performed. If the patient's functional capacity exceeds 4 METs, the patient may proceed to surgery without further testing. Cardiac stress testing should be considered in patients at elevated risk for MACE with a functional capacity of less than 4 METs or if functional capacity cannot be determined, but only if the results of stress testing will change perioperative management. In this case, the patient's RCRI score is 4 (pathologic Q waves on electrocardiogram, stroke, insulin-dependent diabetes mellitus, and preoperative creatinine >2.0 mg/dL [176.8 µmol/L]) corresponding to a MACE (cardiac death, nonfatal myocardial infarction, and nonfatal cardiac arrest) risk of greater than 5.4%, and stress testing is indicated. Because of the elective nature of his scheduled surgery, he would be able to proceed with preoperative coronary angiography if indicated based on the results of stress testing.

This patient's exercise capacity is limited by fatigue, dyspnea, and hip pain; therefore, exercise electrocardiography would most likely be nondiagnostic.

Echocardiography to evaluate left ventricular function should not be routinely performed preoperatively. However, it is recommended in certain clinical scenarios, such as in the presence of dyspnea of unknown origin, heart failure with worsening dyspnea or overall change in clinical status, known left ventricular dysfunction without assessment in the last year, and known or suspected moderate to severe valvular stenosis or regurgitation without echocardiographic assessment in the last year or with a change in clinical status. In this patient, transthoracic echocardiography would not provide the necessary evaluation for myocardial ischemia.

KEY POINT

- Preoperative cardiac stress testing should be considered in patients at elevated risk for a major adverse cardiac event or if functional capacity cannot be determined, but only if the results of stress testing will change perioperative management.

Bibliography

Fleisher LA, Fleischmann KE, Auerbach AD, Barnason SA, Beckman JA, Bozkurt B, et al; American College of Cardiology. 2014 ACC/AHA guideline on perioperative cardiovascular evaluation and management of patients undergoing noncardiac surgery: a report of the American College of Cardiology/American Heart Association Task Force on practice guidelines. J Am Coll Cardiol. 2014;64:e77-137. [PMID: 25091544] doi:10.1016/j.jacc.2014.07.944

Item 134   Answer: B

Educational Objective: Manage impairment in a physician colleague.

The most appropriate management is to directly approach the colleague with the concerns of impairment and guide her through a plan to determine whether impairment exists and, if so, how to manage it. Impairment may be caused by medical or psychiatric illness or the use of psychoactive substances; however, the presence of these conditions does not necessarily signify impairment. According to the American College of Physicians *Ethics Manual*, every physician is responsible for protecting patients from an impaired colleague and for assisting an impaired colleague by identifying appropriate sources of help. These responsibilities should not be hampered by personal relationships, shame, or fear of harming a colleague. This physician's colleague, who may be

demonstrating signs of cognitive impairment, would benefit from assistance.

When signs of physician impairment are present, it is preferable to intervene before patient harm occurs, if possible. Therefore, continuing to monitor the colleague is not the best option.

Although the physician may be tempted to offer to perform the colleague's medical evaluation, several risks are associated with caring for patients with whom a previous relationship exists, including impaired objectivity, insufficient history taking (for example, sexual history), incomplete examination, and incomplete or biased assessment. The colleague should undergo a confidential and complete medical assessment with another physician to search for reversible causes of impairment.

There is a clear ethical responsibility to report a physician who appears to be impaired to an appropriate authority, which may include a chief of staff, chief of service, or, if the impairment is serious, a state medical board. The legal requirements and thresholds for reporting impaired physicians vary. Most state medical societies or medical boards have physician health programs for physicians with potentially impairing illnesses that can be accessed through a voluntary or mandatory track; these physician health programs provide confidential assessment and treatment, with the goal of restoration of function. At this point, there is no objective evidence of impairment, and a confidential evaluation would be the most appropriate first step.

KEY POINT

- Every physician is responsible for protecting patients from an impaired colleague and for assisting an impaired colleague by identifying appropriate sources of help.

Bibliography

Snyder L; American College of Physicians Ethics, Professionalism, and Human Rights Committee. American College of Physicians ethics manual: sixth edition. Ann Intern Med. 2012;156:73-104. [PMID: 22213573] doi: 10.7326/0003-4819-156-1-201201031-00001

Item 135   Answer: B

Educational Objective: Treat erectile dysfunction in a patient with multiple comorbid conditions.

The most appropriate treatment for this patient's erectile dysfunction (ED) is psychotherapy. The patient has a history of depression, which can predispose to intermittent ED. Given that the patient is still able to achieve an erection 50% of the time and experiences nocturnal penile tumescence, a diagnosis of ED secondary to his other medical comorbidities or medication usage is far less likely. On the basis of these findings, he likely has situational or mood-related ED. In situations such as this one, it can be beneficial to proceed with therapies such as cognitive behavioral therapy, biofeedback therapy, and sensory awareness exercises.

Answers and Critiques

Alprostadil is considered second-line therapy, as it requires routine intracavernous injections, transurethral injections, or transurethral suppositories. For many patients, this option is poorly tolerated. In patients with depression and intermittent ED, alprostadil would not be recommended before trying psychotherapy, which is much better tolerated.

Sildenafil and other oral phosphodiesterase-5 inhibitors are considered first-line medical therapy for ED. However, sildenafil is contraindicated in patients taking nitrate therapy, such as this one.

Testosterone supplementation is recommended only in patients with ED and confirmed symptomatic androgen deficiency. This patient has a normal total testosterone level and has no alterations in secondary sexual characteristics, which make the diagnosis of clinically relevant androgen deficiency unlikely. Furthermore, testosterone therapy should be avoided in patients with untreated obstructive sleep apnea.

KEY POINT

- Erectile dysfunction in a patient who experiences nocturnal penile tumescence is most likely situational or mood related; cognitive behavioral therapy, biofeedback, or sensory awareness exercises with a psychotherapist are first-line therapies.

Bibliography
Mobley DF, Khera M, Baum N. Recent advances in the treatment of erectile dysfunction. Postgrad Med J. 2017;93:679-685. [PMID: 28751439] doi:10.1136/postgradmedj-2016-134073

Item 136   Answer: C
Educational Objective: Diagnose Morton neuroma.

This patient's symptoms are most likely due to a Morton neuroma, a condition that causes compression of the interdigital nerve. Common symptoms include paresthesias and the sensation of walking on a pebble. On examination, there are usually no obvious abnormalities, but some patients may have tenderness to direct palpation of the involved interspace. The cause is thought to be use of constricting footwear, such as high-heeled shoes. First-line therapy consists of wearing nonconstricting footwear and local padding. In patients who do not respond to these measures, a local glucocorticoid injection can be offered. For recalcitrant cases, sclerosing alcohol injections, radiofrequency ablation, and surgery (neurectomy) have been used with some success.

Bunion (hallux) deformity refers to lateral deviation of the great toe with medial bone deformity. This condition typically causes pain at the site of the deformity due to footwear pressure. The location of this patient's pain and lack of visible deformity on examination make bunion deformity an incorrect diagnosis.

Hammertoe deformity is also associated with constricting footwear; it refers to a proximal interphalangeal joint flexion deformity with dorsal interphalangeal joint extension and extended or neutral position of the metatarsophalangeal joint. This patient's normal foot appearance makes this diagnosis incorrect.

Plantar fasciitis typically causes pain localized to the medial inferior heel at the insertion of the plantar fascia in the medial calcaneal tubercle. Pain is usually present at activity initiation following prolonged rest and improves with further walking (for example, the first few steps in the morning after arising from bed). As the condition progresses, pain may be present with both activity and rest. The location and description of this patient's pain are not consistent with plantar fasciitis.

KEY POINT

- Hallmarks of a Morton neuroma are pain between the metatarsal heads, the sensation of walking on a pebble, and no obvious abnormalities of the foot upon clinical examination or palpation.

Bibliography
Ferkel E, Davis WH, Ellington JK. Entrapment neuropathies of the foot and ankle. Clin Sports Med. 2015;34:791-801. [PMID: 26409596] doi:10.1016/j.csm.2015.06.002

Item 137   Answer: D
Educational Objective: Identify an appropriate quality improvement model to reduce postoperative wound infection.

The most appropriate tool to assist in reducing postoperative wound sepsis at this institution is the Model for Improvement. The Model for Improvement focuses on achieving specific and measurable results in a specified population. This model relies on identifying a goal to be accomplished with a change, determining how the results of a change will be measured, and deciding on the changes that will bring about an improvement. These changes are tested and implemented using the Plan-Do-Study-Act (PDSA) cycle. PDSA cycles are rapid tests of improvement, and additional PDSA cycles are completed until the desired results are achieved. A medical center, for example, may set the specific goal of decreasing central line–associated bloodstream infections and use the PDSA cycle to rapidly implement and assess the impact of changes, such as using a central line bundle.

A clinical audit involves measuring current practices against desirable outcomes, which are usually guideline based. Feedback is often provided at the individual level. The audit can identify deviations from desired care (for example, surgical infection rate) but does not establish a goal, an intervention, or a metric to gauge the success of the intervention for the purposes of systematically improving care.

A control chart is a commonly used quality improvement tool. Control charts graphically display variation in a process over time and can help determine whether variation is related to a predictable or unpredictable cause. Control charts can additionally be used to determine whether an

CONT.

intervention has had a positive change. This tool could be useful in measuring change but does not involve goal setting or selecting and implementing an intervention, which are required elements in quality improvement models.

The Lean model focuses on closely examining a system's processes and eliminating non-value-added activities, or waste, within that system. By using a tool called value stream mapping that graphically displays the steps of a process (and the time required for each step) from beginning to end, inefficient areas (waste) in a process can be identified and addressed. The Lean model would not be particularly helpful in identifying causes of surgical site infection, selecting and implementing an intervention, and measuring the outcome.

KEY POINT

- The Model for Improvement relies on identifying a goal to be accomplished with a change, determining how the results of a change will be measured, and deciding on the changes that will bring about an improvement.

Bibliography

Lau CY. Quality improvement tools and processes. Neurosurg Clin N Am. 2015;26:177-87, viii. [PMID: 25771273] doi: 10.1016/j.nec.2014.11.016

Item 138   Answer: C

Educational Objective: Treat functional incontinence in a cognitively impaired patient.

The most appropriate management is prompted voiding every 2 to 3 hours. There are four main classifications of urinary incontinence: urgency incontinence, stress incontinence, mixed incontinence, and overflow incontinence. Functional incontinence, which occurs in patients who cannot reach and use the toilet in a timely manner, may occur in patients with significant cognitive or mobility impairments. Classifying the type(s) of incontinence helps guide management. This patient demonstrates functional incontinence, in which decreased cognitive function limits her ability to recognize early signs of the need to void, and impaired mobility limits her ability to get to the bathroom when she does recognize the need. Providing assistance and scheduled toileting through prompting are effective for patients who have impaired cognition or mobility.

Oxybutynin is appropriate therapy for urgency incontinence, but only after behavioral therapy has been implemented and found to be inadequate to control symptoms. Additionally, in this elderly woman, anticholinergic therapy would be associated with increased risk for confusion.

This patient does not report stress incontinence, which occurs with increased intra-abdominal pressure (coughing, laughing, sneezing). Stress incontinence is best treated with pelvic muscle floor training. In addition, the ability of a cognitively impaired patient to comprehend the instructions for pelvic floor muscle training and to remember to perform the maneuvers is likely to be limited.

Sling cystourethropexy is used to treat stress urinary incontinence when behavioral therapy (pelvic floor muscle training) has failed. Carefully balancing surgical risk against potential for benefit would have to be considered. This patient does not have stress urinary incontinence, and surgery is not indicated.

KEY POINT

- Functional incontinence, which occurs in patients who cannot reach and use the toilet in a timely manner, is treated with prompted voiding.

Bibliography

Griebling TL. Urinary incontinence in the elderly. Clin Geriatr Med. 2009;25:445-57. [PMID: 19765492] doi:10.1016/j.cger.2009.06.004

Item 139   Answer: C

Educational Objective: Treat posttraumatic stress disorder.

This patient with posttraumatic stress disorder (PTSD) would benefit most from psychotherapy provided by a specialist with experience in treating the disorder. PTSD is a disorder triggered by the experience of a traumatic event. The experience can be personal, through a loved one, or by repeated exposure to details or footage of such an event. Patients have intrusive memories of the event, such as nightmares and flashbacks, and avoid situations that remind them of the event. PTSD also causes functional impairment, hypervigilance, irritability, and sleep disturbance. In addition to psychotherapy, antidepressants are useful adjunctive therapies.

Clonazepam and other benzodiazepines are not effective in the treatment of PTSD and have significant potential for adverse effects given the high rates of concomitant substance use and suicidality in this condition.

Because of the high prevalence of hyperarousal symptoms associated with PTSD, β-blocker therapy with propranolol would seem to be a reasonable therapeutic option. However, evidence suggests that β-blocker therapy is ineffective in patients with PTSD.

Anticonvulsant medications with mood-stabilizing properties, such as topiramate, have been studied as potential therapies to improve symptoms of impulsive behavior, hyperarousal, and flashbacks in patients with PTSD. However, studies have been small and largely negative, and this class of drugs is not considered first-line therapy for PTSD.

KEY POINT

- Treatment of posttraumatic stress disorder requires psychotherapy from a specialist with experience in treating the disorder; antidepressants are useful adjunctive therapies.

Bibliography

Shalev A, Liberzon I, Marmar C. Post-traumatic stress disorder. N Engl J Med. 2017;376:2459-2469. [PMID: 28636846] doi:10.1056/NEJMra1612499

Item 140   Answer: A

Educational Objective: Diagnose acute angle-closure glaucoma.

In this patient with an acute onset of headache and visual changes with nausea and vomiting, the most likely diagnosis is acute angle-closure glaucoma (AACG). Risk factors for AACG include age older than 60 years, family history, and female sex. Several medications may precipitate an attack or worsen the condition, including anticholinergics; antihistamines; diuretics; and antidepressants, including selective serotonin reuptake inhibitors. Characteristic features include the description of halos around lights, as well as a mid-dilated, nonreactive pupil. An acute attack may be precipitated by dilation of the pupil, which may cause the iris to adhere to the lens, blocking the draining of aqueous humor; the blockage results in increased intraocular pressure. Other situations that can precipitate attacks include excitement, stress, or watching television in a dark room. AACG is an ophthalmologic emergency. Prompt intervention may prevent vision loss.

Bacterial endophthalmitis is inflammation of the aqueous and vitreous humors. It is typically associated with ocular surgery, especially cataract surgery. Patients usually have a subacute history of decreasing vision and eye pain, often mild in intensity. Visual acuity is decreased, and a hypopyon (layering of white blood cells in the anterior chamber) is typically present. Treatment includes intravitreal antibiotics.

Central retinal vein occlusion, which is often caused by a thrombus in the retinal vein, presents as painless onset of blurry vision or vision loss. It is not usually associated with redness or pupillary changes; however, if it is severe, patients may have a relative afferent pupillary defect.

Scleritis can present with severe eye pain that radiates to the periorbital region and watery discharge. Pain may occur with eye movement due to inflammation of the extraocular muscles. The sclera appears violaceous with notable edema. Severe local tenderness can be elicited by exerting pressure on the overlying closed eyelid. In approximately half of scleritis cases, an associated systemic rheumatic or inflammatory disorder is present. The local tenderness to touch and the violaceous and edematous sclera differentiate scleritis from AACG.

KEY POINT

- Characteristic features of acute angle-closure glaucoma include the sudden onset of headache, nausea, vomiting, and vision changes; the appearance of halos around lights; and the presence of a mid-dilated, nonreactive pupil.

Bibliography

Tarff A, Behrens A. Ocular emergencies: red eye. Med Clin North Am. 2017;101:615-639. [PMID: 28372717] doi:10.1016/j.mcna.2016.12.013

Item 141   Answer: B

Educational Objective: Manage a request for genetic testing by first taking a family history.

The most appropriate management of this patient is to obtain a three-generation family history. Obtaining a family history is an inexpensive and important risk assessment tool that allows clinicians to identify persons at increased risk for developing certain conditions. Up to 40% of genetic risk factors that would otherwise be missed can be detected with a family history. Features that suggest the presence of a genetically inherited condition include earlier age of onset than expected for a common disease; two or more relatives with the same disorder, especially if the disorder is uncommon or known to be caused by a single gene mutation; and the presence of a disease in the less-often-afflicted gender, such as breast cancer in a man. Obtaining a comprehensive family history in this patient will help determine her risk for developing Huntington disease, a neurodegenerative condition most commonly inherited in an autosomal-dominant pattern. Huntington disease has a very high penetrance, meaning that nearly all persons with a mutation in the *huntingtin* protein gene will ultimately develop the disease.

Although persons affected with Huntington disease have various abnormalities on MRI, including cortical atrophy and ventriculomegaly, obtaining MRI in this patient would not be helpful given the absence of symptoms and neurologic deficits on physical examination.

Genetic testing should be reserved for patients at increased risk for developing a disease who have received appropriate genetic counseling. Genetic testing raises many ethical questions, as the results affect not only the patient but also other members of the family. Testing can also lead to possible discrimination. The Genetic Information Nondiscrimination Act of 2008 protects against genetic discrimination in regard to both health insurance and employment but does not protect against discrimination involving disability, life, or long-term care insurance.

Genetic counseling is indicated in all patients for whom genetic testing is being considered. The basic components of genetic counseling are education on the condition being tested, including the natural history, possible treatments, and preventive measures; the risks and benefits of genetic testing; alternatives to testing, including the option to forgo testing; and the implications for the patient and family members. A referral for genetic counseling would be indicated if this patient's family history is positive for family members with Huntington disease. Genetic counseling for this disease is unnecessary in the absence of an affected family member.

KEY POINT

- The three-generation family history is an inexpensive and important risk assessment tool that allows clinicians to identify persons at increased risk for developing certain conditions.

Bibliography

Pyeritz RE. The family history: the first genetic test, and still useful after all those years? Genet Med. 2012;14:3-9. [PMID: 22237427] doi:10.1038/gim.0b013e3182310bcf

Item 142   Answer: C

Educational Objective: Treat abnormal uterine bleeding with a levonorgestrel-containing intrauterine device.

The most appropriate management of abnormal uterine bleeding in this patient is a levonorgestrel-containing intrauterine device (IUD). Abnormal uterine bleeding can generally be categorized into ovulatory and anovulatory patterns. Ovulatory abnormal uterine bleeding (menorrhagia) occurs at normal regular intervals but is excessive in volume or duration. Women with ovulatory bleeding have estrogen-mediated endometrial proliferation, produce progesterone, slough the endometrium regularly following progesterone withdrawal, and have a minimal risk for uterine cancer. Anovulatory cycles are characterized by unpredictable bleeding of variable flow and duration caused by the absence of normal cyclic hormonal flux. Without cyclic progesterone, the estrogen-mediated endometrium proliferates excessively, resulting in endometrial instability, erratic bleeding, and an increased risk for uterine cancer. For this perimenopausal patient who is anemic secondary to excessive menstrual blood loss and has contraindications to combination oral contraceptive use (previous deep venous thrombosis and current smoking), using a progestin-containing IUD would likely result in amenorrhea and prevent future blood loss. Managing anovulatory cycles involves the use of progestin to maintain endometrial stability to reduce the risk for endometrial cancer, which a levonorgestrel-containing IUD would do.

An estrogen-progestin oral contraceptive protects against unplanned pregnancy and regulates the menstrual cycle to prevent bleeding between cycles. However, this patient has contraindications to combination hormone therapy, leaving a progestin-containing IUD as the most appropriate choice.

Endometrial ablation or hysterectomy may be considered for patients who do not respond to medical treatment or in whom anatomic causes are identified as the cause of the bleeding. These interventions are not indicated for this patient at this time.

Treatment of anovulatory bleeding is directed toward restoring hormonal balance and stabilizing the endometrium. A progestin such as medroxyprogesterone acetate may be used to promote withdrawal bleeding for women who wish to become pregnant. However, this patient has not expressed a desire to become pregnant, and such treatment is unlikely to prevent future abnormal bleeding in a patient with continued anovulatory cycles.

KEY POINT

- For women with anovulatory abnormal uterine bleeding and contraindications to combination oral contraceptive use, a progestin-containing intrauterine device will likely reduce blood loss and maintain the stability of the endometrium, thereby reducing the risk for uterine cancer.

Bibliography

Bacon JL. Abnormal uterine bleeding: current classification and clinical management. Obstet Gynecol Clin North Am. 2017;44:179-193. [PMID: 28499529] doi:10.1016/j.ogc.2017.02.012

Item 143   Answer: D

Educational Objective: Treat persistent postural-perceptual dizziness.

The most appropriate treatment in addition to vestibular and balance rehabilitation therapy (VBRT) is sertraline. Dizziness that remains nonspecific despite a thorough history, examination, and evaluation is referred to as persistent postural-perceptual dizziness (PPPD; formerly known as chronic subjective dizziness). PPPD is described as persistent, nonvertiginous dizziness or imbalance that worsens with personal motion, upright positioning, and movement of objects in the surrounding environment. Symptoms must be present on most days for at least 3 months. PPPD is most often preceded by another vestibular process (benign paroxysmal positional vertigo, vestibular neuronitis, vestibular migraine, stroke), trauma (concussion, traumatic brain injury), infection, or certain psychiatric conditions (anxiety, panic disorder, major depression). Approximately 75% of patients with PPPD have concomitant anxiety or depressive symptoms. The treatments of choice are VBRT and medical therapy, including selective serotonin reuptake inhibitors (SSRIs) or serotonin-norepinephrine reuptake inhibitors (SNRIs). VBRT focuses on balance training, core stabilization, and desensitization exercises; it is often performed by physical and occupational therapists. SSRIs and SNRIs take 8 to 12 weeks to produce a clinical response; if effective, treatment for at least 1 year is recommended. A positive response to these medications does not depend on the presence of psychiatric symptoms. In this patient with a history of concussion, a cause of dizziness has not been identified after thorough evaluation, and he should be treated with VBRT and an SSRI (such as sertraline) or SNRI.

Treatment response with other classes of antidepressants has been disappointing, and amitriptyline has not been found to be effective in the treatment of PPPD.

The canalith repositioning maneuver (Epley maneuver) is used to treat benign paroxysmal positional vertigo (BPPV). Patients with BPPV have brief episodes of vertigo (10-30 seconds) precipitated by abrupt head movement. This patient's symptoms are not compatible with BPPV, and the canalith repositioning maneuver is not indicated.

Lorazepam and other benzodiazepines have been used in the treatment of acute vertigo. This patient does not have vertigo, which is characterized by a spinning, swaying, or tilting sensation that is often accompanied by nausea and vomiting. In addition, long-term treatment with lorazepam can lead to dependence and may suppress vestibular feedback and central compensation mechanisms, resulting in worsening of PPPD symptoms.

KEY POINT

- The treatments of choice for persistent postural-perceptual dizziness are vestibular and balance rehabilitation therapy and medical therapy with selective serotonin reuptake inhibitors or serotonin-norepinephrine reuptake inhibitors.

Bibliography

Popkirov S, Staab JP, Stone J. Persistent postural-perceptual dizziness (PPPD): a common, characteristic and treatable cause of chronic dizziness. Pract Neurol. 2018;18:5-13. [PMID: 29208729] doi: 10.1136/practneurol-2017-001809

Item 144   Answer: C

Educational Objective: Identify the appropriate level of postdischarge care.

The most appropriate discharge plan for this patient is rehabilitation at a long-term acute care hospital (LTACH). The patient requires continued mechanical ventilation but otherwise no longer requires hospitalization. LTACHs provide longer-term, higher-intensity medical treatment, such as complex wound care, mechanical ventilation weaning, and treatment with intravenous medications. Patients can also receive physical rehabilitation at such facilities.

Acute rehabilitation in a specialized rehabilitation facility is an appropriate choice for patients who require short-term rehabilitation (typically <4 weeks). To ensure reimbursement of services, such facilities require that a patient be able to participate in therapy at least 3 hours per day, 5 days per week. This patient clearly does not meet these criteria.

In-home rehabilitation services are useful for patients who may safely return home but still require physical or occupational therapy to continue optimizing return to their previous level of functioning. In-home rehabilitation services would not be a safe option for this patient who still requires mechanical ventilation and has significant physical deconditioning.

Subacute rehabilitation at a skilled nursing facility is a good option for patients who are not physically ready to return to their previous living situation but cannot tolerate at least 3 hours of therapy per day, 5 days per week. Skilled nursing facilities have physician directors but do not have the physician or staff resources to provide the complex medical care this patient requires.

KEY POINT

- Long-term acute care hospitals provide longer-term, higher-intensity medical treatment, such as complex wound care, mechanical ventilation weaning, and treatment with intravenous medications; such facilities also provide physical rehabilitation services.

Bibliography

Kane RL. Finding the right level of posthospital care: "We didn't realize there was any other option for him." JAMA. 2011;305:284-93. [PMID: 21245184] doi:10.1001/jama.2010.2015

Item 145   Answer: A

Educational Objective: Recognize the types of bias that affect screening tests.

Lead-time bias is most likely to threaten the validity of the authors' conclusions. Lead-time bias occurs when survival time (time from diagnosis to death) appears to be lengthened because the screened patient is diagnosed earlier during the preclinical phase but does not live longer in actuality. To guard against this bias, disease-specific mortality rates rather than survival time should be used as an outcome derived from randomized clinical trials.

Screening is also more likely to detect indolent disease, which has a long latent period, than aggressive disease, which has a short latent period and is most often detected with onset of symptoms. This causes length-time bias, in which a screen-detected cohort will have overrepresentation of indolent disease, whereas a symptom-detected cohort will have overrepresentation of aggressive disease. Consequently, the screen-detected cohort falsely appears to have a better prognosis. Length-time bias is unlikely in studies of ovarian cancer because ovarian cancer is an aggressive disease with a poor survival rate. The cancer has spread beyond the ovary at the time of detection in 75% of patients. This may be the result of rapid progression from unifocal disease to diffuse disease or to multiple foci of cancer within the abdomen, as carcinomatosis has been shown to develop after the removal of normal ovaries in high-risk patients.

Recall bias occurs when patients with a disease of interest are more likely to recall past exposures compared with controls. Recall bias primarily affects observational retrospective study designs. In this case, the screening protocol was a prospective observation study, and those being screened are not being asked to recall exposures; therefore, recall bias would not affect the study authors' conclusions.

Selection bias occurs when the study participants do not accurately reflect the population being studied, usually because the choice to participate is influenced by the clinical question. A national study of randomly selected women with a high participation rate would not be expected to be influenced by selection bias.

KEY POINT

- Lead-time bias occurs when early detection of a disease with a screening test leads to an increase in measured survival but not overall survival time.

Bibliography

Berry DA. Failure of researchers, reviewers, editors, and the media to understand flaws in cancer screening studies: application to an article in Cancer. Cancer. 2014;120:2784-91. [PMID: 24925345] doi:10.1002/cncr.28795

Item 146   Answer: D

Educational Objective: Treat a patient with alcohol use disorder with naltrexone.

The most appropriate treatment is naltrexone. Recent developments in the pharmacologic treatment of alcohol use disorder focus on modifying the reinforcing effects of alcohol use. Physicians underprescribe medications to treat alcohol use disorder and prevent relapse, despite their demonstrated efficacy. This patient, with hypertension and stage 3 chronic kidney disease, would likely benefit most from naltrexone. Available in both oral and long-acting injectable forms, naltrexone has been associated with a substantial decrease in 30-day readmission and emergency department visits when prescribed to patients with alcohol dependence at the time of hospital discharge. Multiple systematic reviews and meta-analyses of clinical trials have found naltrexone to reduce alcohol consumption compared with placebo. Naltrexone carries a risk for hepatotoxicity, for which the patient should be monitored; however, hepatotoxicity is rare with the dosages used for alcohol use disorder. Because naltrexone is an opioid receptor antagonist, opioids are contraindicated while the patient is taking naltrexone. Caution should also be used in patients with depression, due to an increased risk for suicidal ideation.

Acamprosate is FDA approved for the maintenance of abstinence in alcohol use disorder. This medication likely works through the N-methyl-D-aspartate receptor to modulate γ-aminobutyric acid and glutamate levels. In patients with moderate kidney disease, dosage should be adjusted; acamprosate is contraindicated in cases of severe kidney disease (estimated glomerular filtration rate <30 mL/min/1.73 m^2). Recently, conflicting evidence regarding its effectiveness has been published, with some studies finding that acamprosate is no more effective than placebo. Although methodological differences may explain these discrepant results, many experts now recommend naltrexone as preferred therapy in patients without contraindications. Additionally, the thrice-daily dosage regimen can hinder adherence to acamprosate.

Although chlordiazepoxide can be used to treat alcohol withdrawal, it is not indicated for relapse prevention because of its addiction potential and ineffectiveness.

Disulfiram inhibits acetaldehyde dehydrogenase, causing buildup of aldehyde after alcohol consumption; the associated flushing, nausea, and vomiting act as a deterrent to further alcohol use. Unlike naltrexone and acamprosate, disulfiram does not directly diminish the motivation to drink, but it is an aversion therapy causing an unpleasant physiologic reaction when alcohol is consumed. Disulfiram is now considered second-line therapy.

KEY POINT

- Naltrexone, which is available in both oral and long-acting injectable forms, is associated with a substantial decrease in 30-day readmission and emergency department visits when prescribed to patients with alcohol dependence at the time of hospital discharge.

Bibliography
Akbar M, Egli M, Cho YE, Song BJ, Noronha A. Medications for alcohol use disorders: an overview. Pharmacol Ther. 2017. [PMID: 29191394] doi:10.1016/j.pharmthera.2017.11.007

Item 147   Answer: C

Educational Objective: Effectively elicit goals, preferences, and values in a patient with terminal illnesses.

The most appropriate initial strategy to develop goals of care is to ask the patient what he understands about his illnesses. This patient has multisystem organ dysfunction, recurrent hospitalizations, and a poor prognosis. He is at high risk for readmission and dying within the next 12 months, and assessing his understanding of his current illnesses is the first step in starting a conversation about the patient's goals, preferences, and values, after which the clinical care team can make recommendations on how best to meet those goals.

Discussions regarding hospice should occur only after the clinician has assessed the patient's understanding of the prognosis and after the patient's goals, hopes, and worries have been established.

Asking questions regarding resuscitation preferences is often important during a hospitalization, but a meaningful conversation regarding resuscitation preferences must be grounded in a patient's prognostic awareness, as well as their hopes and worries.

The patient's prognosis must be shared before a conversation regarding care preferences can occur. Before sharing the prognosis, however, evaluating the patient's understanding of his illnesses will allow for appropriate and efficient information sharing.

KEY POINT

- For seriously ill patients, understanding of their health and prognosis must be assessed before a conversation regarding care preferences and pathways can occur.

Bibliography
Bernacki RE, Block SD; American College of Physicians High Value Care Task Force. Communication about serious illness care goals: a review and synthesis of best practices. JAMA Intern Med. 2014;174:1994-2003. [PMID: 25330167] doi:10.1001/jamainternmed.2014.5271

Item 148   Answer: A

Educational Objective: Evaluate liver function before initiating statin therapy.

The most appropriate diagnostic testing to perform before initiating high-intensity statin therapy in this patient is alanine aminotransferase level measurement. This patient with clinical atherosclerotic cardiovascular disease (defined as acute coronary syndrome, or a history of myocardial infarction, stable or unstable angina, coronary or other arterial revascularization, stroke/transient ischemic attack, or peripheral artery disease attributable to atherosclerosis) meets the criteria for high-intensity statin therapy for secondary prevention of cardiovascular events. In patients in whom statin therapy is being considered, an initial fasting lipid panel (including total cholesterol, triglycerides, HDL cholesterol, and calculated LDL cholesterol levels) is recommended. A lipid panel should also be obtained 4 to 12 weeks after initiation of therapy to determine treatment adherence and response. Because statin therapy may infrequently cause liver dysfunction, the 2013 American College of Cardiology/American Heart Association cholesterol treatment guideline recommends measuring the alanine aminotransferase level at baseline before initiating statin therapy. Further hepatic monitoring is unnecessary if the baseline alanine aminotransferase level is normal, unless the patient develops symptoms suggestive of liver dysfunction.

In patients who are at risk for adverse muscle events because of personal history of a muscle disease, current muscle symptoms, or concomitant drug therapy that might increase the risk for myopathy, it is reasonable to obtain a creatine kinase level before beginning statin therapy. Routine baseline measurement of creatine kinase, however, is not recommended.

During statin therapy, routine measurement of liver aminotransferases and creatine kinase is not recommended. However, if the patient develops symptoms of hepatotoxicity (such as jaundice, fatigue, weight loss, or abdominal pain), liver aminotransferases should be measured. Likewise, if a patient develops muscle symptoms (such as pain, weakness, generalized fatigue, or tenderness), creatine kinase level measurement is indicated.

KEY POINT

• In patients in whom statin therapy is being considered, an alanine aminotransferase level should be obtained at baseline to evaluate for liver dysfunction; further hepatic monitoring is unnecessary if the baseline level is normal.

Bibliography

Stone NJ, Robinson JG, Lichtenstein AH, Bairey Merz CN, Blum CB, Eckel RH, et al; American College of Cardiology/American Heart Association Task Force on Practice Guidelines. 2013 ACC/AHA guideline on the treatment of blood cholesterol to reduce atherosclerotic cardiovascular risk in adults: a report of the American College of Cardiology/American Heart Association Task Force on Practice Guidelines. Circulation. 2014;129:S1-45. [PMID: 24222016] doi:10.1161/01.cir.0000437738.63853.7a

Item 149   Answer: B

Educational Objective: Screen for diabetes mellitus in a patient with risk factors.

Screening for diabetes mellitus should occur at this visit. The U.S. Preventive Services Task Force (USPSTF) recommends routine screening for abnormal blood glucose and diabetes in asymptomatic adults aged 40 to 70 years who are overweight or obese. Clinicians should offer or refer patients with an abnormal blood glucose level to intensive behavioral counseling interventions to promote a healthful diet and physical activity. In contrast to the USPSTF, the American Diabetes Association (ADA) recommends that screening be performed in obese or overweight patients of any age with one or more additional risk factors for diabetes. Risk factors

include a first-degree relative with diabetes; high-risk race or ethnicity (African American, Latino, Native American, Asian American, Pacific Islander); history of cardiovascular disease; hypertension; HDL cholesterol level less than 35 mg/dL (0.91 mmol/L) and/or triglyceride level greater than 250 mg/dL (2.82 mmol/L); polycystic ovary syndrome; physical inactivity; and other conditions associated with insulin resistance (such as acanthosis nigricans and severe obesity). In patients with normal results, the ADA recommends repeat screening at 3-year intervals. This 40-year old obese patient meets the screening criteria of both the USPSTF and the ADA and should be screened for diabetes now.

In the absence of risk factors for diabetes, the ADA recommends that all patients be screened for diabetes at age 45 years. The USPSTF recommends screening only in asymptomatic adults aged 40 to 70 years who are overweight or obese. This patient, who has risk factors for diabetes (age 40 years, sedentary lifestyle, obesity), should be screened now, not at age 45 years or upon development of an additional diabetes risk factor.

KEY POINT

• Screening for diabetes mellitus is recommended for patients who are overweight or obese and have other risk factors for diabetes.

Bibliography

Selph S, Dana T, Blazina I, Bougatsos C, Patel H, Chou R. Screening for type 2 diabetes mellitus: a systematic review for the U.S. Preventive Services Task Force. Ann Intern Med. 2015;162:765-76. [PMID: 25867111] doi: 10.7326/M14-2221

Item 150   Answer: D

Educational Objective: Diagnose schizophrenia.

This patient's clinical presentation is most consistent with schizophrenia. This heterogeneous disorder is characterized by a combination of positive symptoms (delusions, disorganized thought, hallucinations) and negative symptoms (decreased activity, flattened affect). Typical age of onset is early adulthood. Diagnosis also requires at least one area of functional impairment (occupation, social interactions, or self-care) and duration of at least 6 months (including 1 month of active symptoms).

Bipolar disorder is characterized by major depressive episodes and periods of mania or hypomania. During manic episodes, patients experience increased energy and risk-taking behaviors, as well as inflated self-worth. Patients with major depressive disorder have depressed mood and/or anhedonia, plus other symptoms of depression, including difficulty concentrating, fatigue, feelings of worthlessness, psychomotor agitation or retardation, sleep disturbance, thoughts of suicide, and weight or appetite changes. Although patients may have major depressive disorder or bipolar disorder with psychotic features, this patient does not meet the criteria for either depression (depressed mode and/or anhedonia) or mania (abnormally expansive, euphoric, or irritable mood).

In paranoid personality disorder, patients are distrustful of others, including loved ones, and misperceive social interactions as personal attacks. However, disorganized thoughts, hallucinations, and negative symptoms are not present in patients with paranoid personality disorder.

KEY POINT

- Schizophrenia is a heterogeneous disorder characterized by at least two of the following symptoms: delusions, hallucinations, disorganized speech, disorganized or catatonic behavior, and negative symptoms; the typical age of onset is early adulthood.

Bibliography
Owen MJ, Sawa A, Mortensen PB. Schizophrenia. Lancet. 2016;388:86-97. [PMID: 26777917] doi:10.1016/S0140-6736(15)01121-6

Item 151   Answer: D

Educational Objective: Diagnose bacterial vaginosis.

Bacterial vaginosis can be diagnosed in this patient with detection of at least 20% clue cells on saline microscopy. Bacterial vaginosis is the most common cause of vaginal discharge and results from an imbalance in the normal vaginal bacterial flora—loss of the normal hydrogen-producing lactobacilli in the vagina and subsequent overgrowth of *Gardnerella vaginalis, Mycoplasma* species, and other anaerobes. Clinical diagnosis is made when three of the following features are present: vaginal pH greater than 4.5, thin and homogenous vaginal discharge, positive result on a whiff test (application of 10% potassium hydroxide to vaginal secretions resulting in a fishy odor), and clue cells comprising at least 20% of all squamous cells on saline microscopy. Clue cells are vaginal epithelial cells with ill-defined cell borders on microscopy as a result of adherent coccobacilli. The patient has vaginal pH greater than 4.5 and a homogenous thin discharge but a negative whiff test result. A saline wet mount that demonstrates at least 20% clue cells on microscopy will establish the diagnosis of bacterial vaginosis. Treatment is metronidazole or clindamycin.

Because bacterial vaginosis represents changes in the vaginal flora, vaginal culture has no role in diagnosis. Although cultures for *G. vaginalis* will be positive in almost all women with bacterial vaginosis, cultures lack specificity—the organism is found in over 50% of healthy asymptomatic women. Therefore, culture is not a reasonable test to confirm the diagnosis of bacterial vaginosis and would also be costly and inefficient compared with an office-based diagnosis.

The nucleic acid amplification test (NAAT) is a highly sensitive test for diagnosis of trichomoniasis and other sexually transmitted infections, such as chlamydia and gonorrhea. Although NAAT can detect *G. vaginalis,* it is time consuming, expensive, and unnecessary, and simple office-based diagnosis is preferred in straightforward cases such as this one. When office microscopy is not available, NAAT is a reasonable test to perform.

Vulvovaginal candidiasis is typically characterized by vaginal itching, irritation, and discharge and may be associated with dysuria and dyspareunia. Examination reveals vulvar edema and excoriation, with thick, white, curdy vaginal discharge. The diagnosis can be made when a saline or 10% potassium hydroxide wet mount of vaginal discharge shows yeast, hyphae, or pseudohyphae. This patient's clinical presentation is not consistent with vaginal candidiasis; a 10% potassium hydroxide wet mount is unnecessary and will not establish the most likely diagnosis.

KEY POINT

- Clinical diagnosis of bacterial vaginosis requires three of the following four features: vaginal pH greater than 4.5, thin and homogenous vaginal discharge, positive whiff test result, and clue cells comprising at least 20% of all squamous cells on saline microscopy; culture is not a reasonable test to confirm the diagnosis of bacterial vaginosis and would also be costly and inefficient compared with an office-based diagnosis.

Bibliography
Mills BB. Vaginitis: beyond the basics. Obstet Gynecol Clin North Am. 2017;44:159-177. [PMID: 28499528] doi:10.1016/j.ogc.2017.02.010

Item 152   Answer: C

Educational Objective: Treat benign prostatic hyperplasia and erectile dysfunction with tadalafil.

The most appropriate treatment for this patient with benign prostatic hyperplasia and erectile dysfunction is tadalafil. This patient has lower urinary tract symptoms (LUTS) due to benign prostatic hyperplasia (BPH), with both obstructive symptoms (decreased stream, incomplete emptying, hesitancy) and irritative symptoms (nocturia, frequency, urgency). Diagnosing BPH can be challenging because of the many causes of LUTS; furthermore, there is poor correlation between prostate size on examination and urinary symptoms. Nonetheless, a careful history and examination can usually render the diagnosis. Men older than 50 years are likely to have BPH as a cause of LUTS, whereas men younger than 40 years are likely to have other causes of LUTS. Furthermore, the patient has a history of untreated erectile dysfunction; in cases of BPH and erectile dysfunction, a trial of tadalafil, a phosphodiesterase-5 inhibitor, is recommended. In this setting, tadalafil has been shown to be clinically and symptomatically effective and is the only FDA-approved option to treat the symptoms of both conditions.

Finasteride and other 5α-reductase inhibitors are considered second-line medical therapy for BPH. The American Urological Association recommends the addition of 5α-reductase inhibitors in cases of BPH refractory to α-blocker monotherapy, not as a first-line monotherapy choice. Furthermore, this medication class has been known to lead to erectile and ejaculatory dysfunction.

Oxybutynin and other anticholinergic agents are effective in treating irritative LUTS of BPH. However, given their mechanism of action, anticholinergic agents can lead to worsening obstructive symptoms and could also lead to worsening erectile dysfunction.

Answers and Critiques

Tamsulosin and other α-blocking agents are first-line medical therapy for symptomatic BPH. However, α-blockers have numerous side effects, including hypotension, orthostasis, and sexual dysfunction. Tamsulosin could worsen this patient's erectile dysfunction and thus would not be the most appropriate treatment choice.

KEY POINT

- For patients with concomitant benign prostatic hyperplasia and erectile dysfunction, a trial of tadalafil (a phosphodiesterase-5 inhibitor) has been shown to be effective and is the only FDA-approved option to treat both conditions.

Bibliography

Albisinni S, Biaou I, Marcelis Q, Aoun F, De Nunzio C, Roumeguère T. New medical treatments for lower urinary tract symptoms due to benign prostatic hyperplasia and future perspectives. BMC Urol. 2016;16:58. [PMID: 27629059] doi:10.1186/s12894-016-0176-0

Item 153   Answer: D

Educational Objective: Manage long-term medications in the perioperative setting.

This patient should continue all medications the morning of surgery. In general, many medications are well tolerated throughout the perioperative period. The 2014 American College of Cardiology/American Heart Association guideline on perioperative cardiovascular evaluation and management of patients undergoing noncardiac surgery includes recommendations for the management of statins, β-blockers, and antiplatelet agents.

Statins should be continued in patients who have been taking statins long term. In patients undergoing vascular surgery, initiation of statins is reasonable, and perioperative statin initiation can also be considered in patients who would otherwise qualify for statin therapy based on current guideline-directed medical therapy.

Likewise, β-blockers should be continued in patients who have been taking β-blockers long term, especially those with coronary artery disease. Preoperative initiation of β-blockers may be indicated for some patients undergoing nonurgent surgery, including those with intermediate- or high-risk myocardial ischemia on preoperative stress testing, those with three or more Revised Cardiac Risk Index risk factors (diabetes mellitus, heart failure, coronary artery disease, chronic kidney disease, cerebrovascular disease), or those who otherwise have a compelling indication for β-blockade. However, β-blockers should never be started on the day of surgery, but rather with enough time preoperatively to assess safety and tolerability.

There are very few data available regarding the benefits versus risks of continuing calcium channel blockers such as amlodipine. There are no known interactions with anesthetic agents, and continuing calcium channel blockers is not associated with hemodynamic instability. Most experts, in the absence of data, recommend continuing this class of medication for patients already taking them.

In general, patients with coronary stents should be continued on aspirin throughout the perioperative period unless the bleeding risk is prohibitively high, as is the case with many neurosurgical procedures. It is important to discuss perioperative management of aspirin and $P2Y_{12}$ inhibitors with the surgical team to reach a consensus recommendation.

KEY POINT

- In patients undergoing noncardiac surgery, β-blockers and statins should be continued in those who have been taking the drugs long term, and aspirin generally should be continued in patients with coronary stents unless the bleeding risk is prohibitively high.

Bibliography

Fleisher LA, Fleischmann KE, Auerbach AD, Barnason SA, Beckman JA, Bozkurt B, et al; American College of Cardiology. 2014 ACC/AHA guideline on perioperative cardiovascular evaluation and management of patients undergoing noncardiac surgery: a report of the American College of Cardiology/American Heart Association Task Force on practice guidelines. J Am Coll Cardiol. 2014;64:e77-137. [PMID: 25091544]

Item 154   Answer: D

Educational Objective: Avoid adjunctive breast cancer screening in a low-risk patient with dense breast tissue.

This patient should not undergo adjunctive screening. Breast density is an increasingly recognized risk factor for breast cancer. It is categorized by the Breast Imaging Reporting and Data System (BI-RADS) as (a) almost entirely fatty, (b) scattered areas of fibroglandular tissue, (c) heterogeneously dense, or (d) extremely dense. Women with dense breasts should be informed that high breast density is common (present in up to 50% of women) and increases breast cancer risk but not breast cancer–related mortality. Dense breasts also decrease the sensitivity of mammography. However, women with high breast density without additional risk factors may experience more harms than benefits from supplemental breast imaging. Although supplemental screening with ultrasonography or MRI may increase the cancer detection rate, the impact on important clinical outcomes is unknown. Up to 90% of positive results on supplemental ultrasonography and 66% to 97% of positive results on supplemental MRI are false-positive findings, which may result in additional testing or invasive procedures. Despite this, nearly a quarter of state legislatures mandate that patients be notified of breast density findings, and some specifically recommend adjunctive screening with ultrasonography.

Women with dense breasts and other risk factors that impart a lifetime risk for breast cancer of 20% to 25% or higher, as calculated by models largely dependent on family history, should also undergo breast MRI in addition to screening mammography. The use of supplemental breast MRI in women who have less than a 20% lifetime risk for breast cancer is not currently supported by guidelines.

Digital breast tomosynthesis creates a three-dimensional image of the breast. Clinical studies suggest that tomosynthesis may have a sensitivity equal to or exceeding the sensitivity of digital mammography in the detection of breast cancer in women with dense breasts and that tomosynthesis may decrease the recall rate from screening mammography. Despite these promising findings that may improve screening accuracy, there are no randomized trials or long-term follow-up data.

Most major breast cancer screening guidelines promote biennial screening from age 50 to 75 years. No guideline recommends biannual digital mammography for patients whose only risk factor is high breast density.

KEY POINT

- High breast density alone does not necessitate adjunctive breast imaging other than routine screening mammography.

Bibliography

Melnikow J, Fenton JJ, Whitlock EP, Miglioretti DL, Weyrich MS, Thompson JH, et al. Supplemental screening for breast cancer in women with dense breasts: a systematic review for the U.S. Preventive Services Task Force. Ann Intern Med. 2016;164:268-78. [PMID: 26757021] doi:10.7326/M15-1789

Item 155   Answer: B

Educational Objective: Treat chronic noncancer pain with medical cannabis.

A trial of oral medical cannabis oil would be a reasonable treatment in the management of this patient's chronic pain. Medical cannabis, although classified as a scheduled agent by the U.S. Drug Enforcement Administration on a federal level, has been approved by many states as a treatment for chronic pain. Current data on the effectiveness of medical cannabis for chronic pain are characterized by significant heterogeneity in both patient populations and cannabis preparations, although recent systematic reviews have demonstrated that cannabis has some efficacy in the treatment of chronic noncancer pain. Only two cannabinoid drugs (dronabinol and nabilone) are licensed for sale in the United States, and both drugs are available only in oral form. The pharmacokinetics of oral cannabis differ greatly from those of smoked cannabis, which has varying implications. Oral cannabis is slow in onset of action but produces more pronounced, and often unfavorable, psychoactive effects that last much longer than those experienced with smoking. On the other hand, smoked cannabis is quickly absorbed into the blood, and effects are immediate. However, examining the effects of smoked marijuana can be difficult because the absorption and efficacy of cannabis on symptom relief depend on subject familiarity with smoking and inhaling. This patient with end-stage kidney disease has a complex chronic pain syndrome that is unresponsive to multiple trials of nonpharmacologic and nonopioid analgesic therapies. If she resides in a state in which medical cannabis is available, oral medical cannabis oil would be a reasonable treatment option.

Oral immediate-release morphine sulfate should be avoided in this patient with end-stage kidney disease who is receiving dialysis because it could cause opioid-induced neurotoxicity with repeated use.

Oral methadone is a potent opioid agonist and N-methyl-D-aspartate receptor antagonist. Its complex pharmacokinetics and variable half-life restrict its general use, and it should not be prescribed by clinicians who lack experience in its management.

Topical lidocaine does not penetrate into the deep myofascial tissues and would not be an effective agent for this patient with pelvic pain.

KEY POINT

- Medical cannabis has demonstrated some efficacy in the treatment of chronic noncancer pain.

Bibliography

Whiting PF, Wolff RF, Deshpande S, Di Nisio M, Duffy S, Hernandez AV, et al. Cannabinoids for medical use: a systematic review and meta-analysis. JAMA. 2015;313:2456-73. [PMID: 26103030] doi: 10.1001/jama.2015.6358

Item 156   Answer: E

Educational Objective: Treat a patient with a popliteal cyst.

The most appropriate management is no treatment. This patient has a popliteal (Baker) cyst. Popliteal cysts are synovial fluid–containing extensions of the knee joint space and generally occur as a result of inflammatory arthritis, osteoarthritis, or trauma of the knee. Swelling is seen in the popliteal fossa on physical examination. The cyst is usually asymptomatic but may become painful as it enlarges or ruptures, which may cause significant pain and swelling of the calf, mimicking thrombophlebitis. The knee should be examined for signs of meniscal pathology, effusion, or mechanical signs that indicate an intra-articular irritant causing excessive joint fluid. Treatment is usually directed at the underlying cause of the cyst (such as repair of a torn meniscus). Given this patient's lack of symptoms, no treatment is required.

In this asymptomatic patient, fluid aspiration is not necessary; it should be performed solely for symptom relief, which is unnecessary in this patient. Although the procedure is considered extremely safe, it does carry a small risk for infection.

When arthritis-related popliteal cysts cause symptoms, joint aspiration of the fluid with a subsequent glucocorticoid injection can often relieve the symptoms. Given that this patient lacks symptoms, the procedure is not indicated.

Ibuprofen or another NSAID can be offered to patients with popliteal cysts to treat pain from the underlying cause of the cyst (such as trauma or osteoarthritis), but these analgesics are not considered first-line therapy for the cysts themselves. In patients with asymptomatic popliteal cysts, NSAIDs have no role.

Plain radiographs can be obtained in patients with trauma when there is concern for fracture or to confirm the diagnosis of osteoarthritis. There is no role for plain radiography in patients with an asymptomatic popliteal cyst.

KEY POINT

- Asymptomatic popliteal cysts do not require treatment; in symptomatic cases, treatment is usually directed at the underlying cause.

Bibliography
Herman AM, Marzo JM. Popliteal cysts: a current review. Orthopedics. 2014;37:e678-84. [PMID: 25102502] doi:10.3928/01477447-20140728-52

Item 157   Answer: D

Educational Objective: Exclude a diagnosis of a female sexual disorder in a postmenopausal woman.

This patient does not currently meet the diagnostic criteria for any sexual disorder. Female sexual dysfunction describes sexual difficulties that are persistent, personally distressing to the patient, and not explained by a nonsexual mental disorder. The patient reports that she is only occasionally distressed by these symptoms. Intervention may still be appropriate for patients reporting significant distress, such as sexual health education and/or referral to a sex therapist.

Female orgasmic disorder is the persistent or recurrent absence, delay, or diminished intensity of orgasm following a normal excitement phase with at least 75% of sexual encounters. The patient does not describe symptoms compatible with this disorder.

Genitopelvic pain/penetration disorder is diagnosed when there is persistent or recurrent difficulty in vaginal penetration during intercourse, marked vulvovaginal or pelvic pain during penetration, fear of pain or anxiety about pain in anticipation of or during penetration, or tightening or tensing of pelvic floor muscles during attempted penetration. For this diagnosis, symptoms must occur more than 75% of the time for at least 6 months and cause clinically significant distress. These symptoms are not present in this patient.

Female sexual interest/arousal disorder includes hypoactive sexual desire or arousal dysfunction that is present for a minimum of 6 months and causes significant distress. It is diagnosed if the patient reports at least three of the following symptoms: lack of sexual interest, lack of sexual thoughts or fantasies, decreased initiation of sexual activity or decreased responsiveness to the partner's initiation attempts, reduced excitement or pleasure during sexual activity, reduced response to sexual cues, or decreased genital or nongenital sensations during sexual activity. This patient reports only occasional distress that has been present for 3 months.

KEY POINT

- The diagnosis of a female sexual disorder requires both significant distress and the persistence of symptoms not explained by a nonsexual mental disorder.

Bibliography
Faubion SS, Rullo JE. Sexual dysfunction in women: a practical approach. Am Fam Physician. 2015;92:281-8. [PMID: 26280233]

Item 158   Answer: B

Educational Objective: Evaluate a patient with suspected central vertigo with MRI.

The most appropriate diagnostic test to perform next in this patient with risk factors for stroke is MRI of the brain. Patients with central vertigo secondary to vertebrobasilar stroke (posterior circulation ischemic or hemorrhagic events) frequently display concomitant neurologic findings in addition to vertigo. However, roughly 20% of patients with vertebrobasilar stroke present with isolated vertigo, and studies have shown that up to one third of cases of vertebrobasilar stroke that manifest as isolated vertigo are misclassified as peripheral vertigo, leading to considerable morbidity and mortality. In patients with findings concerning for centrally mediated vertigo (nystagmus, dysphagia, dysarthria, diplopia, ataxia, postural instability, hemiparesis, or mental status changes), or in patients with acute sustained vertigo and risk factors for vertebrobasilar stroke (advanced age, hypertension, hyperlipidemia, diabetes mellitus, peripheral vascular disease, atrial fibrillation), urgent evaluation with MRI is strongly recommended. MRI can detect infarction in the posterior fossa on the first day and is typically performed with magnetic resonance angiography (MRA). MRA is both sensitive and specific in the identification of stenosis or occlusion of the posterior cerebral circulation.

CT can provide an effective and expedited evaluation of hemorrhagic stroke, although hemorrhagic vertebrobasilar stroke accounts for a very small minority of cases of centrally mediated vertigo. MRI is far more sensitive for the early detection of ischemic stroke in these patients.

Vestibular laboratory testing using electronystagmography and videonystagmography can be helpful in distinguishing between peripheral and central vertigo. Electronystagmography and videonystagmography use electrodes and video cameras, respectively, to record eye movements. These techniques record and quantify both spontaneous and induced nystagmus. Vestibular laboratory testing should not take precedence over urgent brain imaging for a potentially life-threatening condition, such as a cerebellar stroke.

Imaging studies are generally unnecessary in the diagnosis of peripheral vertigo. However, because this patient is at high risk for posterior circulation stroke (cardiovascular disease risk factors; acute, sustained vertigo; gait ataxia), further evaluation is urgently required.

KEY POINT

- In patients with findings concerning for centrally mediated vertigo or patients with acute sustained vertigo and risk factors for vertebrobasilar stroke, urgent evaluation with MRI and posterior circulation magnetic resonance angiography are strongly recommended.

Bibliography
Venhovens J, Meulstee J, Verhagen WI. Acute vestibular syndrome: a critical review and diagnostic algorithm concerning the clinical differentiation of peripheral versus central aetiologies in the emergency department. J Neurol. 2016;263:2151-2157. [PMID: 26984607]

Item 159   Answer: B

Educational Objective: Treat an obese patient with comprehensive behavioral therapy.

The initial recommendation to achieve weight loss is lifestyle modification, which includes reducing calorie intake by at least 500 kcal/day, physical activity exceeding 150 minutes weekly, and comprehensive behavioral therapy. High-intensity behavioral therapy programs (≥14 sessions of at least 6 months' duration) delivered by a trained interventionist and including regular self-monitoring of weight and calorie intake are associated with successful weight loss. Although face-to-face interventions most reliably result in weight loss, success has also been demonstrated with phone- or electronic-based interventions. Comprehensive programs lasting 1 year or longer and with at least monthly contact are associated with more successful maintenance of lifestyle change, and they are usually a reimbursable service.

Bariatric surgery for obesity is reserved for when a trial of comprehensive lifestyle intervention does not succeed. Additionally, surgical therapy is recommended only for patients with a BMI of 40 or greater, or with a BMI of 35 or greater and obesity-related comorbid conditions; this patient does not meet these criteria.

This patient is already exercising at the recommended level of at least 150 minutes of moderate to vigorous physical activity per week. Although increasing her physical activity may reduce the caloric restriction required to achieve weight loss, the impact of exercise is thought to be less important in initial weight loss than that of calorie restriction.

This patient admits that she has difficulty adhering to a diet plan; there is no reason to suspect that her adherence to a different plan (whether low-carbohydrate, Mediterranean, or another diet) would improve without the behavioral intervention components of regular calorie tracking and weight monitoring.

Combination low-dose phentermine (a sympathomimetic drug) and low-dose topiramate (an antiepileptic drug) has demonstrated efficacy in reducing weight, possibly by suppressing appetite, altering taste, and increasing metabolism. As with bariatric surgery, pharmacologic therapy is recommended only if a trial of lifestyle intervention is not successful. This patient has not yet truly engaged in a program of behavioral intervention.

KEY POINT

- Weight loss is best achieved with a high-intensity behavioral therapy program (≥14 sessions of ≥6 months' duration) delivered by a trained interventionist and including regular self-monitoring of weight and calorie intake.

Bibliography
Jensen MD, Ryan DH, Apovian CM, Ard JD, Comuzzie AG, Donato KA, et al; American College of Cardiology/American Heart Association Task Force on Practice Guidelines. 2013 AHA/ACC/TOS guideline for the management of overweight and obesity in adults: a report of the American College of Cardiology/American Heart Association Task Force on Practice Guidelines and The Obesity Society. Circulation. 2014;129:S102-38. [PMID: 24222017] doi:10.1161/01.cir.0000437739.71477.ee

Item 160   Answer: C

Educational Objective: Manage surrogate decision making in a patient without an advance directive.

The most appropriate basis for the decision regarding the patient's management is the patient's previously expressed wishes, otherwise known as substituted judgment. The strongest evidence of a patient's preferences derives from a living will, in which a patient can outline specific preferences for treatment decisions (for example, use of dialysis or mechanical ventilation). A patient could also formally designate a health care proxy through a durable power of attorney. Unfortunately, few patients have completed an advance directive, and when one is not available, it is important to be familiar with the local state laws regarding surrogate decision making. Many states have a health consent statute that designates the order in which family members are selected to provide surrogate decisions. The patient's spouse usually takes precedence over parents or adult children.

Decisions based on the patient's best interests should be reserved for situations in which there are no previously expressed oral or written statements of preferences or values from the patient. Family members and physicians may have divergent opinions of what is in the patient's best interests, which may not correlate with what the patient would want for himself.

Although this patient's medical condition is a crucial consideration, proper management of complex cases such as this one depend upon knowledge of the values and ethical principles at play. These decisions should be made in accord with local legal standards; risk management should not be the driving factor. Practicing according to ethical standards of care should reduce legal risk.

KEY POINT

- When decisions are made on behalf of a patient who lacks decision-making capacity, they should be based on previously expressed oral or written statements of preferences or values, also known as substituted judgment.

Bibliography
Snyder L; American College of Physicians Ethics, Professionalism, and Human Rights Committee. American College of Physicians ethics manual: sixth edition. Ann Intern Med. 2012;156:73-104. [PMID: 22213573] doi: 10.7326/0003-4819-156-1-201201031-00001

Item 161   Answer: B

Educational Objective: Treat opioid-induced constipation in a patient with serious illness.

The most appropriate treatment of this patient's constipation is methylnaltrexone. This patient presents with significant constipation refractory to enema therapy, osmotic laxatives (lactulose), and stimulants (bisacodyl, senna). There are several causes of this patient's constipation, but special attention must be paid to his opioid use for dyspnea palliation. Methylnaltrexone is a peripherally acting μ-opioid receptor

CONT.

antagonist, which is rapid acting and effective in the treatment of opioid-induced constipation. By reversing μ-opioid receptor activation in the gut, methylnaltrexone can cause laxation in less than 60 minutes and does not reverse analgesic or antidyspneic effects of systemically administered opioids. It is contraindicated in patients with bowel obstruction.

When constipation symptoms do not respond to osmotic and stimulant laxative therapy, the chloride channel activator lubiprostone can be considered. Two randomized clinical trials in patients with opioid-induced constipation have demonstrated that patients receiving lubiprostone had significant improvement in spontaneous bowel movements, abdominal discomfort, and constipation severity. Lubiprostone is FDA approved for the treatment of opioid-induced constipation; however, it can cause shortness of breath and is likely a poor choice for a patient taking opioids to palliate dyspnea.

Polyethylene glycol is an osmotic laxative that increases the water content of stools to improve bowel motility. This patient is already taking an osmotic laxative (lactulose), and the addition of polyethylene glycol is unlikely to have any effect in the setting of opioid-induced bowel dysmotility refractory to stimulants and enema therapy.

Sodium phosphate enemas are contraindicated in older adult patients and in patients with kidney failure or heart failure because of the risks for dangerous electrolyte shifts and renal toxicity.

KEY POINT

- If maximal medical therapy has failed to achieve laxation in patients taking opioids, peripheral opioid antagonists, such as methylnaltrexone, can be considered; methylnaltrexone does not reverse the analgesic or antidyspneic effects of systemically administered opioids.

Bibliography

Streicher JM, Bilsky EJ. Peripherally acting μ-opioid receptor antagonists for the treatment of opioid-related side effects: mechanism of action and clinical implications. J Pharm Pract. 2017:897190017732263. [PMID: 28946783] doi:10.1177/0897190017732263

Item 162   Answer: B

Educational Objective: Diagnose autism spectrum disorder.

This patient demonstrates behaviors most consistent with autism spectrum disorder. This is a heterogeneous group of disorders that share two diagnostic features: (1) repetitive, nonpurposeful behaviors and (2) deficiencies in communication and social interaction. Although the disorder may not be diagnosed until adulthood, the abnormal behaviors begin in childhood. The exact prevalence is debated, but it is estimated to affect 0.5% to 1% of the U.S. population. Early intervention with behavioral and educational interventions improves long-term functioning, but most patients require lifelong assistance.

Antisocial personality disorder is characterized by lack of empathy for others and engaging in socially unacceptable activities (such as stealing or cheating) without remorse. Patients with this personality disorder do not engage in repetitive behaviors and do not have communication difficulties.

Obsessive-compulsive disorder is characterized by obsessions (persistent and intrusive thoughts, images, or impulses that are associated with distress) and compulsions (repetitive behaviors [such as counting, hand washing, and inspecting] that are performed to decrease anxiety caused by the obsession) that result in marked distress, wasted time, or impaired social function. Although patients with obsessive-compulsive disorder may engage in repetitive behaviors such as those exhibited by this patient, they do not have difficulties with communication or social interaction.

Social anxiety disorder is characterized by severe, persistent anxiety or fear of social or performance situations (public speaking, meeting unfamiliar people) lasting 6 months or longer. In these situations, affected patients experience anxiety and physical symptoms, such as palpitations, dyspnea, and flushing. Patients recognize their anxiety is excessive but nonetheless avoid trigger situations (or endure them with extreme anxiety), resulting in impairments at home, work, and other settings. This patient's repetitive behaviors and difficulty with social interactions are not consistent with social anxiety disorder.

KEY POINT

- Autism spectrum disorder is a heterogeneous group of disorders that share two diagnostic features: (1) repetitive, nonpurposeful behaviors and (2) deficiencies in communication and social interaction.

Bibliography

Nicolaidis C, Kripke CC, Raymaker D. Primary care for adults on the autism spectrum. Med Clin North Am. 2014;98:1169-91. [PMID: 25134878] doi:10.1016/j.mcna.2014.06.011

Item 163   Answer: D

Educational Objective: Treat hyperlipidemia in a patient at low risk for atherosclerotic cardiovascular disease.

This patient with hyperlipidemia and low risk for atherosclerotic cardiovascular disease (ASCVD) should be counseled regarding therapeutic lifestyle changes and followed to monitor progress. Key components of therapeutic lifestyle changes include dietary modification, regular physical activity, weight loss, smoking cessation (if applicable), and addressing risk factors associated with the metabolic syndrome. Patients should be encouraged to adhere to a dietary pattern that focuses on consumption of fruits, vegetables, fiber, and monounsaturated fats and minimizes intake of saturated and *trans* fats, simple carbohydrates, and red meats. Replacing saturated fats with polyunsaturated fats has been shown to reduce LDL cholesterol levels and cardiovascular mortality. Recommended diets include the American Heart Association (AHA) diet and the DASH (Dietary Approaches to Stop Hypertension) diet. The AHA/American College of Cardiology (ACC) lifestyle management guideline additionally recommends that patients engage in 40 minutes of moderate to vigorous activity 3 to 4 days per week to lower LDL and non-HDL cholesterol levels.

According to the ACC/AHA cholesterol treatment guideline, the two groups for which a strong body of evidence supports statin initiation for the primary prevention of ASCVD are patients with an LDL cholesterol level of 190 mg/dL (4.92 mmol/L) or higher and patients aged 40 to 75 years with a 10-year ASCVD risk of 7.5% or higher. In this patient with an ASCVD risk of 3.4% and LDL cholesterol level less than 190 mg/dL (4.92 mmol/L), statin therapy would not be appropriate.

The U.S. Preventive Services Task Force recommends low- to moderate-intensity statin therapy in asymptomatic adults aged 40 to 75 years without ASCVD who have at least one ASCVD risk factor (dyslipidemia, diabetes mellitus, hypertension, or smoking) and a calculated 10-year ASCVD event risk of 10% or higher. Although this patient has hyperlipidemia, his 10-year ASCVD event risk is 3.4%, and neither low- nor moderate-intensity statin therapy is indicated.

KEY POINT

- Therapeutic lifestyle changes, including dietary modification, regular physical activity, weight loss, and smoking cessation, are the initial treatment for hyperlipidemia.

Bibliography

Eckel RH, Jakicic JM, Ard JD, de Jesus JM, Houston Miller N, Hubbard VS, et al; American College of Cardiology/American Heart Association Task Force on Practice Guidelines. 2013 AHA/ACC guideline on lifestyle management to reduce cardiovascular risk: a report of the American College of Cardiology/American Heart Association Task Force on Practice Guidelines. Circulation. 2014;129:S76-99. [PMID: 24222015] doi:10.1161/01.cir.0000437740.48606.d1

Item 164   Answer: A

Educational Objective: Treat a patient with greater trochanteric pain syndrome (trochanteric bursitis).

This patient's clinical presentation is consistent with greater trochanteric pain syndrome (GTPS; formerly trochanteric bursitis), and first-line therapy is pain relief with acetaminophen or an oral NSAID, such as ibuprofen. Patients with GTPS typically have pain localized to the greater trochanter that may radiate down the lateral leg to the knee. The pain is often exacerbated by lying on the affected side and climbing stairs. Pain onset is usually insidious. GTPS can be differentiated from hip joint pain in that GTPS does not usually radiate to the groin or limit hip range of motion. Diagnosis is made by history and by eliciting pain with palpation over the greater trochanter or reproduction of the pain when the patient takes a step up. Use of pain-relieving agents should accompany activity modification, such as avoiding or min-

imizing painful activities. Physical therapy to strengthen the muscles of the hip may help with reducing friction and therefore pain.

Glucocorticoid injections (frequently combined with a local anesthetic) are reserved for patients with GTPS with persistent symptoms and for those who do not respond to acetaminophen or an oral NSAID. Because this patient has not yet received any therapy, it would be most appropriate to start with an oral agent such as ibuprofen instead of progressing directly to glucocorticoid injection.

Most patients respond to acetaminophen, NSAIDs, or glucocorticoid injections. Opioid pain medications are typically unnecessary, have a significant risk profile, and do not have a role in the management of GTPS. Therefore, hydrocodone/acetaminophen would not be an appropriate management option.

GTPS is diagnosed clinically based on a consistent clinical presentation. Plain radiographs are typically normal in patients suspected of having GTPS. The role of imaging studies is to evaluate for alternative diagnoses when the diagnosis of GTPS is unclear. In this patient, plain radiography is unnecessary.

KEY POINT

- Patients with greater trochanteric pain syndrome (trochanteric bursitis) typically have pain localized to the greater trochanter, which may radiate down the lateral leg to the knee, and pain to palpation over the greater trochanter; treatment includes avoiding painful activities, acetaminophen or NSAIDs, and muscle strengthening.

Bibliography

Redmond JM, Chen AW, Domb BG. Greater trochanteric pain syndrome. J Am Acad Orthop Surg. 2016;24:231-40. [PMID: 26990713] doi:10.5435/JAAOS-D-14-00406

Item 165   Answer: B

Educational Objective: Diagnose genitourinary syndrome of menopause.

The most likely diagnosis is genitourinary syndrome of menopause (vaginal atrophy). The clinical history and physical examination are most helpful for diagnosing genitourinary syndrome of menopause. Approximately 10% to 40% of menopausal women experience symptoms related to vaginal atrophy, including vulvar itching, vaginal dryness, and dyspareunia. On physical examination, pale and shiny vaginal walls, decreased rugae, and petechiae are characteristic findings. In contrast to menopausal vasomotor symptoms, which may last for a few years and resolve spontaneously, genitourinary syndrome of menopause is frequently progressive and often requires treatment. Mild to moderate symptoms can be treated with vaginal moisturizers and lubricants, but more severe symptoms, as experienced by this patient, are best treated with vaginal estrogen.

Like genitourinary syndrome of menopause, acute allergic contact dermatitis presents with intense pruritus, often worse at night, as well as burning and stinging. Defining characteristics on physical examination include a discrete, well-demarcated area of erythema and edema. Fissures may be present along the labial folds. Excoriations are common and may become secondarily infected. The course of acute contact dermatitis progresses over days, not months as experienced by this patient. The most commonly implicated culprits are fragrances, medications, and preservatives in medications, such as glucocorticoids. Diagnosis is typically made on clinical grounds; biopsy is rarely necessary. Treatment generally consists of allergen avoidance and soaking in warm water (bathtub or sitz bath), followed by application of an emollient, such as petrolatum or a low-potency glucocorticoid.

Lichen planus is an inflammatory condition that can affect the skin, nails, or mucosa. Clinical presentation includes white lines and patches (Wickham striae) or painful erythema and erosions (erosive variant). Therapies are glucocorticoids (systemic and topical) and immunosuppressive agents in severe disease.

Lichen sclerosus is an inflammatory condition that often presents as white, atrophic patches on the genital and perianal skin. It differs from lichen planus in its clinical presentation of white patches that circumferentially involve the vaginal introitus and perianal area ("figure 8" appearance). Prepubertal girls and postmenopausal women are at highest risk. Biopsy establishes the diagnosis and can differentiate it from other inflammatory disorders. Treatment is with potent topical glucocorticoids.

KEY POINT

- Genitourinary syndrome of menopause is a clinical diagnosis characterized by vulvar itching, vaginal dryness, and dyspareunia; pelvic examination findings include pale, shiny vaginal walls; decreased rugae; and petechiae.

Bibliography
Faubion SS, Sood R, Kapoor E. Genitourinary syndrome of menopause: management strategies for the clinician. Mayo Clin Proc. 2017;92:1842-1849. [PMID: 29202940] doi:10.1016/j.mayocp.2017.08.019

Item 166   Answer: C

Educational Objective: Screen a patient for opioid-related risk.

The recommended next step in management before prescribing opioid therapy is to perform an opioid risk assessment. Opioid therapy may be reasonably prescribed to this patient with pain that has not responded to nonpharmacologic and nonopioid therapies as part of a multimodal treatment plan, which may also include cognitive behavioral therapy and/or physical therapy. The Centers for Disease Control and Prevention Guideline for Prescribing Opioids for Chronic Pain recommends that before starting and periodically during continuation of opioid therapy, clinicians should evaluate risk factors for opioid-related harms. Clinicians should incorporate into the management plan strategies to mitigate risk, including considering offering

naloxone when factors that increase risk for opioid overdose (such as history of overdose, history of substance use disorder, higher opioid dosages [≥50 morphine milligram equivalents per day], or concurrent benzodiazepine use) are present. Other recommended risk-mitigation strategies include reviewing the patient's history of controlled substance use with state prescription monitoring program data and urine drug testing before initiation of therapy and at least annually thereafter.

The Current Opioid Misuse Measure is a brief self-report survey of current aberrant drug-related behavior. It is intended for use in patients currently receiving long-term opioid therapy who may be misusing opioid medications. Its value in improving outcomes related to misuse or overuse of opioids is unknown, and it would not be the next management step in this patient who has yet to be prescribed opioid therapy.

Coprescription of naloxone is recommended in patients at high risk for opioid overdose, such as those receiving daily doses of 50 mg of oral morphine equivalents or more. In this patient, opioid risk assessment would further delineate the patient's risk and may prompt consideration of naloxone, but until the risk assessment is completed, prescribing naloxone is premature.

In patients with no apparent mental health diagnoses, psychiatry referral is not routinely needed before prescribing long-term opioid therapy. Psychiatry referral may be appropriate for patients with a comorbid psychiatric diagnosis and, in those circumstances, could be part of a multimodal treatment plan. However, it is not the next recommended step in the management of this patient's opioid therapy.

KEY POINT

- In patients with chronic pain, risk assessment should be performed before initiating or continuing opioid therapy.

Bibliography
Dowell D, Haegerich TM, Chou R. CDC guideline for prescribing opioids for chronic pain—United States, 2016. JAMA. 2016;315:1624-45. [PMID: 26977696] doi:10.1001/jama.2016.1464

Item 167   Answer: B   H

Educational Objective: Manage perioperative anticoagulation in a patient receiving non–vitamin K antagonist oral anticoagulant therapy.

Apixaban should be discontinued 3 days before surgery because there is a moderate to high bleeding risk with partial colectomy. Perioperative management of non–vitamin K antagonist oral anticoagulant (NOAC) therapy, such as with the factor Xa inhibitors (apixaban, edoxaban, rivaroxaban), is based on the patient's creatinine clearance and bleeding risk. When it is necessary to discontinue anticoagulation for surgery, NOACs can generally be stopped 2 to 3 days preoperatively because of their short half-lives. The shorter period is considered for patients undergoing procedures with low bleeding risk, and the longer period is considered for patients

H
CONT.

undergoing procedures with moderate or high bleeding risk. This applies to patients with normal kidney function or mild to moderate kidney disease (creatinine clearance ≥30 mL/min). For patients with creatinine clearance less than 30 mL/min, there are no data to guide recommendations; clinicians are advised to obtain an anti-Xa level or discontinue anticoagulation at least 72 hours before surgery. In patients taking the direct thrombin inhibitor dabigatran with creatinine clearance greater than 80 mL/min, dabigatran can be discontinued 2 to 3 days before surgery, with the longer period considered for moderate to high bleeding risk; for creatinine clearance less than 80 mL/min, dabigatran should be withheld at least 3 days preoperatively. The lower the creatinine clearance, the longer it must be withheld preoperatively.

For procedures with low bleeding risk, withholding apixaban 2 days preoperatively is usually sufficient; however, withholding apixaban only 1 day before surgery is insufficient for all procedures. Discontinuing apixaban 5 or 7 days before surgery would expose this patient to a small but increased thrombotic risk during that time frame.

In patients taking NOACs, bridging anticoagulation is unnecessary because of the rapid onset and short half-life associated with these drugs. Postoperative timing of NOAC reinstitution depends on the bleeding risk associated with the surgery, as NOACs reach therapeutic levels in 1 to 3 hours, at which point the patient is presumed to be fully anticoagulated. NOACs may be resumed once adequate hemostasis is ensured, usually 24 to 72 hours after surgery. Close collaboration with the surgeon is advised.

KEY POINT

- When it is necessary to discontinue anticoagulant therapy for surgery, non–vitamin K antagonist oral anticoagulants can be stopped 2 to 3 days preoperatively because of their short half-lives.

Bibliography

Doherty JU, Gluckman TJ, Hucker WJ, Januzzi JL Jr, Ortel TL, Saxonhouse SJ, et al. 2017 ACC expert consensus decision pathway for periprocedural management of anticoagulation in patients with nonvalvular atrial fibrillation: a report of the American College of Cardiology Clinical Expert Consensus Document Task Force. J Am Coll Cardiol. 2017;69:871-898. [PMID: 28081965] doi:10.1016/j.jacc.2016.11.024

Item 168   Answer: B

Educational Objective: Treat major depressive disorder with cognitive behavioral therapy.

Cognitive behavioral therapy (CBT) is the most appropriate initial therapy for this patient with major depressive disorder. Most patients with mild or moderate depression (PHQ-9 score <15) are treated in the primary care setting. Referral to a psychiatrist is indicated for patients with severe depression, failure of initial therapy, complex psychiatric comorbidities, and high suicide risk. In a 2016 clinical practice guideline, the American College of Physicians recommends that clinicians treat patients with major depressive disorder with CBT or second-generation antidepressants (selective serotonin reuptake inhibitors, serotonin-norepinephrine reuptake inhibitors, serotonin modulators, or atypical antidepressants) after discussing adverse effect profiles, accessibility, cost, and preferences with the patient. On the basis of moderate-quality evidence, CBT and second-generation antidepressants were equally effective treatments for major depressive disorder, with similar rates of discontinuation. For this patient who is opposed to the use of psychotropic medications, CBT is the best initial treatment.

Amitriptyline and other tricyclic antidepressants can be used to treat major depressive disorder, but these agents are second-line therapy because of the higher rate of associated side effects.

Paroxetine is a second-generation antidepressant that is a reasonable choice for initial management of major depressive disorder. However, there is a particularly high incidence of side effects with paroxetine use. This patient is wary of psychotropic medications, and if one were to be tried, a different second-generation antidepressant with a lower incidence of side effects would be preferred to improve patient adherence.

Quetiapine is FDA approved for use in combination with an antidepressant for the treatment of depression that does not respond to initial therapy. First-line treatment has not yet been attempted in this patient, and quetiapine is not appropriate as monotherapy for major depressive disorder.

KEY POINT

- Cognitive behavioral therapy and second-generation antidepressants have proved equally effective for treatment of major depressive disorder, with similar rates of discontinuation; treatment selection should be made after discussion of adverse effect profiles, accessibility, cost, and preferences with the patient.

Bibliography

Qaseem A, Barry MJ, Kansagara D; Clinical Guidelines Committee of the American College of Physicians. Nonpharmacologic versus pharmacologic treatment of adult patients with major depressive disorder: a clinical practice guideline from the American College of Physicians. Ann Intern Med. 2016;164:350-9. [PMID: 26857948] doi:10.7326/M15-2570

Index

Note: Page numbers followed by f and t indicates figure and table respectively. Test questions are indicated by Q.

A
NAME AND ADDRESS (Please complete.)

_____
Last Name   First Name   Middle Initial

_____
Address

_____
Address cont.

_____
City   State   ZIP Code

_____
Country

_____
Email address

ACP®
American College of Physicians
Leading Internal Medicine, Improving Lives

Medical Knowledge Self-Assessment Program® **18**

TO EARN *CME Credits and/or MOC Points* YOU MUST:

1. Answer all questions.
2. Score a minimum of 50% correct.

===

TO EARN *FREE* INSTANTANEOUS *CME Credits and/or MOC Points* ONLINE:

1. Answer all of your questions.
2. Go to **mksap.acponline.org** and enter your ACP Online username and password to access an online answer sheet.
3. Enter your answers.
4. You can also enter your answers directly at **mksap.acponline.org** without first using this answer sheet.

To Submit Your Answer Sheet by Mail or FAX for a $20 Administrative Fee per Answer Sheet:

1. Answer all of your questions and calculate your score.
2. Complete boxes A-H.
3. Complete payment information.
4. Send the answer sheet and payment information to ACP, using the FAX number/address listed below.

B
Order Number
(Use the 10-digit Order Number on your MKSAP materials packing slip.)

C
ACP ID Number
(Refer to packing slip in your MKSAP materials for your 8-digit ACP ID Number.)

D
Required Submission Information if Applying for MOC

Birth Month and Day | | | | |
M M   D D

ABIM Candidate Number | | | | | | |

COMPLETE FORM BELOW ONLY IF YOU SUBMIT BY MAIL OR FAX

Last Name   First Name   MI

Payment Information. Must remit in US funds, drawn on a US bank.
The processing fee for each paper answer sheet is $20.

☐ Check, made payable to ACP, enclosed

Charge to   ☐ **VISA**   ☐ **MasterCard**   ☐ **AMERICAN EXPRESS**   ☐ **DISCOVER**

Card Number _____

Expiration Date _____ / _____   Security code (3 or 4 digit #s) _____
                      MM   YY

Signature _____

Fax to: 215-351-2799

Mail to:
Member and Customer Service
American College of Physicians
190 N. Independence Mall West
Philadelphia, PA 19106-1572

E

TEST TYPE

TEST TYPE	Maximum Number of CME Credits
○ Cardiovascular Medicine	30
○ Dermatology	16
○ Gastroenterology and Hepatology	22
○ Hematology and Oncology	33
○ Neurology	22
○ Rheumatology	22
○ Endocrinology and Metabolism	19
○ General Internal Medicine	36
○ Infectious Disease	25
○ Nephrology	25
○ Pulmonary and Critical Care Medicine	25

F

CREDITS OR POINTS CLAIMED ON SECTION
1 hour = 1 credit or 1 point

Enter the number of credits earned on the test to the nearest quarter hour. Physicians should claim only the credit commensurate with the extent of their participation in the activity.

G

Enter your score here.

Instructions for calculating your own score are found in front of the self-assessment test in each book. You must receive a minimum score of 50% correct.

_____ %

Credit Submission Date:_____

H

☐ I want to submit for CME credits

☐ I want to submit for CME credits and MOC points.

1 (A)(B)(C)(D)(E)
2 (A)(B)(C)(D)(E)
3 (A)(B)(C)(D)(E)
4 (A)(B)(C)(D)(E)
5 (A)(B)(C)(D)(E)

6 (A)(B)(C)(D)(E)
7 (A)(B)(C)(D)(E)
8 (A)(B)(C)(D)(E)
9 (A)(B)(C)(D)(E)
10 (A)(B)(C)(D)(E)

11 (A)(B)(C)(D)(E)
12 (A)(B)(C)(D)(E)
13 (A)(B)(C)(D)(E)
14 (A)(B)(C)(D)(E)
15 (A)(B)(C)(D)(E)

16 (A)(B)(C)(D)(E)
17 (A)(B)(C)(D)(E)
18 (A)(B)(C)(D)(E)
19 (A)(B)(C)(D)(E)
20 (A)(B)(C)(D)(E)

21 (A)(B)(C)(D)(E)
22 (A)(B)(C)(D)(E)
23 (A)(B)(C)(D)(E)
24 (A)(B)(C)(D)(E)
25 (A)(B)(C)(D)(E)

26 (A)(B)(C)(D)(E)
27 (A)(B)(C)(D)(E)
28 (A)(B)(C)(D)(E)
29 (A)(B)(C)(D)(E)
30 (A)(B)(C)(D)(E)

31 (A)(B)(C)(D)(E)
32 (A)(B)(C)(D)(E)
33 (A)(B)(C)(D)(E)
34 (A)(B)(C)(D)(E)
35 (A)(B)(C)(D)(E)

36 (A)(B)(C)(D)(E)
37 (A)(B)(C)(D)(E)
38 (A)(B)(C)(D)(E)
39 (A)(B)(C)(D)(E)
40 (A)(B)(C)(D)(E)

41 (A)(B)(C)(D)(E)
42 (A)(B)(C)(D)(E)
43 (A)(B)(C)(D)(E)
44 (A)(B)(C)(D)(E)
45 (A)(B)(C)(D)(E)

46 (A)(B)(C)(D)(E)
47 (A)(B)(C)(D)(E)
48 (A)(B)(C)(D)(E)
49 (A)(B)(C)(D)(E)
50 (A)(B)(C)(D)(E)

51 (A)(B)(C)(D)(E)
52 (A)(B)(C)(D)(E)
53 (A)(B)(C)(D)(E)
54 (A)(B)(C)(D)(E)
55 (A)(B)(C)(D)(E)

56 (A)(B)(C)(D)(E)
57 (A)(B)(C)(D)(E)
58 (A)(B)(C)(D)(E)
59 (A)(B)(C)(D)(E)
60 (A)(B)(C)(D)(E)

61 (A)(B)(C)(D)(E)
62 (A)(B)(C)(D)(E)
63 (A)(B)(C)(D)(E)
64 (A)(B)(C)(D)(E)
65 (A)(B)(C)(D)(E)

66 (A)(B)(C)(D)(E)
67 (A)(B)(C)(D)(E)
68 (A)(B)(C)(D)(E)
69 (A)(B)(C)(D)(E)
70 (A)(B)(C)(D)(E)

71 (A)(B)(C)(D)(E)
72 (A)(B)(C)(D)(E)
73 (A)(B)(C)(D)(E)
74 (A)(B)(C)(D)(E)
75 (A)(B)(C)(D)(E)

76 (A)(B)(C)(D)(E)
77 (A)(B)(C)(D)(E)
78 (A)(B)(C)(D)(E)
79 (A)(B)(C)(D)(E)
80 (A)(B)(C)(D)(E)

81 (A)(B)(C)(D)(E)
82 (A)(B)(C)(D)(E)
83 (A)(B)(C)(D)(E)
84 (A)(B)(C)(D)(E)
85 (A)(B)(C)(D)(E)

86 (A)(B)(C)(D)(E)
87 (A)(B)(C)(D)(E)
88 (A)(B)(C)(D)(E)
89 (A)(B)(C)(D)(E)
90 (A)(B)(C)(D)(E)

91 (A)(B)(C)(D)(E)
92 (A)(B)(C)(D)(E)
93 (A)(B)(C)(D)(E)
94 (A)(B)(C)(D)(E)
95 (A)(B)(C)(D)(E)

96 (A)(B)(C)(D)(E)
97 (A)(B)(C)(D)(E)
98 (A)(B)(C)(D)(E)
99 (A)(B)(C)(D)(E)
100 (A)(B)(C)(D)(E)

101 (A)(B)(C)(D)(E)
102 (A)(B)(C)(D)(E)
103 (A)(B)(C)(D)(E)
104 (A)(B)(C)(D)(E)
105 (A)(B)(C)(D)(E)

106 (A)(B)(C)(D)(E)
107 (A)(B)(C)(D)(E)
108 (A)(B)(C)(D)(E)
109 (A)(B)(C)(D)(E)
110 (A)(B)(C)(D)(E)

111 (A)(B)(C)(D)(E)
112 (A)(B)(C)(D)(E)
113 (A)(B)(C)(D)(E)
114 (A)(B)(C)(D)(E)
115 (A)(B)(C)(D)(E)

116 (A)(B)(C)(D)(E)
117 (A)(B)(C)(D)(E)
118 (A)(B)(C)(D)(E)
119 (A)(B)(C)(D)(E)
120 (A)(B)(C)(D)(E)

121 (A)(B)(C)(D)(E)
122 (A)(B)(C)(D)(E)
123 (A)(B)(C)(D)(E)
124 (A)(B)(C)(D)(E)
125 (A)(B)(C)(D)(E)

126 (A)(B)(C)(D)(E)
127 (A)(B)(C)(D)(E)
128 (A)(B)(C)(D)(E)
129 (A)(B)(C)(D)(E)
130 (A)(B)(C)(D)(E)

131 (A)(B)(C)(D)(E)
132 (A)(B)(C)(D)(E)
133 (A)(B)(C)(D)(E)
134 (A)(B)(C)(D)(E)
135 (A)(B)(C)(D)(E)

136 (A)(B)(C)(D)(E)
137 (A)(B)(C)(D)(E)
138 (A)(B)(C)(D)(E)
139 (A)(B)(C)(D)(E)
140 (A)(B)(C)(D)(E)

141 (A)(B)(C)(D)(E)
142 (A)(B)(C)(D)(E)
143 (A)(B)(C)(D)(E)
144 (A)(B)(C)(D)(E)
145 (A)(B)(C)(D)(E)

146 (A)(B)(C)(D)(E)
147 (A)(B)(C)(D)(E)
148 (A)(B)(C)(D)(E)
149 (A)(B)(C)(D)(E)
150 (A)(B)(C)(D)(E)

151 (A)(B)(C)(D)(E)
152 (A)(B)(C)(D)(E)
153 (A)(B)(C)(D)(E)
154 (A)(B)(C)(D)(E)
155 (A)(B)(C)(D)(E)

156 (A)(B)(C)(D)(E)
157 (A)(B)(C)(D)(E)
158 (A)(B)(C)(D)(E)
159 (A)(B)(C)(D)(E)
160 (A)(B)(C)(D)(E)

161 (A)(B)(C)(D)(E)
162 (A)(B)(C)(D)(E)
163 (A)(B)(C)(D)(E)
164 (A)(B)(C)(D)(E)
165 (A)(B)(C)(D)(E)

166 (A)(B)(C)(D)(E)
167 (A)(B)(C)(D)(E)
168 (A)(B)(C)(D)(E)
169 (A)(B)(C)(D)(E)
170 (A)(B)(C)(D)(E)

171 (A)(B)(C)(D)(E)
172 (A)(B)(C)(D)(E)
173 (A)(B)(C)(D)(E)
174 (A)(B)(C)(D)(E)
175 (A)(B)(C)(D)(E)

176 (A)(B)(C)(D)(E)
177 (A)(B)(C)(D)(E)
178 (A)(B)(C)(D)(E)
179 (A)(B)(C)(D)(E)
180 (A)(B)(C)(D)(E)